GLUCOCORTICOIDS – NEW RECOGNITION OF OUR FAMILIAR FRIEND

Edited by **Xiaoxiao Qian**

Glucocorticoids – New Recognition of Our Familiar Friend
http://dx.doi.org/10.5772/2915
Edited by Xiaoxiao Qian

Contributors

Rosalie M. Uht, Mingxi Tang, Anu Joseph, Qian Chen, Jianwei Jiao, Ya-Ping Tang, Xing-Ming Shi, Norman Chutkan, Mark W. Hamrick, Carlos M. Isales, Feodora I. Kostadinova, Nina Hostettler, Pamela Bianchi, Thomas Brunner, Anna-Mart Engelbrecht, Benjamin Loos, Hümeyra Ünsal, Muharrem Balkaya, Ilhem Berrou, Marija Krstic-Demonacos, Constantinos Demonacos, Huapeng Fan, Eric F. Morand, Fhionna R. Moore, Carine Smith, Silvia Graciela Ruginsk, Rodrigo Cesar Rorato, Beatriz de Carvalho Borges, Ernane Torres Uchoa, Lucila Leico Kagohara Elias, Jose Antunes-Rodrigues, Liliya Nadolnik, Emin Turkay Korgun, Aslı Ozmen, Gozde Unek, Inanc Mendilcioglu, Milica Manojlović-Stojanoski, Nataša Nestorović, Verica Milošević, Hayley Dickinson, Bree A. O'Connell, David W. Walker, Karen M. Moritz, Fortunato Vesce, Emilio Giugliano, Elisa Cagnazzo, Stefania Bignardi, Elena Mossuto, Tarcisio Servello, Roberto Marci, Aml Mohammed Erhuma, Hiroshi Hashimoto, Abdullah A. Alangari, Fabiana C.P. Valera, Edwin Tamashiro, Wilma T. Anselmo-Lima, Mohammad Zandi, Amr Amin, Zeinab Nawito, Mahboub Bassam, Vats Mayank, Taner Senyigit, Ozgen Ozer, Pritish Chowdhury, Juri Moni Borah

Published by InTech

Janeza Trdine 9, 51000 Rijeka, Croatia

Publishing Process Manager Tanja Skorupan
Technical Editor InTech Prepress, Novi Sad
Cover InTech Design team

Additional hard copies can be obtained from orders@intechopen.com

Glucocorticoids – New Recognition of Our Familiar Friend, Edited by Xiaoxiao Qian
p. cm.
ISBN 978-953-51-0872-6

For EU product safety concerns:
IN TECH d.o.o., Prolaz Marije Krucifikse Kozulić 3, 51000 Rijeka, Croatia,
info@intechopen.com or visit our website at intechopen.com.

Meet the editor

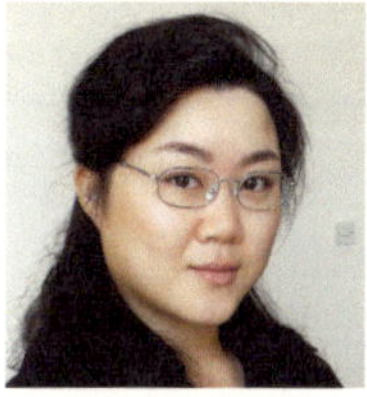

Dr. Xiaoxiao Qian, a neuroscientist/neurobiologist working in the field of stress and depression. After earned her BSc's degree in Pharmacology and Pharmacy from Peking University (Beijing, China) in 2003, she went to the University of Bristol (Bristol, United Kingdom) to pursue her MSc study in Molecular Neuroendocrinology. After that she went to the University of Oxford (Oxfordshire, United Kingdom) to investigate the brain circuits involved in the pathology of schizophrenia and was rewarded with a D. Phil (PhD) in Neuropharmacology in 2007. Being fascinated by the unknown questions remained in mental diseases, she went back to the University of Bristol and has been investigating the relationship between stress and depression, especially the relationship between hypothalamus-pituitary-adrenal axis and stress response-induced glucocorticoid changes in the body.

Contents

Preface

Unlike many other laborious professional names and terms that are used by scientists in the academic world, the word "glucocorticoids" is not that unfamiliar to the general public. The clinical use of glucocorticoids is widely covering treatment for various diseases, ranging from as common as an inhaled asthma spray to after-surgery anti-inflammation treatment. The most commonly mentioned roles of glucocorticoids are their metabolism-mediating and anti-inflammatory effects, meanwhile the occurrence of side effects and resistance during glucocorticoid treatment is not ignorable. However, the therapeutic effects of glucocorticoids in many diseases have yet been replaced by any other compounds, which has made this type of steroids still unique. How much do we really understand about glucocorticoids? Have we thoroughly unveiled the curtain behind the effects of glucocorticoids in either physiological or pathological processes? Why instead of designing a replacing compound to be safely used in clinic, physicians still have to prescribe glucocorticoids to patients but at the same time pay great attention to the dosage and duration of treatment to avoid side effects or glucocorticoid-resistance? Although glucocorticoids have been known for more than a century, the aforementioned questions remain obscure.

As a class of steroid hormones secreted by the adrenal gland and circulating in the blood, glucocorticoids spread almost all over the essential organs of the body. Therefore, it is hard to avoid mentioning glucocorticoids when discussing one particular system. For example, glucocorticoids regulate many processes in the body including the mobilization of energy stores, immune functions, gene expression, and maintenance of the homeostasis as well as the stress response. Furthermore, glucocorticoids play key roles in consolidation of memories of a stressful event. Consequently in a typical medical text book, glucocorticoids and their use in clinical therapy against specific disease have been described in various chapters themed "the cardiovascular system", "the central nervous system", "the immune system" and so on. However, there has been lack of reference that systemically gives a relatively thorough introduction of glucocorticoids as a specific topic. It is really influential of InTech publisher to endeavour to invite scientists from worldwide, sharing their unique specialties and knowledge to fill in the gap and I feel extremely honoured to contribute my part in the processing of this book.

Around the world, exciting research programmes on mechanisms of glucocorticoids' effects on specific system are underway, especially combining modern molecular technologies, we are building up more understanding of glucocorticoids. The first part of the book Glucocorticoids - New Recognition of Our Familiar Friend aims to cover the main systems that are influenced by glucocorticoids. How glucocorticoids mediate the gene expression of key molecules that are heavily involved in the function of hypothalamus-pituitary-adrenal axis has been reviewed, which gives implication on how glucocorticoids affect the neuroendocrine system. The mechanisms of how glucocorticoids influence tumour development, osteoporosis process, cardioprotection, and intestinal environment are also reviewed and discussed. The second part of the book introduces the animal models that are commonly used in recent studies of glucocorticoids. In the third part, the glucocorticoids' role in regulating the metabolism balance and energy homeostasis is reviewed, the recently found molecular pathways that are involved in physiopathology of Addison's and Cushing's diseases are discussed. Part Four focuses on how prenatal glucocorticoids affect the placental development and the consequent long-term impacts on the adulthood.

As mentioned earlier, although endocrinologists have been searching for the replacement for glucocorticoid therapy in order to eliminate unwanted side effects, glucocorticoids are still widely used clinically for various diseases. In Part Five, comprehensive overview is carried out, focusing on the clinical use of glucocorticoids in the treatment for systemic lupus erythematosus, acute asthma, rheumatic inflammatory disorders and oral/maxillofacial surgery. Using latest clinical case studies and reports, the chapters in this part systemically review the background of the disease, therapeutic effects introduced by glucocorticoids as well as side effects, recommended dosage and duration of the treatment, and the cause of the glucocorticoid resistance.

In summary, as one type of the most important steroid hormones, undoubtedly glucocorticoids' role in mediating physiology of multiple organs and systems is well recognised and has been widely introduced into clinical practice. However, using glucocorticoids is similar to holding a double-edged sword - while benefiting from the therapeutic effects brought in by glucocorticoids, patients also suffer from painful side effects produced by glucocorticoids. Certainly replacement compounds or medical treatment can supply new alternatives to the glucocorticoid treatment, however it is equally essential for endocrinologists and scientists to build up more knowledge, based on the tremendous findings about glucocorticoids over the last few decades, about the mechanisms that underlie the phenomenons and finally achieve the ideal balance between the beneficial therapeutic effects and side effects of glucocorticoids.

Finally, I would like to acknowledge all of the authors who have contributed tremendously to the publishing of this book. Their kindness of sharing their expertise and knowledge in the relevant field is truly appreciated. Also, I would like to express my appreciation to Ms. Tanja Skorupan, the Publishing Process Manager at InTech (Europe), for her diligent coordination work that guarantees the publication of this book.

Dr. Xiaoxiao Qian
Henry Wellcome Laboratories for Integrative Neuroscience and Endocrinology,
University of Bristol,
United Kingdom

Section 1

Behind the Curtain: The Mechanisms of the Impacts of Glucocorticoids

Chapter 1

Mechanisms of Glucocorticoid Receptor (GR) Mediated Corticotropin Releasing Hormone Gene Expression

Rosalie M. Uht

Additional information is available at the end of the chapter

http://dx.doi.org/10.5772/54844

1. Introduction

Normal physiologic functioning is dependent on the maintenance of homeostasis in the face of numerous stressors. Responses to stress include the fight or flight reaction and activation of the sympathetic nervous and endocrine systems. The central component of the endocrine response is the hypothalamic-pituitary-adrenal (HPA) axis, which when activated leads to increased levels of circulating glucocorticoids. Indeed, an increase in glucocorticoids has been used as an operational definition of stress.

The HPA axis is activated by a wide range of stimuli which includes perception of danger, pain, sepsis, and others. These stimuli are integrated at points throughout the central nervous system and ultimately impinge on the HPA axis motor neurons in the paraventricular nucleus of the hypothalamus (PVH). HPA neurons synthesize and secrete corticotropin releasing factors (crfs), the best known of which is the 41 amino acid peptide corticotropin releasing hormone (CRH);(Vale et al 1981)). CRH travels through the hypothalamic portal circulation to the anterior pituitary where it binds CRH receptors. This in turn leads to adrenocorticotrophic hormone (ACTH) secretion into the systemic circulation which stimulates the adrenal cortex to secrete glucocorticoids.

Glucocorticoids elicit gluconeogenesis, which increases circulating levels of glucose. Although this mechanism is adaptive in the face of a homeostatic challenge, glucocorticoids can also have deleterious effects. Dysregulation of the HPA axis underlies classic endocrine disorders, such as Cushing's disease, and is highly correlated with a number of psychiatric disorders, including post-traumatic stress disorder, anorexia nervosa, and depression. In addition, high circulating levels of glucocorticoids lead to osteopenia and immunosuppression. Thus, regulation of the HPA axis must be exquisitely controlled.

There are numerous components to HPA axis down-regulation; one of the most significant of these is the end product of HPA axis regulation itself – glucocorticoids. Glucocorticoids down-regulate axis activity by acting at numerous loci in the HPA axis and in extra-hypothalamic regions of the brain, such as the hippocampus(de Kloet et al 2005, (Sapolsky et al 1984). Glucocorticoid regulation in the hippocampus, extra-hypothalamic sites and pituitary are reviewed below.

1.1. Glucocorticoidregulation of the hippocampal-hypothalamic pathway

Glucocorticoid receptors (GRs) are most densely concentrated in the hippocampus of the central nervous system (CNS), and in fact it is in the hippocampus where glucocorticoid binding sites were first detected(McEwen et al 1979). GRs were first classified by their binding characteristics. Two types were identified, distinguished in part by their binding characteristics to corticosterone and the synthetic glucocorticoid dexamethasone (Dex) (de Kloet et al 1975). After steroid receptor cloning it became apparent that the two receptors correlate to the mineralocorticoid receptor (MR) and the GR. The GR is recruited in the presence of high levels of circulating glucocorticoids elicited in the face of stress (de Kloet et al 2005).

Down-regulatory signals from the hippocampus are processed through a multisynaptic pathway. Hippocampal projections to the subiculum elicit excititory signals in the form of glutamatergic synapses in the basal nucleus of the stria terminalis (BNST). These stimulate inhibitory output from the BNST, which in turn down regulates the HPA axis. Thus, damage to the hippocampus leads to loss of HPA axis inhibition (Choi et al 2007, Herman et al 2003).

1.2. Glucocorticoid regulation at the level of the pituitary

One of the best studied components of glucocorticoid down-regulation of the HPA axis is ligand-bound GR-mediated down-regulation of the gene that codes for the ACTH precursor, pre-pro-opiomenlanocortin (POMC)(Bicknell 2008). As is the case in other cells, glucocorticoids gain entry to the cyptoplasm and bind the cytoplasmic GR. Ligand binding activates the receptor, a process that includes dissociation from the heat shock protein 90 (hsp90) as reviewed by Pratt and Dittmar(Pratt & Dittmar 1998). The ligand-bound receptor is transported into the nucleus where it interacts with numerous nuclear proteins and chromatin to regulate transcription. Prototypically, the GR binds to glucocorticoid response elements that are inverted palindromes; however, the regulatory region of *pomc* does not have such elements. Rather, it has a negative glucocorticoid response elements (nGREs) – hybrid elements also called composite elements. GRs bind these sites as monomers and interact with monomers of other transcription factors to down-regulate *pomc* transcription. GRs also repress transcription in the absence of direct DNA binding by modulating the activity of other transcription factors. In these aspects *pomc* regulation is similar to regulation of *crh*.

A significant difference between the synthesis of CRH and ACTH is the relative contribution of post-translational enzymatic processing. In the case of CRH synthesis, one peptide is produced, thus, the majority of regulatory steps are pre-translational. Conversely, numerous peptides are generated from *pomc.* These include ACTH, beta-endorphin, and alpha-melanocyte stimulating hormone. Thus, pre-pro-POMC enzymatic processing plays a major role in determining levels of functional ACTH.

1.3. Hypothalamic crfs

CRH-expressing parvocellular neurons are the final common integrators of humeral and synaptic input. Located in the mpPVH, they receive inputs from numerous sites in the CNS: the hippocampus, brainstem, amygdala, intrahypothalamic sites, and PVH interneurons. (Swanson & Sawchenko 1980).

Although CRH is the most potent and best known crf, it is only one of several. Prior to the biochemical characterization of CRH(Vale et al 1981), arginine vasopressin (AVP) and oxytocin were also known to have crf properties(Gibbs 1986). Perhaps the most studied of these is AVP, best known for its activity as an anti-diuretic hormone. AVP arises from PVH magnocellular neurons whose terminals secrete AVP directly into the systemic circulation.The AVP that acts as a crf is synthesized in parvocellular neurons of the PVH. Interestingly, all parvocellular neurons that express AVP also express CRH. Furthermore, all of these express GRs(Cintra et al 1987, Uht et al 1988), and their function is measured by the ability to translocate into the nucleus in the presence of Dex(Uht et al 1988).

2. Glucocorticoid receptors

Many biochemical and pharmacologic properties of GRs were characterized prior to cloning (Gustafsson et al 1987). The existence of the MR and the GR was determined pharmacologically. In the absence of ligand the GR was present in a cytoplasmic complex. In the presence of ligand, the GR was present in the nucleus. Furthermore, ligand bound GR had been shown to bind specific sites in DNA, which came to be known as glucocorticoid response elements (GREs). Thus, before cloning, the fundamental differences between a steroid receptor and receptors for other hormones had been determined. The GR was an intracellular receptor rather than a plasma membrane bound receptor and its mechanism of action involved binding DNA. Hence the term that evolved -- ligand activated nuclear receptors.

2.1. Glucocorticoid receptor cloning and identification of functional domain

The initial cloning of the GR revealed two GRs: alpha and beta. Oakley *et al* discovered that GR beta did not bind ligand(Oakley et al. 1996) -- biological functions of GR-beta are still in the early stages of discovery(Yudt & Cidlowski 2002). This review focuses on GR-alpha, which will be referred to as GR.

2.2. GR as a founding member of the nuclear receptor (NR) superfamily

The GR and the estrogen receptor (ER) are founding members of the NR superfamily, and were cloned within the same time period(Green et al 1986, Greene et al 1986). They are highly homologous and are composed of domains that retain much of their function when dissociated from each other. Both GR and ER have three major domains, the NTD, DBD and LBD, as do all steroid receptors (Fig 1). The domains are dissociable and for certain functions are also interchangeable. For example, an ER chimera, which contains a GR binding domain, activates transcription in the presence of estradiol but does so by binding a GRE(Green & Chambon 1987).

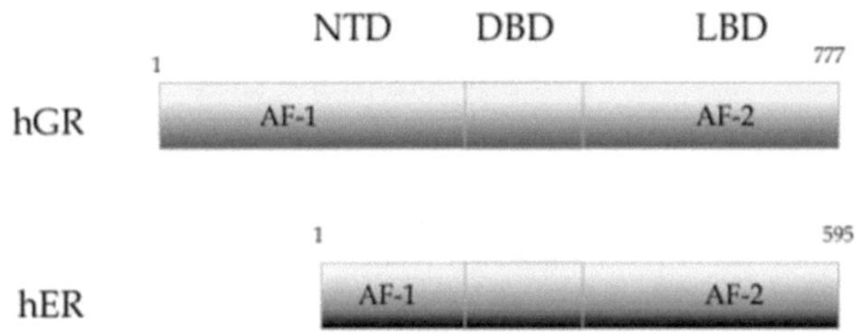

Figure 1. Domains of the GR and ER. (hGR) human glucocorticoid receptor, (hER) human estrogen receptor, (AF-1 and AF-2) activation functions 1 and 2, respectively

3. GR-regulated gene repression: response elements

Prior to the late 1980s, a prevailing view of GR-mediated repression was that it would require a palindromic DNA binding site. This assumption could not explain the fact that glucocorticoids repress a number of genes in the absence of a prototypic GRE. The discovery of composite elements and the discovery that elements for other transcription factors could sustain GR-mediated inhibition of gene activation were major advances in the understanding of GR-mediated repression.

3.1. Repression mediated by composite elements

Composite elements are hybrids (Lefstin & Yamamoto 1998). In the case of GR regulation they consist of half sites, one for a GR monomer and one for a monomer of a distinct transcription factor -- *e.g.* a monomer of an activator protein-1 (AP-1) family member. They are found in numerous genes, including those directly involved in regulating the HPA-axis -- *crh* and *pomc*.

Much of the initial molecular analysis of composite elements was performed using the proliferin gene (*proliferin*).The *proliferin* composite element consists of half sites for GRE and AP-1 binding and confers both activation and repression, dictated by the specific AP-1 family member bound (Diamond et al 1990, Pearce et al 1998). AP-1 family members include c-Jun, cFos and similar proteins. A GR monomer bound in the presence of a c-Jun monomer will stimulate activation from the *proliferin* element, whereas high levels of c-Fos inhibit activation(Diamond et al 1990). Like the *proliferin* element, the *crh* nGRE is composed of GRE and AP-1 half sites. In addition, the extent to which the nGRE directs repression is dependent on the AP-1 family member bound to the composite element (Malkoski & Dorin 1999).

3.2. Repression mediated through other transcription factors and components of the basal transcriptional activity

Three papers published simultaneously in 1990 reported that glucocorticoid-bound GR could down-regulate AP-1 stimulated gene expression (Jonat et al 1990, Schule et al 1990, Yang-Yen et al 1990). Mechanisms by which the GR down-regulates AP-1 activity and activity of other transcription factors are still being elucidated -- some interact with coregulators and others interact directly with components of the general transcription machinery. An example of the latter is GR down-regulation of nuclear factor-kappa B (NF-kB) activity. In the context of the interleukin-8 gene(*il-8*), GR is a physical and functional intermediary between the RelA (p65) component of NF-kB and the C′-terminal domain of polymerase II (pol II). GR alters the phosphorylation state of the C′-terminal domain of pol II and thus regulates its activity(Nissen & Yamamoto 2000). The GR also down-regulates *il-8* expression by interfering with the activity of the transcription elongation factor-b (Luecke & Yamamoto 2005). Thus, GR targets both initiation and elongation steps in the context of the *il-8* promoter. It is unknown whether or not GR works through either of these mechanisms in the context of *crh.*

4. Identification of NR coregulators

By the 1990s it was clear that NRs required additional factors to regulate gene expression. The discovery of NR co-regulators — coactivators and corepressors — permitted a quantum leap in the elucidation of NR mechanisms of gene regulation.

4.1. NR coactivators

Although there are numerous coactivators, this review focuses on the three members of the p160 family commonly referred to as SRCs-1, -2, and -3. In addition, a nomenclature group has codified the names of these coactivators as NCoA 1-3. Here they will be referred to collectively as the p160 family and individually the names first reported will be used with the agreed upon nomenclature indicated, *e.g.* SRC-1 (NCoA 1).

The first p160 was discovered by O'Malley as a coactivator for a progesterone receptor -- the steroid receptor co-activator-1, SRC-1 (NCoA 1)(Onate et al 1995). Subsequently, Stallcup reported a p160 coactivator for the mouse GR, Glucocorticoid Receptor Interacting Protein 1 GRIP1(Hong et al 1997, Hong et al 1996), also designated NCoA 2. The third p160, reported by several investigators, bears many names, including AIB1(Anzick et al 1997) and RAC3(Li et al 1997) but it is often referred to as SRC-3 (NCoA 3).

Each p160 contains two highly conserved regions. In the center of the protein is a cluster of three Leucine-X-X-Leucine-Leucine (LXXLL) motifs, in which X denotes any amino acid(Ding et al 1998, Heery et al 1997). These are also referred to as NR-boxes. The motifs are a requisite site of interaction with nuclear receptors; mutations of these sites abrogate NR activation functions (Feng et al 1998). p160s also contain a domain that binds to histone acetylases, *e.g.* the cAMP regulatory element binding protein (CREB)-binding protein (CBP), which remodel chromatin by acetylating specific lysines in histones(Marmorstein 2001).

Mechanisms by which p160s regulate *crh* expression are not well understood. The best studied of these is SRC-1. The SRC-1a isoform mRNA has been mapped to the PVH, and CRH mRNA levels have been evaluated in SRC-1 knockout mice (Lachize et al 2009). Paradoxically, SRC-1 is associated with *crh* repression(van der Laan et al 2008). There is precedent for this -- Rogatsky and colleagues reported that GRIP1 has a repressive function(Rogatsky et al 2001). The GRIP1 domain that supports this function, however, is unique to the GRIP1 p160. Thus, the mechanisms of SRC-1a down-regulation have yet to be identified.

4.1.1. Coactivator interaction with histone acetyl transferases (HATs)

The discovery of the p160s and the discovery of a coactivator for the cAMP regulatory element binding protein (CREB) - binding protein (CBP) and its homologue p300 occurred contemporaneously. In addition to a p160 binding domain the two coactivators contain a histone acetylase domain. CBP is a coactivator for numerous transcription factors that include a number of nuclear receptors and factors involved in inflammation, *e.g.* STAT1 (Horvai et al 1997). In addition to CBP and p300, other acetylases such as the p300/CBP-associated factor (p/CAF;(Yang et al 1996)play a role in nuclear receptor regulation; however, their role in GR regulated *crh* expression is poorly understood.

4.2. Nuclear receptor co-repressors

Some members of the NR family, such as the thyroid hormone receptor (TR), maintain a constitutively silent state of gene expression. The search for a co-repressor for TR led to the discovery of the Nuclear Receptor Corepressor (NCoR), whose homologue is known as the silencing mediator of retinoic acid receptor and the thyroid receptor (SMRT). The NR interaction site in NCoR is remarkably similar to the NR-boxes in the p160 coactivator family. The corepressor motif is L/I XXI/V-I, compared to the p160 coactivator motif, LXXLL. The corepressor motif is referred to as a CoRNR box. These features of coactivator and corepressor regulated gene expression are summarized in Table 1.

Coregulator	Interaction Site	Associated Enzyme	Enzymatic Action	Effect on Chromatin	Effect on Transcription
Coactivator	NR box LXXLL	HAT	Histone Acetylation	Decondensation	Activation
Corepressor	CoRNR box L/I XXI/V-I	HDAC	Histone Deacetylation	Condensation	Deactivation or Repression

Table 1. The chain of events for activation parallels that for repression.

The mechanisms by which co-repressors interact with GR to down-regulate *crh* expression are largely uncharacterized. Using transient transfection/reporter assays, van der Laan *et al.* reported that cotransfection of NCoR and SMRT did not accentuate glucocorticoid mediated *crh* repression. Instead, these repressors accentuated corticosterone inhibition of forskolin-stimulated expression(van der Laan et al 2008).

The corepressors NCoR and SMRT bind to histone deacetylases (HDACs). The specificity of an HDAC for a given receptor has been elucidated in some studies. An early report revealed that HDAC3 but not HDAC1 is involved in TR repression (Guenther et al 2001). Given the conserved nature of many functions across nuclear receptors one might predict that like the TR, GR- repressed transcription of *crh* expression would involve HDAC3 but not HDAC1. In the context of the *crh* promoter, however, the reverse is true(Miller et al 2011).

5. Structural analysis of GR

Structural analysis of GR permits identification not only of a single protein structure but also of protein interfaces involved in specific inter-molecular interactions.

5.1. The DNA binding domain

Crystallographic analysis of a GR dimer bound to its DNA recognition site revealed that GR zinc fingers intercalate with DNA (Freedman et al 1988, Luisi et al 1991). Subsequent NMR analysis of the DBD structure revealed inherent stability in the absence of DNA (Berglund et al 1992). The DBD is now known to have several functions in addition to binding DNA, and it may be that the inherent structure supports these functions.

5.2. The ligand binding domain

A characteristic of all NRs is that the LBD is longer and less structured than the DBD. This partially explains why the crystal structure of two smaller nuclear receptors, RXR-alpha and TR were the first to be solved (Bourguet et al 1995, Wagner et al 1995). The TR was the first ligand-bound NR to be crystallized; even so, it took years to optimize LBD purification in sufficient quantities to permit crystallization (Apriletti et al 1995, Apriletti et al 1988) (McGrath et al 1994). This process was facilitated by use of a radioactively labeled ligand (Apriletti et al 1995, Apriletti et al 1988), which allowed LBD to be tracked throughout purification. The discovery of NR boxes was taking place simultaneously with efforts to crystalize the TR LBD. Thus, crystallization of the ligand-bound TR bound to a GRIP1NR box followed shortly thereafter (Darimont et al 1998, Wagner et al 1995).

The next LBD structure to be solved was ER-alpha, again bound to ligand and an NR box. As a member of the steroid receptor branch of the NR superfamily it has a longer, more complex LBD than the TR. Thus, the protein is inherently more difficult to crystalize, and its crystal structure more difficult to solve. Coordinates used to solve the TR structure permitted ER modeling (Shiau et al 1998). Indeed, in the absence of TR crystal structure coordinates, solution of the ER crystal structure may have been intractable at the time.

The GR LBD is even less structured than either TR or ER-alpha. In fact, a mutation in the GR LBD was required to generate crystals. Co-crystallization of GR LBD bound to Dex and to an NR box revealed that the overall structure of the receptor LBD is the same as the TR and ER-alpha with three key differences: an additional dimerization function, a second set of charge clamps, and an additional pocket (Bledsoe et al 2002, Bledsoe et al 2004). These distinctive features underscore the complexity of GR (Bledsoe et al 2004).

6. Epigenetics and chromatin modification

Strictly defined, the term epigenetics refers to an inheritable factor composed of something other than unmodified genomic DNA— this is distinct from chromatin modifications that regulate processes that are not inherited. Thus, most of the processes referred to here are not truly epigenetic, but rather consist of chromatin modifications that modulate gene expression.

6.1. Histone acetylation

Although typically associated with transcriptional activation, histone acetylation is also associated with repressed states of gene expression (Shahbazian & Grunstein 2007). The initial focus of study in this field was on chromatin acetylation via recruitment of histone acetyl transferases (HATs). The addition of an acetyl to a lysine (Lys) neutralizes the acid-base interaction with DNA. This neutralization, as well as the steric hindrance conferred by Lys acetylation, destabilizes histone:DNA interactions, and allows proteins such as transcription factors, transcription initiators, and elongation factors access to DNA binding sites.

6.2. Histone Deacetylation

Deacetylation is the counterpart to acetylation. Histone Deacetylases (HDACs) are comprised of a family of enzymes with three subdivisions. The nomenclature of mammalian HDACs is somewhat confounding, having arisen from sequential numbering as the enzymes were discovered. Class I includes HDAC 1-3, 8 and 11. They have one catalytic domain and for the most part are nuclear. Class II HDACs are larger than Class I and are divided into two subclasses, IIa and IIb. Class IIa HDACs include HDAC 4, 5, 7and have an N′-terminal domain unique to this class. In addition, Class IIa HDACs shuttle between the nucleus and cytoplasm. Class IIb HDACs, 6 and 10, have two HDAC domains instead of a unique N′-terminus, and are predominantly found in the cytoplasm (Verdin et al 2003). Class III HDACs are distinguished by their requirement for NAD^+. They are named sirtuins due to similarity to the yeast Sir2. Like Sir2, they are targets of intense study given their association with aging and neurodegenerative processes. Because HDACs are tightly correlated with repression they have been examined in the context of GR-repressed *crh* expression (Miller et al 2011).

7. Corticotropin Releasing Hormone (CRH)

Although CRH is widely expressed in the mammalian CNS, the focus here is on regulation of *crh* in the medial parvocellular region of the PVH (mpPVH).

7.1. CRH cloning

In 1983, a fragment of the human *crh* was cloned that contained the proximal promoter and coding region. The predicted amino acid sequence differs from the ovine by seven residues (Shibahara et al 1983). Cloning the rat cDNA and a portion of the promoter were reported in 1987(Thompson et al 1987). The rat cDNA has high sequence homology to human cDNA, and in fact the peptide sequences are identical. Rat and human proximal promoter sequences are also highly conserved (Thompson et al 1987).

7.2. *crh* regulation

A cAMP regulatory element (CRE) at approximately -200 in the proximal promoter plays a pivotal role in activating *crh* expression by recruitment of (CREB)(Seasholtz et al 1988, Thompson et al 1987). Interestingty this site not only mediates activation but also mediates repression by recruiting the inducible cAMP early repressor(Aguilera & Liu 2012). In addition, a negative GRE in the 200 base span contributes to *crh* down-regulation (Malkoski & Dorin 1999,(Malkoski et al 1997). Indeed the entire first 200 bases of the proximal promoter are highly conserved, underscoring the importance of this region to regulation of the stress response(Yao et al 2007).

Specific mechanisms of GR-mediated *crh* down-regulation have been difficult to parse, as is case for most glucocorticoid down-regulated genes. At the most basic level it is unclear whether glucocorticoids suppress *crh*-activated expression only, or if they also suppress basal levels of expression. This distinction is important in that recruitment of signal-specific co-activators would be required prior to GR inhibition. Repressionof basal activity, however, would entail recruiting a corepressor.

Most studies of inhibited *crh* regulation have used transient transfection assays or isolated DNA. In neither case is DNA in its natural state of chromatinization. More recent studies of *crh* expression underscore the importance of considering the chromatin environment.

8. Impact of chromatin modifications on analysis of GR-mediated *crh* down-regulation

A number of factors regulate the *crh* chromatin environment. Inhibition of activated *crh* expression involves both the CRE and the nGRE, and maintenance of basal activity involves histone acetylation and DNA methylation. Numerous steps in mechanisms of inhibition and repression have yet to be elucidated.

8.1.1. Repression of cAMP activated crh expression

CRE is required for regulation of *crh* expression through signal transduction. Phosphorylated CREB (pCREB) can interact with an inhibitory member of the CREB family, the inducible cAMP early repressor (ICER). ICER is a dominant negative of pCREB and decreases cAMP activated expression. Further details on the role of pCREB and its family members in regulating *crh* expression can be found in the Aguilera and Liu review(Aguilera & Liu 2012).

8.1.2. Regulation through the nGRE

Repression mediated through the nGRE in the proximal *crh* promoter is similar to repression mediated through the *proliferin* nGRE. A monomer of GR and a monomer of the AP-1 family bind the composite element. The prototypic coactivator for pCREB is CBP, which is also a coactivator for AP-1(Bannister & Kouzarides 1995, Bannister et al 1995). Thus, in the context of *crh,* CBP might permit a functional interaction between the GR:AP-1 dimer and a dimer of CREB family members bound to the CRE.

8.2. Maintenance of basal levels of activation

Basal levels of activation involve a balance of activation and repression. There are numerous ways in which this balance may be maintained -- one is to maintain a constant state of chromatin modification. Two modification types that play a role in *crh* regulation are histone acetylation and methylation of CpG islands.

8.2.1. Histone acetylation

Activated *crh* expression involves CBP recruitment to the proximal promoter. CBP is a HAT coactivator for both pCREB and c-Jun, so activation of either the pKA pathway or the pKC pathway could be involved in CBP recruitment.

Analysis of global histone 3 and 4 (H3 and H4) acetylation in the context of estradiol-regulated *crh* expression has been reported(Lalmansingh & Uht 2008). As is the case in estradiol regulation, Dex regulates H3 and H4 acetylation differentially, as measured by chromatin immunoprecipitation followed by PCR amplification(Miller et al 2011). Dex increases H4 acetylation, a finding that underscores the fact that acetylation may be associated a state of repression as well as activation.

The level of histone acetylation is a function of the presence of enzymatically active HATs and HDACs. In the case of Dex-regulated *crh* expression, the amount of ligand bound GR is increased in the region of the promoter(Miller et al 2011). When measured at the same time, HDAC levels are also increased. Furthermore, GR binds HDAC1 in a Dex-dependent manner, suggesting the possibility that GR recruits HDAC1 to the *crh* promoter (Figure 2).

Like the differential acetylation of H3 and H4, the Dex associated increase in HDACs displays a degree of specificity — although HDAC1 is increased at the promoter, HDAC3 is not (Miller et al 2011). The mechanisms by which these enzymes leave and are recruited to chromatin are poorly understood and merit further study.

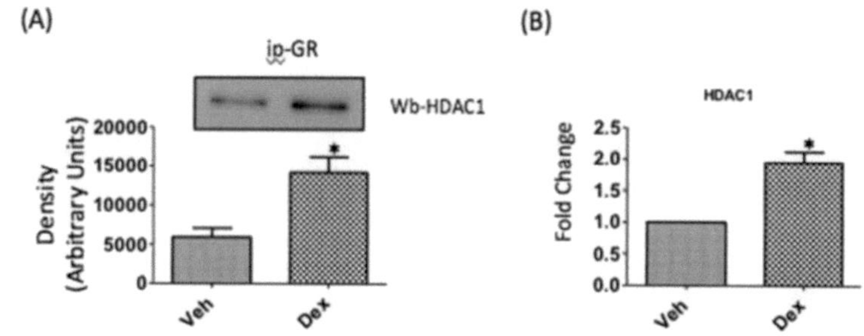

Figure 2. Dex treatment leads to increased HDAC1:GR complexes and increased HDAC1 at the *crh* promoter. (A) Co-immunoprecipitation analysis; nuclear extract was immunoprecipitated with a polyclonal antibody against GR. Western blot analysis of the immune-precipitate revealed an increase in the co-immunoprecipitation of HDAC1. n=3; Bars represent the mean ± SEM and are represented as the fold difference of the Veh *, $P < 0.05$. (B) ChIP analysis of the CRH promoter; cells were treated with Dex and chromatin was immune-precipitated with an anti HDAC1 antibody. Quantitative RT-PCR analysis of the immune-precipitated DNA indicates enrichment of HDAC1 at the promoter. n=3; Bars represent the mean ± SEM and are represented as the fold difference of the Veh *, $P < 0.05$.

8.2.2. DNA methylation

Methylation of CpG islands of the GR promoter was one of the earliest reported true epigenetic phenomena in that it was associated with inheritance -- in this case a behavioral phenotype(Weaver et al 2004). More recently, CpG island methylated *crh* has been described in the context of social defeat(Elliott et al 2010).

The first report of CpG island methylation in the context of *crh* regulation was an offshoot from a study of a mouse model of Rett Syndrome. This syndrome occurs in girls and manifests as diminished intelligence, repetitive motor movements, and anxiety — all of which have variable penetrance. The genetic lesion in Rett Syndrome is a mutation in the methyl CpG (meCpG) binding protein 2 (MeCP2). This protein binds to meCpG islands and represses the expression of bound genes. McGill and colleagues found that one of these genes is *crh.* Remarkably, mice bearing the MeCP2 mutation have a hyperactive HPA axis associated with elevated levels of CRH mRNA in the PVH, central amygdala, and BNST— all regions that express GRs and which are associated with HPA axis regulation. In addition, meCpG sites have been mapped in the *crh* proximal promoter region and were found to be present in the same region as the CRE and nGRE(McGill et al 2006). These findings underscore the importance of this region in *crh* regulation.

9. A role for bioinformatics in GR-regulated *crh* expression

Dalwadi and Uht recently investigated expression patterns of two neuronal cell lines, which were derived from embryonic PVH and amygdala. Paradoxically, even though neurons in these populations express CRH and contain GRs, they differ in the response to glucocorticoid treatment. In the mpPVH, glucocorticoids down-regulate *crh* expression whereas in the amygdala they up-regulate it. Expression microarrays are currently being analyzed using the expression pattern of two neuronal cell lines, amygdalar AR-5 and hypothalamic IVB - both differentially express *crh* in response to Dex treatment. The number of genes associated with development of projections is similar between the two cell lines, whereas the number of genes involved in steroid hormone responsiveness is two-fold greater in the hypothalamic line compared to the amygdalar line. Given the importance of the hypothalamus relative to amygdala in regulation of steroid hormone physiology, these results are not unexpected. However, the two lines also differ in the relative expression of genes associated with response to oxidative stress and to DNA binding, as categorized in the Gene Ontology database (GO; Figure 3). These differences are intriguing and have spurred further investigation.

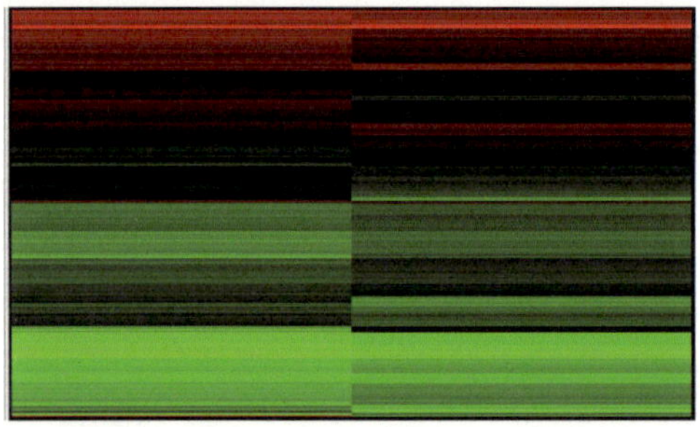

GO Term	AR-5	IVB
DNA Binding	36	21
Neuron Projection Development	9	8
Response to Oxidative Stress	10	6
Response to Steroid Hormone Stimulus	6	12

Figure 3. Hierarchal cluster showing relative abundance of genes between the AR-5 and IVB cell lines (red - abundant, green - less abundant). (GO) Gene Ontology as defined by the DAVID analysis program. (AR-5) Amygdalar cell line, (IVB) Hypothalamic cell line.

More refined techniques are now available for bioinformatics analysis of gene expression. One of those is the combination of chromatin immunoprecipitation and microarray assays (ChIP-chip). In this approach, DNA isolated from ChIPs is used to probe a genomic microarray. ChIP-chip has been used to analyze GR binding sites. So and colleagues used a combination of conventional expression array analysis followed by ChIP-chip. When glucocorticoid-induced genes were compared to glucocorticoid-repressed genes, analysis revealed that the GR-holoreceptor induced all genes that were regulated via a conventional palindrome. In distinction, none of the genes repressed contained such an element (So et al 2007). Such a clear-cut distinction is rare in biology.

A second example of a bioinformatics approach useful in the analysis of NR mediated gene regulation is global run-on and sequencing (GRO-seq)(Core et al 2008). This technique permits unbiased analysis of all RNA transcripts, which allows detection of both mRNA and non-coding RNAs. It has been used in a number of biological systems, including use of this technique to determine the nature of transcripts induced by 17estradiol treatment of MCF-7 cells, a prototypic breast cancer cell line. To date, however, there are no reports of GRO-seq analysis of glucocorticoid regulated genes.

10. Summary

In the last fifteen years an explosion of new information has facilitated novel ways of looking at GR mediated gene expression. The seminal findings by Yamamoto in the early 1980s —that GRs bind to specific palindromic glucocorticoid response elements(Payvar et al 1983)— is now frequently referred to as the classic mechanism of gene regulation. At present, numerous alternate mechanisms of gene regulation are being elucidated. Many of these involve interactions with coregulatory factors. Such interactions have helped bridge the gap between transcription and chromatin remodeling, which in turn has resulted in the intersection of the NR field with the field of epigenetics.

This review has focused on glucocorticoid regulation of genomic effects via the GR. Other areas currently being investigated include the actions of GR splice variants, and the role of glucocorticoid regulation of heat shock proteins. Lastly, the effects of glucocorticoids at the cell membrane (non-genomic events), mechanisms of cell membrane transport of glucocorticoids, and nuclear import of the GR holoreceptors are all steps in regulation that merit further analysis.

Author details

Rosalie M. Uht
Institute for Aging and Alzheimer's Disease Research and Department of Pharmacology and Neuroscience University of North Texas Health Science Center, USA

Acknowledgement

Dedicated to the Memory of Wylie Vale 1941 - 2012.

The data for figures were generated by Dharmendra Sharma (Fig 2) and Dhwanil Dalwadi (Fig 3).

The author thanks Teresa Olsen for editing the manuscript.

Funding obtained from UNTHSC startup funds and NIHR01 RMH082900A (RMU).

11. References

Aguilera G, Liu Y. 2012. The molecular physiology of CRH neurons. *Frontiers in neuroendocrinology* 33: 67-84

Anzick SL, Kononen J, Walker RL, Azorsa DO, Tanner MM, et al. 1997. AIB1, a steroid receptor coactivator amplified in breast and ovarian cancer. *Science* 277: 965-8

Apriletti JW, Baxter JD, Lau KH, West BL. 1995. Expression of the rat alpha 1 thyroid hormone receptor ligand binding domain in Escherichia coli and the use of a ligand-induced conformation change as a method for its purification to homogeneity. *Protein expression and purification* 6: 363-70

Apriletti JW, Baxter JD, Lavin TN. 1988. Large scale purification of the nuclear thyroid hormone receptor from rat liver and sequence-specific binding of the receptor to DNA. *The Journal of biological chemistry* 263: 9409-17

Bannister AJ, Kouzarides T. 1995. CBP-induced stimulation of c-Fos activity is abrogated by E1A. *The EMBO journal* 14: 4758-62

Bannister AJ, Oehler T, Wilhelm D, Angel P, Kouzarides T. 1995. Stimulation of c-Jun activity by CBP: c-Jun residues Ser63/73 are required for CBP induced stimulation in vivo and CBP binding in vitro. *Oncogene* 11: 2509-14

Berglund H, Kovacs H, Dahlman-Wright K, Gustafsson JA, Hard T. 1992. Backbone dynamics of the glucocorticoid receptor DNA-binding domain. *Biochemistry* 31: 12001-11

Bicknell AB. 2008. The tissue-specific processing of pro-opiomelanocortin. *Journal of neuroendocrinology* 20: 692-9

Bledsoe RK, Montana VG, Stanley TB, Delves CJ, Apolito CJ, et al. 2002. Crystal structure of the glucocorticoid receptor ligand binding domain reveals a novel mode of receptor dimerization and coactivator recognition. *Cell* 110: 93-105

Bledsoe RK, Stewart EL, Pearce KH. 2004. Structure and function of the glucocorticoid receptor ligand binding domain. *Vitamins and hormones* 68: 49-91

Bourguet W, Ruff M, Chambon P, Gronemeyer H, Moras D. 1995. Crystal structure of the ligand-binding domain of the human nuclear receptor RXR-alpha. *Nature* 375: 377-82

Choi DC, Furay AR, Evanson NK, Ostrander MM, Ulrich-Lai YM, Herman JP. 2007. Bed nucleus of the stria terminalis subregions differentially regulate hypothalamic-pituitary-adrenal axis activity: implications for the integration of limbic inputs. *The Journal of neuroscience : the official journal of the Society for Neuroscience* 27: 2025-34

Cintra A, Fuxe K, Harfstrand A, Agnati LF, Wikstrom AC, et al. 1987. Presence of glucocorticoid receptor immunoreactivity in corticotrophin releasing factor and in growth hormone releasing factor immunoreactive neurons of the rat di- and telencephalon. *Neuroscience letters* 77: 25-30

Core LJ, Waterfall JJ, Lis JT. 2008. Nascent RNA sequencing reveals widespread pausing and divergent initiation at human promoters. *Science* 322: 1845-8

Darimont BD, Wagner RL, Apriletti JW, Stallcup MR, Kushner PJ, et al. 1998. Structure and specificity of nuclear receptor-coactivator interactions. *Genes & development* 12: 3343-56

de Kloet ER, Joels M, Holsboer F. 2005. Stress and the brain: from adaptation to disease. *Nature reviews. Neuroscience* 6: 463-75

de Kloet R, Wallach G, Mc EBS. 1975. Differences in Corticosterone and Dexamethasone Binding to Rat Brain and Pituitary. *Endocrinology* 96: 598-609

Diamond MI, Miner JN, Yoshinaga SK, Yamamoto KR. 1990. Transcription factor interactions: selectors of positive or negative regulation from a single DNA element. *Science* 249: 1266-72

Ding XF, Anderson CM, Ma H, Hong H, Uht RM, et al. 1998. Nuclear receptor-binding sites of coactivators glucocorticoid receptor interacting protein 1 (GRIP1) and steroid receptor coactivator 1 (SRC-1): multiple motifs with different binding specificities. *Mol Endocrinol* 12: 302-13

Elliott E, Ezra-Nevo G, Regev L, Neufeld-Cohen A, Chen A. 2010. Resilience to social stress coincides with functional DNA methylation of the Crf gene in adult mice. *Nature neuroscience* 13: 1351-3

Feng W, Ribeiro RC, Wagner RL, Nguyen H, Apriletti JW, et al. 1998. Hormone-dependent coactivator binding to a hydrophobic cleft on nuclear receptors. *Science* 280: 1747-9

Freedman LP, Luisi BF, Korszun ZR, Basavappa R, Sigler PB, Yamamoto KR. 1988. The function and structure of the metal coordination sites within the glucocorticoid receptor DNA binding domain. *Nature* 334: 543-6

Gibbs DM. 1986. Vasopressin and oxytocin: hypothalamic modulators of the stress response: a review. *Psychoneuroendocrinology* 11: 131-9

Green S, Chambon P. 1987. Oestradiol induction of a glucocorticoid-responsive gene by a chimaeric receptor. *Nature* 325: 75-8

Green S, Walter P, Kumar V, Krust A, Bornert J-M, et al. 1986. Human oestrogen receptor cDNA: sequence, expression and homology to v-*erb-A*. *Nature* 320: 134-39

Greene GL, Gilna P, Waterfield M, Baker A, Hort Y, Shine J. 1986. Sequence and expression of human estrogen receptor complementary DNA. *Science* 231: 1150-4

Guenther MG, Barak O, Lazar MA. 2001. The SMRT and N-CoR corepressors are activating cofactors for histone deacetylase 3. *Molecular and cellular biology* 21: 6091-101

Gustafsson JA, Carlstedt-Duke J, Poellinger L, Okret S, Wikstrom AC, et al. 1987. Biochemistry, molecular biology, and physiology of the glucocorticoid receptor. *Endocrine reviews* 8: 185-234

Heery DM, Kalkhoven E, Hoare S, Parker MG. 1997. A signature motif in transcriptional co-activators mediates binding to nuclear receptors. *Nature* 387: 733-6

Herman JP, Figueiredo H, Mueller NK, Ulrich-Lai Y, Ostrander MM, et al. 2003. Central mechanisms of stress integration: hierarchical circuitry controlling hypothalamo-pituitary-adrenocortical responsiveness. *Frontiers in neuroendocrinology* 24: 151-80

Hong H, Kohli K, Garabedian MJ, Stallcup MR. 1997. GRIP1, a transcriptional coactivator for the AF-2 transactivation domain of steroid, thyroid, retinoid, and vitamin D receptors. *Molecular and cellular biology* 17: 2735-44

Hong H, Kohli K, Trivedi A, Johnson DL, Stallcup MR. 1996. GRIP1, a novel mouse protein that serves as a transcriptional coactivator in yeast for the hormone binding domains of steroid receptors. *Proceedings of the National Academy of Sciences of the United States of America* 93: 4948-52

Horvai AE, Xu L, Korzus E, Brard G, Kalafus D, et al. 1997. Nuclear integration of JAK/STAT and Ras/AP-1 signaling by CBP and p300. *Proceedings of the National Academy of Sciences of the United States of America* 94: 1074-9

Jonat C, Rahmsdorf HJ, Park K-K, Cato ACB, Gebel S, et al. 1990. Antitumor promotion and antiinflammation: down-modulation of AP-1 (fos/jun) activity by glucocorticoid hormone. *Cell* 62: 1189-204

Lachize S, Apostolakis EM, van der Laan S, Tijssen AM, Xu J, et al. 2009. Steroid receptor coactivator-1 is necessary for regulation of corticotropin-releasing hormone by chronic stress and glucocorticoids. *Proceedings of the National Academy of Sciences of the United States of America* 106: 8038-42

Lalmansingh AS, Uht RM. 2008. Estradiol regulates corticotropin-releasing hormone gene (crh) expression in a rapid and phasic manner that parallels estrogen receptor-alpha and -beta recruitment to a 3',5'-cyclic adenosine 5'-monophosphate regulatory region of the proximal crh promoter. *Endocrinology* 149: 346-57

Lefstin JA, Yamamoto KR. 1998. Allosteric effects of DNA on transcriptional regulators. *Nature* 392: 885-8

Li H, Gomes PJ, Chen JD. 1997. RAC3, a steroid/nuclear receptor-associated coactivator that is related to SRC-1 and TIF2. *Proceedings of the National Academy of Sciences of the United States of America* 94: 8479-84

Luecke HF, Yamamoto KR. 2005. The glucocorticoid receptor blocks P-TEFb recruitment by NFkappaB to effect promoter-specific transcriptional repression. *Genes & development* 19: 1116-27

Luisi BF, Xu WX, Otwinowski Z, Freedman LP, Yamamoto KR, Sigler PB. 1991. Crystallographic analysis of the interaction of the glucocorticoid receptor with DNA. *Nature* 352: 497-505

Malkoski SP, Dorin RI. 1999. Composite glucocorticoid regulation at a functionally defined negative glucocorticoid response element of the human corticotropin-releasing hormone gene. *Mol Endocrinol* 13: 1629-44

Malkoski SP, Handanos CM, Dorin RI. 1997. Localization of a negative glucocorticoid response element of the human corticotropin releasing hormone gene. *Molecular and cellular endocrinology* 127: 189-99

Marmorstein R. 2001. Structure and function of histone acetyltransferases. *Cellular and molecular life sciences : CMLS* 58: 693-703

McEwen BS, Davis PG, Parsons B, Pfaff DW. 1979. The brain as a target for steroid hormone action. *Annual review of neuroscience* 2: 65-112

McGill BE, Bundle SF, Yaylaoglu MB, Carson JP, Thaller C, Zoghbi HY. 2006. Enhanced anxiety and stress-induced corticosterone release are associated with increased Crh expression in a mouse model of Rett syndrome. *Proceedings of the National Academy of Sciences of the United States of America* 103: 18267-72

McGrath ME, Wagner RL, Apriletti JW, West BL, Ramalingam V, et al. 1994. Preliminary crystallographic studies of the ligand-binding domain of the thyroid hormone receptor complexed with triiodothyronine. *Journal of molecular biology* 237: 236-9

Miller L, Foradori CD, Lalmansingh AS, Sharma D, Handa RJ, Uht RM. 2011. Histone deacetylase 1 (HDAC1) participates in the down-regulation of corticotropin releasing hormone gene (crh) expression. *Physiology & behavior* 104: 312-20

Nissen RM, Yamamoto KR. 2000. The glucocorticoid receptor inhibits NFkappaB by interfering with serine-2 phosphorylation of the RNA polymerase II carboxy-terminal domain. *Genes & development* 14: 2314-29

Oakley RH, Sar M, Cidlowski JA. 1996. The human glucocorticoid receptor beta isoform. Expression, biochemical properties, and putative function. *The Journal of biological chemistry* 271: 9550-9

Onate SA, Tsai SY, Tsai MJ, O'Malley BW. 1995. Sequence and characterization of a coactivator for the steroid hormone receptor superfamily. *Science* 270: 1354-7

Payvar F, DeFranco D, Firestone GL, Edgar B, Wrange O, et al. 1983. Sequence-specific binding of glucocorticoid receptor to MTV DNA at sites within and upstream of the transcribed region. *Cell* 35: 381-92

Pearce D, Matsui W, Miner JN, Yamamoto KR. 1998. Glucocorticoid receptor transcriptional activity determined by spacing of receptor and nonreceptor DNA sites. *The Journal of biological chemistry* 273: 30081-5

Pratt WB, Dittmar KD. 1998. Studies with Purified Chaperones Advance the Understanding of the Mechanism of Glucocorticoid Receptor-hsp90 Heterocomplex Assembly. *Trends in endocrinology and metabolism: TEM* 9: 244-52

Rogatsky I, Zarember KA, Yamamoto KR. 2001. Factor recruitment and TIF2/GRIP1 corepressor activity at a collagenase-3 response element that mediates regulation by phorbol esters and hormones. *The EMBO journal* 20: 6071-83

Sapolsky RM, Krey LC, McEwen BS. 1984. Stress down-regulates corticosterone receptors in a site-specific manner in the brain. *Endocrinology* 114: 287-92

Schule R, Rangarajan P, Kliewer S, Ransone LJ, Bolado J, et al. 1990. Functional antagonism between oncoprotein c-jun and the glucocorticoid receptor. *Cell* 62: 1217-26

Seasholtz AF, Thompson RC, Douglass JO. 1988. Identification of a cyclic adenosine monophosphate-responsive element in the rat corticotropin-releasing hormone gene. *Molec Endocrinol* 2: 1311-19

Shahbazian MD, Grunstein M. 2007. Functions of site-specific histone acetylation and deacetylation. *Annual review of biochemistry* 76: 75-100

Shiau AK, Barstad D, Loria PM, Cheng L, Kushner PJ, et al. 1998. The structural basis of estrogen receptor/coactivator recognition and the antagonism of this interaction by tamoxifen. *Cell* 95: 927-37

Shibahara S, Morimoto Y, Furutani Y, Notake M, Takahashi H, et al. 1983. Isolation and sequence analysis of the human corticotropin-releasing factor precursor gene. *The EMBO journal* 2: 775-9

So AY, Chaivorapol C, Bolton EC, Li H, Yamamoto KR. 2007. Determinants of cell- and gene-specific transcriptional regulation by the glucocorticoid receptor. *PLoS genetics* 3: e94

Swanson L, Sawchenko P. 1980. Paraventricular nucleus: a site for the integration of neuroendocrine and autonomic mechanisms. *Neuroendocrinol* 31: 410-17

Swanson LW, Sawchenko PE, Lind RW, Rho JH. 1987. The CRH motoneuron: differential peptide regulation in neurons with possible synaptic, paracrine, and endocrine outputs. *Annals of the New York Academy of Sciences* 512: 12-23

Thompson RC, Seasholtz AF, Douglass JO, Herbert E. 1987. *The rat corticotropin releasing hormone gene*. New York: New York Academy of Sciences. 1-11 pp.

Uht RM, McKelvy JF, Harrison RW, Bohn MC. 1988. Demonstration of glucocorticoid receptor-like immunoreactivity in glucocorticoid-sensitive vasopressin and corticotropin-releasing factor neurons in the hypothalamic paraventricular nucleus. *Journal of neuroscience research* 19: 405-11, 68-9

Vale W, Spiess J, Rivier C, Rivier J. 1981. Characterization of a 41-residue ovine hypothalamic peptide that stimulates secretion of corticotropin and beta-endorphin. *Science* 213: 1394-7

van der Laan S, Lachize SB, Vreugdenhil E, de Kloet ER, Meijer OC. 2008. Nuclear receptor coregulators differentially modulate induction and glucocorticoid receptor-mediated repression of the corticotropin-releasing hormone gene. *Endocrinology* 149: 725-32

Verdin E, Dequiedt F, Kasler HG. 2003. Class II histone deacetylases: versatile regulators. *Trends in genetics : TIG* 19: 286-93

Wagner RL, Apriletti JW, McGrath ME, West BL, Baxter JD, Fletterick RJ. 1995. A structural role for hormone in the thyroid hormone receptor. *Nature* 378: 690-7

Weaver IC, Cervoni N, Champagne FA, D'Alessio AC, Sharma S, et al. 2004. Epigenetic programming by maternal behavior. *Nature neuroscience* 7: 847-54

Yang XJ, Ogryzko VV, Nishikawa J, Howard BH, Nakatani Y. 1996. A p300/CBP-associated factor that competes with the adenoviral oncoprotein E1A. *Nature* 382: 319-24

Yang-Yen H-F, Chambard J-C, Sun Y-L, Smeal T, Schmidt TJ, et al. 1990. Transcriptional interference between c-Jun and the glucocorticoid receptor: mutual inhibition of DNA binding due to direct protein-protein interaction. *Cell* 62: 1205-15

Yao M, Stenzel-Poore M, Denver RJ. 2007. Structural and functional conservation of vertebrate corticotropin-releasing factor genes: evidence for a critical role for a conserved cyclic AMP response element. *Endocrinology* 148: 2518-31

Yudt MR, Cidlowski JA. 2002. The glucocorticoid receptor: coding a diversity of proteins and responses through a single gene. *Mol Endocrinol* 16: 1719-26

Chapter 2

CCKergic System, Hypothalamus-Pituitary-Adrenal (HPA) Axis, and Early-Life Stress (ELS)

Mingxi Tang, Anu Joseph, Qian Chen, Jianwei Jiao and Ya-Ping Tang

Additional information is available at the end of the chapter

http://dx.doi.org/10.5772/52042

1. Introduction

Early-life exposure to adverse experience or stress, simply termed early-life stress (ELS), is a worldwide problem that has a significantly negative impact in human health [1, 2]. In the United States, about 50% of adults had experienced some kind of stress before age 18 [3], and up to 15-25% of adults had traumatic ELS such as sexual abuse [4]. Most ELS is parents-originated, such as neglect, maltreatment, and abuse [5, 6]. In addition to the immediate, dreadful, and destructive effects on a child's life, ELS may produce a series of mental [7, 8], cardiovascular [9, 10], metabolic [11, 12], and many other types of disease [13, 14], at a later life stage. For example, adults who were sexually abused during childhood have a 5.7-fold increase in risk for drug abuse over those without ELS [7], and the prevalence of posttraumatic stress disorder (PTSD), a predominant form of anxiety disorders (ADs), is highly associated with ELS, with a 4-5 fold difference between adults with ELS and those without ELS [15]. Moreover, cognitive dysfunctions [16-18] such as learning and memory impairment [19-21] are also highly associated with ELS. Given that children, especially early adolescents, have a higher possibility to expose to a traumatic insult [22], adolescent trauma (AT) is an important risk factor for these post-ELS disorders.

Over the past decades, considerable insights have been gained into the molecular/neuronal mechanisms regarding how ELS impacts brain function and behavior [23-26]. Generally, it is now accepted that ELS can produce changes, most permanently, at multiple levels [25, 27]. Following ELS, for example, the overall volume of the hippocampus [28-30], corpus callosum [31-33], and cortex [34-36] all becomes smaller, compared to that of those brain regions in age-matched subjects. Besides these neuroanatomical changes, the neuronal activity and the synaptic function in the brain in ELS-victims are impaired [37-39], and most neurotransmitter systems are significantly affected too. By using positron emission tomography or fMRI, it has been found that a significantly increased release of dopamine in the ventral striatum is associated to ELS [40, 41]. The turnover rate of the serotonin (5-HT) metabolism or the 5-HT receptor density [42, 43] is altered following ELS. Similarly, the activity of the glutamatergic system [44, 45] and the cholinergic system [46, 47] are also altered in the brain of individuals following ELS. However, it should be emphasized that the changes in the hypothalamic-pituitary-adrenal (HPA) axis activity is of the most interest [48-52].

As the most important stress-related neuroendocrine system in the body, the HPA axis is anatomically and functionally composed of three major structures: the paraventricular nucleus of the hypothalamus (PVN), the anterior lobe of the pituitary gland, and the adrenal gland [53, 54]. The PVN contains magnocellular neurosecretory neurons that synthesize and release a corticotropin-releasing factor (CRF). CRF is a 41 amino acid peptide [55, 56], and can bind to three types of G-protein-coupled receptors: CRFR1, CRFR2, and CRFR3 [57-59]. In the mammalian brain, both CRF and CRFR1 are mainly distributed in the limbic system, while CRFR-2 is in the hypothalamus [60-62]. The essential role for the CRF system is to maintain the basal HPA axis activity as well as to trigger the HPA axis in response to stresses. After released from the PVN, the CRF binds to CRFR1 at the anterior pituitary and increase the release of adrenocorticotropic hormone (ACTH). The ACTH consequently stimulates the release of glucocorticoids from the adrenal gland [63]. Once released, glucocorticoids bind both high-affinity mineralocorticoid receptors and lower-affinity glucocorticoid receptors. The glucocorticoids, or cortisol in humans and corticosterone in rodents, play an essential role in energy metabolism, growth processes, immune function, and brain functions [63, 64].

In response to stress, CRF system plays an essential role in modifying peripheral physiological response to support "fight or flight" reactions, such as mobilizing energy stores, increasing blood sugar and heart rate, inhibiting digestive functions etc [65,66]. In addition, CRF itself may act on CRFR2 in the brain to directly regulate adaptive behavioral changes encountering stress [67-69]. Taken together, the CRF/HPA system plays a primary role in coordinating the endocrine, autonomic, immune, and behavioral response to stress. As stress, either real or imaged, is a necessary inducer for ADs, the CRF/HPA system must play a unique role in anxiety-related behaviors. Indeed, a huge body of evidence has documented this notion. For example, administration of CRF [70-72] or CRFR1 agonists [69,73,74] or overexpression of the CRF gene [75-77] produces Anxiety-like behaviors (ALBs) in the animals. On the other hand, CRFR1 antagonists exert significantly anxiolytic effects [78-80]. Knockout of CRF or CRFR1 in mice significantly reduces ALBs to stress and dramatically blunts stress-induced HPA axis activity [61,81,82]. Remarkably, previous chronic stress is able to enhance HPA axis activity in response to a novel acute stress, despite the negative feedback effects of increased glucocorticoids produced by the chronic stress [83-85]. For example, CCK-4-induced panic status in healthy volunteers significantly increases HPA axis activities [86]. Even the effects of early-life stress on HPA axis function are found to be associated with CCK sensitivity [130]. Most interestingly, interactions between the CCKergic system and the CRF/HPA system exist [88-90]. For example, the CCKergic system was found to be involved in this chronic stress-enhanced responsiveness, since chronic stress can specifically facilitate the release of CCK into the PVN, which directly projects to the pituitary, in response to acute stress [125]. All these findings have not only established the role of the CRF/HPA system in initiating behavioral responses to stresses, but also indicate that a significant interaction may exist between the CRF/HPA system and CCKergic system to regulate stress-related behaviors.

However, the vulnerability among different individuals to AT is different. This variability may at least partially attribute to a genetic variability [91]. A twin study of Vietnam veterans revealed that about 37.9% of vulnerability to PTSD was genetically related [92]. Further genetic evidence comes from clinical association studies, by which several candidate genes for ADs including PTSD have been associated, although a causative gene has not been yet established [91]. Among those candidate genes, cholecystokinin (CCK) receptor-2 (CCKR-2) has been linked to panic disorder, another major form of ADs [93,94].

As the most abundant neuropeptides, CCK distributes broadly in the brain and mainly in the limbic system [95,96]. CCK binds to CCK receptor-1 (CCKR-1) and CCKR-2, of which the CCKR-2 is predominantly found in the brain with the highest level in cortical area and the limbic system [97], a brain region that is critically involved in emotion response and behavior. Virtually, the CCKergic system has long been recognized as an anxiogenic factor for the animals [98], and this effect has been well validated in human populations as well [89,99,100]. Our recent study also showed that overexpression of CCKR2 in neurons of the forebrain of mice significantly enhanced ALBs [101]. At the same time, some candidate genes that are linked to ADs are also associated with HPA axis activity. For example, a common polymorphism at the serotonin transporter (5-HTT) gene, namely 5HTTLPR, is a strong candidate genetic variation for ADs and depression [102-103], and also is significantly implicated in HPA axis activity [104]. Similar to the CCKergic system, the HPA axis system has long been recognized as a stress hormone [105,106], and plays a critical role in the pathogenesis of ADs [107,108]. Indeed, following ELS, the activity of the HPA axis system is dysfunctional [109-111]. Moreover, given the overall role of both the HPA axis system [112-114] and the CCKergic system [115-117] in regulating neuronal, cardiovascular, and metabolic functions in the body, these two systems may play an integrative role in the pathogenesis of post-ELS disorders.

In this study, by using our previously engineered inducible forebrain-specific CCKR-2 transgenic (IF-CCKR-2 tg) mice [101], we demonstrated that the elevated CCKergic tone in the brain significantly facilitated the effect of AT on the impairment of the glucocorticoid negative feedback inhibition in response to a novel acute stressor during the adult stage in the mouse, providing direct evidence that reveals a molecular basis for this co-effect.

2. Materials and methods

2.1. Experimental animals

The procedures for the generation of IF-CCKR-2 tg (simply dtg) mice were described in our previous publication [101]. Briefly, we used the tTA/tetO-inducible gene expression system to produce these dtg mice. This system requires two independent transgenic mouse strains, tTA transgenic and tetO/CCKR-2 transgenic mice. Accordingly, two constructs were made. The first was for tTA transgenic mice, in which the expression of the tTA was under the control of an alpha-Ca^{2+} calmodulin kinase II (CaMKII) promoter. The tTA transgene cassette consists of

0.6 kb of exon-intron splicing signal (pNN265), 1.0 kb of tTA encoding sequence (pTet-Off, Clontech), and 0.5 kb of SV-40 poly-A signals (pTet-Off, CLONTECH). The other construct is for CCKR-2 transgenic mice, in which the expression of the CCKR-2 transgene was under the control of the tetO promoter. The CCKR-2 transgene cassette consisted of 1.3 kb of mouse CCKR-2 cDNA, an upstream 0.6 kb of splicing signal (pNN265), and a downstream 1.1 kb of b-globin poly-A signals. All these components were subcloned into the pTRE2 vector (CLONTECH). CCKR-2 cDNA was cloned by RT-PCR from the total RNA extracted from the brain of a male B6/CBA F_1 mouse (The Jackson Laboratory) with the primers of 5'-CGG GAT CCA TGG ATC TGC TCA AGC TG-3' and 5'-GCT CTA GAT CAG CCA GGT CCC AGC GT-3'. A commercial RNA extraction kit (Invitrogen) and a reverse transcription kit (Stratagene) were used. The cloned cDNA was confirmed by sequencing. The plasmid constructs were then linearized with suitable enzymes and separately injected into the pronucleoli of B6/CBA F_1 zygotes, as described [118]. Transgenic founders and the transgene copy numbers were determined by Southern blot analyses of the tail DNA. Founder mice with suitable gene copy numbers were backcrossed into B6/CBA F_1 mice first to produce hemizygous single transgenic mice and then to produce double hemizygous transgenic mice. We have totally generated nine CaMKII-tTA transgenic founders and seven tetO-CCKR-2 transgenic founders. Southern blot analyses indicated that the gene copy numbers were from 2 to 70 for tTA transgenic founders and 2-150 for CCKR-2 transgenic founders (data not shown). To map the tTA expression pattern in the brain, we crossed a tetO-Lac-Z reporter mouse line (SJL-TgN-tetoplacZ, the Jackson Laboratory) into different independent CaMKII-tTA mouse lines to produce different tTA-LacZ double transgenic mouse lines. For Lac-Z staining, a commercial X-Gal staining kit (Invitrogen) and the recommended staining protocol were used with sagittal brain sections (30 μm), by which we identified a tTA transgenic line that was of the capacity to drive tetO/gene expression in almost all the neurons in the forebrain region (data not shown). Genotyping was determined by PCR analyses of both tTA (5'-AGG CTT GAG ATC TGG CCA TAC-3' and 5'-AGG AAA AGT GAG TAT GGT G-3') and the CCKR-2 (5'-ACG GTG GGA GGC CTA TAT AA-3' and 5'-GAG TGT GAA GGG CATG CAA-3') transgenes. Dtg mice used here were around 12-16 generations since they were generated, during which duration dtg mice were backcrossed into B6/CBA F_1 mice in every 5-6 generations, in order to avoid an inbreed effect. Single transgenic (tTA or tetO-CCKR-2 only) and wild-type (wt) littermates of dtg mice were used as controls, and are collectively and simply called wt mice hereafter. Mice used here were kept in standard laboratory mouse cages under the standard condition (12 hours light/dark cycle, temperature at 22 ± 1 °C, humility at 75%) with food and water *ad libitum*. All experimental procedures for the use of animals were previously reviewed and approved by the institutional animal care and use committee at the Louisiana State University Heath Sciences Center at New Orleans, and all of the experiments were conducted in accordance with the Guide for the Care and Use of Laboratory Animals published by the US National Institutes of Health.

2.2. *In situ* hybridization

The hybridization was used to detect the expression level and pattern of the CCKR-2 transgene in the brain. Brains from both wt and dtg mice were collected by decapitation, and were frozen with powered dry ice immediately. Sagittal sections (20 μm) were made with a Cryostat (Leica, CM 1900, Richmond, IL). An oligo probe for tTA and a cRNA probe for the total CCKR-2 mRNAs were labeled with ^{35}S UTP (>1,000 Ci/mmol; NEN, Boston, MA) by a random labeling kit and *in vitro* transcription kit (Invitrogen, Carlsbad, CA), respectively. The hybridization was performed overnight at 55°C, and after washing, slides were exposed to Kodak BioMax film (NEN) for the same time.

2.3. Adolescent trauma (AT)

Both wt and dtg mice at the age of P25 were individually put into a small shock-box (4 X 4 X 10 inch in high) that was modified from the shock box from a fear-conditioning system (Coulbourn Instruments, Whitehall, PA), in order to ensure that the mice did not have much space for escaping during shocking. The current of the footshock was higher (1.0 mA) than it was commonly used in the fear-conditioning test (0.6-0.8 mA). The footshock was conducted for 5 times (trials), in total, during a period of 1 minute, and each trial lasted for 2 seconds, with an interval of 10 seconds between trials.

2.4. Acute stressor (AS)

Additional acute stressor (AS; 0.8 mA for 2 seconds for one trial) with a standard fear-conditioning paradigm as described previously [119], was used to trigger HPA axis reaction at the age of P60 (2 months).

2.5. ELISA

Commercially available kits for both the adrenocorticotropic hormone (ACTH) (MD Bioproducts, St. Paul, MN) and corticosteroid hormone (CORT) (R&D systems, Minneapolis, MN) were used to determine the serum level of these hormones. Experimental procedures followed the recommended steps. In order to have samples enough for triplicate measurements, blood was collected with a retroorbital eye bleeding method. In order to minimize non-specific effects, blood collection was conducted at 9:00 Am, and the procedure was completed within 30 seconds, by which time any possible change that might be produced by the sampling procedure was not yet measurable.

2.6. Statistical analysis

Both female and male mice were almost equally distributed in each group. Data were analyzed with one-way ANOVA, followed by post-hoc tests. The p value less than 0.05 is considered significant.

3. Results

3.1. Expression of the CCKR-2 transgene in the brain of dtg mice

As shown in Fig 1, *in situ* hybridization revealed that the expression of the tTA was forebrain-specific in dtg mice (Fig. 1B), but was not detectable in wt mice (Fig. 1A). The expression pattern of the CCKR-2 transgene (data not shown) was the same as both the pattern of the tTA expression and the CCKR-2 transgene expression reported in our previous study [101].

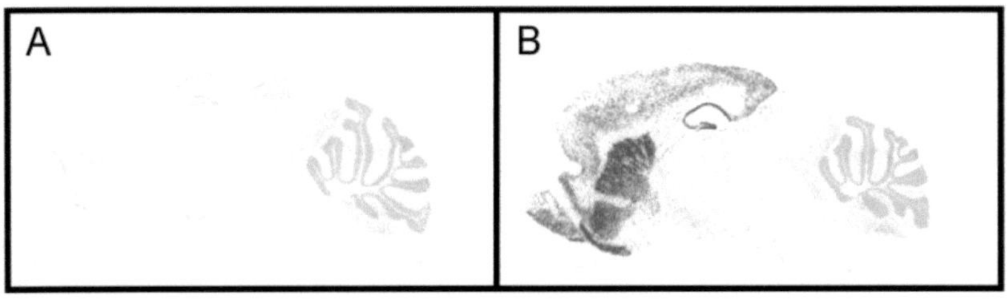

Figure 1. Expression pattern of the tTA mRNA detected by *in situ* hybridization with saggital brain sections in wt (A) and dtg (B) mice.

3.2. Dtg mice with AT exhibit an increased HPA axis activity in response to AS

Either wt (n = 60) or dtg mice (n = 60) were subjected to AT, and then were divided into 5 groups (n = 12) for a time-course study, in which both ACTH and CORT were examined before the AS for the basal level, and 1, 2, 4, and 8 hours following the AS. As shown in Fig. 2, although the difference in the basal level of ACTH (Fig. 2A) or CORT (Fig. 2C) between these mice was not significant, a tendency of a lower level ACTH ($p = 0.0741$) and CORT ($p = 0.0648$) was observed in dtg groups, compared to wt groups. Following the AS, an one-way ANOVA revealed a significant effect of the AT and CCKR-2 transgene on ACTH [$F(1,8) = 6.781$, $p < 0.01$] and CORT [$F(1,8) = 9.201$, $p < 0.01$]. Detailed post-hoc tests revealed that both ACTH (Fig. 2B) and CORT (Fig. 2D) in either wt or dtg mice reached the peak level at 1 hr after the AS, while a significant difference was observed at 1 and 2 hr in ACTH between wt and dtg groups ($p > 0.05$), and at 1 and 2 hr in CORT between wt and dtg groups ($p > 0.05$). In both wt and dtg mice, ACTH returned to the basal level at 4 hr (Fig. 2B), while CORT returned to the basal level at 4 hr (Fig. 2D). All these results indicate that the interaction between the AT and CCKR-2 transgene does not only increase the activity of the HPA axis following a novel stressor, but also impairs the CORT negative feedback in response this stressor.

3.3. Disassociation of the CCKR2 transgene expression and AT largely diminishes the effect of AT on HPA axis activity in response to AS

In this study, both wt and dtg mice were treated with doxycycline (doxy, 2 mg/100 ml in drinking water) for 5 days prior to AT, so that the transgene expression in dtg mice was inhibited during the episode of AT, and this inhibition lasted for about 3-5 days after the doxy treatment. At 2 months old, these mice were subjected to AS, and 1 hr later, which is the peak time of HPA axis response, as described in Fig. 2, the HPA axis activity was measured. Surprisedly, the levels of both ACTH and CORT were indistinguishable between wt and dtg mice, indicating that the coupling of AT and the transgene expression is critical for the AT to produce impaired glucocorticoid negative feedback inhibition in the animals.

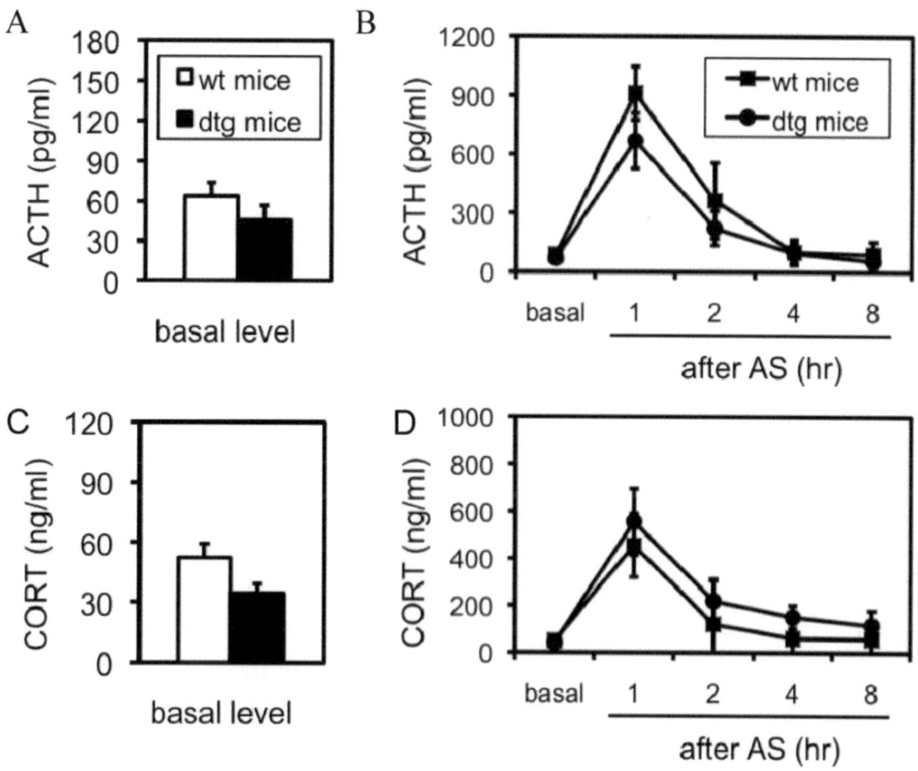

Figure 2. Increased HPA axis activity in dtg mice with AT/AS. A. Basal serum level of ACTH in naïve wt mice and naïve dtg mice. A tendency of a difference is shown, but it is not significant. Data are expressed as mean ± SEM. **B.** Time-course of ACTH response following the AS. **C.** Basal serum level of CORT in naïve wt mice and naïve dtg mice. A tendency of a difference is shown, but it is not significant. Data are expressed as mean ± SEM. **D.** Time-course of CORT response following the AS. The same groups of mice above were examined.

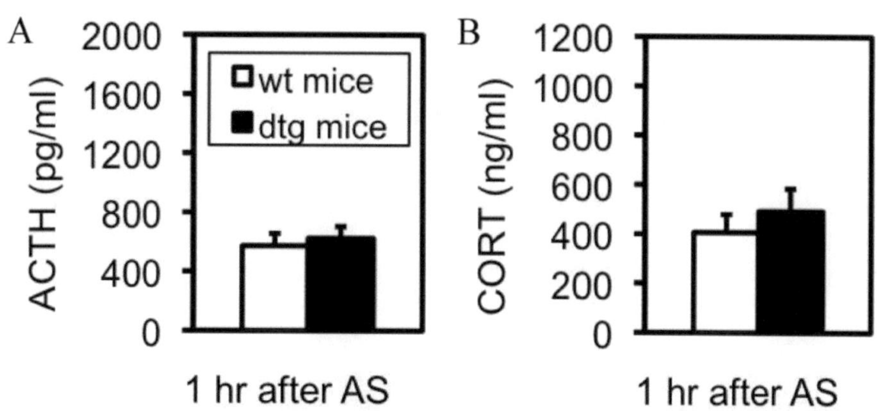

Figure 3. Level of ACTH (A) and CORT (B) in the mice after AT/AS. No significant difference was found between wt and dtg mice when the expression of the CCKR-2 transgene was suppressed during AT.

4. Discussion

We have for the first time demonstrated that a coupling of a higher CCKergic tone with an ELS event is a causative factor for the development of an impairment of glucocorticoid negative feedback inhibition in the animals in response to additional acute stressor at a later life stage.

This demonstration is achieved based on the technical merit in our transgenic mice, in which the transgene expression is inducible/reversible. The time resolution for this inducible/reversible feature is within 1 week, which is high enough for this time-coupling analysis. However, it is still not clear how this real-time coupling occurs, partially due to the fact that the functional significance of the CCKergic system is still not fully understood. As G protein-coupled receptors, CCKR are associated with Ca^{2+} release, PKC activation, PLA2 activity, and cAMP production [120]. In addition, there are robust interactions between the CCKergic system and other neurotransmitter systems including dopaminergic, serotonergic, and GABAergic systems at both the structural and functional levels [121,122], and therefore, the mechanism underlying this associative effect should be complicated, and need to be further studied.

An important finding in this study is the discovery of the change in the HPA axis activity, and these changes include (1) a slightly lower basal level of the HPA axis activity in dtg mice, compared to wt mice, (2) a synergistic effect of AT and the CCKR-2 transgene on the peak level of the HPA axis activity in response to the AS; (3) a prolonged decay time of the HPA axis activity following the AS in dtg mice with AT, and (4) a requirement of real-time coupling of the transgene expression and TA. It should be mentioned that it has been well established that a previous chronic stress in the animals down-regulates the HPA axis activity, but enhances their response to a novel acute stress, despite the negative feedback effects [83,123,124]. Because chronic stress can specifically facilitate the release of CCK into the PVN, which directly projects to the pituitary, in response to acute stress [88], the elevated CCKergic tone in our dtg mice may mimic the effect of a chronic stress by working as an "intrinsic stressor" for the animals. Therefore, this intrinsic stressor constitutes a basis for the higher vulnerability of dtg mice to AT. At the same time, the impaired AS-induced CORT negative feedback response may, in tern, significantly alter many other physiological functions, and eventually lead to a pathological condition.

As described above, following ELS, neuroanatomical changes were found in different brain regions. In addition, neuronal activity is altered too {125}. Consistent to the current study, the activity of the HPA axis system in the subject who experienced ELS was dysregulated [48-52]. Moreover, many other neurotransmitter systems were also affected by ELS [40, 126-128]. Therefore, the finding from the current study has provided additional evidence regarding how the CCKergic system and the HPA axis system are involved in the pathogenesis of post-ELS disorders.

The most important finding in this study is the demonstration of that if the transgene was temporally suppressed during the time of AT exposure, this impaired HPA axis inhibition in response to another acute stressor was largely diminished, indicating that the temporal association of the elevated CCKergic tone with AT is critically pathogenic. This finding has a potential translational significance. It is well know that the endogenous CCKergic activity, or the CCKR-2 level in the brain, plays a dominant role in the expression of anxiety. For example, the expression of anxiety was correlated with the increased CCKergic tone, which was evidenced by a higher CCK receptor-binding capacity in the brain of anxious animals, in comparison with non-anxious animals [129-131]. Different fear responses among different strains of the same animal species were attributed to different expression levels of CCKR-2 [132-134]. On the other hand, evidence also indicates that the CCKergic tone in the brain is dynamically regulated by stress. Following stress, for example, both CCK peptide immunoreactivity and CCK receptor density in the brain were significantly increased [135-139]. Social isolation, an anxiogenic stress, increased the CCK mRNA expression in the brain [140]. Especially, the effect of ELS on the HPA axis activity was associated with CCK activity [87]. Chronic stress could specifically facilitate the release of CCK into the PNV in response to acute stress [84,141]. Consistently, CCKR-2 agonists could only produce, or produce more pronounced, anxiogenic effect in stressed animals, but not in un-stressed animals [88, 142-144]. Patients with ADs were more sensitive to CCKR-2 agonists than normal controls [145-148]. Together with all these findings, it seems conclusive that the CCKergic system is dynamically involved in ELS-triggered mental disorders, and thus, an inhibition of the CCKergic tone timely associated with an ELS event might be useful to prevent the development of post-ELS disorder, especially ADs.

In summary, our study has revealed a Novel molecular underpinning for the development of post-ESL disorders, especially for mental disorders, and provide insightful information regarding how can we develop a preventive strategy for these post-ESL disorders in the humans.

Author details

Mingxi Tang
Department of Pathology, Luzhou Medical College, Sichuan, P. R. China

Anu Joseph , Qian Chen , Jianwei Jiao and Ya-Ping Tang *
Department of Cell Biology and Anatomy, Louisiana State University Health Sciences Center, New Orleans, LA, USA

Acknowledgement

This work was partially conducted in the University of Chicago. This study was partially supported by grants from National Institute of Mental Health (MH066243), Alzheimer's Association (NIRG-02-4368), National Science Foundation (0213112), and NARSAD, all to YPT.

---

* Corresponding Author

5. References

[1] Turecki G, Ernst C, Jollant F, Labonte B, & Mechawar N (2012) The neurodevelopmental origins of suicidal behavior. *Trends Neurosci* 35(1):14-23.

[2] McGowan PO & Szyf M (2110) The epigenetics of social adversity in early life: implications for mental health outcomes. *Neurobiol Dis* 39(1):66-72 .

[3] Green JG, *et al.* (2010) Childhood adversities and adult psychiatric disorders in the national comorbidity survey replication I: associations with first onset of DSM-IV disorders. *Arch Gen Psychiatry* 67(2):113-123 .

[4] Vogeltanz ND, *et al.* (1999) Prevalence and risk factors for childhood sexual abuse in women: national survey findings. *Child Abuse Negl* 23(6):579-592.

[5] Luecken LJ & Lemery KS (2004) Early caregiving and physiological stress responses. *Clin Psychol Rev* 24(2):171-191.

[6] Weich S, Patterson J, Shaw R, & Stewart-Brown S (2009) Family relationships in childhood and common psychiatric disorders in later life: systematic review of prospective studies. *Br J Psychiatry* 194(5):392-398.

[7] Kendler KS, *et al.* (2000) Childhood sexual abuse and adult psychiatric and substance use disorders in women: an epidemiological and cotwin control analysis. *Arch Gen Psychiatry* 57(10):953-959.

[8] Howell BR & Sanchez MM (2011) Understanding behavioral effects of early life stress using the reactive scope and allostatic load models. *Dev Psychopathol* 23(4):1001-1016 .

[9] Schooling CM, *et al.* (2011) Parental death during childhood and adult cardiovascular risk in a developing country: the Guangzhou Biobank Cohort Study. *PLoS One* 6(5):e19675.

[10] Nuyt AM & Alexander BT (2009) Developmental programming and hypertension. *Curr Opin Nephrol Hypertens* 18(2):144-152.

[11] Tarry-Adkins JL & Ozanne SE (2011) Mechanisms of early life programming: current knowledge and future directions. *Am J Clin Nutr* 94(6):1765S-1771S

[12] Portha B, Chavey A, & Movassat J (2011) Early-life origins of type 2 diabetes: fetal programming of the beta-cell mass. *Exp Diabetes Res* 2011:105076

[13] Rooks C, Veledar E, Goldberg J, Bremner JD, & Vaccarino V (2012) Early trauma and inflammation: role of familial factors in a study of twins. *Psychosom Med* 74(2):146-152.

[14] Entringer S, *et al.* (2011) Stress exposure in intrauterine life is associated with shorter telomere length in young adulthood. *Proc Natl Acad Sci U S A* 108(33):E513-518.

[15] Breslau N, Davis GC, & Schultz LR (2003) Posttraumatic stress disorder and the incidence of nicotine, alcohol, and other drug disorders in persons who have experienced trauma. *Arch Gen Psychiatry* 60(3):289-294.

[16] Pechtel P & Pizzagalli DA (2010) Effects of early life stress on cognitive and affective function: an integrated review of human literature. *Psychopharmacology (Berl).*

[17] Majer M, Nater UM, Lin JM, Capuron L, & Reeves WC (2010) Association of childhood trauma with cognitive function in healthy adults: a pilot study. *BMC Neurol* 10:61.

[18] Hedges DW & Woon FL (2010) Early-life stress and cognitive outcome. (Translated from Eng) *Psychopharmacology (Berl)*

[19] Chu JA, Frey LM, Ganzel BL, & Matthews JA (1999) Memories of childhood abuse: dissociation, amnesia, and corroboration. *Am J Psychiatry* 156(5):749-755.

[20] Goodman GS, Quas JA, & Ogle CM (2010) Child maltreatment and memory. *Annu Rev Psychol* 61:325-351

[21] McCormick CM & Mathews IZ (2010) Adolescent development, hypothalamic-pituitary-adrenal function, and programming of adult learning and memory. (Translated from eng) *Prog Neuropsychopharmacol Biol Psychiatry* 34(5):756-765 (in eng).

[22] Costello EJ, Erkanli A, Fairbank JA, & Angold A (2002) The prevalence of potentially traumatic events in childhood and adolescence. (Translated from eng) *J Trauma Stress* 15(2):99-112 (in eng).

[23] Loman MM & Gunnar MR (2010) Early experience and the development of stress reactivity and regulation in children. (Translated from eng) *Neurosci Biobehav Rev* 34(6):867-876 (in eng).

[24] Fenoglio KA, Brunson KL, & Baram TZ (2006) Hippocampal neuroplasticity induced by early-life stress: functional and molecular aspects. (Translated from eng) *Front Neuroendocrinol* 27(2):180-192 (in eng).

[25] Gunnar M & Quevedo K (2007) The neurobiology of stress and development. (Translated from eng) *Annu Rev Psychol* 58:145-173 (in eng).

[26] Glaser R & Kiecolt-Glaser J (2005) How stress damages immune system and health. (Translated from eng) *Discov Med* 5(26):165-169 (in eng).

[27] Kiecolt-Glaser JK, *et al.* (2011) Childhood adversity heightens the impact of later-life caregiving stress on telomere length and inflammation. (Translated from eng) *Psychosom Med* 73(1):16-22 (in eng).

[28] Rao U, *et al.* (2010) Hippocampal changes associated with early-life adversity and vulnerability to depression. (Translated from eng) *Biol Psychiatry* 67(4):357-364 (in eng).

[29] Cohen RA, *et al.* (2006) Early life stress and morphometry of the adult anterior cingulate cortex and caudate nuclei. (Translated from eng) *Biol Psychiatry* 59(10):975-982 (in eng).

[30] Rao H, *et al.* (2010) Early parental care is important for hippocampal maturation: evidence from brain morphology in humans. (Translated from eng) *Neuroimage* 49(1):1144-1150 (in eng).

[31] Kitayama N, *et al.* (2007) Morphologic alterations in the corpus callosum in abuse-related posttraumatic stress disorder: a preliminary study. (Translated from eng) *J Nerv Ment Dis* 195(12):1027-1029 (in eng).

[32] Teicher MH, *et al.* (2004) Childhood neglect is associated with reduced corpus callosum area. (Translated from eng) *Biol Psychiatry* 56(2):80-85 (in eng).

[33] Jackowski A, *et al.* (2011) Early-life stress, corpus callosum development, hippocampal volumetrics, and anxious behavior in male nonhuman primates. (Translated from eng) *Psychiatry Res* 192(1):37-44 (in eng).

[34] van Harmelen AL, *et al.* (2010) Reduced medial prefrontal cortex volume in adults reporting childhood emotional maltreatment. (Translated from eng) *Biol Psychiatry* 68(9):832-838 (in eng).
[35] Tomoda A, *et al.* (2009) Reduced prefrontal cortical gray matter volume in young adults exposed to harsh corporal punishment. (Translated from eng) *Neuroimage* 47 Suppl 2:T66-71 (in eng).
[36] Hohmann CF, Beard NA, Kari-Kari P, Jarvis N, & Simmons Q (2012) Effects of brief stress exposure during early postnatal development in Balb/CByJ mice: II. Altered cortical morphology. (Translated from Eng) *Dev Psychobiol* (in Eng).
[37] Judo C, *et al.* (2010) Early stress exposure impairs synaptic potentiation in the rat medial prefrontal cortex underlying contextual fear extinction. (Translated from eng) *Neuroscience* 169(4):1705-1714 (in eng).
[38] Carrion VG, Haas BW, Garrett A, Song S, & Reiss AL (2010) Reduced hippocampal activity in youth with posttraumatic stress symptoms: an FMRI study. (Translated from eng) *J Pediatr Psychol* 35(5):559-569 (in eng).
[39] Korosi A, *et al.* (2010) Early-life experience reduces excitation to stress-responsive hypothalamic neurons and reprograms the expression of corticotropin-releasing hormone. (Translated from eng) *J Neurosci* 30(2):703-713 (in eng).
[40] Pruessner JC, Champagne F, Meaney MJ, & Dagher A (2004) Dopamine release in response to a psychological stress in humans and its relationship to early life maternal care: a positron emission tomography study using [11C]raclopride. (Translated from eng) *J Neurosci* 24(11):2825-2831 (in eng).
[41] Soliman A, *et al.* (2011) Limbic response to psychosocial stress in schizotypy: a functional magnetic resonance imaging study. (Translated from eng) *Schizophr Res* 131(1-3):184-191 (in eng).
[42] Huggins KN, *et al.* (2012) Effects of early life stress on drinking and serotonin system activity in rhesus macaques: 5-hydroxyindoleacetic acid in cerebrospinal fluid predicts brain tissue levels. (Translated from Eng) *Alcohol* (in Eng).
[43] Matsuzaki H, *et al.* (2011) Juvenile stress attenuates the dorsal hippocampal postsynaptic 5-HT1A receptor function in adult rats. (Translated from eng) *Psychopharmacology (Berl)* 214(1):329-337 (in eng).
[44] Martisova E, *et al.* (2012) Long lasting effects of early-life stress on glutamatergic/GABAergic circuitry in the rat hippocampus. (Translated from eng) *Neuropharmacology* 62(5-6):1944-1953 (in eng).
[45] Alexander GM, *et al.* (2012) Disruptions in serotonergic regulation of cortical glutamate release in primate insular cortex in response to chronic ethanol and nursery rearing. (Translated from eng) *Neuroscience* 207:167-181 (in eng).
[46] Aisa B, *et al.* (2009) Neonatal stress affects vulnerability of cholinergic neurons and cognition in the rat: involvement of the HPA axis. (Translated from eng) *Psychoneuroendocrinology* 34(10):1495-1505 (in eng).

[47] Lapiz MD, *et al.* (2003) Influence of postweaning social isolation in the rat on brain development, conditioned behavior, and neurotransmission. (Translated from eng) *Neurosci Behav Physiol* 33(1):13-29 (in eng).
[48] Carpenter LL, Shattuck TT, Tyrka AR, Geracioti TD, & Price LH (2010) Effect of childhood physical abuse on cortisol stress response. (Translated from Eng) *Psychopharmacology (Berl)* (in Eng).
[49] Gillespie CF, Phifer J, Bradley B, & Ressler KJ (2009) Risk and resilience: genetic and environmental influences on development of the stress response. (Translated from eng) *Depress Anxiety* 26(11):984-992 (in eng).
[50] Mirescu C, Peters JD, & Gould E (2004) Early life experience alters response of adult neurogenesis to stress. (Translated from eng) *Nat Neurosci* 7(8):841-846 (in eng).
[51] Cicchetti D, Rogosch FA, Gunnar MR, & Toth SL (2010) The differential impacts of early physical and sexual abuse and internalizing problems on daytime cortisol rhythm in school-aged children. (Translated from eng) *Child Dev* 81(1):252-269 (in eng).
[52] Gunnar MR, Frenn K, Wewerka SS, & Van Ryzin MJ (2009) Moderate versus severe early life stress: associations with stress reactivity and regulation in 10-12-year-old children. (Translated from eng) *Psychoneuroendocrinology* 34(1):62-75 (in eng).
[53] Smith SM & Vale WW (2006) The role of the hypothalamic-pituitary-adrenal axis in neuroendocrine responses to stress. (Translated from eng) *Dialogues Clin Neurosci* 8(4):383-395 (in eng).
[54] Koob GF (2010) The role of CRF and CRF-related peptides in the dark side of addiction. (Translated from eng) *Brain Res* 1314:3-14 (in eng).
[55] Vale W, Spiess J, Rivier C, & Rivier J (1981) Characterization of a 41-residue ovine hypothalamic peptide that stimulates secretion of corticotropin and beta-endorphin. (Translated from eng) *Science* 213(4514):1394-1397 (in eng).
[56] Liu J, *et al.* (2004) Corticotropin-releasing factor and Urocortin I modulate excitatory glutamatergic synaptic transmission. (Translated from eng) *J Neurosci* 24(16):4020-4029 (in eng).
[57] Dautzenberg FM & Hauger RL (2002) The CRF peptide family and their receptors: yet more partners discovered. (Translated from eng) *Trends Pharmacol Sci* 23(2):71-77 (in eng).
[58] Lewis K, *et al.* (2001) Identification of urocortin III, an additional member of the corticotropin-releasing factor (CRF) family with high affinity for the CRF2 receptor. (Translated from eng) *Proc Natl Acad Sci U S A* 98(13):7570-7575 (in eng).
[59] Perrin MH & Vale WW (1999) Corticotropin releasing factor receptors and their ligand family. (Translated from eng) *Ann N Y Acad Sci* 885:312-328 (in eng).
[60] Kostich WA, Grzanna R, Lu NZ, & Largent BL (2004) Immunohistochemical visualization of corticotropin-releasing factor type 1 (CRF1) receptors in monkey brain. (Translated from eng) *J Comp Neurol* 478(2):111-125 (in eng).

[61] Potter E, *et al.* (1994) Distribution of corticotropin-releasing factor receptor mRNA expression in the rat brain and pituitary. (Translated from eng) *Proc Natl Acad Sci U S A* 91(19):8777-8781 (in eng).

[62] Van Pett K, *et al.* (2000) Distribution of mRNAs encoding CRF receptors in brain and pituitary of rat and mouse. (Translated from eng) *J Comp Neurol* 428(2):191-212 (in eng).

[63] Dallman MF, Akana SF, Strack AM, Hanson ES, & Sebastian RJ (1995) The neural network that regulates energy balance is responsive to glucocorticoids and insulin and also regulates HPA axis responsivity at a site proximal to CRF neurons. (Translated from eng) *Ann N Y Acad Sci* 771:730-742 (in eng).

[64] Feek CM, Marante DJ, & Edwards CR (1983) The hypothalamic-pituitary-adrenal axis. (Translated from eng) *Clin Endocrinol Metab* 12(3):597-618 (in eng).

[65] Pecoraro N, Gomez F, & Dallman MF (2005) Glucocorticoids dose-dependently remodel energy stores and amplify incentive relativity effects. (Translated from eng) *Psychoneuroendocrinology* 30(9):815-825 (in eng).

[66] Dunn AJ & Berridge CW (1990) Physiological and behavioral responses to corticotropin-releasing factor administration: is CRF a mediator of anxiety or stress responses? (Translated from eng) *Brain Res Brain Res Rev* 15(2):71-100 (in eng).

[67] Kishimoto T, *et al.* (2000) Deletion of crhr2 reveals an anxiolytic role for corticotropin-releasing hormone receptor-2. (Translated from eng) *Nat Genet* 24(4):415-419 (in eng).

[68] Matys T, *et al.* (2004) Tissue plasminogen activator promotes the effects of corticotropin-releasing factor on the amygdala and anxiety-like behavior. (Translated from eng) *Proc Natl Acad Sci U S A* 101(46):16345-16350 (in eng).

[69] Rainnie DG, *et al.* (2004) Corticotrophin releasing factor-induced synaptic plasticity in the amygdala translates stress into emotional disorders. (Translated from eng) *J Neurosci* 24(14):3471-3479 (in eng).

[70] Butler PD, Weiss JM, Stout JC, & Nemeroff CB (1990) Corticotropin-releasing factor produces fear-enhancing and behavioral activating effects following infusion into the locus coeruleus. (Translated from eng) *J Neurosci* 10(1):176-183 (in eng).

[71] Sutton RE, Koob GF, Le Moal M, Rivier J, & Vale W (1982) Corticotropin releasing factor produces behavioural activation in rats. (Translated from eng) *Nature* 297(5864):331-333 (in eng).

[72] Salak-Johnson JL, Anderson DL, & McGlone JJ (2004) Differential dose effects of central CRF and effects of CRF astressin on pig behavior. (Translated from eng) *Physiol Behav* 83(1):143-150 (in eng).

[73] Valdez GR, Zorrilla EP, Rivier J, Vale WW, & Koob GF (2003) Locomotor suppressive and anxiolytic-like effects of urocortin 3, a highly selective type 2 corticotropin-releasing factor agonist. (Translated from eng) *Brain Res* 980(2):206-212 (in eng).

[74] Bale TL (2005) Sensitivity to stress: dysregulation of CRF pathways and disease development. (Translated from eng) *Horm Behav* 48(1):1-10 (in eng).

[75] Heinrichs SC, *et al.* (1997) Anti-sexual and anxiogenic behavioral consequences of corticotropin-releasing factor overexpression are centrally mediated. (Translated from eng) *Psychoneuroendocrinology* 22(4):215-224 (in eng).

[76] van Gaalen MM, Stenzel-Poore MP, Holsboer F, & Steckler T (2002) Effects of transgenic overproduction of CRH on anxiety-like behaviour. (Translated from eng) *Eur J Neurosci* 15(12):2007-2015 (in eng).

[77] Kasahara M, Groenink L, Breuer M, Olivier B, & Sarnyai Z (2007) Altered behavioural adaptation in mice with neural corticotrophin-releasing factor overexpression. (Translated from eng) *Genes Brain Behav* 6(7):598-607 (in eng).

[78] Rassnick S, Heinrichs SC, Britton KT, & Koob GF (1993) Microinjection of a corticotropin-releasing factor antagonist into the central nucleus of the amygdala reverses anxiogenic-like effects of ethanol withdrawal. (Translated from eng) *Brain Res* 605(1):25-32 (in eng).

[79] Takahashi LK (2001) Role of CRF(1) and CRF(2) receptors in fear and anxiety. (Translated from eng) *Neurosci Biobehav Rev* 25(7-8):627-636 (in eng).

[80] Kehne J & De Lombaert S (2002) Non-peptidic CRF1 receptor antagonists for the treatment of anxiety, depression and stress disorders. (Translated from eng) *Curr Drug Targets CNS Neurol Disord* 1(5):467-493 (in eng).

[81] Timpl P, *et al.* (1998) Impaired stress response and reduced anxiety in mice lacking a functional corticotropin-releasing hormone receptor 1. (Translated from eng) *Nat Genet* 19(2):162-166 (in eng).

[82] Nguyen NK, *et al.* (2006) Conditional CRF receptor 1 knockout mice show altered neuronal activation pattern to mild anxiogenic challenge. (Translated from eng) *Psychopharmacology (Berl)* 188(3):374-385 (in eng).

[83] Akana SF, *et al.* (1996) Clamped Corticosterone (B) Reveals the Effect of Endogenous B on Both Facilitated Responsivity to Acute Restraint and Metabolic Responses to Chronic Stress. (Translated from Eng) *Stress* 1(1):33-49 (in Eng).

[84] Bhatnagar S, *et al.* (2000) A cholecystokinin-mediated pathway to the paraventricular thalamus is recruited in chronically stressed rats and regulates hypothalamic-pituitary-adrenal function. (Translated from eng) *J Neurosci* 20(14):5564-5573 (in eng).

[85] Young EA, Akana S, & Dallman MF (1990) Decreased sensitivity to glucocorticoid fast feedback in chronically stressed rats. (Translated from eng) *Neuroendocrinology* 51(5):536-542 (in eng).

[86] Eser D, *et al.* (2005) Panic induction with cholecystokinin-tetrapeptide (CCK-4) Increases plasma concentrations of the neuroactive steroid 3alpha, 5alpha tetrahydrodeoxycorticosterone (3alpha, 5alpha-THDOC) in healthy volunteers. (Translated from eng) *Neuropsychopharmacology* 30(1):192-195 (in eng).

[87] Greisen MH, Bolwig TG, & Wortwein G (2005) Cholecystokinin tetrapeptide effects on HPA axis function and elevated plus maze behaviour in maternally separated and handled rats. (Translated from eng) *Behav Brain Res* 161(2):204-212 (in eng).

[88] Abelson JL, Khan S, Liberzon I, & Young EA (2007) HPA axis activity in patients with panic disorder: review and synthesis of four studies. (Translated from eng) *Depress Anxiety* 24(1):66-76 (in eng).
[89] Raedler TJ, *et al.* (2006) Megestrol attenuates the hormonal response to CCK-4-induced panic attacks. (Translated from eng) *Depress Anxiety* 23(3):139-144 (in eng).
[90] Abelson JL & Young EA (2003) Hypothalamic-pituitary adrenal response to cholecystokinin-B receptor agonism is resistant to cortisol feedback inhibition. (Translated from eng) *Psychoneuroendocrinology* 28(2):169-180 (in eng).
[91] Cornelis MC, Nugent NR, Amstadter AB, & Koenen KC (2010) Genetics of post-traumatic stress disorder: review and recommendations for genome-wide association studies. (Translated from eng) *Curr Psychiatry Rep* 12(4):313-326 (in eng).
[92] Chantarujikapong SI, *et al.* (2001) A twin study of generalized anxiety disorder symptoms, panic disorder symptoms and post-traumatic stress disorder in men. (Translated from eng) *Psychiatry Res* 103(2-3):133-145 (in eng).
[93] Kennedy JL, *et al.* (1999) Investigation of cholecystokinin system genes in panic disorder. (Translated from eng) *Mol Psychiatry* 4(3):284-285 (in eng).
[94] Maron E, *et al.* (2005) Association study of 90 candidate gene polymorphisms in panic disorder. (Translated from eng) *Psychiatr Genet* 15(1):17-24 (in eng).
[95] Dockray GJ (1976) Immunochemical evidence of cholecystokinin-like peptides in brain. (Translated from eng) *Nature* 264(5586):568-570 (in eng).
[96] Lotstra F & Vanderhaeghen JJ (1987) Distribution of immunoreactive cholecystokinin in the human hippocampus. (Translated from eng) *Peptides* 8(5):911-920 (in eng).
[97] Hill DR, Campbell NJ, Shaw TM, & Woodruff GN (1987) Autoradiographic localization and biochemical characterization of peripheral type CCK receptors in rat CNS using highly selective nonpeptide CCK antagonists. (Translated from eng) *J Neurosci* 7(9):2967-2976 (in eng).
[98] Della-Fera MA & Baile CA (1979) Cholecystokinin octapeptide: continuous picomole injections into the cerebral ventricles of sheep suppress feeding. (Translated from eng) *Science* 206(4417):471-473 (in eng).
[99] Katzman MA, Koszycki D, & Bradwejn J (2004) Effects of CCK-tetrapeptide in patients with social phobia and obsessive-compulsive disorder. (Translated from eng) *Depress Anxiety* 20(2):51-58 (in eng).
[100] Hebb AL, Poulin JF, Roach SP, Zacharko RM, & Drolet G (2005) Cholecystokinin and endogenous opioid peptides: interactive influence on pain, cognition, and emotion. (Translated from eng) *Prog Neuropsychopharmacol Biol Psychiatry* 29(8):1225-1238 (in eng).
[101] Chen Q, Nakajima A, Meacham C, & Tang YP (2006) Elevated cholecystokininergic tone constitutes an important molecular/neuronal mechanism for the expression of anxiety in the mouse. *Proc Natl Acad Sci U S A* 103(10):3881-3886.
[102] Gonda X, Rihmer Z, Juhasz G, Zsombok T, & Bagdy G (2007) High anxiety and migraine are associated with the s allele of the 5HTTLPR gene polymorphism. (Translated from eng) *Psychiatry Res* 149(1-3):261-266 (in eng).

[103] Neumeister A, *et al.* (2002) Association between serotonin transporter gene promoter polymorphism (5HTTLPR) and behavioral responses to tryptophan depletion in healthy women with and without family history of depression. (Translated from eng) *Arch Gen Psychiatry* 59(7):613-620 (in eng).

[104] Wust S, *et al.* (2009) Sex-specific association between the 5-HTT gene-linked polymorphic region and basal cortisol secretion. (Translated from eng) *Psychoneuroendocrinology* 34(7):972-982 (in eng).

[105] Udelsman R & Chrousos GP (1988) Hormonal responses to surgical stress. (Translated from eng) *Adv Exp Med Biol* 245:265-272 (in eng).

[106] Armario A, *et al.* (2012) What can We Know from Pituitary-Adrenal Hormones About the Nature and Consequences of Exposure to Emotional Stressors? (Translated from Eng) *Cell Mol Neurobiol* (in Eng).

[107] Tronche F, *et al.* (1999) Disruption of the glucocorticoid receptor gene in the nervous system results in reduced anxiety. (Translated from eng) *Nat Genet* 23(1):99-103 (in eng).

[108] van Santen A, *et al.* (2010) Psychological traits and the cortisol awakening response: results from the Netherlands Study of Depression and Anxiety. (Translated from eng) *Psychoneuroendocrinology* 36(2):240-248 (in eng).

[109] Essex MJ, *et al.* (2011) Influence of early life stress on later hypothalamic-pituitary-adrenal axis functioning and its covariation with mental health symptoms: a study of the allostatic process from childhood into adolescence. (Translated from eng) *Dev Psychopathol* 23(4):1039-1058 (in eng).

[110] Wilkinson PO & Goodyer IM (2011) Childhood adversity and allostatic overload of the hypothalamic-pituitary-adrenal axis: a vulnerability model for depressive disorders. (Translated from eng) *Dev Psychopathol* 23(4):1017-1037 (in eng).

[111] Murgatroyd C & Spengler D (2011) Epigenetic programming of the HPA axis: early life decides. (Translated from eng) *Stress* 14(6):581-589 (in eng).

[112] Kudielka BM & Wust S (2011) Human models in acute and chronic stress: assessing determinants of individual hypothalamus-pituitary-adrenal axis activity and reactivity. (Translated from eng) *Stress* 13(1):1-14 (in eng).

[113] Nieuwenhuizen AG & Rutters F (2008) The hypothalamic-pituitary-adrenal-axis in the regulation of energy balance. (Translated from eng) *Physiol Behav* 94(2):169-177 (in eng).

[114] Walker BR (2007) Glucocorticoids and cardiovascular disease. (Translated from eng) *Eur J Endocrinol* 157(5):545-559 (in eng).

[115] Benedetti F, Amanzio M, Vighetti S, & Asteggiano G (2006) The biochemical and neuroendocrine bases of the hyperalgesic nocebo effect. (Translated from eng) *J Neurosci* 26(46):12014-12022 (in eng).

[116] Lovick TA (2009) CCK as a modulator of cardiovascular function. (Translated from eng) *J Chem Neuroanat* 38(3):176-184 (in eng).

[117] Lee SY & Soltesz I (2011) Cholecystokinin: a multi-functional molecular switch of neuronal circuits. (Translated from eng) *Dev Neurobiol* 71(1):83-91 (in eng).

[118] Hogan B, Beddington R, Costantini F, & Lacy E (1994) Manipulating the mouse embryo, a laboratory manual. *(in eng).*

[119] Im HI, *et al.* (2009) Post-training dephosphorylation of eEF-2 promotes protein synthesis for memory consolidation. (Translated from eng) *PLoS One* 4(10):e7424 (in eng).

[120] Wank SA (1995) Cholecystokinin receptors. (Translated from eng) *Am J Physiol* 269(5 Pt 1):G628-646 (in eng).

[121] Bradwejn J & de Montigny C (1984) Benzodiazepines antagonize cholecystokinin-induced activation of rat hippocampal neurones. (Translated from eng) *Nature* 312(5992):363-364 (in eng).

[122] Rasmussen K, Helton DR, Berger JE, & Scearce E (1993) The CCK-B antagonist LY288513 blocks effects of diazepam withdrawal on auditory startle. (Translated from eng) *Neuroreport* 5(2):154-156 (in eng).

[123] Hauger RL, Lorang M, Irwin M, & Aguilera G (1990) CRF receptor regulation and sensitization of ACTH responses to acute ether stress during chronic intermittent immobilization stress. (Translated from eng) *Brain Res* 532(1-2):34-40 (in eng).

[124] Ma S & Morilak DA (2005) Chronic intermittent cold stress sensitises the hypothalamic-pituitary-adrenal response to a novel acute stress by enhancing noradrenergic influence in the rat paraventricular nucleus. (Translated from eng) *J Neuroendocrinol* 17(11):761-769 (in eng).

[125] Mueller SC, *et al.* (2010) Early-life stress is associated with impairment in cognitive control in adolescence: an fMRI study. (Translated from eng) *Neuropsychologia* 48(10):3037-3044 (in eng).

[126] Ryan B, *et al.* (2009) Remodelling by early-life stress of NMDA receptor-dependent synaptic plasticity in a gene-environment rat model of depression. (Translated from eng) *Int J Neuropsychopharmacol* 12(4):553-559 (in eng).

[127] Coplan JD, *et al.* (2010) Early-life stress and neurometabolites of the hippocampus. (Translated from eng) *Brain Res* 1358:191-199 (in eng).

[128] Gatt JM, *et al.* (2010) Early Life Stress Combined with Serotonin 3A Receptor and Brain-Derived Neurotrophic Factor Valine 66 to Methionine Genotypes Impacts Emotional Brain and Arousal Correlates of Risk for Depression. (Translated from Eng) *Biol Psychiatry* (in Eng).

[129] Harro J, Kiivet RA, Lang A, & Vasar E (1990) Rats with anxious or non-anxious type of exploratory behaviour differ in their brain CCK-8 and benzodiazepine receptor characteristics. (Translated from eng) *Behav Brain Res* 39(1):63-71 (in eng).

[130] MacNeil G, Sela Y, McIntosh J, & Zacharko RM (1997) Anxiogenic behavior in the light-dark paradigm follwoing intraventricular administration of cholecystokinin-8S, restraint stress, or uncontrollable footshock in the CD-1 mouse. (Translated from eng) *Pharmacol Biochem Behav* 58(3):737-746 (in eng).

[131] Pavlasevic S, Bednar I, Qureshi GA, & Sodersten P (1993) Brain cholecystokinin tetrapeptide levels are increased in a rat model of anxiety. (Translated from eng) *Neuroreport* 5(3):225-228 (in eng).

[132] Farook JM, *et al.* (2004) The CCK2 agonist BC264 reverses freezing behavior habituation in PVG hooded rats on repeated exposures to a cat. (Translated from eng) *Neurosci Lett* 355(3):205-208 (in eng).

[133] Farook JM, *et al.* (2001) Strain differences in freezing behavior of PVG hooded and Sprague-Dawley rats: differential cortical expression of cholecystokinin2 receptors. (Translated from eng) *Neuroreport* 12(12):2717-2720 (in eng).

[134] Wang H, *et al.* (2003) Genetic variations in CCK2 receptor in PVG hooded and Sprague-Dawley rats and its mRNA expression on cat exposure. (Translated from eng) *Behav Neurosci* 117(2):385-390 (in eng).

[135] Harro J, Lofberg C, Rehfeld JF, & Oreland L (1996) Cholecystokinin peptides and receptors in the rat brain during stress. (Translated from eng) *Naunyn Schmiedebergs Arch Pharmacol* 354(1):59-66 (in eng).

[136] Harro J, Marcusson J, & Oreland L (1992) Alterations in brain cholecystokinin receptors in suicide victims. (Translated from eng) *Eur Neuropsychopharmacol* 2(1):57-63 (in eng).

[137] Nevo I, Becker C, Hamon M, & Benoliel JJ (1996) Stress- and yohimbine-induced release of cholecystokinin in the frontal cortex of the freely moving rat: prevention by diazepam but not ondansetron. (Translated from eng) *J Neurochem* 66(5):2041-2049 (in eng).

[138] Siegel RA, Duker EM, Pahnke U, & Wuttke W (1987) Stress-induced changes in cholecystokinin and substance P concentrations in discrete regions of the rat hypothalamus. (Translated from eng) *Neuroendocrinology* 46(1):75-81 (in eng).

[139] Zhang LX, *et al.* (1996) Changes in cholecystokinin mRNA expression after amygdala kindled seizures: an in situ hybridization study. (Translated from eng) *Brain Res Mol Brain Res* 35(1-2):278-284 (in eng).

[140] Del Bel EA & Guimaraes FS (1997) Social isolation increases cholecystokinin mRNA in the central nervous system of rats. (Translated from eng) *Neuroreport* 8(16):3597-3600 (in eng).

[141] Herman JP, Flak J, & Jankord R (2008) Chronic stress plasticity in the hypothalamic paraventricular nucleus. (Translated from eng) *Prog Brain Res* 170:353-364 (in eng).

[142] Widom CS (1999) Posttraumatic stress disorder in abused and neglected children grown up. (Translated from eng) *Am J Psychiatry* 156(8):1223-1229 (in eng).

[143] Cohen H, Kaplan Z, & Kotler M (1999) CCK-antagonists in a rat exposed to acute stress: implication for anxiety associated with post-traumatic stress disorder. (Translated from eng) *Depress Anxiety* 10(1):8-17 (in eng).

[144] Koks S, *et al.* (2000) Cholecystokinin-induced anxiety in rats: relevance of pre-experimental stress and seasonal variations. (Translated from eng) *J Psychiatry Neurosci* 25(1):33-42 (in eng).

[145] Bradwejn J, Koszycki D, & Shriqui C (1991) Enhanced sensitivity to cholecystokinin tetrapeptide in panic disorder. Clinical and behavioral findings. (Translated from eng) *Arch Gen Psychiatry* 48(7):603-610 (in eng).

[146] Brawman-Mintzer O, *et al.* (1997) Effects of the cholecystokinin agonist pentagastrin in patients with generalized anxiety disorder. (Translated from eng) *Am J Psychiatry* 154(5):700-702 (in eng).

[147] Kellner M, *et al.* (2000) Behavioral and endocrine response to cholecystokinin tetrapeptide in patients with posttraumatic stress disorder. (Translated from eng) *Biol Psychiatry* 47(2):107-111 (in eng).

[148] van Vliet IM, Westenberg HG, Slaap BR, den Boer JA, & Ho Pian KL (1997) Anxiogenic effects of pentagastrin in patients with social phobia and healthy controls. (Translated from eng) *Biol Psychiatry* 42(1):76-78 (in eng).

Chapter 3

Mechanism of Glucocorticoid-Induced Osteoporosis: An Update

Xing-Ming Shi, Norman Chutkan, Mark W. Hamrick and Carlos M. Isales

Additional information is available at the end of the chapter

http://dx.doi.org/10.5772/53978

1. Introduction

Synthetic oral steroids were initially developed in the 1940-1950's. Although their use was initially limited by their high cost, as they became more affordable and began to be used for treatment of a wide variety of conditions, side effects associated with their use became much more prevalent. In fact, glucocorticoid-induced osteoporosis is now the most common secondary cause of osteoporosis. Until relatively recently, the mechanism of action of these drugs and the mechanisms involved in the development of side effects such as osteoporosis and the higher incidence of bone fractures was not known. Although steroids are widely viewed as mainly catabolic for bone a distinction needs to be made between physiologic and pharmacologic doses of steroids. Recent evidence demonstrates that steroids can clearly be anabolic for bone. In this chapter we review recent findings and mechanisms of glucocorticoid action on bone and some of the clinical consequences of pharmacologic doses of these compounds on bone.

2. Glucocorticoids and osteoporosis

Glucocorticoids are among the most potent anti-inflammatory and immunosuppressive agents and are key therapeutic agents for the management of chronic inflammatory diseases, including rheumatic diseases [1-4], pulmonary disease [5;6], asthma [7-11] and post transplantation immunotherapy [12]. However, long-term glucocorticoid therapy (>3 months) causes bone loss resulting in osteoporosis (glucocorticoid-induced osteoporosis or GIOP) [3;4;13-15], a severe-side effect that occurs in 30 – 50% of patients [16-18]. The incidence of GIOP is indiscriminate of race, age and gender [19;20]. Children, as young as 4 years of age, and adolescents who are on glucocorticoid therapy for various pediatric disorders, including asthma [20-22], juvenile rheumatoid arthritis [23;24], Crohn's disease [25], systemic lupus erythematosus [26;27], and inflammatory bowel disease [28;29] have been reported to endure significant bone density decrease. There is no clearly defined threshold for safe use of glucocorticoids. In practice, a dose equal to or greater than 5mg/day of prednisone is considered as low, and 10mg/day or more is high. The severity of bone loss in GIOP is both time- and dose-dependent. GIOP occurs in two phases: a rapid, early phase in which bone mineral density is reduced, within the first 5 to 7 months of therapy, possibly as a result of excessive bone resorption, and a slower, progressive phase in which bone mineral density declines because of impaired bone formation [30]. Bone loss continues as long as treatment is maintained.

3. Glucocorticoid mechanism of action as anti-inflammatory and immunosuppressant drugs

Glucocorticoids exert their actions via intracellular glucocorticoid receptors (GRs) [31;32]. The GR belongs to the ligand-regulated nuclear receptor superfamily [33]. Like other members in this superfamily, GR contains three major functional domains: a N-terminal activation domain required for transcriptional activation and association with basal transcription factors; a central DNA-binding domain (DBD) consisting of two highly conserved zinc finger regions that are critical for dimerization, DNA binding, transcriptional activation and repression; and a C-terminal ligand-binding domain (LBD) that serves as the binding site for glucocorticoids, chaperone proteins, and coactivators [34;35]. In the absence of ligand, GR is predominantly retained in the cytoplasm as an inactive multi-protein complex consisting of heat shock protein (hsp90) and a number of other proteins, including the immunophilins. The binding of glucocorticoid triggers a conformational change in the GR and leads to dissociation of the multi-protein complex and exposure of a nuclear localization sequence resulting in its nuclear translocation. Once in the nucleus, GR, in the form of a homodimer, binds to a palindromic glucocorticoid-response element (GRE) in the target gene promoter and activates transcription (*e.g.*, of the tyrosine amino transferase gene), or it can bind to a negative GRE (nGRE) to repress transcription (*e.g.*, of the osteocalcin gene) [36].

Glucocorticoids suppress the expression of a panel of inflammatory-relevant genes including cytokines [interleukins (IL) and tumor necrosis factors (TNF-α,β], chemokines (Regulated upon Activation Normal T-cell Expressed and Secreted or RANTES, Macrophage Inflammatory Protein-1-alpha or MIP-1α, Monocyte Chemotactic Protein or MCP-1, -3, and -4], inflammatory enzymes (COX-2, iNOS), and adhesion molecules (Intercellular Adhesion Molecule 1 or ICAM-1, E-selectin) that play a key role in the recruitment of inflammatory cells to the inflammation sites [37-39]. However, most of these genes do not have negative GREs in their promoter regions, and therefore, they are not directly regulated by the binding of GRs to such regulatory elements. These genes do contain NF-κB- and/or AP-1-binding sites and are activated through these sites by NF-κB and/or AP-1 in response to stimuli (cytokines). Thus, one mechanism by which glucocorticoids could regulate transcription would be modulation of NF-κB or AP-1 DNA-binding activity. In 1990, three independent groups found cross-talk between GR and AP-1 [40-42]. In these studies, it was found that activated GR can interact with c-Jun/AP-1 and that the formation of a GR-c-Jun complex prevents c-Jun/AP-1 DNA-binding, resulting in the inhibition of gene expression. Later, it was found that the activated GR can associate with the p65 subunit of NF-κB and inhibit gene activation mediated by NF-κB [43;44]. These findings led to the establishment of the **protein-protein interaction model**.

In 1995, it was found that glucocorticoids induce the expression of a cytoplasmic inhibitor of NF-κB, the IκB-α [45;46]. These studies led to the establishment of a second model, **the IκB-α upregulation model**. This model proposes that glucocorticoids induce the expression of IκB-α and that the newly synthesized IκB-α sequesters the p65 subunit of the NF-κB in the cytoplasm and thereby inhibits NF-κB nuclear functions. However, this mechanism has been challenged by a number of studies. It has now been established that the effect of glucocorticoids on IκB-α expression, and subsequently NF-κB nuclear translocation, is cell-type specific. In some cell types glucocorticoid inhibition of proinflammatory stimuli-induced p65 nuclear translocation is coupled with the induction of IκB-α [45-48]. In other cell types, however, these two events are uncoupled [49;50]. Moreover, a GR mutant that does not enhance IκB-α expression, is still able to repress NF-κB activity [51].

4. Glucocorticoid effects on bone cells

Glucocorticoids have both anabolic and catabolic effects on bone. However, the outcome of glucocorticoid therapy is a net loss of bone [4;52;53]. Corticosteroid 11β-hydroxysteroid dehydrogenase 2 [11β-HSD2] is an enzyme that oxidizes the active form of glucocorticoid cortisol to the inactive metabolite cortisone, thus the levels of expression and activity of this enzyme is critical for glucocorticoid signaling. *In vivo* studies show that bone-specific transgenic overexpression of 11β-HSD2, under the control of type I collagen promoter, impairs osteoblast differentiation and bone acquisition [54-56]. These studies demonstrate that the endogenous glucocorticoid signaling is essential for normal skeletal development. However, glucocorticoid in excess such as patients with Cushing's syndrome [22] or the patients on glucocorticoid therapy rapidly lose bone mass resulting in osteoporosis. The direct effects of glucocorticoids on bone cells are illustrated in Figure 1.

5. Glucocorticoid effects on bone marrow Mesenchymal Stem Cells (MSCs)

Bone marrow MSCs are multipotent cells that can give rise to several distinct cell lineages, including osteoblasts, adipocytes, and chondrocytes [57-60]. Patients on glucocorticoid therapy not only lose bone but also accumulate large amounts of marrow fat (fatty marrow), indicating that glucocorticoid has altered lineage commitment of MSC to adipocytes at the expense of osteoblasts because these two pathways have a reciprocal relationship [61-64]. Thus, one possible mechanism by which glucocorticoids alter MSC fate determination is through the induction of the master adipogenic regulator peroxisome proliferator-activated receptor gamma (PPARγ) [65;66], which is transcriptionally activated by the CCAAT/enhancer binding protein (C/EBP) family transcription factors in response to glucocorticoid [67-70] (Figure 2). Indeed, Weinstein and colleagues showed that administration of glucocorticoids to mice reduces the numbers of osteoprogenitor cells [71].

This could be achieved through induction of PPARγ since under the same condition bone marrow adipogenesis is enhanced [72], and that a reduction in PPARγ dosage (haploinsufficiency) in mice results in reduced adipogenesis and enhanced osteogenesis from bone marrow progenitors [73].

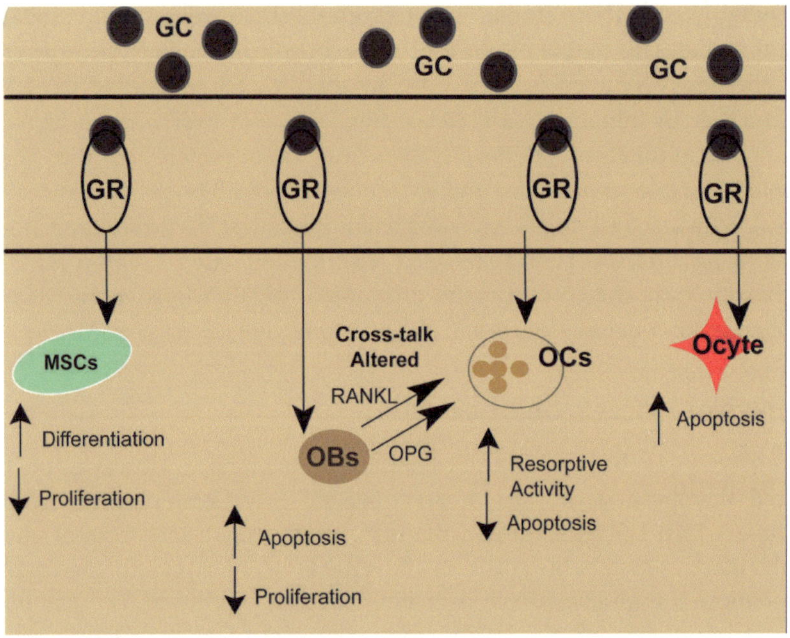

Figure 1. Glucocorticoids bind to the glucocorticoid receptor (GR) and affect mesenchymal stem cell (MSC), osteoblast (OB), osteoclast (OC) and osteocyte (Ocyte) function. The net result is decreased bone formation and increased bone resorption. ↑increase; ↓decrease.

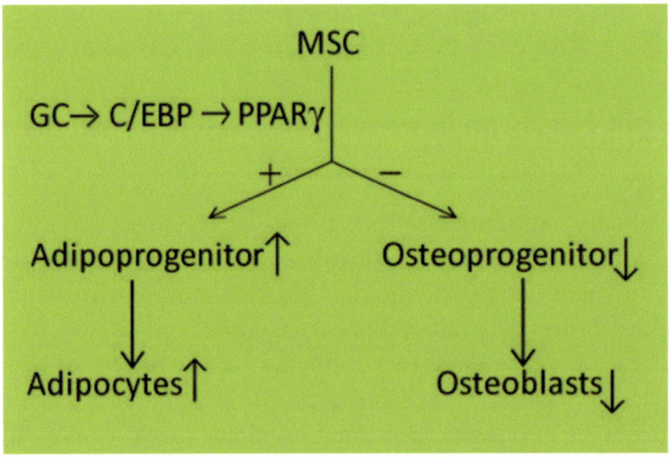

Figure 2. Glucocorticoid reduces the number of osteoprogenitors from MSC by promoting adipogenic differentiation pathway. Glucocorticoid induces the expression of C/EBP family transcription factors that directly activate the transcription of PPARγ, the master regulator of adipogenesis, and shifts the lineage commitment of MSCs to adipocyte pathway, thus reducing the number of osteoprogenitor cells.

6. Glucocorticoid effects on osteoblasts and osteocytes

It has been known for decades that glucocorticoid inhibits bone formation [52;74], but only recently have we realized that glucocorticoids directly target bone cells. By administering a high dose of prednisolone to mice, Weinstein and colleagues found that glucocorticoid induces the death of mature osteoblasts and osteocytes [71;75]. In the same study, the authors also showed that the same is true in bone biopsy samples obtained from patients with glucocorticoid-induced osteoporosis. These results were further strengthened in a transgenic mouse model, in which the glucocorticoid signaling is disrupted by overexpression of 11β-HSD2 specifically in osteoblasts. The study showed that the 11β-HSD2 transgenic mice are protected from glucocorticoid-induced osteoblasts and osteocytes apoptosis and suppression of bone formation [76]. These studies demonstrate that glucocorticoids cause bone loss by restricting the supply of bone building cells, the osteoblasts, and by interfering with the communication network within bone environment via osteocyte death. The osteocytes are the mechanosensory cells that detect and send signals for bone formation in response to damages caused by mechanical loading and unloading [77;78].

7. Glucocorticoid effects on osteoclasts

Osteoclasts are bone resorbing cells and play a key role in the maintenance of bone homeostasis through bone remodeling. In patients, glucocorticoid-induced osteoporosis features a rapid early phase increase in bone resorption, followed by a slow progressive decrease in bone formation [52]. Earlier studies showed that glucocorticoids stimulate osteoclast differentiation and increase their activity [72;79;80]. It is now recognized that glucocorticoids increase the longevity of osteoclasts but may inhibit their bone resorptive activity [81;82]. Moreover, a recent study suggests that glucocorticoids do not inhibit, but modify osteoclast resorptive behavior, making osteoclasts erode bone surfaces over long distances without interruption [83].

8. Glucocorticoid-induced Leucine Zipper (GILZ): A new glucocorticoid anti-inflammatory effect mediator

The protein-protein interaction and the IκB-α upregulation models described earlier in this chapter were established prior to the discovery of a glucocorticoid-inducible protein named glucocorticoid-induced leucine zipper (GILZ), which was identified in 1997 [84]. GILZ is a member of the leucine zipper protein family [84;85] and belongs to the transforming growth factor-beta (TGF-β)-stimulated clone-22 (TSC-22d3) family of transcription factors [86;87]. Members of this family of proteins contain three distinct domains; an N-terminal domain containing a TSC box (N-Ter), a middle leucine zipper domain (LZ), and a C-terminal poly-proline rich domain (PRR).

Unlike IκB-α, which is induced by glucocorticoids in certain cell types [49;50;88], GILZ is induced by glucocorticoids virtually in all cell types examined so far, including bone marrow mesenchymal stem cells, osteoblasts, adipocytes, macrophages and epithelial cells [89]. *In vitro* studies show that overexpression of GILZ protects T-cells from apoptosis induced by anti-CD3 monoclonal antibody, but not other apoptosis-inducing agents such as dexamethasone, ultraviolet irradiation, starvation, or triggered by cross-linked anti-Fas mAb [84]. T-cell-specific transgenic overexpression of GILZ results in thymocyte apoptosis *ex vivo*, possibly through down-regulation of Bcl-xL [90]. The *in vitro* actions of GILZ have been shown to be mediated through direct protein-protein interactions between GILZ and NF-κB, and between GILZ and AP-1 [86;91;92]. The interaction between GILZ and NF-κB blocks NF-κB nuclear translocation and DNA-binding, and the interaction with AP-1 inhibits the binding of AP-1 to its DNA elements [91;92]. GILZ also interacts directly with the mitogen-activated protein kinase (MAPK) family members, Ras and Raf-1, resulting in inhibition of Raf-1 phosphorylation and subsequently, inhibition of MEK/ERK-1/2 phosphorylation and AP-1-dependent transcription [86;93]. Moreover, GILZ can deactivate macrophages [94], inhibit proinflammatory cytokine-induced inflammatory enzymes such as cyclooxygenase-2 [95], inhibit IL-2/IL-2 receptor and IL-5 expression [91;96], and stimulate the production of anti-inflammatory IL-10 by immature dendritic cells, thereby, preventing the production of inflammatory chemokines by CD40L-activated dendritic cells [97]. These studies demonstrate that GILZ is a glucocorticoid anti-inflammatory effect mediator and utilizes very similar mechanisms, to those GR uses [98].

9. GILZ mediates the anabolic effect of glucocorticoids

GILZ is a direct GR target gene with several GREs present in its promoter region [99]. In the absence of glucocorticoid stimulation GILZ is expressed at a very low basal level. However, in the presence of glucocorticoid, GILZ expression is rapidly induced (Figure 3] but GR is also activated, and the activated GR negatively impacts bone, both directly (i.e., inhibits osteocalcin gene transcription) and indirectly through other pathways as illustrated (Figure 4]. Because of that, it is impossible to determine the role of GILZ in osteoblast differentiation and bone formation without the influence of GR, which plays a negative role and may override GILZ actions. To further study this problem, a retrovirus-mediated GILZ overexpression system was established in bone marrow MSCs/osteoprogenitor cells. Studies carried out in this system showed that GILZ has potent pro-osteogenic activity as demonstrated by significantly increased alkaline phosphatase activity, enhanced mineralized bone nodule formation, and the expression of osteoblast-associated genes such as Runx2, type I collagen, alkaline phosphatase, and osteocalcin [100]. Furthermore, our recent studies have shown that overexpression of GILZ can antagonize the inhibitory effect of TNF-α on MSC osteogenic differentiation [101]. Possible mechanisms underlying this antagonism may include GILZ inhibition of TNF-α-induced ERK/MAP kinase activation, which has been shown to be responsible for TNF-α down-regulation of a key osteogenic factor Osx [102;103], and inhibition of TNF-α-induced expression of E3 ubiquitin ligase Smurf proteins, which have been shown to accelerate the degradation of Runx2 protein [104-106].

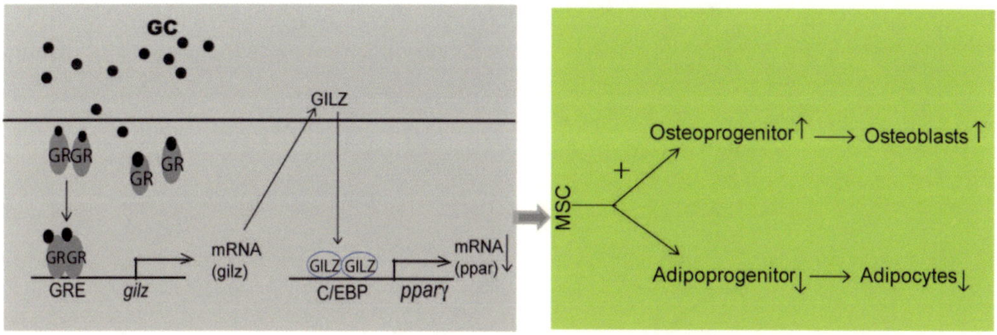

Figure 3. GILZ enhances MSC osteogenic differentiation by shifting MSC lineage preference to osteogenic pathway.

10. GR mediates the catabolic effects of glucocorticoids

There are many glucocorticoid effectors involved in the regulation of bone development or metabolism through different pathways. However, it was only recently demonstrated that the GR was directly responsible for glucocorticoid-induced bone loss *in vivo*. Using a bone-specific GR knockout mouse model, Rauch et al showed that glucocorticoids are unable to induce bone loss or to inhibit bone formation in these mice because the GR-deficient osteoblasts become refractory to glucocorticoid-induced apoptosis, inhibition of proliferation, and differentiation [107]. Interestingly, data from this study also demonstrated that GR-deficiency results in a low bone mass phenotype, confirming the previous studies that the endogenous glucocorticoid signaling is critical for normal bone acquisition [54-56]. Other evidence supporting the role of GR in glucocorticoid-induced bone loss includes: 1] the glucocorticoid-activated GR binds directly to the negative glucocorticoid response elements (nGREs) in the promoter region of the osteocalcin (*Ocn*) gene, an osteoblast-specific gene that plays an important role in bone mineralization, and inhibit its transcription [36;108]; 2] GR transcriptionally activates the expression of MAP kinase phosphatase-1 (MKP-1] [109], which inactivates MAP kinase and thus inhibits osteogenic differentiation [64;110;111]; and 3] GR can physically interact with and inhibit the transcriptional functions of Smad3, an intracellular signaling mediator of transforming growth factor-beta (TGF-β) [112] (Figure 4]. Glucocorticoids have been known to antagonize TGF-β action in bone [113-115] and TGF-β stimulates osteoprogenitor cell proliferation [116-119] and attract osteoprogenitor cells to the remodeling sites during bone remodeling [120]. It is important to note that while the catabolic effects of glucocorticoids are often associated with long-term glucocorticoid excess [1-4;7], a short term exposure to glucocorticoid seems beneficial; for example, treatment of bone marrow stromal cells or osteoblasts with dexamethasone enhances, rather than inhibits, alkaline phosphatase (ALP) activity. The ALP is expressed at the early stage of osteoblast differentiation program and the increase of ALP expression or activity marks the entry of cells into the osteoblast lineage.

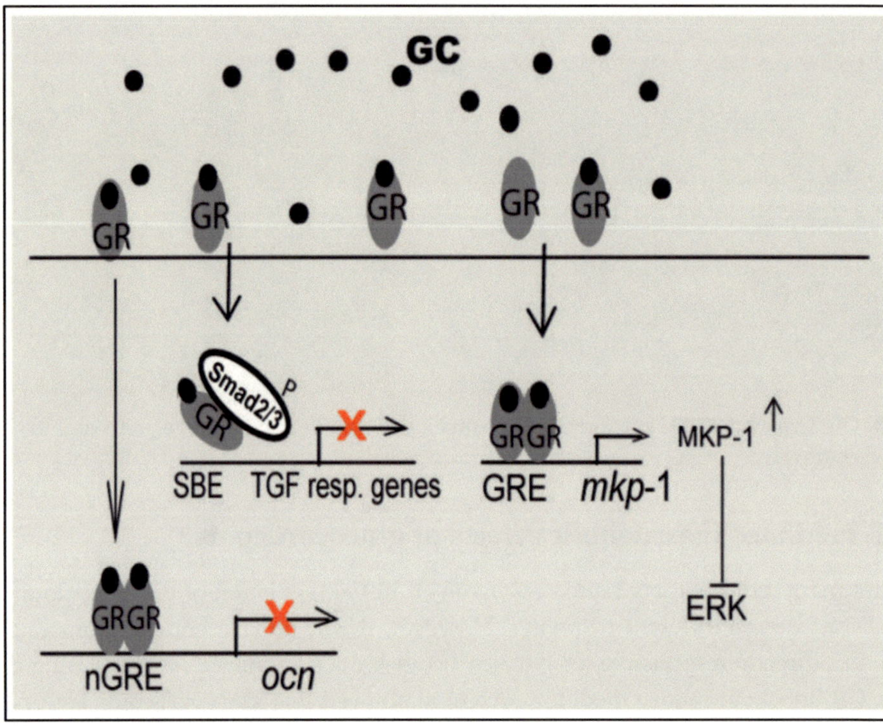

Figure 4. GR inhibits MSC proliferation, ERK activation and Ocn expression. Ligand-bound GR physically interacts with: 1] TGF-β signaling mediator Smad3 and disrupts its transcriptional activity; 2] Activates mkp-1 transcription, by binding to GRE in the mkp-1 promoter region, resulting inhibition of ERK activation; and 3] Suppresses Ocn expression by binding to nGRE in the Ocn promoter region.

11. Glucocorticoid-Induced Osteoporosis (GIOP)

Although glucocorticoids are an essential hormone for survival and normal function, when present in excess (pharmacologic doses) lead to a number of serious side effects including bone loss and fractures. In fact, it is estimated that 30-50% of patients chronically exposed to high levels of glucocorticoids will develop a bone fracture [121]. Glucocorticoid excess can result from either endogenous (Cushing's) or exogenous (iatrogenic) sources. Glucocorticoids are widely used for the treatment of a variety of inflammatory and autoimmune conditions. It is estimated that 0.5% of the population receives steroid therapy and exogenous steroids are thus the most common cause of secondary osteoporosis [122]. There has been a lot of discussion on the dose, duration and mode of administration of steroids and the impact on the development of osteoporosis. There has been a lot of debate on a "safe" dose for glucocorticoid replacement. Doses as low as 2.5 mg of prednisolone have been reported to result in osteoporosis [122]. Even patients on "physiologic" glucocorticoid replacement for Addison's disease have been reported to have lower bone density than controls, although clearly many of these patients were overreplaced with steroid therapy [123]. Further, steroids even when given in an intermittent, rather than continuous fashion, or in an inhaled rather than oral fashion, are still associated with an increased risk of fracture. In treatment guidelines by the American College of Rheumatology in 2010, it was recommended that for patients with low fracture risk receiving more than 7.5 mg of prednisolone equivalents for more than 3 months receive some form of therapy for fracture prevention. In contrast for patients at high fracture risk it was recommended that they receive some form of therapy even at glucocorticoid doses lower than 5 mg and even for periods for less than one month [124].

12. Mechanism

Glucocorticoids have multiple effects on bone and bone cells. In addition, in cases where the glucocorticoids are given to treat systemic inflammatory conditions (e.g. rheumatoid arthritis), the underlying condition also contributes to bone loss. Glucocorticoids also inhibit endogenous production of sex steroids (testosterone and estrogen) in addition to production of adrenal androgens, all of which may have protective effects against bone loss [125]. Further, prolonged high dose glucocorticoid use results in both muscle weakness thus predisposing to an increased number of falls and muscle wasting. Bone-muscle interactions may also contribute to maintaining bone health. Glucocorticoids also decrease intestinal calcium absorption thus further predisposing to osteoporosis. Recently, effects of glucocorticoids on decreasing bone vasculature, has also been implicated as a potential mechanism for glucocorticoid effects on bone [126]. There also seems to be an age-dependence of glucocorticoid effects on bone. The likelihood of fractures with glucocorticoids appears to increase with increasing patient age. Glucocorticoid-induced bone loss appears to be biphasic with an initial rapid phase of bone loss of 5-15% /year followed by a more sustained bone loss rate of 2% [121].

Glucocorticoids affect all bone cells, they result in osteocytic and osteoblastic apoptosis and decreased function of both osteoclasts and osteoblasts. However, they decrease osteoclastic apoptosis. Thus, the net effect is reduced bone formation and increased bone breakdown. Trabecular bone seems to be particularly sensitive to the detrimental effects of steroids resulting in a higher incidence of vertebral and femoral neck fractures [121]. Vertebral compression fractures are commonly missed since only about 30% of them are symptomatic. A study by Angeli et al [127] which examined the prevalence of vertebral fractures in patients receiving glucocorticoids for a variety of autoimmune conditions determined that over 37% of patients had at least one asymptomatic vertebral compression fracture and more than 14% had two or more asymptomatic fractures.

Glucocorticoid effects on bone appear to be generally reversible and once therapy is stopped bone repair occurs over the year following drug cessation. Thus, if feasible, steroid cessation may be the therapy of choice for GIOP.

13. Diagnosis

Determining fracture risk for patients on steroids is difficult since even patients with normal bone densitometry on steroids have a higher fracture risk. Current use of steroids is one of the risk factors used in the calculation of the FRAX (Fracture Risk Assessment) score.

However a recent joint position statement by the International Society for Clinical Densitometry and the International Osteoporosis Foundation concluded that when using the FRAX tool there probably was an underestimation of fracture risk with daily prednisone doses greater than 7.5 mg and an overestimation of fracture risk with daily prednisone doses of less than 2.5 mg. In addition, FRAX probably underestimated fracture risk when high dose inhaled steroids were used. Finally, it was concluded that for patients with adrenal insufficiency receiving appropriate replacement steroid doses this not be included in the FRAX calculation [128].

The American College of Rheumatology recommends that some form of therapy be considered for all patients receiving prolonged steroid therapy and that for those who have a bone densitometry test (Dual energy x-ray absorptiometry or DXA), a T-score of less than -1.0 be considered abnormal [125].

14. Therapy

Since glucocorticoids interfere with intestinal calcium absorption, all patients about to start glucocorticoid therapy should be placed on calcium and vitamin D replacement. Antiresorptive agents such as bisphosphonates (both oral and IV) have been used for the therapy of GIOP, are effective in decreasing the increased fracture risk associated with steroids and are approved for this indication. However, as discussed by Teitelbaum et al. [129], although initial use of steroids is associated with increased bone resorption (osteoclast mediated and related to decreased osteoclastic apoptosis and a situation in which antiresorptive use makes sense), more prolonged steroid use is associated with decreased bone formation and antiresorptive agents have the theoretical possibility of making things worse by further suppressing a low bone turnover state. Thus, use of an anabolic agent such as teriparatide (synthetic parathyroid hormone) for treatment of GIOP would appear more appropriate. In fact in a clinical trial, comparing alendronate vs. teriparatide for 18 months in 428 men/women with established osteoporosis and who had received at least 5mg of prednisone for at least 3 months, teriparatide was significantly more effective in both increasing bone mineral density at the spine [7.2 vs 3.4%) and in decreasing new vertebral fractures [0.6% vs 6.1%) [130]. Of note, this was a secondary instead of a primary osteoporosis prevention trial and there was a greater incidence of side effects associated with teriparatide use as compared to controls [131]. In addition, use of teriparatide by patients is currently limited to two years, thus alternative and better forms of therapy for GIOP need to be developed.

15. Conclusion

Although adverse side effects of glucocorticoids on bone have been long recognized, both from endogenous sources as described by Harvey Cushing in the 1930's or from exogenous sources after development of glucocorticoids in the 1950's the mechanisms involved in this process have only recently began to be understood. It is clear that although physiologic levels of glucocorticoids are important in normal bone development, pharmacologic doses result in a high level of fractures, particularly of vertebral bone. Thus, it would seem that glucocorticoids have both anabolic and catabolic actions on bone. Data from our labs and from others suggest that GILZ may be an important mediator of GR's anabolic actions and thus may be an attractive therapeutic target for drug development.

Author details

Xing-Ming Shi
Institute of Molecular Medicine and Genetics, Department of Pathology
Georgia Health Sciences University, Augusta, GA, USA

Norman Chutkan
Department of Orthopaedic Surgery, Georgia Health Sciences University, Augusta, GA, USA

Mark W. Hamrick
Departments of Cellular Biology & Anatomy and Orthopaedic Surgery, Georgia Health Sciences University, Augusta, GA, USA

Carlos M. Isales
Institute of Molecular Medicine and Genetics, Departments of Orthopaedic Surgery and Medicine, Georgia Health Sciences University, Augusta, GA, USA

Acknowledgement

This work was supported by grants from the National Institutes of Health (DK76045] and National Institute on Aging (P01AG036675].

16. References

[1] Harris, E.D., Jr., Emkey, R.D., Nichols, J.E., and Newberg, A. 1983. Low dose prednisone therapy in rheumatoid arthritis: a double blind study. *J.Rheumatol.* 10:713-721.

[2] Conn, D.L. 2001. Resolved: Low-dose prednisone is indicated as a standard treatment in patients with rheumatoid arthritis. *Arthritis Rheum.* 45:462-467.

[3] Locascio, V., Bonucci, E., Imbimbo, B., Ballanti, P., Adami, S., Milani, S., Tartarotti, D., and DellaRocca, C. 1990. Bone loss in response to long-term glucocorticoid therapy. *Bone Miner.* 8:39-51.

[4] Nishimura, J. and Ikuyama, S. 2000. Glucocorticoid-induced osteoporosis: pathogenesis and management. *J.Bone Miner.Metab* 18:350-352.

[5] The Lung Health Study Research Group. 2000. Effect of inhaled triamcinolone on the decline in pulmonary function in chronic obstructive pulmonary disease. *N.Engl.J.Med.* 343:1902-1909.

[6] Walsh, L.J., Wong, C.A., Oborne, J., Cooper, S., Lewis, S.A., Pringle, M., Hubbard, R., and Tattersfield, A.E. 2001. Adverse effects of oral corticosteroids in relation to dose in patients with lung disease. *Thorax* 56:279-284.

[7] Ruegsegger, P., Medici, T.C., and Anliker, M. 1983. Corticosteroid-induced bone loss. A longitudinal study of alternate day therapy in patients with bronchial asthma using quantitative computed tomography. *Eur.J.Clin.Pharmacol.* 25:615-620.

[8] Bazzy-Asaad, A. 2001. Safety of inhaled corticosteroids in children with asthma. *Curr.Opin.Pediatr.* 13:523-527.

[9] Corren, J., Nelson, H., Greos, L.S., Bensch, G., Goldstein, M., Wu, J., Wang, S., and Newman, K. 2001. Effective control of asthma with hydrofluoroalkane flunisolide delivered as an extrafine aerosol in asthma patients. *Ann.Allergy Asthma Immunol.* 87:405-411.

[10] Fernandes, A.L., Faresin, S.M., Amorim, M.M., Fritscher, C.C., Pereira, C.A., and Jardim, J.R. 2001. Inhaled budesonide for adults with mild-to-moderate asthma: a randomized placebo-controlled, double-blind clinical trial. *Sao Paulo Med.J.* 119:169-174.

[11] Adinoff, A.D. and Hollister, J.R. 1983. Steroid-induced fractures and bone loss in patients with asthma. *N.Engl.J.Med.* 309:265-268.

[12] Park, S.J., Nguyen, D.Q., Savik, K., Hertz, M.I., and Bolman, R.M., III. 2001. Pre-transplant corticosteroid use and outcome in lung transplantation. *J.Heart Lung Transplant.* 20:304-309.

[13] Dequeker, J. and Westhovens, R. 1995. Low dose corticosteroid associated osteoporosis in rheumatoid arthritis and its prophylaxis and treatment: bones of contention. *J.Rheumatol.* 22:1013-1019.

[14] Adachi, J.D., Olszynski, W.P., Hanley, D.A., Hodsman, A.B., Kendler, D.L., Siminoski, K.G., Brown, J., Cowden, E.A., Goltzman, D., Ioannidis, G. *et al.* 2000. Management of corticosteroid-induced osteoporosis. *Semin.Arthritis Rheum.* 29:228-251.

[15] Saag, K.G., Koehnke, R., Caldwell, J.R., Brasington, R., Burmeister, L.F., Zimmerman, B., Kohler, J.A., and Furst, D.E. 1994. Low dose long-term corticosteroid therapy in rheumatoid arthritis: an analysis of serious adverse events. *Am.J.Med.* 96:115-123.

[16] Braun, J. and Sieper, J. 2001. [Glucocorticoid-induced osteoporosis]. *Orthopade* 30:444-450.

[17] Clowes, J.A., Peel, N., and Eastell, R. 2001. Glucocorticoid-induced osteoporosis. *Curr.Opin.Rheumatol.* 13:326-332.

[18] Lukert, B.P. and Raisz, L.G. 1990. Glucocorticoid-induced osteoporosis: pathogenesis and management. *Ann.Intern.Med.* 112:352-364.

[19] Klein, G. 2004. Glucocorticoid-induced bone loss in children. *Clinical Reviews in Bone and Mineral Metabolism* 2:37-52.

[20] VAN STAA, T.P., COOPER, C., Leufkens, H., and Bishop, N. 2003. Children and the Risk of Fractures Caused by Oral Corticosteroids. *Journal of Bone and Mineral Research* 18:913-918.

[21] Boot, A.M., de Jongste, J.C., Verberne, A.A.P.H., Pols, H.A.P., and de Muinck Keizer-Schrama, S. 1997. Bone mineral density and bone metabolism of prepubertal children with asthma after long-term treatment with inhaled corticosteroids. *Pediatr.Pulmonol.* 24:379-384.

[22] Covar, R.A., Leung, D.Y., McCormick, D., Steelman, J., Zeitler, P., and Spahn, J.D. 2000. Risk factors associated with glucocorticoid-induced adverse effects in children with severe asthma. *J Allergy Clin Immunol* 106:651-659.

[23] Burnham, J.M. and Leonard, M.B. 2004. Bone disease in pediatric rheumatologic disorders. *Curr.Rheumatol.Rep.* 6:70-78.

[24] Viswanathan, A. and Sylvester, F. 2008. Chronic pediatric inflammatory diseases: Effects on bone. *Reviews in Endocrine & Metabolic Disorders* 9:107-122.

[25] Burnham, J.M., Shults, J., Semeao, E., Foster, B., Zemel, B.S., Stallings, V.A., and Leonard, M.B. 2004. Whole Body BMC in Pediatric Crohn Disease: Independent Effects of Altered Growth, Maturation, and Body Composition. *Journal of Bone and Mineral Research* 19:1961-1968.

[26] Lilleby, V., Lien, G., Frey Fr_Ėslie, K., Haugen, M., Flat_Ė, B., and F_Ėrre, ś. 2005. Frequency of osteopenia in children and young adults with childhood-onset systemic lupus erythematosus. *Arthritis & Rheumatism* 52:2051-2059.

[27] Compeyrot-Lacassagne, S., Tyrrell, P.N., Atenafu, E., Doria, A.S., Stephens, D., Gilday, D., and Silverman, E.D. 2007. Prevalence and etiology of low bone mineral density in juvenile systemic lupus erythematosus. *Arthritis & Rheumatism* 56:1966-1973.

[28] Walther, F., Fusch, C., Radke, M., Beckert, S., and Findeisen, A. 2006. Osteoporosis in pediatric patients suffering from chronic inflammatory bowel disease with and without steroid treatment. *J Pediatr.Gastroenterol.Nutr.* 43:42-51.

[29] Boot, A.M., Bouquet, J., Krenning, E.P., and Muinck Keizer-Schrama, S.M.P.F. 1998. Bone mineral density and nutritional status in children with chronic inflammatory bowel disease. *Gut* 42:188-194.

[30] Mazziotti, G., Angeli, A., Bilezikian, J.P., Canalis, E., and Giustina, A. 2006. Glucocorticoid-induced osteoporosis: an update. *Trends in Endocrinology & Metabolism* 17:144-149.

[31] Webster, J.C. and Cidlowski, J.A. 1999. Mechanisms of Glucocorticoid-receptor-mediated Repression of Gene Expression. *Trends in Endocrinology and Metabolism* 10:396-402.

[32] Kumar, R. and Thompson, E.B. 2005. Gene regulation by the glucocorticoid receptor: Structure:function relationship. *The Journal of Steroid Biochemistry and Molecular Biology* 94:383-394.

[33] Kallio, P.J., Palvimo, J., and Janne, O.A. 1994. [Nuclear hormone receptors]. *Duodecim* 110:383-394.

[34] Giguere, V., Hollenberg, S.M., Rosenfeld, M.G., and Evans, R.M. 1986. Functional domains of the human glucocorticoid receptor. *Cell* 46:645-652.

[35] Parker, M.G. 1990. Structure and function of nuclear hormone receptors. *Semin.Cancer Biol* 1:81-87.

[36] Morrison, N. and Eisman, J. 1993. Role of the negative glucocorticoid regulatory element in glucocorticoid repression of the human osteocalcin promoter. *J Bone Miner.Res.* 8:969-975.

[37] De Bosscher, K., Vanden Berghe, W., and Haegeman, G. 2003. The Interplay between the Glucocorticoid Receptor and Nuclear Factor-{kappa}B or Activator Protein-1: Molecular Mechanisms for Gene Repression. *Endocr Rev* 24:488-522.

[38] De Bosscher, K., Vanden Berghe, W., and Haegeman, G. 2000. Mechanisms of anti-inflammatory action and of immunosuppression by glucocorticoids: negative

interference of activated glucocorticoid receptor with transcription factors. *J Neuroimmunol.* 109:16-22.

[39] Zitnik, R.J., Whiting, N.L., and Elias, J.A. 1994. Glucocorticoid inhibition of interleukin-1-induced interleukin-6 production by human lung fibroblasts: evidence for transcriptional and post-transcriptional regulatory mechanisms. *Am J Respir.Cell Mol Biol* 10:643-650.

[40] Yang-Yen, H.F., Chambard, J.C., Sun, Y.L., Smeal, T., Schmidt, T.J., Drouin, J., and Karin, M. 1990. Transcriptional interference between c-Jun and the glucocorticoid receptor: mutual inhibition of DNA binding due to direct protein-protein interaction. *Cell* 62:1205-1215.

[41] Jonat, C., Rahmsdorf, H.J., Park, K.K., Cato, A.C., Gebel, S., Ponta, H., and Herrlich, P. 1990. Antitumor promotion and antiinflammation: down-modulation of AP-1 (Fos/Jun) activity by glucocorticoid hormone. *Cell* 62:1189-1204.

[42] Schule, R., Rangarajan, P., Kliewer, S., Ransone, L.J., Bolado, J., Yang, N., Verma, I.M., and Evans, R.M. 1990. Functional antagonism between oncoprotein c-Jun and the glucocorticoid receptor. *Cell* 62:1217-1226.

[43] Ray, A. and Prefontaine, K.E. 1994. Physical association and functional antagonism between the p65 subunit of transcription factor NF-kappa B and the glucocorticoid receptor. *Proc.Natl.Acad.Sci.U.S.A* 91:752-756.

[44] Scheinman, R.I., Gualberto, A., Jewell, C.M., Cidlowski, J.A., and Baldwin, A.S., Jr. 1995. Characterization of mechanisms involved in transrepression of NF-kappa B by activated glucocorticoid receptors. *Mol.Cell.Biol.* 15:943-953.

[45] Auphan, N., DiDonato, J.A., Rosette, C., Helmberg, A., and Karin, M. 1995. Immunosuppression by glucocorticoids: inhibition of NF-kappa B activity through induction of I kappa B synthesis. *Science* 270:286-290.

[46] Scheinman, R.I., Cogswell, P.C., Lofquist, A.K., and Baldwin, A.S., Jr. 1995. Role of transcriptional activation of I kappa B alpha in mediation of immunosuppression by glucocorticoids. *Science* 270:283-286.

[47] Crinelli, R., Antonelli, A., Bianchi, M., Gentilini, L., Scaramucci, S., and Magnani, M. 2000. Selective inhibition of NF-kB activation and TNF-alpha production in macrophages by red blood cell-mediated delivery of dexamethasone. *Blood Cells Mol Dis* 26:211-222.

[48] Thiele, K., Bierhaus, A., Autschbach, F., Hofmann, M., Stremmel, W., Thiele, H., Ziegler, R., and Nawroth, P.P. 1999. Cell specific effects of glucocorticoid treatment on the NF-kappaBp65/IkappaBalpha system in patients with Crohn's disease. *Gut* 45:693-704.

[49] De Bosscher, K., Schmitz, M.L., Vanden Berghe, W., Plaisance, S.p., Fiers, W., and Haegeman, G. 1997. Glucocorticoid-mediated repression of nuclear factor-__Bdependent transcription involves direct interference withΓĆētransactivation. *PNAS* 94:13504-13509.

[50] Brostjan, C., Anrather, J., Csizmadia, V., Stroka, D., Soares, M., Bach, F.H., and Winkler, H. 1996. Glucocorticoid-mediated Repression of NF__B Activity in Endothelial Cells Does Not Involve Induction of I__B__ Synthesis. *J.Biol.Chem.* 271:19612-19616.

[51] Heck, S., Bender, K., Kullmann, M., Gottlicher, M., Herrlich, P., and Cato, A.C. 1997. I kappaB alpha-independent downregulation of NF-kappaB activity by glucocorticoid receptor. *EMBO J* 16:4698-4707.

[52] Canalis, E., Mazziotti, G., Giustina, A., and Bilezikian, J.P. 2007. Glucocorticoid-induced osteoporosis: pathophysiology and therapy. *Osteoporos.Int* 18:1319-1328.

[53] Lukert, B.P. and Raisz, L.G. 1994. Glucocorticoid-induced osteoporosis. *Rheum. Dis. Clin. North Am.* 20:629-650.

[54] Sher, L.B., Woitge, H.W., Adams, D.J., Gronowicz, G.A., Krozowski, Z., Harrison, J.R., and Kream, B.E. 2004. Transgenic Expression of 11__-Hydroxysteroid Dehydrogenase Type 2 in Osteoblasts Reveals an Anabolic Role for Endogenous Glucocorticoids in Bone. *Endocrinology* 145:922-929.

[55] Sher, L.B., Harrison, J.R., Adams, D.J., and Kream, B.E. 2006. Impaired cortical bone acquisition and osteoblast differentiation in mice with osteoblast-targeted disruption of glucocorticoid signaling. *Calcif.Tissue Int* 79:118-125.

[56] Yang, M., Trettel, L.B., Adams, D.J., Harrison, J.R., Canalis, E., and Kream, B.E. 2010. Col3.6-HSD2 transgenic mice: A glucocorticoid loss-of-function model spanning early and late osteoblast differentiation. *Bone* 47:573-582.

[57] Bruder, S.P., Jaiswal, N., and Haynesworth, S.E. 1997. Growth kinetics, self-renewal, and the osteogenic potential of purified human mesenchymal stem cells during extensive subcultivation and following cryopreservation. *J.Cell Biochem.* 64:278-294.

[58] Engler, A.J., Sen, S., Sweeney, H.L., and Discher, D.E. 2006. Matrix Elasticity Directs Stem Cell Lineage Specification. *Cell* 126:677-689.

[59] Pittenger, M.F., Mackay, A.M., Beck, S.C., Jaiswal, R.K., Douglas, R., Mosca, J.D., Moorman, M.A., Simonetti, D.W., Craig, S., and Marshak, D.R. 1999. Multilineage Potential of Adult Human Mesenchymal Stem Cells. *Science* 284:143-147.

[60] Prockop, D.J. 1997. Marrow stromal cells as stem cells for nonhematopoietic tissues. *Science* 276:71-74.

[61] Ahdjoudj, S., Lasmoles, F., Oyajobi, B.O., Lomri, A., Delannoy, P., and Marie, P.J. 2001. Reciprocal control of osteoblast/chondroblast and osteoblast/adipocyte differentiation of multipotential clonal human marrow stromal F/STRO-1(+) cells. *J Cell Biochem.* 81:23-38.

[62] Beresford, J.N., Bennett, J.H., Devlin, C., Leboy, P.S., and Owen, M.E. 1992. Evidence for an inverse relationship between the differentiation of adipocytic and osteogenic cells in rat marrow stromal cell cultures. *J.Cell Sci.* 102 (Pt 2]:341-351.

[63] Gori, F., Thomas, T., Hicok, K.C., Spelsberg, T.C., and Riggs, B.L. 1999. Differentiation of human marrow stromal precursor cells: bone morphogenetic protein-2 increases OSF2/CBFA1, enhances osteoblast commitment, and inhibits late adipocyte maturation. *J.Bone Miner.Res.* 14:1522-1535.

[64] Jaiswal, R.K., Jaiswal, N., Bruder, S.P., Mbalaviele, G., Marshak, D.R., and Pittenger, M.F. 2000. Adult human mesenchymal stem cell differentiation to the osteogenic or adipogenic lineage is regulated by mitogen-activated protein kinase. *J.Biol.Chem.* 275:9645-9652.

[65] Barak, Y., Nelson, M.C., Ong, E.S., Jones, Y.Z., Ruiz-Lozano, P., Chien, K.R., Koder, A., and Evans, R.M. 1999. PPAR gamma is required for placental, cardiac, and adipose tissue development. *Mol.Cell* 4:585-595.

[66] Rosen, E.D., Sarraf, P., Troy, A.E., Bradwin, G., Moore, K., Milstone, D.S., Spiegelman, B.M., and Mortensen, R.M. 1999. PPAR gamma is required for the differentiation of adipose tissue in vivo and in vitro. *Mol.Cell* 4:611-617.

[67] Shi, X.M., Blair, H.C., Yang, X., McDonald, J.M., and Cao, X. 2000. Tandem repeat of C/EBP binding sites mediates PPARgamma2 gene transcription in glucocorticoid-induced adipocyte differentiation. *J.Cell Biochem.* 76:518-527.

[68] Wu, Z., Bucher, N.L., and Farmer, S.R. 1996. Induction of peroxisome proliferator-activated receptor gamma during the conversion of 3T3 fibroblasts into adipocytes is mediated by C/EBPbeta, C/EBPdelta, and glucocorticoids. *Mol.Cell.Biol.* 16:4128-4136.

[69] Tang, Q.Q., Zhang, J.W., and Daniel Lane, M. 2004. Sequential gene promoter interactions by C/EBP[beta], C/EBP[alpha], and PPAR[gamma] during adipogenesis. *Biochemical and Biophysical Research Communications* 318:213-218.

[70] Clarke, S.L., Robinson, C.E., and Gimble, J.M. 1997. CAAT/Enhancer Binding Proteins Directly Modulate Transcription from the Peroxisome Proliferator- Activated Receptor [gamma]2 Promoter. *Biochemical and Biophysical Research Communications* 240:99-103.

[71] Weinstein, R.S., Jilka, R.L., Parfitt, A.M., and Manolagas, S.C. 1998. Inhibition of osteoblastogenesis and promotion of apoptosis of osteoblasts and osteocytes by glucocorticoids. Potential mechanisms of their deleterious effects on bone. *J Clin.Invest* 102:274-282.

[72] Yao, W., Cheng, Z., Busse, C., Pham, A., Nakamura, M.C., and Lane, N.E. 2008. Glucocorticoid excess in mice results in early activation of osteoclastogenesis and adipogenesis and prolonged suppression of osteogenesis: A longitudinal study of gene expression in bone tissue from glucocorticoid-treated mice. *Arthritis & Rheumatism* 58:1674-1686.

[73] Akune, T., Ohba, S., Kamekura, S., Yamaguchi, M., Chung, U.I., Kubota, N., Terauchi, Y., Harada, Y., Azuma, Y., Nakamura, K. *et al.* 2004. PPARgamma insufficiency enhances osteogenesis through osteoblast formation from bone marrow progenitors. *J.Clin.Invest* 113:846-855.

[74] Canalis, E. 2005. Mechanisms of glucocorticoid action in bone. *Curr.Osteoporos.Rep.* 3:98-102.

[75] Weinstein, R.S. 2001. Glucocorticoid-induced osteoporosis. *Rev.Endocr.Metab Disord.* 2:65-73.

[76] O'Brien, C.A., Jia, D., Plotkin, L.I., Bellido, T., Powers, C.C., Stewart, S.A., Manolagas, S.C., and Weinstein, R.S. 2004. Glucocorticoids Act Directly on Osteoblasts and Osteocytes to Induce Their Apoptosis and Reduce Bone Formation and Strength. *Endocrinology* 145:1835-1841.

[77] Robling, A.G., Niziolek, P.J., Baldridge, L.A., Condon, K.W., Allen, M.R., Alam, I., Mantila, S.M., Gluhak-Heinrich, J., Bellido, T.M., Harris, S.E. *et al.* 2008. Mechanical Stimulation of Bone in Vivo Reduces Osteocyte Expression of Sost/Sclerostin. *J.Biol.Chem.* 283:5866-5875.

[78] Gluhak-Heinrich, J., Ye, L., Bonewald, L.F., Feng, J.Q., MacDougall, M., Harris, S.E., and Pavlin, D. 2003. Mechanical Loading Stimulates Dentin Matrix Protein 1 (DMP1] Expression in Osteocytes In Vivo. *Journal of Bone and Mineral Research* 18:807-817.

[79] Hirayama, T., Sabokbar, A., and Athanasou, N.A. 2002. Effect of corticosteroids on human osteoclast formation and activity. *J Endocrinol* 175:155-163.

[80] Sivagurunathan, S., Muir, M.M., Brennan, T.C., Seale, J.P., and Mason, R.S. 2005. Influence of Glucocorticoids on Human Osteoclast Generation and Activity. *Journal of Bone and Mineral Research* 20:390-398.

[81] Jia, D., O'Brien, C.A., Stewart, S.A., Manolagas, S.C., and Weinstein, R.S. 2006. Glucocorticoids Act Directly on Osteoclasts to Increase Their Life Span and Reduce Bone Density. *Endocrinology* 147:5592-5599.

[82] Kim, H.J., Zhao, H., Kitaura, H., Bhattacharyya, S., Brewer, J.A., Muglia, L.J., Ross, F.P., and Teitelbaum, S.L. 2006. Glucocorticoids suppress bone formation via the osteoclast. *J Clin Invest* 116:2152-2160.

[83] S_Ėe, K. and Delaiss_®, J.M. 2010. Glucocorticoids maintain human osteoclasts in the active mode of their resorption cycle. *Journal of Bone and Mineral Research* 25:2184-2192.

[84] D'Adamio, F., Zollo, O., Moraca, R., Ayroldi, E., Bruscoli, S., Bartoli, A., Cannarile, L., Migliorati, G., and Riccardi, C. 1997. A new dexamethasone-induced gene of the leucine zipper family protects T lymphocytes from TCR/CD3-activated cell death. *Immunity.* 7:803-812.

[85] Cannarile, L., Zollo, O., D'Adamio, F., Ayroldi, E., Marchetti, C., Tabilio, A., Bruscoli, S., and Riccardi, C. 2001. Cloning, chromosomal assignment and tissue distribution of human GILZ, a glucocorticoid hormone-induced gene. *Cell Death.Differ.* 8:201-203.

[86] Ayroldi, E., Zollo, O., Macchiarulo, A., Di Marco, B., Marchetti, C., and Riccardi, C. 2002. Glucocorticoid-induced leucine zipper inhibits the Raf-extracellular signal-regulated kinase pathway by binding to Raf-1. *Mol.Cell Biol.* 22:7929-7941.

[87] Shibanuma, M., Kuroki, T., and Nose, K. 1992. Isolation of a gene encoding a putative leucine zipper structure that is induced by transforming growth factor beta 1 and other growth factors. *J.Biol.Chem.* 267:10219-10224.

[88] Newton, R., Hart, L.A., Stevens, D.A., Bergmann, M., Donnelly, L.E., Adcock, I.M., and Barnes, P.J. 1998. Effect of dexamethasone on interleukin-1beta-(IL-1beta)-induced nuclear factor-kappaB (NF-kappaB) and kappaB-dependent transcription in epithelial cells. *Eur J Biochem* 254:81-89.

[89] Eddleston, J., Herschbach, J., Wagelie-Steffen, A.L., Christiansen, S.C., and Zuraw, B.L. 2007. The anti-inflammatory effect of glucocorticoids is mediated by glucocorticoid-induced leucine zipper in epithelial cells. *J Allergy Clin Immunol* 119:115-122.

[90] Delfino, D.V., Agostini, M., Spinicelli, S., Vito, P., and Riccardi, C. 2004. Decrease of Bcl-xL and augmentation of thymocyte apoptosis in GILZ overexpressing transgenic mice. *Blood.*

[91] Ayroldi, E., Migliorati, G., Bruscoli, S., Marchetti, C., Zollo, O., Cannarile, L., D'Adamio, F., and Riccardi, C. 2001. Modulation of T-cell activation by the glucocorticoid-induced leucine zipper factor via inhibition of nuclear factor kappaB. *Blood* 98:743-753.

[92] Mittelstadt, P.R. and Ashwell, J.D. 2001. Inhibition of AP-1 by the glucocorticoid-inducible protein GILZ. *J.Biol.Chem.* 276:29603-29610.

[93] Ayroldi, E., Zollo, O., Bastianelli, A., Marchetti, C., Agostini, M., Di Virgilio, R., and Riccardi, C. 2007. GILZ mediates the antiproliferative activity of glucocorticoids by negative regulation of Ras signaling. *J Clin Invest* 117:1605-1615.

[94] Berrebi, D., Bruscoli, S., Cohen, N., Foussat, A., Migliorati, G., Bouchet-Delbos, L., Maillot, M.C., Portier, A., Couderc, J., Galanaud, P. *et al.* 2003. Synthesis of glucocorticoid-induced leucine zipper (GILZ) by macrophages: an anti-inflammatory and immunosuppressive mechanism shared by glucocorticoids and IL-10. *Blood* 101:729-738.

[95] Yang, N., Zhang, W., and Shi, X.M. 2007. Glucocorticoid-induced leucine zipper (GILZ) mediates glucocorticoid action and inhibits inflammatory cytokine-induced COX-2 expression. *J Cell Biochem* 103:1760-1771.

[96] Arthaningtyas, E., Kok, C.C., Mordvinov, V.A., and Sanderson, C.J. 2005. The conserved lymphokine element 0 is a powerful activator and target for corticosteroid inhibition in human interleukin-5 transcription. *Growth Factors* 23:211-221.

[97] Cohen, N., Mouly, E., Hamdi, H., Maillot, M.C., Pallardy, M., Godot, V., Capel, F., Balian, A., Naveau, S., Galanaud, P. *et al.* 2005. GILZ expression in human dendritic cells redirects their maturation and prevents antigen-specific T lymphocyte response. *Blood*2005-2007.

[98] Ayroldi, E. and Riccardi, C. 2009. Glucocorticoid-induced leucine zipper (GILZ): a new important mediator of glucocorticoid action. *FASEB J.* 23:1-10.

[99] Asselin-Labat, M.L., Biola-Vidamment, A., Kerbrat, S., Lombes, M., Bertoglio, J., and Pallardy, M. 2005. FoxO3 Mediates Antagonistic Effects of Glucocorticoids and Interleukin-2 on Glucocorticoid-Induced Leucine Zipper Expression. *Mol Endocrinol* 19:1752-1764.

[100] Zhang, W., Yang, N., and Shi, X.M. 2008. Regulation of Mesenchymal Stem Cell Osteogenic Differentiation by Glucocorticoid-induced Leucine Zipper (GILZ). *J.Biol.Chem.* 283:4723-4729.

[101] He, L., Yang, N., Isales, C.M., and Shi, X.M. 2012. Glucocorticoid-Induced Leucine Zipper (GILZ) Antagonizes TNF-__ Inhibition of Mesenchymal Stem Cell Osteogenic Differentiation. *PLoS ONE* 7:e31717.

[102] Nakashima, K., Zhou, X., Kunkel, G., Zhang, Z.P., Deng, J.M., Behringer, R.R., and de Crombrugghe, B. 2002. The novel zinc finger-containing transcription factor Osterix is required for osteoblast differentiation and bone formation. *Cell* 108:17-29.

[103] Lu, X., Gilbert, L., He, X., Rubin, J., and Nanes, M.S. 2006. Transcriptional Regulation of the Osterix (Osx, Sp7] Promoter by Tumor Necrosis Factor Identifies Disparate Effects of Mitogen-activated Protein Kinase and NF+¦B Pathways. *J.Biol.Chem.* 281:6297-6306.

[104] Gilbert, L., He, X., Farmer, P., Rubin, J., Drissi, H., van Wijnen, A.J., Lian, J.B., Stein, G.S., and Nanes, M.S. 2002. Expression of the Osteoblast Differentiation Factor RUNX2 (Cbfa1/AML3/Pebp2alpha A) Is Inhibited by Tumor Necrosis Factor-alpha. *J.Biol.Chem.* 277:2695-2701.

[105] Kaneki, H., Guo, R., Chen, D., Yao, Z., Schwarz, E.M., Zhang, Y.E., Boyce, B.F., and Xing, L. 2006. Tumor Necrosis Factor Promotes Runx2 Degradation through Up-regulation of Smurf1 and Smurf2 in Osteoblasts. *J.Biol.Chem.* 281:4326-4333.

[106] Zhao, M., Qiao, M., Oyajobi, B.O., Mundy, G.R., and Chen, D. 2003. E3 ubiquitin ligase Smurf1 mediates core-binding factor alpha1/Runx2 degradation and plays a specific role in osteoblast differentiation. *J.Biol.Chem.* 278:27939-27944.

[107] Rauch, A., Seitz, S., Baschant, U., Schilling, A.F., Illing, A., Stride, B., Kirilov, M., Mandic, V., Takacz, A., Schmidt-Ullrich, R. *et al.* 2010. Glucocorticoids Suppress Bone Formation by Attenuating Osteoblast Differentiation via the Monomeric Glucocorticoid Receptor. *Cell Metabolism* 11:517-531.

[108] Yao, W., Cheng, Z., Busse, C., Pham, A., Nakamura, M.C., and Lane, N.E. 2008. Glucocorticoid excess in mice results in early activation of osteoclastogenesis and adipogenesis and prolonged suppression of osteogenesis: A longitudinal study of gene expression in bone tissue from glucocorticoid-treated mice. *Arthritis & Rheumatism* 58:1674-1686.

[109] Kassel, O., Sancono, A., Kratzschmar, J., Kreft, B., Stassen, M., and Cato, A.C.B. 2001. Glucocorticoids inhibit MAP kinase via increased expression and decreased degradation of MKP-1. *EMBO J* 20:7108-7116.

[110] Suzuki, A., Guicheux, J., Palmer, G., Miura, Y., Oiso, Y., Bonjour, J.P., and Caverzasio, J. 2002. Evidence for a role of p38 MAP kinase in expression of alkaline phosphatase during osteoblastic cell differentiation. *Bone* 30:91-98.

[111] Park, O.J., Kim, H.J., Woo, K.M., Baek, J.H., and Ryoo, H.M. 2010. FGF2-activated ERK Mitogen-activated Protein Kinase Enhances Runx2 Acetylation and Stabilization. *J.Biol.Chem.* 285:3568-3574.

[112] Song, C.Z., Tian, X., and Gelehrter, T.D. 1999. Glucocorticoid receptor inhibits transforming growth factor-beta signaling by directly targeting the transcriptional activation function of Smad3. *Proc Natl Acad Sci U.S.A* 96:11776-11781.

[113] Iu, M.F., Kaji, H., Sowa, H., Naito, J., Sugimoto, T., and Chihara, K. 2005. Dexamethasone suppresses Smad3 pathway in osteoblastic cells. *J Endocrinol* 185:131-138.

[114] Periyasamy, S. and Sβnchez, E.R. 2002. Antagonism of glucocorticoid receptor transactivity and cell growth inhibition by transforming growth factor-[beta] through AP-1-mediated transcriptional repression. *The International Journal of Biochemistry & Cell Biology* 34:1571-1585.

[115] Song, C.Z., Tian, X., and Gelehrter, T.D. 1999. Glucocorticoid receptor inhibits transforming growth factor-beta signaling by directly targeting the transcriptional activation function of Smad3. *Proc Natl Acad Sci U.S.A* 96:11776-11781.

[116] Locklin, R.M., Oreffo, R.O.C., and Triffitt, J.T. 1999. Effects of TGF[beta] and BFGF on the differentiation of human bone marrow stromal fibroblasts. *Cell Biology International* 23:185-194.

[117] Alliston, T., Choy, L., Ducy, P., Karsenty, G., and Derynck, R. 2001. TGF-[beta]-induced repression of CBFA1 by Smad3 decreases cbfa1 and osteocalcin expression and inhibits osteoblast differentiation. *EMBO J* 20:2254-2272.

[118] Kassem, Kveiborg, and Eriksen. 2000. Production and action of transforming growth factor-__ in human osteoblast cultures: dependence on cell differentiation and modulation by calcitriol. *European Journal of Clinical Investigation* 30:429-437.

[119] Edwards, J.R., Nyman, J.S., Lwin, S.T., Moore, M.M., Esparza, J., O'Quinn, E.C., Hart, A.J., Biswas, S., Patil, C.A., Lonning, S. *et al.* 2010. Inhibition of TGF-beta signaling by 1D11 antibody treatment increases bone mass and quality in vivo. *jbmr*n-a.

[120] Tang, Y., Wu, X., Lei, W., Pang, L., Wan, C., Shi, Z., Zhao, L., Nagy, T.R., Peng, X., Hu, J. *et al.* 2009. TGF-beta1-induced migration of bone mesenchymal stem cells couples bone resorption with formation. *Nat.Med.* 15:757-765.

[121] Bouvard, B., Audran, M., Legrand, E., and Chappard, D. 2009. Ultrastructural characteristics of glucocorticoid-induced osteoporosis. *Osteoporosis International* 20:1089-1092.

[122] Berris, K.K., Repp, A.L., and Kleerekoper, M. 2007. Glucocorticoid-induced osteoporosis. *Current Opinion in Endocrinology, Diabetes and Obesity* 14.

[123] L_Ėv_źs, K., Gjesdal, C.G., Christensen, M., Wolff, A.B., Alm_źs, B.Ė., Svartberg, J., Fougner, K.J., Syversen, U., Bollerslev, J., Falch, J.A. *et al.* 2009. Glucocorticoid replacement therapy and pharmacogenetics in Addison's disease: effects on bone. *Eur J Endocrinol* 160:993-1002.

[124] Grossman, J.M., Gordon, R., Ranganath, V.K., Deal, C., Caplan, L., Chen, W., Curtis, J.R., Furst, D.E., McMahon, M., Patkar, N.M. *et al.* 2010. American College of Rheumatology 2010 recommendations for the prevention and treatment of glucocorticoid-induced osteoporosis. *Arthritis Care Res* 62:1515-1526.

[125] van Staa, T. 2006. The Pathogenesis, Epidemiology and Management of Glucocorticoid-Induced Osteoporosis. *Calcified Tissue International* 79:129-137.

[126] Weinstein, R.S. 2010. Glucocorticoids, osteocytes, and skeletal fragility: The role of bone vascularity. *Bone* 46:564-570.

[127] Angeli, A., Guglielmi, G., Dovio, A., Capelli, G., de Feo, D., Giannini, S., Giorgino, R., Moro, L., and Giustina, A. 2006. High prevalence of asymptomatic vertebral fractures in post-menopausal women receiving chronic glucocorticoid therapy: A cross-sectional outpatient study. *Bone* 39:253-259.

[128] Leib, E.S., Saag, K.G., Adachi, J.D., Geusens, P.P., Binkley, N., McCloskey, E.V., and Hans, D.B. 2011. Official Positions for FRAX_« Clinical Regarding Glucocorticoids: The Impact of the Use of Glucocorticoids on the Estimate by FRAX_« of the 10 Year Risk of Fracture: From Joint Official Positions Development Conference of the International Society for Clinical Densitometry and International Osteoporosis Foundation on FRAX_«. *Journal of Clinical Densitometry* 14:212-219.

[129] Teitelbaum, S.L., Seton, M.P., and Saag, K.G. 2011. Should bisphosphonates be used for long-term treatment of glucocorticoid-induced osteoporosis? *Arthritis & Rheumatism* 63:325-328.

[130] Saag, K.G., Shane, E., Boonen, S., Mar_Łn, F., Donley, D.W., Taylor, K.A., Dalsky, G.P., and Marcus, R. 2007. Teriparatide or Alendronate in Glucocorticoid-Induced Osteoporosis. *New England Journal of Medicine* 357:2028-2039.

[131] Sambrook, P.N. 2007. Anabolic Therapy in Glucocorticoid-Induced Osteoporosis. *New England Journal of Medicine* 357:2084-2086.

Chapter 4

Extra-Adrenal Glucocorticoid Synthesis in Mucosal Tissues and Its Implication in Mucosal Immune Homeostasis and Tumor Development

Feodora I. Kostadinova, Nina Hostettler,
Pamela Bianchi and Thomas Brunner

Additional information is available at the end of the chapter

http://dx.doi.org/10.5772/52788

1. Introduction

While glucocorticoids (GC) exert broad effects on metabolism, behavior and immunity, local production of even small amounts of GC, which may act in a paracrine or even autocrine manner, enable a specific site of the body to regulate their exposure to GC according to their specific needs. Mucosal tissues, for example, are at the borderline to the outside world, and are therefore in constant contact with either harmless foreign particles or potentially pathogenic microorganisms, which might provoke devastating inflammatory disorders due to chronic stimulation of the mucosal immune system. Increasing the local concentration of immunoregulatory GC by extra-adrenal de novo GC synthesis or local reactivation of inactive serum metabolites provides a protective mechanism to either restore homeostasis after clearance of infection or to regulate the critical balance between immunity and tolerance.

2. Adrenal versus extra-adrenal GC synthesis

Production of GC in the adrenal glands is regulated by hypothalamic-pituitary-adrenal (HPA) axis and follows under normal conditions the circadian rhythm. However, GC are also a major humoral response to various types of stress. [1]. Immunological stress by excessive activation of immune cells rapidly results in elevated plasma levels of tumor necrosis factor alpha (TNFα), interleukin (IL) -1 and IL-6, which then stimulate the HPA axis and lead to an increase of systemic GC [2]. These and similar signals stimulate also the local GC synthesis in mucosal tissues, as will be discussed later (Table 1).

Local GC synthesis	Cellular source	Special features	Described functions	References
Thymus	Epithelial cells in cortex	Mutual antagonism	Thymic selection	[3-7]
Skin Hair follicle	Keratinocytes, melanocytes, fibroblasts etc.	Autonomous HPA-axis	Integrity and growth; response to stress factors	[8-19]
Cardiovascular system	Vessel walls, Heart	Together with mineralocorticoids	Vascular contractility and remodeling	[20-29]
Central Nervous system	Neurons, glia	Various neurosteroids	Sensitizing GABA and other receptors; feed-back on HPA-axis; cognitive functions	[30-45]
Intestine	Crypt cells	Regulation via LRH-1	Immune regulation	[46-53]
Lung	unknown	Reactivation by 11β-HSD	Immune regulation	[54]
Colon carcinoma	Tumor cells	Regulation via LRH-1	Immunosuppression	[55]

Table 1. Extra-adrenal GC sources and their functions.

Because most data published so far on local GC synthesis has been generated in animal models a brief overview of steroidogenic processes in rodents compared to humans must be made (Figure 1). A major difference is the implication of the enzyme 17α-hydroxylase in the GC synthesis in humans, but not in rodents. Pregnenolone is transformed directly into progesterone in most rodents, and in other mammalians and humans it is first hydroxylated and then metabolized into 17-OH-progesterone [56]. 11β-hydroxylase (P450C11) is an enzyme expressed in the zonae fasciculata et reticularis and is a product of the gene CYP11B1. Thus, in rodents this enzyme uses 11-deoxycorticosterone as a substrate and turns it into corticosterone, which is the active GC in these species. In humans 11β-hydroxylase metabolizes mainly 11-deoxycortisol into cortisol and to a lesser degree 11-deoxycorticosterone into corticosterone. Hence, cortisol is the major active GC in the human. 11-Deoxyorticosterone and corticosterone are important metabolites in both species, which can be hydroxylised and oxidised in the zona glomerulosa of the adrenals, subsequently leading to the mineralcorticosteroid aldosterone [57].

It is well established that the adrenal glands are the major source of systemic GC. Surgical removal of the adrenal glands results in a rapid drop of serum GC levels, which after a couple of days become undetectable, illustrating that the adrenals are primarily responsible for the GC levels detected in the circulation [46, 58]. However, in recent years there has been accumulating evidence that several other tissues are capable of producing GC and thereby regulate local processes in an adrenal-independent manner [7, 59].

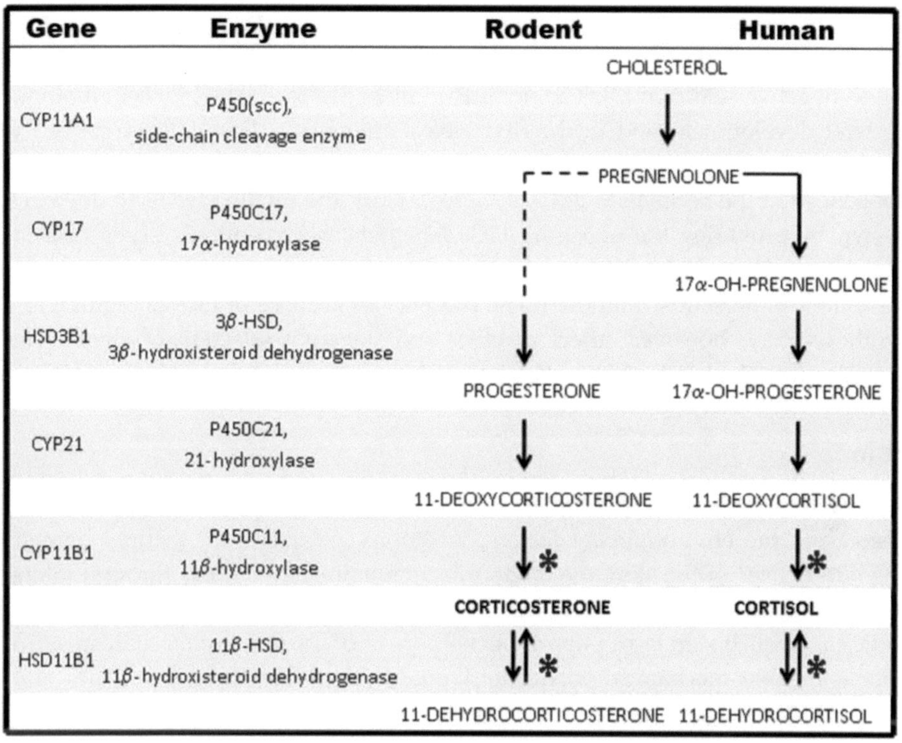

Legend: ▫ enzymes; □ metabolites: → metabolic pathway; - - - absent in rodents; * inhibitory effect of metyrapone.

Figure 1. Differences in the GC synthesis pathway in rodents and humans.

3. Extra-adrenal sources of GC synthesis

3.1. Thymus

The Thymus plays a central role in the development of the immune system. Thymocyte development and differentiation is shaped and regulated by the interaction with the thymic epithelial cells and the factors secreted by them [60, 61].

Initial characterizations of extra-adrenal GC synthesis started in the thymus. In the mid to late 90ties of the last century it was described that the non-immune cells in the thymic cortex are capable of producing various steroid metabolites. Accordingly, the expression of various enzymes of the corticosteroid synthesis pathway has been demonstrated in thymic epithelial cells [3-5]. While the function of thymic GC has been a matter of scientific debate for some time [62, 63], particularly the work of Ashwell and co-workers illustrated that GC production in the thymus has an important role in the regulation of thymocyte development and selection. Interestingly, while thymocytes are exquisitely sensitive to GC and rapidly die by apoptosis, the in situ produced corticosterone seems to oppose the signals induced by the T cell receptor and thereby lower T cell receptor-induced apoptosis (negative selection). On the other hand T cell receptor activation also inhibits the apoptosis-inducing activity of GC in thymocytes [64]. Thus, the "mutual antagonism" between T cell receptor and glucocorticoid receptor (GR) signaling seems overall to enhance survival and thereby positive selection of thymocytes by increasing the threshold of T cell receptor signals leading to negative selection [3]. The thymus in mice produces the highest amounts of GC during fetal development and in the first weeks after birth. This is the time of the most extensive lymphocyte development and differentiation, and it occurs at a time when the steroidogenesis in the adrenals is not fully active. Thus, the thymus seems to depend largely on its own by providing the necessary GC. Whether thymic epithelial cells constitutively produce GC or whether this is dependent on the interaction with activated thymocytes or soluble factors, is presently unknown. The presence or absence of factors regulating thymic GC synthesis may, however, affect positive and negative selection of thymocytes, and thereby also affect the levels of potentially autoreactive T cells in the periphery. [6, 7].

3.2. Skin

The skin is an organ with a complex structure and its purpose is to protect the inner organism from the environmental factors, infections, dehydration, thermal deregulations etc. The outer cover of the skin, the epidermis, maintains its integrity through intense self-renewing by the proliferating keratinocytes in the basal layer and the dividing cells in the hair follicles. As such skin is an important component of the defense mechanisms providing not only a reliable mechanical barrier and producing antimicrobial enzymes and other substances, but also being populated with many specialized immune cells, e.g. dendritic cells (Langerhans cells) within the epidermis, as well as resident macrophages, dendritic cells and lymphocytes in the derma [65]. The skin also displays active metabolic and endocrine functions. Along with the synthesis of vitamin D, the skin was shown to produce various hormones and regulatory factors, like parathyroid-related protein, melanocyte-stimulating hormone (MSH), β-endorphin peptides, urocortin, neurotransmitters and others (for review [10, 11]). With regard of this chapter's topic of interest is the ability of the skin to produce all components of the HPA axis. A great contribution to the understanding of GC metabolism and regulation in the skin has been made by the extensive research of Slominski and co-workers [10]. In human keratinocytes and cells of the hair follicles expression of corticotropin-releasing factor (CRF) has been demonstrated at the mRNA and protein level, whereas in mice the local synthesis of CRF has not been proven yet. The observed local increased concentration of CRF in the skin could be possibly explained by its release from neuronal cells and its active transport into the skin along the local nerve endings [12, 15]. Many cell types found in the skin, e.g. keratinocytes [66], melanocytes [13], dermal fibroblasts [67], immune cells and endothelial cells in the derma, as well as hair follicles [16] and skin tissue cultures, are able to respond to CRF stimulation and to produce proopiomelanocortin, which can be further processed into adrenocorticotropic hormone (ACTH), MSH and β -endorphin. Moreover, GC-synthesizing enzymes and active GC have been demonstrated in human and rodent skin. Metabolic assays demonstrated that ex vivo cultured normal rat skin could transform progesterone into deoxycorticosterone and corticosterone, and further to 11-dehydrocorticosterone [9]. Human skin has been demonstrated to respond to ACTH, to express various steroidogenic enzymes, and to be capable of synthesizing cortisol [8, 18]. Local steroidogenesis was demonstrated in human keratinocytes [19], sebaceous cells [18], fibroblasts [14], and melanocytes [13]. Hair follicles, also known as pilosebaceus units, appear to function as fully autonomous peripheral equivalents of the HPA axis. The CRF/ACTH-induced cortisol production appears to provide also a negative feedback on the local CRF synthesis and thereby terminate local steroidogenesis [15]. It has been suggested that this local HPA axis is implemented in the regulation of hair growth, pigmentation and modulation of local immune response [17]. Components of the HPA axis, mainly CRF, are proposed to affect the epithelial cell proliferation, apoptosis and differentiation [15]. Recent findings describe the role of local cortisol synthesis in a model of tissue injury. Up-regulation of CYP11B1 and subsequent enhanced production of cortisol was induced by the proinflammatory cytokine IL-1β and depressed by insulin-like growth factor 1 (IGF-1) [19]. In the same study elevation of cortisol synthesis was observed approximately 48 hours after acute injury and maintained the proper wound healing.

In conclusion, the skin possesses an autonomous HPA axis, regulating the normal integrity and growth, and is able to respond to stress factors. At the same time the GC-synthesizing machinery of the skin can be stimulated by inflammatory mediators in order to provide an adequate local self-limitation of immune responses.

3.3. Central nervous system

The term neurosteroids was defined after the discovery that various steroid metabolites can be detected in the brain of simultaneously adrenalectomized and gonadectomized rats [30]. Among the locally synthesized and active steroids are pregnenolone and pregnenolone sulphate, progesterone, allopregnanolone, dehydroepiandrosterone and dehydroepiandrosterone sulphate. These steroids can exert their effects in neurogenesis, development, myelinization, memory, reactions to stress through engaging nuclear receptors and modulating transcription, as well as affecting neurotransmission by modifying the activity of gamma-aminobutiric acid ($GABA_A$), N-methyl-D-aspartic acid (NMDA), and sigma receptors (for review [31, 32, 68]). Low levels of transcripts for CYP11A1, CYP11B1 and the other enzymes of corticosterone synthesis were detected in normal rat brain, in cerebral cortex and cerebellum [33], and 11β-hydroxylase protein expression was later demonstrated in the Purkinje cells and other cells of the hippocampus [35]. In vitro conversion of precursors into corticosterone has also been demonstrated in rat fetal hippocampal neurons [34]. The extremely low levels of CYP21 transcripts and enzyme (deoxycorticosterone synthetase, P450C21) detected [36] gave raise to many doubts whether complete GC synthesis can be sustained in the brain. Nevertheless, the activity of brain tissue to convert progesterone to 11-deoxycorticosterone (resp. 17α-OH-progesterone to 11-deoxycortisol) pointed out that steroid metabolism in the brain exists. Recently, the expression of isoforms of CYP2D4 and CYP2D6 in rat and human brains, respectively, as well as demonstration of their 21-hydroxylation activity confirmed the capacity of rodent and human brain to produce GC locally [37, 69], though suggesting a slightly different enzymatic pathway compared to that of the adrenals. Nonetheless, CRF and ACTH, likely released by the hypothalamus, resp. pituitary gland, seem to regulate GC synthesis in the brain in a similar manner as in the adrenals. Interestingly, adrenalectomy even increases the expression of CYP11B1 in the rat brain [70].

Peripheral reactivation of 11-dehydrocorticosterone to corticosterone, resp. cortisone to cortisol via 11β-hydroxysteroid dehydrogenase type 1 (11β-HSD1) activity contributes considerably not only to the local concentrations and effects of GC, but also to the plasma level of GC, as shown by an almost 30% increase in corticosterone levels in the portal vein compared to the incoming arterial circulation [38, 39, 71]. In the brain 11β-HSD1 expression was found in various areas. Local levels of corticosterone in the cerebral cortex, hippocampus, hypothalamus and pituitary gland modulate the activity of the HPA axis. This effect is particularly apparent in 11β-HSD1 knockout mice. The lack of 11β-HSD1 activity in the brain of these mice leads to considerably reduced local levels of corticosterone. Hence, the HPA axis is hyperactivated and higher amounts of ACTH are produced, which in turn causes adrenal hypertrophy. Normal or even elevated systemic GC fail to transmit proper feedback responses to the hypothalamus [40-42]. Other curious effects of the local levels of GC attributed to the activity of 11β-HSD1 in the hippocampus are cognitive disorders during aging. Experiments in 11β-HSD1-deficient mice showed that these animals are protected from the decline of the learning abilities [43, 72]. 11β-HSD1 is expressed in the human prefrontal cortex, cerebellum and hippocampus, and its expression, as well as local GC levels, has also been correlated to the cognitive decline in elderly patients [44, 45], [42]. Furthermore, some clinical studies showed an improvement in verbal fluency and memory in patients treated with the specific 11β-HSD1 inhibitor carbenoxolone [44].

3.4. Cardiovascular system

The impact of mineralocorticoids and glucocorticoids on the heart and blood vessels is well known and described. Yet, the capacity of these structures to sustain their own supplies is not understood in detail. Data obtained mainly in rats indicate that vascular tissue expresses steroidogenic factors, such as StAR, CYP11A1, CYP11B1 and CYP11B2 [20, 21, 73]. Ex vivo cultured rat blood vessels were able to produce corticosterone and aldosterone [23, 73]. Expression of various steroidogenic enzymes has been shown also in the human heart and blood vessels [26, 27]. However, CYP11B1 and CYP11B2 expression was only demonstrated in patients with myocardial infarction and heart failure [28], but barely under steady state conditions or in cultured endothelial cells [29], suggesting that local GC synthesis may be triggered during pathological conditions. Presence of CYP11B2 (aldosterone synthetase) and the fact that steroidogenesis in the cardiovascular system is triggered by the angiotensin signaling system [24] points out that local steroidogensis in the vascular systems is connected to the renin-angiotensin-aldosterone regulatory mechanisms [25]. Local reactivation of 11-dehydrocorticosterone was also observed in the smooth muscle cells in arteries, where it may contribute to vascular contractility and remodeling [74], [75]. Despite a clear demonstration of steroidogenesis in the vasculature detailed studies on the anti-inflammatory role of local GC synthesis in blood vessels are still missing.

In addition to the different tissues described above local GC synthesis was also reported in the placenta [76], the ovaries [77], the testis [78], the uterus [79], and the mammary gland [80].

4. GC synthesis in mucosal tissues

Mucosal surfaces in the gastrointestinal, respiratory and urinal tract represent important contact zones between the body and the outside world. They exert important functions in the exchange of nutrients, gases and other substances between the organism and the surrounding world. They comprise an enormous interactive surface and are thereby also constantly exposed to various antigens and microorganisms. Though, most of them are harmless, and thus the body has developed mechanisms to tolerate these harmless antigens. Yet, dangerous infections of the lung and the intestine occur, in which case the local defense machinery must be engaged to protect the host from invasion. The barrier between inside and outside is primarily formed of a simple one-layered epithelium with the respective specialized functions. Beneath the epithelial layer in the lamina propria of the intestine or in the interstitium of the lung resides a large number of immune cells. Clearly the huge mucosal surface must be protected from invading pathogens, and thus these epithelial tissues are home of the largest immune system in our body. Inappropriate activation of these local immune cells by environmental antigens, though, can result in uncontrolled inflammation and associated tissue destruction. Several lines of evidence discussed in detail below indicate that locally produced GC significantly contribute to the regulation of local immune responses and the maintenance of immune homeostasis in these epithelial tissues.

4.1. GC synthesis in the intestinal epithelium

In the intestinal mucosa two super-systems collide. The intestinal lumen hosts ten times more bacteria than cells in our body are found. At the same time, the intestinal epithelium and lamina propria are also home of the largest number of B and T cells, and are also densely populated by macrophages and dendritic cells. Accidental and uncontrolled activation of these cells and/or other infiltrating immune cells by harmless commensal bacteria or food antigens is the underlying cause of a variety of inflammatory disorders, such as inflammatory bowel disease and food allergies [81]

There is accumulating evidence that local production of immunoregulatory GC significantly contributes to the control of intestinal immune homeostasis and prevents a clash between immune cells and commensal bacteria. The notion that the intestinal mucosa could be a steroidogenic organ has been already suggested some time ago, when it was found that genetic deletion of the nuclear receptor SF-1 (steroidogenic factor-1, NR5a1), largely responsible for the transcriptional control of the adrenal development and GC synthesis, could not abrogate intestinal CYP11A1 expression in the mouse embryonic gut [82]. At the same time remaining GC levels were observed in the circulation of prenatal mice, indicating that an extra-adrenal source of GC synthesis must exist [83]. Our own research started to explicitly investigate the possibility that the intestinal mucosa is an important source of immunoregulatory GC some ten years ago. Investigating the function of so-called intraepithelial lymphocytes, T cells that reside within the intestinal epithelial layer, it was found that these cells rapidly died upon isolation and ex vivo culture, but could be partially rescued when the GR was blocked by the receptor antagonist RU-486 [84]. This observation suggested that these intestinal T cells were constantly exposed to GC, and that removal of survival signals, e.g. by detachment from the epithelial layer, would promote GR-dependent apoptosis.

Subsequent studies revealed that the intestinal mucosa is home of a complex steroidogenic system, likely adapted to cope with the specialized environment of the gut. Many of the steroidogenic enzymes required for the synthesis of corticosterone from cholesterol or the reactivation of corticosterone from dehydrocorticosterone are constitutively expressed in the intestinal epithelium, whereas other enzymes become strongly induced upon immunological stress [46, 52, 53]. The ability of the intestinal tissue to synthesize corticosterone in mice [46] and humans [55] indicates that the intestinal mucosa expresses the complete and functional enzymatic machinery. This steroidogenic capacity is further confirmed by the use of metyrapone, a potent 11β-hydroxylase inhibitor with some inhibitory effects also on P450scc and 11β-HSD1, which efficiently blocks ex vivo GC synthesis in intestinal organ cultures [46, 55], confirming that GC measured were produced locally in the tissue.

While in most experiments and ex vivo organ cultures basal GC levels are detected, a significant induction is usually observed, when mice are stressed by immune cell-activating agents. Administration of T cell-activating anti-CD3ε antibody, macrophage-activating lipopolysaccharides, or TNFα, infection of mice with viruses or chemically induced intestinal inflammation promotes the expression of certain steroidogenic enzymes, e.g. CYP11A1 and CYP11B1, and strongly stimulates the synthesis of intestinal GC. In some of these in vivo experiments a role of intestinal GC synthesis in the control of intestinal immune cells could also be confirmed. Most pronounced are the effects reported on viral infection and experimental colitis. Infection of mice with the lymphocytic choriomeningitis virus (LCMV) leads to a rapid expansion of the virus, which infects various target organs, including the intestine [46, 85, 86]. The virus promotes a massive expansion of virus-specific cytotoxic T cells, which in turn control the viral expansion by killing virus-infected cells. Employing this experimental system it has been shown that intestinal T cells from mice with deregulated intestinal GC synthesis (using the pharmacological inhibitor of GC synthesis metyrapone) became more profoundly activated by the virus, and expressed activation markers and inflammatory cytokines at much higher levels [46]. Similarly, in experimental models of colitis defective intestinal GC synthesis resulted in a more rapid and more pronounced induction of intestinal inflammation, as monitored by immune cell infiltration, epithelial layer damage, weight loss, etc. [49, 53].

4.2. Regulation of intestinal GC synthesis

The regulation of adrenal GC synthesis has been well documented over many decades of research (reviewed in [87]). The connection between physical, emotional and immunological stress, and the activation of the HPA axis has been well established. Similarly, the role of the hormone ACTH in stimulating adrenal GC synthesis, and the nuclear receptor SF-1 in the transcriptional control of adrenal steroidogenesis is widely accepted [88]. In agreement with this critical role of SF-1 in the induction of steroidogenic enzymes in the adrenal glands is the observation that mice deficient for SF-1 have no detectable corticosterone in the serum. In fact, SF-1-deficient mice even lack adrenal glands, as SF-1 is also required for the embryonic development of the adrenal glands. As discussed above, mice lacking SF-1 expression still express the steroidogenic enzyme gene CYP11A1 in the primitive gut of embryonic mice, supporting the notion that in the intestine steroidogensis is differentially controlled. Along these lines, it was found that SF-1 expression is basically absent in the intestine, but functionally replaced by its close homolog LRH-1 (liver receptor homolog-1, NR5a2). LRH-1 has strong sequence homology with SF-1, and regulates gene expression by binding to identical transcription factor response elements in the promoter of their target genes [47]. In general, SF-1 and LRH-1 have a mutually exclusive expression pattern, with very low LRH-1 expression in the adrenals, but very high expression in epithelial cells from the liver, pancreas, intestine and ovaries [89].

The role of LRH-1 in the regulation of extra-adrenal GC synthesis in the intestine has been investigated in intestinal epithelial cell lines in vitro as well as in vivo models [47, 49]. Overexpression of LRH-1 in intestinal epithelial cells induces the expression of the steroidogenic enzymes CYP11A1 and CYP11B1, and mutation of corresponding response elements in their promoter abrogates their LRH-1- and SF-1-induced activation [47]. Similarly, inhibition of LRH-1 expression or function leads to reduced expression of these steroidogenic enzymes in intestinal epithelial cells. Overexpression of LRH-1 in turn directly promotes detectable levels of corticosterone in the supernatant of intestinal epithelial cell cultures. In vivo the role of LRH-1 has been investigated by the use of LRH-1 haplodeficient as well as conditional LRH-1 knockout mice [48, 49]. LRH-1 haplodeficient mice showed a largely reduced induction of steroidogenic enzymes after anti-CD3ε injection and a complete block in intestinal GC synthesis induction, confirming an important role of LRH-1 in the regulation of intestinal GC synthesis. While induction of DSS (dextran sodium sulfate)- or TNBS (trinitrobenzen sulfonic acid)-mediated colitis stimulates the expression of steroidogenic enzmymes and a transient intestinal GC synthesis [51], deletion of LRH-1 in intestinal epithelial cells largely abrogates intestinal steroidogenesis [49]. More importantly, absence of LRH-1 and associated intestinal GC synthesis also leads to a more pronounced and accelerated colitis, confirming an important role of LRH-1 and intestinal GC synthesis in the regulation of local immune responses. LRH-1 likely regulates intestinal GC synthesis not only via the induction of certain steroidogenic enzymes. Steroid acute regulator (StAR) has an important role in transporting cholesterol within the cell, and thus supplying the steroid synthesizing machinery with the substrate for GC synthesis. As LRH-1 also transcriptionally regulates StAR expression [90], LRH-1 seems to control intestinal GC synthesis at many levels.

Interestingly, LRH-1 appears to have various modes of activation. Though initially defined as orphan nuclear receptor due the lack of known ligands, the crystallization of

LRH-1 and subsequent structural analysis revealed a ligand binding to the ligand-binding domain of LRH-1. This ligand was identified as phosphatidylinositol, however, it is very likely that a larger variety of natural and synthetic ligands may bind to this ligand-binding domain and transactivate LRH-1. Of interest are recent reports demonstrating LRH-1 activation by testosterone [91], the herbizide atrazin [92] as well as several synthetic ligands with selective activities for LRH-1 over SF-1 [93]. However, ligand binding may not be an absolute requirement for LRH-1 activation. In particular, mouse LRH-1 can be activated in a ligand-independent manner, as mutation of the ligand-binding domain does not affect its activity [94].

In marked contrast, phosphorylation by upstream kinases may selectively activate both, human and mouse LRH-1. Two serine residues in the hinge region of LRH-1 have been identified as phosphorylation targets of the MAP kinase ERK1/2, and mutation of these two serine residues strongly affects LRH-1 activity [95]. In line with this idea of LRH-1 activation via the MAP kinase pathway is the observation that the MEK1 inhibitor U0126 also blocks LRH-1 activity ([95]; Bianchi, Brunner, unpublished). Next to ERK1/2 also other yet to be identified kinases may be involved in LRH-1 phosphorylation and activation.

As many other nuclear receptors LRH-1 is also efficiently regulated by cofactors and repressors. For example, SRC-1 (steroid receptor coactivator-1) binds to LRH-1 and enhances its transcriptional activity. On the other hand, various inhibitors of LRH-1, such as DAX-1 (dosage-sensitive sex reversal, adrenal hypoplasia critical region, on chromosome X, gene 1), SHP (small heterodimer partner) and Prox-1 (Prospero homeobox protein 1) have been shown to interact with LRH-1 and inhibit its activity [89, 96, 97]. Of interest is the fact that SHP is a major transcriptional target of LRH-1, and SHP induction likely represents a negative feedback loop terminating the transcriptional activity of LRH-1.

Thus far intestinal GC synthesis has been always described in the context of immunological stress and inflammation. Clearly, factors released by activated immune cells must be able to trigger steroidogenesis in intestinal epithelial cells, likely via the activation of LRH-1. Of major interest in this regard are factors that also promote adrenal GC synthesis. Surprisingly, ACTH or ACTH receptor signaling pathways, such as an increase in cellular cyclic AMP, fail to promote intestinal GC synthesis and rather inhibit it [47] indicating that next to the preferential use of SF-1 and LRH-1 there are other elements in the regulation of adrenal versus intestinal GC synthesis that are different. The pro-inflammatory cytokines IL-6 and TNFα are known as potent triggers of adrenal GC synthesis. While no evidence could be found for a role of IL-6 in the immune cell-mediated induction of intestinal steroid synthesis, TNFα appears to represent a critical mediator of intestinal GC synthesis. TNFα alone promotes the expression of steroidogenic enzymes in intestinal epithelial cells in vitro and in vivo, and stimulates the synthesis of corticosterone. More importantly, induction of intestinal GC synthesis by injection of anti-CD3ε, LPS as well as experimental colitis largely depends on the signaling via TNF receptors [53]. Surprisingly, deletion of either one of the two TNF receptors abrogates immune cell-induced intestinal GC synthesis [52], indicating that simultaneous signaling via both receptors is required.

The important role of TNFα in the induction of intestinal GC synthesis is particularly evident when analyzing different models of experimentally induced colitis. While DSS and the hapten TNBS promote intestinal steroidogenesis, the hapten oxazolone fails to do so, despite very comparable induction of inflammation [53]. Clearly, inflammation alone is insufficient to initiate intestinal steroidogensis, but the type of inflammation may be critical. DSS and TNBS stimulate an immune response with Th1 cytokine predominance, abundant TNFα and IFNγ, whereas oxazolone promotes a Th2 type cytokine response with no TNFα, but IL-4 and IL-5. Supporting the important role of TNFα in these processes, it was found that oxazolone does not trigger intestinal GC synthesis, however injection of recombinant TNFα can restore the expression of steroidogenic enzymes and GC synthesis, and thereby ameliorate intestinal inflammation induced by oxazolone. Thus, TNFα seems to be an important sensor of immunological stress in the intestine and responsible for initiating negative feedback mechanisms via the induction of intestinal GC synthesis. This is inasmuch surprising as TNFα is an important therapeutic target in the pathogenesis of inflammatory bowel disease (IBD), such as Crohn's disease and ulcerative colitis [98-100]. TNFα is an important disease promoting and initiating factor during IBD, and its neutralization inhibits inflammatory processes right from the start. Its role in the regulation of intestinal GC synthesis, however, point also out a thus far unrecognized anti-inflammatory role of TNFα (reviewed in [51]).

4.3. GC synthesis in the lung

The intestinal and the lung epithelium have much in common. Their main function is the absorption of nutrients and gases, respectively, and due to their enormous surface to cope with this task they are also constantly exposed to a plethora of antigens, microbes and potential pathogens. Thus, much alike the intestinal mucosa the lung harbors a large number of resident immune cells, mostly macrophages and dendritic cells, and is rapidly populated by infiltrating immune cells upon infection or stimulation with antigens. Similarly, uncontrolled immune responses in the lung may lead to chronic disorders, such as allergen-induced asthma and chronic obstructive pulmonary disorder (COPD). This illustrates on one hand the need for an efficient immune response in the lung in order to defend this vast epithelial surface from infection and invasion by pathogens, but also points out that local immune responses must be tightly regulated to avoid chronic inflammation, tissue damage and resulting loss of function of the absorptive epithelium.

All these thoughts suggest that similar regulatory mechanisms exist in the lung as in the intestinal mucosa, and local GC synthesis may represent such a homeostatic control mechanism. Indeed, it has been described that genes involved in the GC synthesis pathway are transiently expressed in the developing mouse lung [101]. More recently, our own research has investigated the capacity of the adult lung to express steroidogenic enzymes and to synthesize GC in response to immunological stress [54]. Unlike the intestinal epithelium, the entire enzymatic machinery appears to be constitutively expressed in the adult lung tissue, and only CYP11A1, encoding P450scc, is induced upon immunological stress initiated by injection of T cell-activating anti-CD3ε antibody or macrophage-activating

LPS. Furthermore, particularly CYP11B1, although detectable by quantitative PCR, seems to be expressed at very low levels and not to be induced as in the intestine. When analyzing corticosterone synthesis in ex vivo lung cultures two observations are compelling. The lung tissue constitutively synthesizes considerable amounts of corticosterone in unchallenged mice, and the induced GC levels upon immunological stress are much higher when compared to equal amounts of tissue in the intestine [54]. Importantly, also in the lung ex vivo GC synthesis is efficiently blocked by the pharmacological inhibitor metyrapone, supporting the idea that GC measured are de novo synthesized in the lung tissue, though here its effect may not be via the inhibition of 11β-hydroxylase. This indicates that the lung tissue may be an even more potent extra-adrenal source of immunoregulatory GC than the intestinal epithelium.

Thus far, the cellular source of lung GC synthesis has not been identified yet. Very likely, though, lung epithelial cells, either type I or type II epithelial cells, may be the relevant source of lung GC. In support of this hypothesis is the observation that lung epithelial cell lines express steroidogenic enzymes and are capable of metabolizing steroid precursors to corticosterone (Hostettler, Brunner, unpublished observations). Despite the many similarities between the intestinal and the lung epithelium in terms of response to inflammatory triggers and the synthesis of GC, there are also many differences in the induction of intestinal versus lung GC synthesis. While systemic activation of immune cells by anti-CD3 or LPS injection triggers both, intestinal and lung GC synthesis [52, 54], the response to local inflammation seems to be regulated somewhat differently. A typical model of allergic airway inflammation is the sensitization of mice with the model antigen ovalbumin in the context of alum as adjuvant, and the challenge with the antigen via aerosol. This leads to a T helper 2 type inflammatory response with a major eosinophilic and neutrophilic granulocyte infiltration of the lung tissue and lung lumen within 24 hours. Despite the massive inflammation and infiltration with immune cells only a minimal and not significant transient increase in local GC synthesis is observed, not comparable to the high concentrations measured after stimulation with anti-CD3 or LPS [54]. Given the fact that ovalbumin airway hypersensitivity and oxazolone-induced colitis are both T helper 2-driven immune responses, the idea that lack of TNFα secretion could be the missing stimulator of lung GC synthesis appears very attractive. Indeed, only minimal TNFα levels are measured in the serum and the bronchoalveolar lavage (BAL) after ovalbumin challenge [54]. Similarly, when TNFα is injected into mice local GC synthesis in the lung can be efficiently induced. However, experiments in TNF receptor-deficient mice using anti-CD3 as a trigger clearly showed that TNFα signaling is not required for immune cell-stimulated local GC synthesis in the lung tissue. Thus, very likely other cytokines and/or factors, yet to be identified, may be substituting TNFα as a sensor of immune cell activation and trigger of local GC synthesis. It is feasible to believe that such a sensor of immunological stress is not induced during allergic inflammation of the lung, e.g. asthma, but present during contact with pathogens, such as influenza infection, thereby helping to reestablish local immune homeostasis via the secretion of GC. The identification of this or these critical inducers of local GC synthesis may lead to interesting targets for therapeutic intervention of chronic inflammation of the lung via the induction of local GC synthesis.

4.4. Regulation of lung GC synthesis

Presently, not much is know regarding the molecular mechanisms of lung GC synthesis, and more detailed analysis of the regulatory pathways leading to the induction and activation of steroidogenic enzymes in the lung tissue will be needed. While the presence of all steroidogenic enzymes required for the synthesis of corticosterone from cholesterol suggests identical synthesis pathways in the lung, adrenals and intestine, metabolic assays indicate major differences between the tissues. Interestingly, ex vivo cultured lung tissue failed to convert radioactively labeled deoxycorticosterone into corticosterone, suggesting that the expression levels of CYP11B1/11β-hydroxylase are insufficient to promote this pathway of GC synthesis. In contrast, dehydrocorticosterone is efficiently metabolized by the lung tissue into corticosterone, supporting the idea that reactivation of inactive serum dehydrocorticosterone via an 11β-HDS1-dependent pathway is the primary corticosterone synthesis pathway in the lung. Along these lines is the observation that the lung expresses very low levels of CYP11B1 but very high levels of HSD11B1, and that adrenalectomy completely abolishes lung GC synthesis [54]. Though metyrapone has been reported to be selective for 11β-hydroxylase, inhibition of 11β-HSD1 has also been noted [102], explaining why ex vivo GC synthesis in lung tissue is efficiently blocked by metyrapone. A dominant role for an 11β-HSD1-dependent corticosterone synthesis pathway is also supported by the lack of evidence for a role of LRH-1 in the regulation of lung GC synthesis. While anti-CD3-induced intestinal GC synthesis was significantly reduced in LRH-1 haplodeficient mice [48], lung GC synthesis was found to be normal [54], indicating that other nuclear receptors or transcription factors are involved in the regulation of steroidogenesis in the lung tissue.

5. GC synthesis in colorectal tumors

The role of tumor immunology in the surveillance of transformed cells and the control of tumor development is a highly controversial issue. While tumor-specific immune responses and even tumor-specific T cells can be demonstrated in certain types of tumors, stimulation of tumor-specific T cells by immunization has thus far not been too successful in the prevention or treatment of tumors. A major exception is the vaccination against human papilloma virus, which strongly reduces the incidence of cervical cancer [103, 104]. Despite relatively disappointing results of such immunization protocols, clinical and histological studies support the notion that tumor-infiltrating leukocytes (TIL) are indeed capable of limiting the growth and development of certain types of cancer. An extensive study in patients with colorectal cancer revealed that those patients that had a pronounced infiltration of the tumor with lymphocytes, and in particular with memory T cells, showed a significantly prolonged survival compared to patients with little or no immune cell infiltrate [105]. Though an indirect proof, these studies demonstrate a strong correlation between anti-tumor immune responses, tumor development and patient survival. These findings, however, also suggest that tumors capable of escaping or suppressing immune responses by any means may have a major advantage and kill the patient more rapidly.

Various immune escape mechanisms have been described in different tumors. Tumor cells secrete suppressive cytokines, such as TGFβ and IL-10, express pro-apoptotic ligands (Fas ligand and TRAIL), which kill TIL, or simply reduce their immunogenicity by downregulating MHC molecules and associated antigen presentation on their surface. In this paragraph we will also discuss the proposed role of extra-adrenal GC synthesis in colorectal tumors as a mechanism of immune escape. Though various types of tumors have been shown to be active sources of steroid hormones, most of these tumors derive from steroidogenic tissues, such as the adrenal glands, ovaries or testis. For example, adrenal hyperplasia and tumors often lead to a massive release of GC, resulting in Cushing syndrome [106]. In addition, small cell bronchogenic carcinoma, carcinoids of thymus, pancreas, ovary, as well as medullary carcinoma of thyroid gland etc. have been shown to release ACTH or in rare cases CRH, and thereby to stimulate indirectly the release of systemic GC from the adrenals with subsequent suppression of the immune system [107, 108]. Yet, thus far no direct GC synthesis in tumors from non-steroidogenic tissues has been described.

As discussed in detail above, LRH-1 has a prominent role in the regulation of intestinal GC synthesis [48, 52]. Interestingly, however, LRH-1 has also been implicated in other aspects of intestinal epithelial cell biology. LRH-1 is primarily expressed in the pluripotent and proliferating cells of the intestinal crypts where it regulates the expression of cyclin D1. Furthermore, in collaboration with the Wnt signaling pathway and β-catenin it also controls the expression of cyclin E1 and c-Myc, and thereby the proliferation of crypt cells and the renewal of the intestinal epithelial layer (reviewed in [109, 110]). Not surprisingly, this mitogenic role of LRH-1 appears to be also involved in the development of intestinal tumors. Mice with a mutation in the APC gene ($APC^{min/+}$ mice) spontaneously develop adenomas in both small and large bowel. Interestingly tumor development is significantly reduced in mice with LRH-1 deficiency [111]. Thus, LRH-1 appears to be a proto-oncogene in the development of intestinal tumors. In line with this idea is the observation that different tumors derived from endoderm tissue show LRH-1 overexpression. For example, LRH-1 is overexpressed in colorectal [55] and in pancreatic tumors [112], where it also regulates cell cycle progression.

Given the important role of LRH-1 in cell cycle regulation as well as intestinal GC synthesis LRH-1-mediated synthesis of immunoregulatory GC in colorectal tumors as a mechanism to control anti-tumor immune responses appears to be an attractive idea. Indeed, considerable synthesis of cortisol can be measured in colorectal cancer cell lines as well as primary colorectal tumors using radioimmuno assay, bioassay as well as metabolic assays [55]. In line with this steroidogenic potential of colorectal tumor cells is the widely distributed expression of LRH-1 and steroidogenic enzymes. Furthermore, overexpression of LRH-1 further boost the expression of steroidogenic enyzmes and the synthesis of cortisol, whereas inhibition of LRH-1 expression downregulates these processes. Interestingly, GC synthesis in colorectal tumor cell lines as well as ex vivo cultured primary tumors seems to be constitutive, whereas in normal colonic tissue it is inducible by phorbol ester, likely via the ERK1/2-mediated activation of LRH-1. This suggests that in colorectal tumors LRH-1 may be constitutively active, and suggests that signal transduction pathways leading to tumor development and proliferation also govern the activation of LRH-1 and associated GC synthesis. Of interest in this regard is that LRH-1 not only controls cell cycle progression, but that its activity is also controlled by the cell cycle [50]. Various mitogenic signals controlling tumor cell proliferation may therefore also promote the activation of LRH-1. In line with this idea is the observation that many colorectal tumors have activating mutations of the epidermal growth factor receptor pathway [113] and that epidermal growth factor can stimulate LRH-1 activation in an ERK1/2-dependent manner in Hela cells [95]. However, more detailed analysis of the signaling pathways leading to LRH-1 activation and GC synthesis in colorectal tumors will be required to confirm whether mitogenic stimuli are indeed important triggers of extra-adrenal GC synthesis in tumor cells.

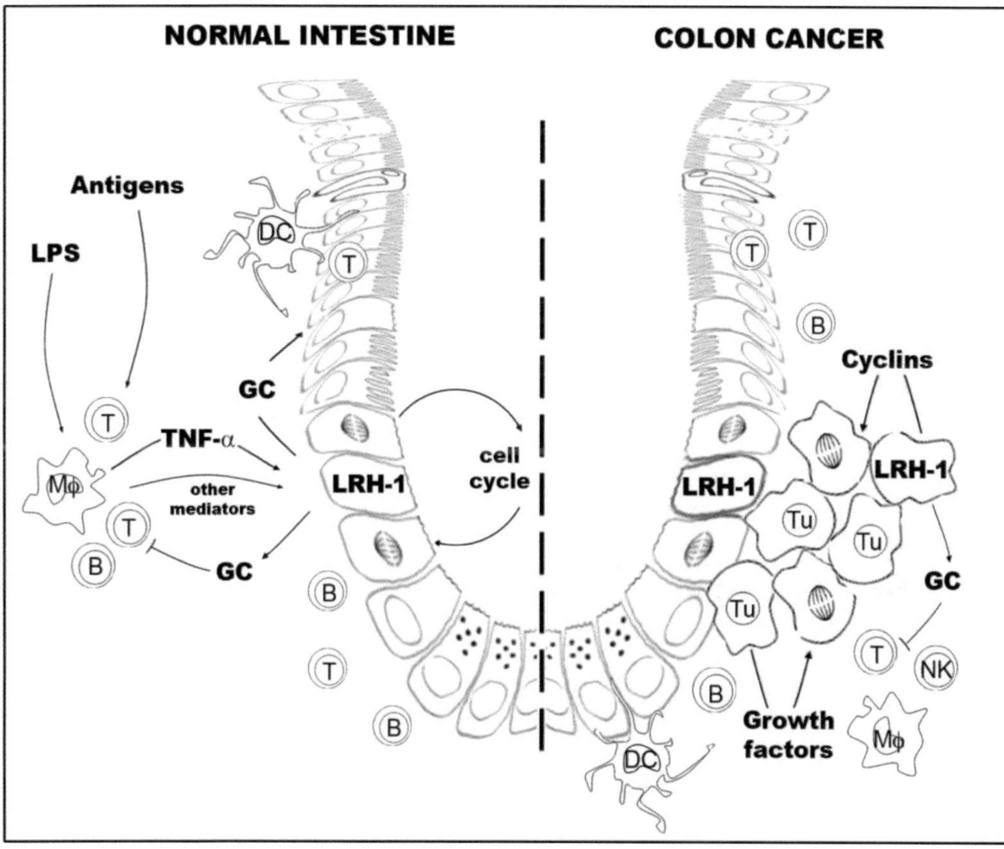

Abbreviations: B – B-Lymphocytes; DC – dendritic cells; LPS – lipopolysaccharides; Mφ – macrophages; NK – natural killer cells; T – T-Lymphocytes; Tu – tumor cells.

Figure 2. Proposed role of intestinal GC synthesis in maintaining immune homeostasis in normal gut mucosa and promoting immune escape in colon cancer.

While the immunoregulatory role of GC synthesis in normal intestinal tissue is quite well established [46, 49, 52, 53], the evidence in colorectal tumors is yet relatively indirect. The supernatant of colorectal tumor cell lines and primary tumors has been found to contain a suppressive activity, which inhibits the activation of primary T cells, as measured by the induction of activation marker CD69 [55]. Similarly, tumor-derived supernatant was able to promote apoptosis in GC sensitive immune cells. Importantly, these suppressive or pro-apoptotic activities were blocked by either interfering with the GC synthesis pathway in tumor cells by metyrapone, or by blocking the GR in immune cells [55]. While colorectal tumor cells may also secrete other immunoregulatory factors, such as TGFβ, these finding demonstrate that GC are present in the supernatant of tumor cells and that their concentration is high enough to promote biological responses and immunosuppression. The secretion of immunoregulatory GC by colorectal tumors may thus represent a novel mechanism how tumor cells escape from destruction by the immune system. Similar mechanisms may also exist in tumors from tissues capable of secreting bioactive GC, e.g. lung cancer.

6. Conclusion

In summary, the extremely potent GC synthesizing activity of the adrenal glands has obscured for a long time the fact that various other extra-adrenal tissues are important sources of immunoregulatory GC. This chapter has highlighted in particular the role of the pulmonary and intestinal mucosa, and its associated tumors, as potent sources of extra-adrenal GC synthesis. Their more recent identification has lead to new interpretations of how locally produced GC may be involved in the maintenance of tissue homeostasis, regulation of inflammatory processes and tumor development. Finally, the detailed analysis of the differential signal transduction pathways controlling GC synthesis in the adrenals versus extra-adrenal tissues may offer novel opportunities for the development of therapeutic interventions.

Author details

Feodora I. Kostadinova and Thomas Brunner*
Division of Biochemical Pharmacology, Department of Biology, University of Konstanz, Germany

Nina Hostettler and Pamela Bianchi
Division of Experimental Pathology, Institute of Pathology, University of Bern, Switzerland

Acknowledgement

The authors thank previous and present members of the Brunner lab, especially Igor Cima, Mathias Müller, Mario Noti, Daniel Sidler and Nadia Corazza, for their contributions to the investigation of extra-adrenal GC synthesis, Kristina Schoonjans and Johan Auwerx for fruitful collaborations and many reagents, and the Swiss National Science Foundation, Swiss Cancer League, the Bangerter Foundation, the Crohn's and Colitis Foundation of America and the German Research Foundation for continuous support of this research area.

* Corresponding Author

7. References

[1] Sapolsky RM, Romero LM, Munck AU (2000) How Do Glucocorticoids Influence Stress Responses? Integrating Permissive, Suppressive, Stimulatory, and Preparative Actions. Endocr Rev. 21: 55-89.

[2] Chrousos GP (1995) The Hypothalamic-Pituitary-Adrenal Axis and Immune-Mediated Inflammation. N Engl J Med. 332: 1351-62.

[3] Vacchio MS, Papadopoulos V, Ashwell JD (1994) Steroid Production in the Thymus: Implications for Thymocyte Selection. J Exp Med. 179: 1835-46.

[4] Lechner O, Wiegers GJ, Oliveira-Dos-Santos AJ, Dietrich H, Recheis H, et al. (2000) Glucocorticoid Production in the Murine Thymus. European journal of immunology. 30: 337-46.

[5] Pazirandeh A, Xue Y, Rafter I, Sjovall J, Jondal M, et al. (1999) Paracrine Glucocorticoid Activity Produced by Mouse Thymic Epithelial Cells. FASEB journal : official publication of the Federation of American Societies for Experimental Biology. 13: 893-901.

[6] Ashwell JD, Lu FW, Vacchio MS (2000) Glucocorticoids in T Cell Development and Function*. Annu Rev Immunol. 18: 309-45.

[7] Taves MD, Gomez-Sanchez CE, Soma KK (2011) Extra-Adrenal Glucocorticoids and Mineralocorticoids: Evidence for Local Synthesis, Regulation, and Function. American journal of physiology. Endocrinology and metabolism. 301: E11-24.

[8] Slominski A, Ermak G, Mihm M (1996) Acth Receptor, Cyp11a1, Cyp17 and Cyp21a2 Genes Are Expressed in Skin. J Clin Endocrinol Metab. 81: 2746-9.

[9] Slominski A, Gomez-Sanchez CE, Foecking MF, Wortsman J (2000) Active Steroidogenesis in the Normal Rat Skin. Biochim Biophys Acta. 1474: 1-4.

[10] Slominski A, Wortsman J (2000) Neuroendocrinology of the Skin. Endocr Rev. 21: 457-87.

[11] Slominski A, Wortsman J, Paus R, Elias PM, Tobin DJ, et al. (2008) Skin as an Endocrine Organ: Implications for Its Function. Drug Discov Today Dis Mech. 5: 137-44.

[12] Slominski A, Wortsman J, Pisarchik A, Zbytek B, Linton EA, et al. (2001) Cutaneous Expression of Corticotropin-Releasing Hormone (Crh), Urocortin, and Crh Receptors. FASEB journal : official publication of the Federation of American Societies for Experimental Biology. 15: 1678-93.

[13] Slominski A, Zbytek B, Szczesniewski A, Semak I, Kaminski J, et al. (2005) Crh Stimulation of Corticosteroids Production in Melanocytes Is Mediated by Acth. American journal of physiology. Endocrinology and metabolism. 288: E701-6.

[14] Slominski A, Zjawiony J, Wortsman J, Semak I, Stewart J, et al. (2004) A Novel Pathway for Sequential Transformation of 7-Dehydrocholesterol and Expression of the P450scc System in Mammalian Skin. Eur J Biochem. 271: 4178-88.

[15] Ito N, Ito T, Kromminga A, Bettermann A, Takigawa M, et al. (2005) Human Hair Follicles Display a Functional Equivalent of the Hypothalamic-Pituitary-Adrenal Axis and Synthesize Cortisol. FASEB journal : official publication of the Federation of American Societies for Experimental Biology. 19: 1332-4.

[16] Paus R, Botchkarev VA, Botchkareva NV, Mecklenburg L, Luger T, et al. (1999) The Skin Pomc System (Sps). Leads and Lessons from the Hair Follicle. Annals of the New York Academy of Sciences. 885: 350-63.

[17] Paus R, Ito N, Takigawa M, Ito T (2003) The Hair Follicle and Immune Privilege. J Investig Dermatol Symp Proc. 8: 188-94.

[18] Thiboutot D, Jabara S, McAllister JM, Sivarajah A, Gilliland K, et al. (2003) Human Skin Is a Steroidogenic Tissue: Steroidogenic Enzymes and Cofactors Are Expressed in Epidermis, Normal Sebocytes, and an Immortalized Sebocyte Cell Line (Seb-1). J Invest Dermatol. 120: 905-14.

[19] Vukelic S, Stojadinovic O, Pastar I, Rabach M, Krzyzanowska A, et al. (2011) Cortisol Synthesis in Epidermis Is Induced by Il-1 and Tissue Injury. The Journal of biological chemistry. 286: 10265-75.

[20] Casal AJ, Silvestre JS, Delcayre C, Capponi AM (2003) Expression and Modulation of Steroidogenic Acute Regulatory Protein Messenger Ribonucleic Acid in Rat Cardiocytes and after Myocardial Infarction. Endocrinology. 144: 1861-8.

[21] Silvestre JS, Robert V, Heymes C, Aupetit-Faisant B, Mouas C, et al. (1998) Myocardial Production of Aldosterone and Corticosterone in the Rat. Physiological Regulation. The Journal of biological chemistry. 273: 4883-91.

[22] Silvestre JS, Heymes C, Oubenaissa A, Robert V, Aupetit-Faisant B, et al. (1999) Activation of Cardiac Aldosterone Production in Rat Myocardial Infarction: Effect of Angiotensin Ii Receptor Blockade and Role in Cardiac Fibrosis. Circulation. 99: 2694-701.

[23] Takeda Y, Miyamori I, Yoneda T, Iki K, Hatakeyama H, et al. (1994) Synthesis of Corticosterone in the Vascular Wall. Endocrinology. 135: 2283-6.

[24] Takeda Y, Miyamori I, Yoneda T, Hatakeyama H, Inaba S, et al. (1996) Regulation of Aldosterone Synthase in Human Vascular Endothelial Cells by Angiotensin Ii and Adrenocorticotropin. J Clin Endocrinol Metab. 81: 2797-800.

[25] Takeda Y (2005) Role of Cardiovascular Aldosterone in Hypertension. Curr Med Chem Cardiovasc Hematol Agents. 3: 261-6.

[26] Hatakeyama H, Miyamori I, Takeda Y, Yamamoto H, Mabuchi H (1996) The Expression of Steroidogenic Enzyme Genes in Human Vascular Cells. Biochem Mol Biol Int. 40: 639-45.

[27] Kayes-Wandover KM, White PC (2000) Steroidogenic Enzyme Gene Expression in the Human Heart. J Clin Endocrinol Metab. 85: 2519-25.

[28] Young MJ, Clyne CD, Cole TJ, Funder JW (2001) Cardiac Steroidogenesis in the Normal and Failing Heart. J Clin Endocrinol Metab. 86: 5121-6.

[29] Ahmad N, Romero DG, Gomez-Sanchez EP, Gomez-Sanchez CE (2004) Do Human Vascular Endothelial Cells Produce Aldosterone? Endocrinology. 145: 3626-9.

[30] Baulieu EE (1998) Neurosteroids: A Novel Function of the Brain. Psychoneuroendocrinology. 23: 963-87.

[31] Mellon SH (2007) Neurosteroid Regulation of Central Nervous System Development. Pharmacol Ther. 116: 107-24.

[32] Gunn BG, Brown AR, Lambert JJ, Belelli D (2011) Neurosteroids and Gaba(a) Receptor Interactions: A Focus on Stress. Front Neurosci. 5: 131.

[33] Stromstedt M, Waterman MR (1995) Messenger Rnas Encoding Steroidogenic Enzymes Are Expressed in Rodent Brain. Brain Res Mol Brain Res. 34: 75-88.

[34] MacKenzie SM, Clark CJ, Ingram MC, Lai M, Seckl J, et al. (2000) Corticosteroid Production by Fetal Rat Hippocampal Neurons. Endocr Res. 26: 531-5.

[35] MacKenzie SM, Clark CJ, Fraser R, Gomez-Sanchez CE, Connell JM, et al. (2000) Expression of 11beta-Hydroxylase and Aldosterone Synthase Genes in the Rat Brain. J Mol Endocrinol. 24: 321-8.

[36] Yu L, Romero DG, Gomez-Sanchez CE, Gomez-Sanchez EP (2002) Steroidogenic Enzyme Gene Expression in the Human Brain. Mol Cell Endocrinol. 190: 9-17.

[37] Higo S, Hojo Y, Ishii H, Komatsuzaki Y, Ooishi Y, et al. (2011) Endogenous Synthesis of Corticosteroids in the Hippocampus. PLoS One. 6: e21631.

[38] Basu R, Singh RJ, Basu A, Chittilapilly EG, Johnson CM, et al. (2004) Splanchnic Cortisol Production Occurs in Humans: Evidence for Conversion of Cortisone to Cortisol Via the 11-Beta Hydroxysteroid Dehydrogenase (11beta-Hsd) Type 1 Pathway. Diabetes. 53: 2051-9.

[39] Andrew R, Westerbacka J, Wahren J, Yki-Jarvinen H, Walker BR (2005) The Contribution of Visceral Adipose Tissue to Splanchnic Cortisol Production in Healthy Humans. Diabetes. 54: 1364-70.

[40] Harris HJ, Kotelevtsev Y, Mullins JJ, Seckl JR, Holmes MC (2001) Intracellular Regeneration of Glucocorticoids by 11beta-Hydroxysteroid Dehydrogenase (11beta-Hsd)-1 Plays a Key Role in Regulation of the Hypothalamic-Pituitary-Adrenal Axis: Analysis of 11beta-Hsd-1-Deficient Mice. Endocrinology. 142: 114-20.

[41] Carter RN, Paterson JM, Tworowska U, Stenvers DJ, Mullins JJ, et al. (2009) Hypothalamic-Pituitary-Adrenal Axis Abnormalities in Response to Deletion of 11beta-Hsd1 Is Strain-Dependent. J Neuroendocrinol. 21: 879-87.

[42] Wyrwoll CS, Holmes MC, Seckl JR (2011) 11beta-Hydroxysteroid Dehydrogenases and the Brain: From Zero to Hero, a Decade of Progress. Front Neuroendocrinol. 32: 265-86.

[43] Holmes MC, Carter RN, Noble J, Chitnis S, Dutia A, et al. (2010) 11beta-Hydroxysteroid Dehydrogenase Type 1 Expression Is Increased in the Aged Mouse Hippocampus and Parietal Cortex and Causes Memory Impairments. J Neurosci. 30: 6916-20.

[44] Sandeep TC, Yau JL, MacLullich AM, Noble J, Deary IJ, et al. (2004) 11beta-Hydroxysteroid Dehydrogenase Inhibition Improves Cognitive Function in Healthy Elderly Men and Type 2 Diabetics. Proceedings of the National Academy of Sciences of the United States of America. 101: 6734-9.

[45] MacLullich AM, Ferguson KJ, Reid LM, Deary IJ, Starr JM, et al. (2012) 11beta-Hydroxysteroid Dehydrogenase Type 1, Brain Atrophy and Cognitive Decline. Neurobiol Aging. 33: 207 e1-8.

[46] Cima I, Corazza N, Dick B, Fuhrer A, Herren S, et al. (2004) Intestinal Epithelial Cells Synthesize Glucocorticoids and Regulate T Cell Activation. The Journal of experimental medicine. 200: 1635-46.

[47] Mueller M, Atanasov A, Cima I, Corazza N, Schoonjans K, et al. (2007) Differential Regulation of Glucocorticoid Synthesis in Murine Intestinal Epithelial Versus Adrenocortical Cell Lines. Endocrinology. 148: 1445-53.

[48] Mueller M, Cima I, Noti M, Fuhrer A, Jakob S, et al. (2006) The Nuclear Receptor Lrh-1 Critically Regulates Extra-Adrenal Glucocorticoid Synthesis in the Intestine. The Journal of experimental medicine. 203: 2057-62.

[49] Coste A, Dubuquoy L, Barnouin R, Annicotte JS, Magnier B, et al. (2007) Lrh-1-Mediated Glucocorticoid Synthesis in Enterocytes Protects against Inflammatory Bowel Disease. Proc Natl Acad Sci U S A. 104: 13098-103.

[50] Atanasov AG, Leiser D, Roesselet C, Noti M, Corazza N, et al. (2008) Cell Cycle-Dependent Regulation of Extra-Adrenal Glucocorticoid Synthesis in Murine Intestinal Epithelial Cells. FASEB journal : official publication of the Federation of American Societies for Experimental Biology. 22: 4117-25.

[51] Noti M, Sidler D, Brunner T (2009) Extra-Adrenal Glucocorticoid Synthesis in the Intestinal Epithelium: More Than a Drop in the Ocean? Semin Immunopathol. 31: 237-48.

[52] Noti M, Corazza N, Tuffin G, Schoonjans K, Brunner T (2010) Lipopolysaccharide Induces Intestinal Glucocorticoid Synthesis in a Tnfalpha-Dependent Manner. FASEB journal : official publication of the Federation of American Societies for Experimental Biology. 24: 1340-6.

[53] Noti M, Corazza N, Mueller C, Berger B, Brunner T (2010) Tnf Suppresses Acute Intestinal Inflammation by Inducing Local Glucocorticoid Synthesis. The Journal of experimental medicine. 207: 1057-66.

[54] Hostettler N, Bianchi P, Gennari-Moser C, Kassahn D, Schoonjans K, et al. (2012) Local Glucocorticoid Production in the Mouse Lung Is Induced by Immune Cell Stimulation. Allergy. 67: 227-34.

[55] Sidler D, Renzulli P, Schnoz C, Berger B, Schneider-Jakob S, et al. (2011) Colon Cancer Cells Produce Immunoregulatory Glucocorticoids. Oncogene. 30: 2411-9.

[56] Keeney DS, Jenkins CM, Waterman MR (1995) Developmentally Regulated Expression of Adrenal 17 Alpha-Hydroxylase Cytochrome P450 in the Mouse Embryo. Endocrinology. 136: 4872-9.

[57] Okamoto M, Nonaka Y, Takemori H, Doi J (2005) Molecular Identity and Gene Expression of Aldosterone Synthase Cytochrome P450. Biochem Biophys Res Commun. 338: 325-30.

[58] Laurent V, Kimble A, Peng B, Zhu P, Pintar JE, et al. (2002) Mortality in 7b2 Null Mice Can Be Rescued by Adrenalectomy: Involvement of Dopamine in Acth Hypersecretion. Proceedings of the National Academy of Sciences of the United States of America. 99: 3087-92.

[59] Davies E, MacKenzie SM (2003) Extra-Adrenal Production of Corticosteroids. Clin Exp Pharmacol Physiol. 30: 437-45.

[60] Blackburn CC, Manley NR (2004) Developing a New Paradigm for Thymus Organogenesis. Nat Rev Immunol. 4: 278-89.

[61] Spits H (2002) Development of Alphabeta T Cells in the Human Thymus. Nat Rev Immunol. 2: 760-72.

[62] Ashwell JD, Vacchio MS, Galon J (2000) Do Glucocorticoids Participate in Thymocyte Development? Immunol Today. 21: 644-6.

[63] Godfrey DI, Purton JF, Boyd RL, Cole TJ (2000) Stress-Free T-Cell Development: Glucocorticoids Are Not Obligatory. Immunol Today. 21: 606-11.

[64] Zacharchuk CM, Mercep M, Chakraborti PK, Simons SS, Jr., Ashwell JD (1990) Programmed T Lymphocyte Death. Cell Activation- and Steroid-Induced Pathways Are Mutually Antagonistic. Journal of immunology. 145: 4037-45.

[65] Kupper TS, Fuhlbrigge RC (2004) Immune Surveillance in the Skin: Mechanisms and Clinical Consequences. Nat Rev Immunol. 4: 211-22.

[66] Rousseau K, Kauser S, Pritchard LE, Warhurst A, Oliver RL, et al. (2007) Proopiomelanocortin (Pomc), the Acth/Melanocortin Precursor, Is Secreted by Human Epidermal Keratinocytes and Melanocytes and Stimulates Melanogenesis. FASEB journal : official publication of the Federation of American Societies for Experimental Biology. 21: 1844-56.

[67] Slominski A, Zbytek B, Semak I, Sweatman T, Wortsman J (2005) Crh Stimulates Pomc Activity and Corticosterone Production in Dermal Fibroblasts. J Neuroimmunol. 162: 97-102.

[68] Mellon SH, Griffin LD (2002) Neurosteroids: Biochemistry and Clinical Significance. Trends Endocrinol Metab. 13: 35-43.

[69] Kishimoto W, Hiroi T, Shiraishi M, Osada M, Imaoka S, et al. (2004) Cytochrome P450 2d Catalyze Steroid 21-Hydroxylation in the Brain. Endocrinology. 145: 699-705.

[70] Ye P, Kenyon CJ, Mackenzie SM, Nichol K, Seckl JR, et al. (2008) Effects of Acth, Dexamethasone, and Adrenalectomy on 11beta-Hydroxylase (Cyp11b1) and Aldosterone Synthase (Cyp11b2) Gene Expression in the Rat Central Nervous System. J Endocrinol. 196: 305-11.

[71] Walker BR, Andrew R (2006) Tissue Production of Cortisol by 11beta-Hydroxysteroid Dehydrogenase Type 1 and Metabolic Disease. Annals of the New York Academy of Sciences. 1083: 165-84.

[72] Yau JL, McNair KM, Noble J, Brownstein D, Hibberd C, et al. (2007) Enhanced Hippocampal Long-Term Potentiation and Spatial Learning in Aged 11beta-Hydroxysteroid Dehydrogenase Type 1 Knock-out Mice. J Neurosci. 27: 10487-96.

[73] Takeda Y, Miyamori I, Yoneda T, Iki K, Hatakeyama H, et al. (1995) Production of Aldosterone in Isolated Rat Blood Vessels. Hypertension. 25: 170-3.

[74] Christy C, Hadoke PW, Paterson JM, Mullins JJ, Seckl JR, et al. (2003) 11beta-Hydroxysteroid Dehydrogenase Type 2 in Mouse Aorta: Localization and Influence on Response to Glucocorticoids. Hypertension. 42: 580-7.

[75] Hadoke PW, Macdonald L, Logie JJ, Small GR, Dover AR, et al. (2006) Intra-Vascular Glucocorticoid Metabolism as a Modulator of Vascular Structure and Function. Cellular and molecular life sciences : CMLS. 63: 565-78.

[76] Goodyer CG, Branchaud CL (1981) Regulation of Hormone Production in the Human Feto-Placental Unit. Ciba Found Symp. 86: 89-123.

[77] Yong PY, Thong KJ, Andrew R, Walker BR, Hillier SG (2000) Development-Related Increase in Cortisol Biosynthesis by Human Granulosa Cells. J Clin Endocrinol Metab. 85: 4728-33.

[78] Wang GM, Ge RS, Latif SA, Morris DJ, Hardy MP (2002) Expression of 11beta-Hydroxylase in Rat Leydig Cells. Endocrinology. 143: 621-6.

[79] Burton PJ, Krozowski ZS, Waddell BJ (1998) Immunolocalization of 11beta-Hydroxysteroid Dehydrogenase Types 1 and 2 in Rat Uterus: Variation across the Estrous Cycle and Regulation by Estrogen and Progesterone. Endocrinology. 139: 376-82.

[80] Quirk SJ, Slattery J, Funder JW (1990) 11 Beta-Hydroxysteroid Dehydrogenase Activity in the Mammary Gland. J Steroid Biochem. 35: 623-5.

[81] Brunner T (2009) Living on the Edge: Immune Cells and Immunopathology in the Intestinal Mucosa. Seminars in immunopathology. 31: 143-4.

[82] Keeney DS, Ikeda Y, Waterman MR, Parker KL (1995) Cholesterol Side-Chain Cleavage Cytochrome P450 Gene Expression in the Primitive Gut of the Mouse Embryo Does Not Require Steroidogenic Factor 1. Mol Endocrinol. 9: 1091-8.

[83] Sadovsky Y, Crawford PA, Woodson KG, Polish JA, Clements MA, et al. (1995) Mice Deficient in the Orphan Receptor Steroidogenic Factor 1 Lack Adrenal Glands and Gonads but Express P450 Side-Chain-Cleavage Enzyme in the Placenta and Have Normal Embryonic Serum Levels of Corticosteroids. Proceedings of the National Academy of Sciences of the United States of America. 92: 10939-43.

[84] Brunner T, Arnold D, Wasem C, Herren S, Frutschi C (2001) Regulation of Cell Death and Survival in Intestinal Intraepithelial Lymphocytes. Cell death and differentiation. 8: 706-14.

[85] Wasem C, Arnold D, Saurer L, Corazza N, Jakob S, et al. (2003) Sensitizing Antigen-Specific Cd8+ T Cells for Accelerated Suicide Causes Immune Incompetence. The Journal of clinical investigation. 111: 1191-9.

[86] Corazza N, Muller S, Brunner T, Kagi D, Mueller C (2000) Differential Contribution of Fas- and Perforin-Mediated Mechanisms to the Cell-Mediated Cytotoxic Activity of Naive and in Vivo-Primed Intestinal Intraepithelial Lymphocytes. Journal of immunology. 164: 398-403.

[87] Parker KL, Rice DA, Lala DS, Ikeda Y, Luo X, et al. (2002) Steroidogenic Factor 1: An Essential Mediator of Endocrine Development. Recent Prog Horm Res. 57: 19-36.

[88] Parker KL (1998) The Roles of Steroidogenic Factor 1 in Endocrine Development and Function. Mol Cell Endocrinol. 145: 15-20.

[89] Fayard E, Auwerx J, Schoonjans K (2004) Lrh-1: An Orphan Nuclear Receptor Involved in Development, Metabolism and Steroidogenesis. Trends Cell Biol. 14: 250-60.

[90] Sirianni R, Seely JB, Attia G, Stocco DM, Carr BR, et al. (2002) Liver Receptor Homologue-1 Is Expressed in Human Steroidogenic Tissues and Activates Transcription of Genes Encoding Steroidogenic Enzymes. J Endocrinol. 174: R13-7.

[91] Wu YG, Bennett J, Talla D, Stocco C (2011) Testosterone, Not 5alpha-Dihydrotestosterone, Stimulates Lrh-1 Leading to Fsh-Independent Expression of Cyp19 and P450scc in Granulosa Cells. Mol Endocrinol. 25: 656-68.

[92] Suzawa M, Ingraham HA (2008) The Herbicide Atrazine Activates Endocrine Gene Networks Via Non-Steroidal Nr5a Nuclear Receptors in Fish and Mammalian Cells. PLoS One. 3: e2117.

[93] Whitby RJ, Stec J, Blind RD, Dixon S, Leesnitzer LM, et al. (2011) Small Molecule Agonists of the Orphan Nuclear Receptors Steroidogenic Factor-1 (Sf-1, Nr5a1) and Liver Receptor Homologue-1 (Lrh-1, Nr5a2). J Med Chem. 54: 2266-81.

[94] Sablin EP, Krylova IN, Fletterick RJ, Ingraham HA (2003) Structural Basis for Ligand-Independent Activation of the Orphan Nuclear Receptor Lrh-1. Molecular cell. 11: 1575-85.

[95] Lee YK, Choi YH, Chua S, Park YJ, Moore DD (2006) Phosphorylation of the Hinge Domain of the Nuclear Hormone Receptor Lrh-1 Stimulates Transactivation. The Journal of biological chemistry. 281: 7850-5.

[96] Sablin EP, Woods A, Krylova IN, Hwang P, Ingraham HA, et al. (2008) The Structure of Corepressor Dax-1 Bound to Its Target Nuclear Receptor Lrh-1. Proceedings of the National Academy of Sciences of the United States of America. 105: 18390-5.

[97] Lee YK, Moore DD (2002) Dual Mechanisms for Repression of the Monomeric Orphan Receptor Liver Receptor Homologous Protein-1 by the Orphan Small Heterodimer Partner. The Journal of biological chemistry. 277: 2463-7.

[98] Reimund JM, Wittersheim C, Dumont S, Muller CD, Baumann R, et al. (1996) Mucosal Inflammatory Cytokine Production by Intestinal Biopsies in Patients with Ulcerative Colitis and Crohn's Disease. J Clin Immunol. 16: 144-50.

[99] Rutgeerts PJ (1999) Review Article: Efficacy of Infliximab in Crohn's Disease--Induction and Maintenance of Remission. Aliment Pharmacol Ther. 13 Suppl 4: 9-15; discussion 38.

[100] Ford AC, Sandborn WJ, Khan KJ, Hanauer SB, Talley NJ, et al. (2011) Efficacy of Biological Therapies in Inflammatory Bowel Disease: Systematic Review and Meta-Analysis. Am J Gastroenterol. 106: 644-59, quiz 60.

[101] Provost PR, Tremblay Y (2005) Genes Involved in the Adrenal Pathway of Glucocorticoid Synthesis Are Transiently Expressed in the Developing Lung. Endocrinology. 146: 2239-45.

[102] Sampath-Kumar R, Yu M, Khalil MW, Yang K (1997) Metyrapone Is a Competitive Inhibitor of 11beta-Hydroxysteroid Dehydrogenase Type 1 Reductase. J Steroid Biochem Mol Biol. 62: 195-9.

[103] Roteli-Martins C, Naud P, De Borba P, Teixeira J, De Carvalho N, et al. (2012) Sustained Immunogenicity and Efficacy of the Hpv-16/18 As04-Adjuvanted Vaccine: Up to 8.4 Years of Follow-Up. Hum Vaccin Immunother. 8.

[104] Lehtinen M, Paavonen J, Wheeler CM, Jaisamrarn U, Garland SM, et al. (2012) Overall Efficacy of Hpv-16/18 As04-Adjuvanted Vaccine against Grade 3 or Greater Cervical Intraepithelial Neoplasia: 4-Year End-of-Study Analysis of the Randomised, Double-Blind Patricia Trial. Lancet Oncol. 13: 89-99.

[105] Galon J, Costes A, Sanchez-Cabo F, Kirilovsky A, Mlecnik B, et al. (2006) Type, Density, and Location of Immune Cells within Human Colorectal Tumors Predict Clinical Outcome. Science. 313: 1960-4.

[106] Newell-Price J, Bertagna X, Grossman AB, Nieman LK (2006) Cushing's Syndrome. Lancet. 367: 1605-17.

[107] Isidori AM, Kaltsas GA, Pozza C, Frajese V, Newell-Price J, et al. (2006) The Ectopic Adrenocorticotropin Syndrome: Clinical Features, Diagnosis, Management, and Long-Term Follow-Up. J Clin Endocrinol Metab. 91: 371-7.

[108] Shahani S, Nudelman RJ, Nalini R, Kim HS, Samson SL (2010) Ectopic Corticotropin-Releasing Hormone (Crh) Syndrome from Metastatic Small Cell Carcinoma: A Case Report and Review of the Literature. Diagn Pathol. 5: 56.

[109] Botrugno OA, Fayard E, Annicotte JS, Haby C, Brennan T, et al. (2004) Synergy between Lrh-1 and Beta-Catenin Induces G1 Cyclin-Mediated Cell Proliferation. Molecular cell. 15: 499-509.

[110] Fernandez-Marcos PJ, Auwerx J, Schoonjans K (2011) Emerging Actions of the Nuclear Receptor Lrh-1 in the Gut. Biochim Biophys Acta. 1812: 947-55.

[111] Schoonjans K, Dubuquoy L, Mebis J, Fayard E, Wendling O, et al. (2005) Liver Receptor Homolog 1 Contributes to Intestinal Tumor Formation through Effects on Cell Cycle and Inflammation. Proceedings of the National Academy of Sciences of the United States of America. 102: 2058-62.

[112] Benod C, Vinogradova MV, Jouravel N, Kim GE, Fletterick RJ, et al. (2011) Nuclear Receptor Liver Receptor Homologue 1 (Lrh-1) Regulates Pancreatic Cancer Cell Growth and Proliferation. Proceedings of the National Academy of Sciences of the United States of America. 108: 16927-31.

[113] Normanno N, Tejpar S, Morgillo F, De Luca A, Van Cutsem E, et al. (2009) Implications for Kras Status and Egfr-Targeted Therapies in Metastatic Crc. Nat Rev Clin Oncol. 6: 519-27.

Chapter 5

Glucocorticoid-Induced Cardioprotection: A Novel Role for Autophagy?

Anna-Mart Engelbrecht and Benjamin Loos

Additional information is available at the end of the chapter

http://dx.doi.org/10.5772/52406

1. Introduction

Glucocorticoids (GC) are commonly used as anti-inflammatory and immunosuppressive therapy by approximately 1% of the total adult population. Glucocorticoid therapy has also been used in non-autoimmune and non-inflammatory conditions such as acute myocardial infarction, angina, endocarditis as well as in invasive cardiology, coronary interventions and cardiopulmonary- bypass surgery. Despite ample evidence for GC's role as a natural, physiologic regulator of the immune system, little is known about the molecular events induced by GCs during a stress response. Autophagy is a survival mechanism which is upregulated in response to stress in the cell. It has been described as the cell's major adaptive strategy in response to a multitude of extracellular stresses, such as nutrient deprivation, mitochondrial damage, endoplasmic reticulum stress or infection. Conserved in all eukaryotes, it is mediated by a unique organelle, the autophagosome, which, under inclusion of cytoplasmic cargo, fuses with lysosomes in order to yield recyclable nutrient metabolites. Basal autophagic activity plays a vital role in maintaining homeostasis during cellular stress. Its malfunction has been implicated with human pathologies such as heart disease, neurological storage disease and cancer.

It is known that GC-triggered autophagy plays a role in cell death during development. However, recent landmark studies also indicate that autophagy operates as a hub, integrating cellular stress, metabolism and glucocorticoid mediated anti-inflammatory action. Importantly, recent lines of evidence suggest that glucocorticoids impact on key signalling components, which control the activity of the autophagic machinery.

In this review we will focus on the connections between these key signaling components and autophagy, describing their central roles as modulators of GC-induced protection during a cellular stress response.

2. Glucocorticoid generation and metabolism

The understanding of the physiological regulation of glucocorticoid activity has considerably improved over the last few decades. The generation of glucocorticoids from cholesterol, which occurs in the zonae fasiculata and reticularis of the adrenal cortex, is tightly regulated by the hypothalamic-pituitary-adrenal (HPA) axis where glucocorticoids regulate its own generation through negative feedback inhibition. Glucocorticoids are produced de novo under this control and are released into the blood as required, with a definite circadian rhythm producing peak concentrations in the early morning [1]. When secreted into the blood, most (90-95%) of glucocorticoids are sequestered to corticosteroid-binding globulin and albumin with the unbound fraction available to interact with their receptors [2]. Metabolic inactivation of glucocorticoids occurs predominantly in the liver, but also in the kidney with inactive metabolites excreted in the urine.

3. Molecular actions of glucocorticoids: Genomic and non-genomic pathways

The classical mode of glucocorticoid-induced gene expression, i.e. the genomic effect involves ligand-dependent activation and release from chaperone proteins (heat shock protein-90 and others), translocation of the receptor-complex to the nucleus where binding of the glucocorticoid receptor to glucocorticoid response element (GRE) in the promoter of the target genes will lead to transcriptional activation of the genes within hours [3, 4]. Activation of glucocorticoid-responsive genes occurs via interaction between the DNA-bound GR and transcriptional co-activator molecules such as CREB-binding protein, which have intrinsic histone acetyltransferase activity and cause acetylation of core histones. This tags histones to recruit chromatin remodeling engines and subsequent association of RNA polymerase II resulting in gene activation [5]. Increasing evidence suggests that glucocorticoids can also cause rapid activation of signaling molecules prior to altering gene expression. These so called non-genomic effects occur within minutes of glucocorticoid exposure and are not affected by inhibiting RNA transcription [5, 6].

Metabolic effects of glucocorticoids represent most of the adverse effects of glucocorticoid therapy and are mainly ascribed to the transcriptional activity of the glucocorticoid receptor, whereas the therapeutically beneficial anti-inflammatory actions are thought to be predominantly caused by the mechanism of transrepression where the activated GR can selectively repress the transcription of specific inflammatory genes without binding to DNA itself but by a number of pleiotropic actions at the promoters of inflammatory genes. Inflammatory genes are regulated by the actions of proinflammatory transcription factors such as nuclear factor-κB (NF-κB), activator protein -1 (AP-1), and signal transducer and transcription proteins. Activated GR binds to these transcription factors, either directly or indirectly, and recruits co-repressor proteins that blunt the ability of these transcription factors to switch on inflammatory genes [7]. Furthermore, many pro-inflammatory genes are repressed by GC at post-transcriptional level via mRNA destabilization or inhibition of translation, however, this phenomenon cannot be accounted for by transrepression, therefore suggest the existence of an additional anti-inflammatory mechanism of GCs [8].

4. Ischemia/reperfusion-induced stress in the heart

Glucocorticoids play a key role in the response to stress in the heart where it can influence the regulation of blood pressure, inflammation, immune function and cellular energy metabolism [9-10]. These acute effects contribute to an adaptive response in the short term. Although the cardioprotective effects of glucocorticoids in the acute setting of ischemia/reperfusion have been experimentally demonstrated in animals [11-13] and humans [14], the molecular mechanisms still need to be fully elucidated.

Ischemia can be defined as an imbalance between the amount of oxygen, glucose and other substrates needed by the heart [15,16]. This leads to anaerobic metabolism and reduced contractile function. A biochemical imbalance occurs as the maintenance of the metabolism cannot be kept at a steady state due to inadequate coronary flow. A reduction in metabolite clearance also occurs during ischemia and intracellular pH levels drop as the acid by-products of glycolysis accumulate. The severity of ischemic injury depends on the duration of ischemia and subsequent reperfusion [15,16]. If, ischemia is maintained, reversible injury gradually transitions to irreversible injury and a myocardial infarct develops. Reperfusion with its reinforced oxygen and substrate availability is thus a prerequisite for myocardial salvage [16]. However, reperfusion after an ischemic period causes generation of free radicals and is associated with detrimental changes such as enzyme release, arrhythmias and intramyocardial haemorrhage which are known as reperfusion injuries [17]. Cardiomyocytes are highly dependent on a continuous supply of oxygen. During ischemia, cardiomyocyte capacity to generate sufficient ATP and creatine phosphate becomes depleted and multiple adaptive processes occur in response to these hypoxic environments created during ischemia. To reduce oxygen consumption, oxidative phosphorylation is limited and glycolysis is stimulated. This aids in ATP production, even under low oxygen supply [18]. Prolonged ischemia leads to cardiac failure which is characterized by the progressive death of myocytes [19]. Three major morphologies of cell death have been described, viz. apoptosis (type I), cell death associated with autophagy (type II) and necrosis (type III).

5. The basic mechanisms of Autophagy

Autophagy, from greek *self eating*, is a conserved degradation and recycling system for long-lived proteins and other sub-cellular constituents. This degradation system is inherent to all eukaryotes and is mediated by a unique organelle, the autophagosome, which, under inclusion of cytoplasmic cargo, fuses with lysosomes in order to yield recyclable nutrient metabolites. Although already described in 1966 by de Duve and Wattiaux [20], Autophagy has received significant renewed attention in the last years. This new interest is primarily based on the recently gained understanding of the molecular components of the autophagic machinery. Genetic analyses in yeast identified more than 30 autophagy-related genes (ATG), and their corresponding proteins (Atg) participating in the autophagic pathway [21].

Multiple mechanisms exist for the mode of delivery of cytoplasmic material to the lysosome, giving rise to different types of autophagy. While microphagy is characterized by cytoplasm engulfment directly at the lysosomal surface by invagination of its membrane, macroautophagy involves the synthesis of double-membrane vesicles, which sequester portions of the cytoplasm [22]. Chaperone mediated autophagy (CMA) on the other hand involves selective motif tagged protein translocation directly through the lysosomal membrane [23]. However, shared by all three mechanisms is the final step of lysosomal cargo degradation by hydrolases, allowing the recycling of degraded material. Here we will focus on macroautophagy (herein referred to as autophagy), as it is the primary mechanism for cytoplasm-to-lysosome delivery.

The autophagic process can be divided into distinct steps, which include the induction, cargo packaging, vesicle nucleation, vesicle expansion and protein retrieval, docking and fusion and finally vesicle degradation [21]. In brief, the first event is the formation of the isolation membrane of the autophagosome. The Atg1 kinase complex governs these early steps in autophagosome formation. Central to this regulation is the nutrient sensor kinase mTOR (TORC). When mTOR is suppressed due to nutrient starvation, Atg1 kinase activity is triggered and affinity for Atg13 increases [24], which leads to the recruiting of other Atg proteins to initiate autophagosome formation. Cellular sources for this autophagosome formation step have been shown to be Golgi, ER, mitochondria and the plasma membrane [25]. During this process, two strongly interdependent conjugation systems are coordinating the events leading to the formation, elongation and sealing of the isolation membrane [26]. In the first conjugation system, Atg proteins 5, 7, 10 and 12 undergo a multimerization step with Atg16, leading to the formation of an Atg16 homotetramer, which assembles with four Atg12-Atg5 conjugates [27]. In the second conjugation system, the protein Atg8 is Atg4 dependently conjugated with phosphatidylethanolamine (PE) [28]. Reactive oxygen species play a role in controlling this step, as Atg4 oxidization enables autophagosome formation to proceed [29]. Next, two kinase complexes, PI3 kinase and Atg1, participate in the late stages of autophagosome formation. Atg6 (the mammalian orthologue, beclin-1) belongs to the PI3 kinase (PI3-K) class III complex. When Atg1 interacts with Atg13, progression towards a complete autophagosome takes place [27]. Cytoplasmic cargo is now confined. Docking and fusion with a lysosome will allow acidification of the autophagosome lumen, leading to the complete and rapid degradation of cargo into constituent components that are released into cytoplasmic space via permeases (Figure 1).

6. Autophagy as a protective response during stress in the heart

The terminally differentiated nature of cardiomyocytes demands a strong molecular reliance upon a functional autophagic degradation system. In cardiomyocytes autophagy has been described already in the late 1970's where it was emphasized as an important repair mechanism of sublethal injury [30]. Sybers and coworkers demonstrated the occurrence of myocyte autophagy in a fetal mouse heart that was kept for 1 h in organ culture. In addition they observed that Autophagy was accelerated by oxygen and glucose deprivation, but the hearts function could be restored following resupply of glucose and oxygen. However, when the period of injury lasted for longer than four hours, necrotic cell death was induced [30]. To date, many models have produced clear evidence that upregulation of autophagy promotes cell survival under conditions of metabolic perturbations and energy deprivation [31-33]. In the ischaemic myocardium, autophagy is upregulated rapidly following 20 minutes of coronary artery occlusion, leading to an increased number in autophagosomes [34]. In isolated cardiomyocytes exposed to anoxia-reoxygenation it was shown that inhibition of autophagy leads to an increase in necrotic cell death, which was further increased by additional inhibition of apoptosis [35]. However, enhancing autophagic flux, as indicated by an increased rate of autophagosomal clearance, protects cardiac myocytes against ischaemic injury by reducing apoptosis [31]. Moreover, the homeostatic role of functional basal autophagic activity in the myocardium has been demonstrated by cardiac specific disruption of Atg5, manifesting in impaired contractility, hypertrophy, dilation and sarcomeric disarray [36-37].

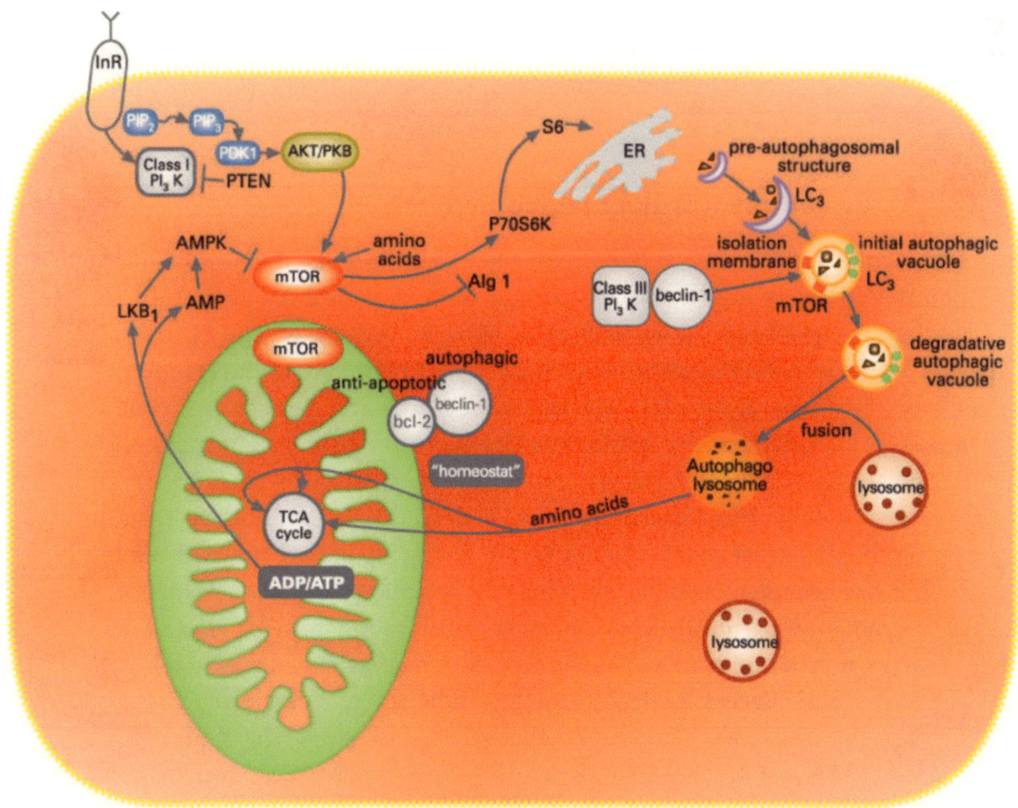

Figure 1. Schematic representation of the autophagic process, indicating the signalling network from induction to permease efflux with amino acid release, providing substrates for the TCA cycle.

7. Detrimental effects of Autophagy in the heart

Literature suggests that autophagy is uniquely controlled during ischemia and reperfusion. A large body of evidence indicates that upregulation of autophagy particularly during the reperfusion phase is detrimental and exacerbates myocyte death. Energy sensing mediated by the 5′-AMP-activated protein kinase (AMPK) appears to be central to this control mechanism. In glucose-deprived cardiac myocytes, autophagy resulting from ischemia has been shown to be accompanied by AMPK activation, and was inhibited by dominant negative AMPK, suggesting an AMPK dependent mechanism [34]. AMPK is rapidly activated during myocardial ischemia, and leads to an increase in glucose uptake and oxidation as well as fatty acid oxidation [38]. Autophagy is enhanced after reperfusion, which is accompanied by an inactivation of AMPK and an increase in beclin-1 [34]. As AMPK switches off ATP-dependent processes, [39] its inactivation at reperfusion may contribute to an unfavorable metabolic environment. Moreover, data indicate that energy sensing mediated by AMPK is also differentially controlled depending on the severity of the ischaemic insult [40]. These reports are strengthened by recent data derived from cultured myoblasts, where a differential induction of cell death was observed, which was dependent on the severity and duration of the ischaemic insult [33]. Only mild ischaemic injury induced autophagy and apoptosis, while severe injury led to primarily necrotic cell death.

8. Autophagy and myocardial metabolism

The total cellular ATP amount in the cardiac myocyte is consumed in less than one minute [41] indicating the very high metabolic demand of the myocardium, and at the same time highlighting the existence of an extremely efficient system of energy conversion. In ischaemic conditions, energy metabolism is disrupted to a level where energy production cannot meet the myocardial energy demand. However, there is a clear role for autophagy in ischemia to influence the cell's energy profile, indicative to maintain metabolic supply-demand homeostasis [33]. ATP levels decrease rapidly with ischemia and recover rapidly after reperfusion [42]. These dynamics of ATP depletion become highly relevant when considering the molecular overlap between autophagy, apoptosis and necrosis [32; 43-44, Figure 2]. It has been demonstrated that an ATP depletion of >50% is needed in order to change the mode of cell death from apoptotic to necrotic [45]. *Vice versa*, a progressive replacement of necrosis with apoptosis has been described, when intracellular ATP becomes available again [46]. Recent evidence strongly indicates the previously underestimated metabolic role of autophagy in generating metabolite substrates by shifting the cellular energetic balance [33; 47-49], suggesting that intracellular ATP availability may be controlled to a significant degree by the autophagic flux (Figure 2). These data strongly suggest that not only the magnitude of autophagic activity but also the cell's metabolic profile and microenvironment are crucial in controlling a favorable cellular response other than necrosis, and delaying apoptosis [32] (Figure 3).

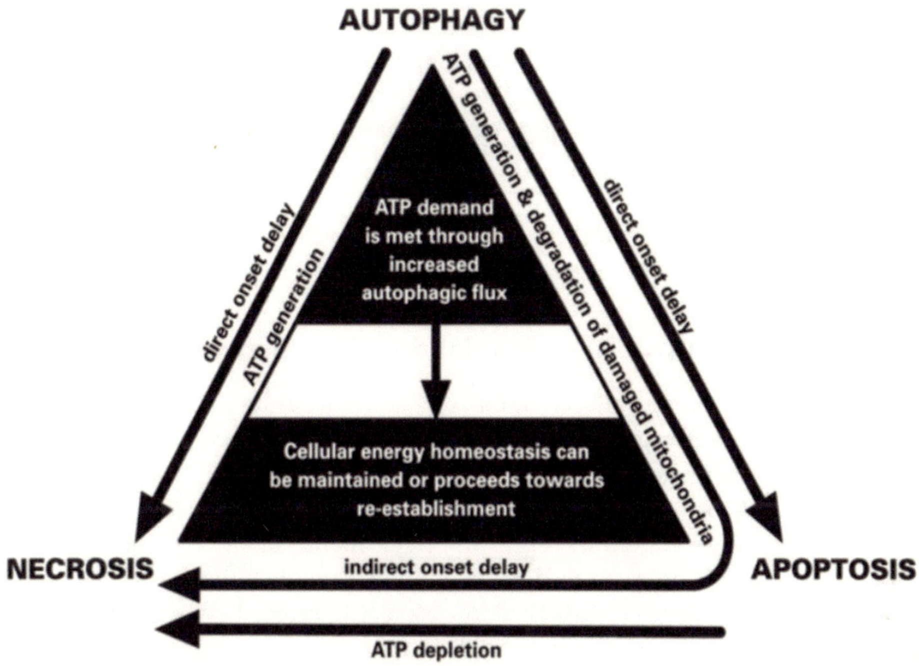

Figure 2. Recent evidence strongly indicates the previously underestimated metabolic role of autophagy in generating metabolite substrates and ATP by shifting the cellular energetic balance, with a direct and indirect effect on apoptosis and necrosis.

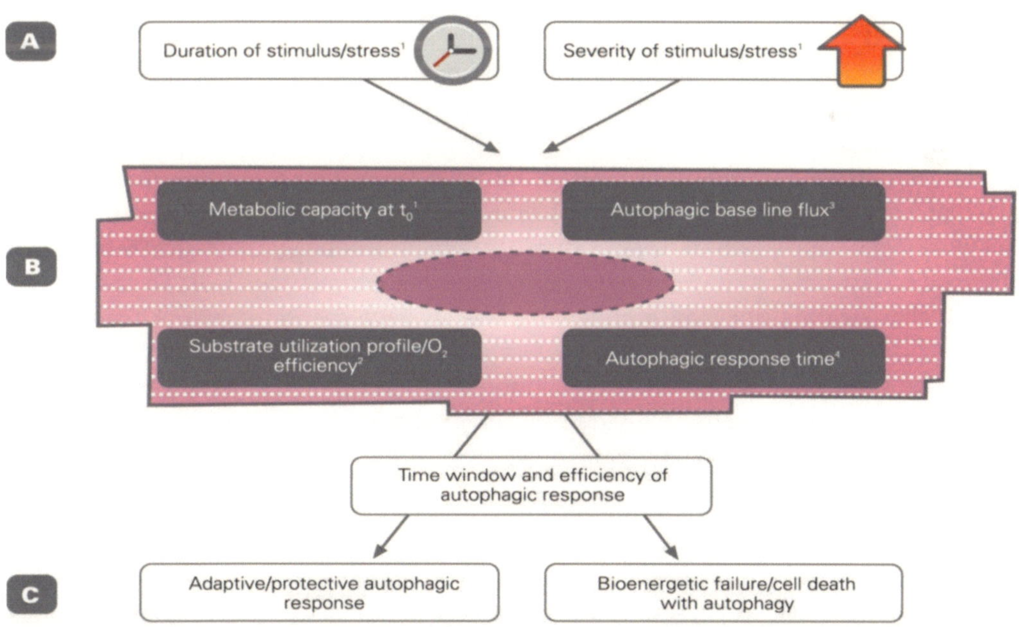

Figure 3. Whether autophagy may manifest in cytoprotection or type II programmed cell death is dependent on the severity and duration of the ischaemic insult, as well as autophagic flux- and metabolic parameters.

The above results also stress the significance of the severity and duration of the ischaemic event, to allow a sufficient induction of the autophagic machinery to take place. In fact, a direct relationship between autophagic flux and myocardial function has recently been proposed [50], indicating the strong need to measure autophagic activity accurately. Further characterization of the autophagic flux in clear context with myocardial injury will help to answer questions when autophagy functions as a primarily destructive pathway, manifesting in type II programmed cell death or when autophagy functions in a cytoprotective manner.

9. Autophagy and glucocorticoids-relationship and metabolic response

The multifaceted relationship between autophagy and glucocorticoids is already indicated in embryogenesis. Recent reports not only demonstrate an important metabolic role for autophagy during embryogenesis and postnatal development [51,52], but also indicate a likely molecular link between autophagic programmed cell death and steroids during development [53]. Embryos from the atg5$^{-/-}$ knockout mouse model die perinatally due to energy depletion, leading to a reduced plasma- and tissue amino acid concentration [54]. Moreover, increased apoptosis is displayed in various embryonic tissues derived from such embryos, supporting a role for autophagy in the removal of apoptotic bodies or in delaying the onset of apoptotic cell death [54]. Targeted disruption of beclin 1 in mice also leads to early death in embryogenesis [55]. Many examples of autophagy as a mode of programmed cell death during embryogenesis exist, suggesting that an important role for autophagic cell death in development. It has been shown that autophagic cell death requires the genes ATG7 as well as beclin 1 and can be induced by caspase-8 inhibition [56]. In addition, embryonic fibroblasts from Bax/Bak double knockout mice undergo autophagic cell death, which can be suppressed by inhibitors of autophagy and which is dependent on ATG5. These data suggest a role for Bcl-2 family proteins controlling also non-apoptotic cell death in addition to regulating apoptosis [57]. Especially in lower eukaryotes, the rise in steroid titers can elicit a transcription regulatory hierarchy that results in synchronous autophagic cell death [53]. Such steroid triggered programmed autophagic cell death has been observed in larval salivary gland cells [53] as well as motorneurons [58]. These findings suggest that steroids can play a governing role in very specific scenarios, controlling autophagic activity and the duration of increased flux, which in turn can control the synchronous induction of cell death. It is however not known, whether a robust increase in cortisol release in humans following psychological stress, trauma, sepsis or starvation can elicit similar effects on autophagic activity during embryogenesis. Such studies deserve a great deal of attention.

Although limited data are available, similarities exist between the role of the autophagic pathway as a response mechanism to metabolic perturbations and glucocorticoids in the regulation of metabolic responses. Chronic excessive activation of glucocorticoid receptors leads to major cellular metabolic rearrangements such as insulin resistance, glucose intolerance and dyslipidaemia. Obesity and metabolic syndrome, which are characterized by a nutrient overload, have been associated with a hyperactivation of tissue mTOR, indicating a blunted autophagic response [59]. The systemic glucocorticoid excess is associated with an increase in cardiovascular risk factors [60]. One of the major causes of impact on these risk factors is thought to be the glucocorticoid mediated intravascular volume overload [60]. As the access of glucocorticoids to their receptors is controlled by the isozymes of 11-β-hydroxysteroid dehydrogenase in a tissue specific manner, makes manipulation of this pathway an attractive therapeutic target. By selective isozyme inhibitors, the glucocorticoid activity can be modulated locally, keeping systemic glucocorticoid concentrations within homeostatic range.

Also in the acute setting a relationship exists between glucocorticoid availability and autophagy induction. In the treatment of acute lymphoblastic leukemia, glucocorticoids are used as crucial therapeutic agent, due to their effect on inducing G1 phase cell cycle arrest and apoptosis. Recently it was shown that dexamethasone treatment induces cell death and involves the induction of autophagy before the onset of apoptosis [61]. Moreover, another level of interaction has been demonstrated as the role of autophagy in innate immunity has recently become clear. Both the ATG16L1 risk allele as well as ATG5 are selectively important for the function of the Paneth cell, a specialized epithelial cell in the small intestine [62]. Through genome-wide association screenings it was shown that the autophagic pathway plays a fundamental role in the predisposition to the inflammatory bowel condition Chron's disease [63]. Taken together, these data indicate the dynamic relationship between glucocorticoid-induced metabolic perturbations, autophagy induction, inflammation and cell death susceptibility. Further investigations are likely to provide new insights into this complex relationship to treat cardiovascular disease more effectively by exploiting the modulation of the autophagic machinery in context with controlling local glucocorticoid activity.

10. The role of the mitogen-activated protein kinases (MAPKs) during ischemia/reperfusion-induced stress in the heart

Great efforts have been made to disentangle the intricate relationship between signalling pathways and the stress response of the heart during ischemia/reperfusion-induced injury. Analysis is complicated due to the fact that several pathways can be activated simultaneously with differential effects. It has become however evident that the MAPKs are major mediators of I/R-induced injury. Recent data pin point the MAPK's as one of the crossroads between autophagy and glucocorticoid signalling events.

Three major classes of MAPKs (Figure 4), which include the extracellular signal regulated protein kinase (ERK)/p42/44, c-Jun NH2-terminal protein kinase (JNK)/stress activated protein kinase (SAPK) and p38 MAPK families have been identified [64,65]. The ERK pathway has been depicted as a pro-survival pathway and is activated by a variety of mitogens and phorbol esters [66,67]. The JNK and p38 MAPK pathways are regarded as pro-apoptotic pathways and are mainly activated by environmental stress and inflammatory cytokines [67,68].

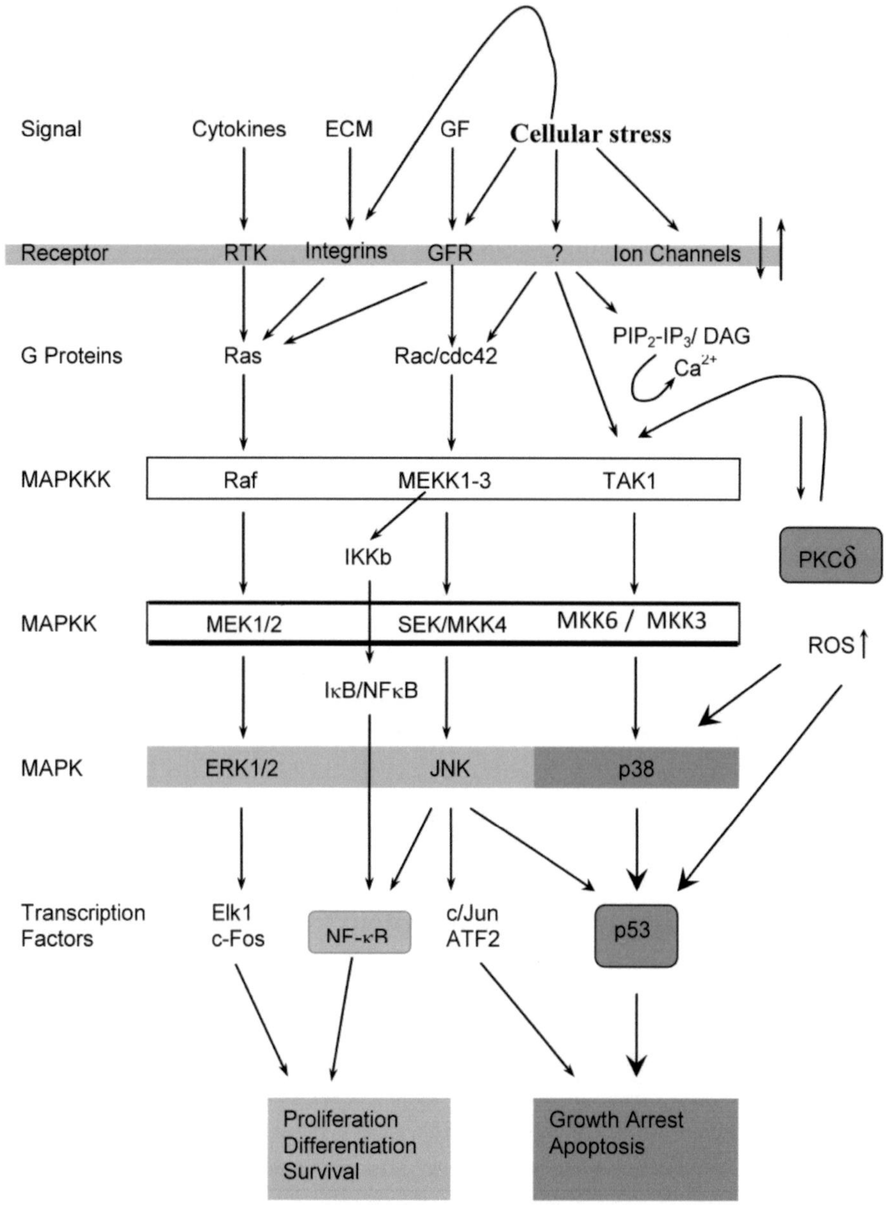

Figure 4. MAPK activation in stress-induced signalling in the heart. A variety of stress signals can activate the MAPKs directly or indirectly. MAPKs comprise a family of tyrosine/threonine kinases. Receptor activation initiates a cascade of phosphorylation events involving sequential activation of G proteins, MAPK kinase kinase (MAPKKK), MAPK kinase (MAPKK) and finally MAPK. Activated MAPK, in turn, is responsible for the phosphorylation and activation of various other regulatory proteins and transcription factors, which induce the expression of genes involved in the regulation of cell proliferation and apoptosis. ERK kinases mediate cell survival and proliferation, whereas JNK and p38 induce growth arrest and apoptosis (modified from Wernig and Xu, 2002).

Studies using chemical inhibitors have led to the conclusion that activation of the p38-MAPK promotes cardiac myocyte death during extended periods of ischemia [69-71]. In a cultured neonatal rat cardiac myocyte model, inhibition of p38-MAPK protects against ischaemic injury by decreasing LDH release [69,70]. In addition, Barancik and co-workers (2000) reported that a specific inhibitor of p38-MAPK, SB203580, protected pig myocardium against ischaemic injury in an *in vivo* model by reducing infarct size [71]. Several studies indicated that p38-MAPK plays a pivotal role in promoting myocardial apoptosis [69,72-73]. Ma and co-workers (1999) demonstrated that in isolated perfused rabbit hearts, ischemia alone caused a moderate but transient increase in p38-MAPK activity [72]. Ten minutes' reperfusion further activated p38-MAPK, which remained elevated throughout reperfusion (20 minutes). Administration of SB203580 before ischemia and during reperfusion completely inhibited p38 MAPK activation and exerted significant cardioprotective effects, characterized by decreased myocardial apoptosis and improved post-ischaemic function, as well as attenuated myocardial necrotic injury. In contrast, administering SB203580 10 minutes after reperfusion (a time point when maximal MAPK activation had already been achieved), failed to convey significant cardioprotection. Mackay and Mochly-Rosen (1999) indicated that in neonatal rat cardiac myocytes, two distinct phases of p38 activation were observed during ischemia: the first phase began within 10 minutes and lasted less than 1 hour, and the second began after 2 hours and lasted throughout the ischaemic period [69]. They demonstrated that SB203580 also protected cardiac myocytes against ischemia by reducing activation of caspase-3, a key event in apoptosis. However, the protective effect was seen even when the inhibitor was present during only the second, sustained phase of p38 MAPK activation. Subsequent studies by Yue and co-workers (2000), exposing rat neonatal cardiomyocytes to ischemia showed a rapid and transient activation of p38-MAPK and JNK [73]. On reoxygenation, further activation of SAPKs was noted. With pretreatment of the cells with SB203580 apoptotic cells were reduced, suggesting p38 MAPK activation mediates apoptosis in rat cardiac myocytes subjected to ischemia/reoxygenation. In addition, Yue and co-workers (2000) also showed that SB203580 improved cardiac contractile function in rat isolated ischaemic hearts. Inhibition of p38 MAPK activation, therefore, correlated with cardioprotection against ischemia/reperfusion injury in cardiac myocytes as well as in isolated hearts [73].

Zechner and co-workers (1998) also reported that overexpression of MKK6 (Figure 4), an upstream activator of p38 MAPK, resulted in protection of cardiac myocytes from apoptosis induced either by anisomycin or MEKK1, an upstream activator of the JNK pathway [74]. In addition, expression of MKK6 elicited a hyperthrophic response, which was enhanced by co-infection of p38β [75]. Therefore, a distinct isoform of p38 MAPK, p38β, may participate in mediating cell survival. In contrast, over expression of MKK3 in mouse cardiomyocytes led to apoptosis, which was increased by co-infection of p38α [75]. Therefore differential activation of p38-MAPK isoforms may exert opposing effects: p38α is implicated in cell death, while p38β may mediate myocardial survival.

To determine whether p38 MAPK activation was isoform selective, rat neonatal cardiomyocytes were infected with adenovirus encoding wild-type p38α or p38β [70]. They showed that transfected p38α and p38β were differentially activated during sustained ischemia, with p38α remaining activated but p38β deactivated. Furthermore, cells expressing a dominant negative p38α, which prevented ischemia-induced p38 MAPK activation, were resistant to sustained ischaemic injury. Therefore, activation of p38α MAPK isoform is detrimental during ischemia.

11. MAPK inactivation by phosphatases

Dephosphorylation of either the threonine or tyrosine residue within the MAPK activation loop T*x*Y motif alone can result in their enzymatic inactivation. In intact cells, dephosphorylation and inactivation of MAPK occur, within minutes to several hours depending on the cell type and activating stimulus. In endothelial cells, exposure to serum leads to ERK activation that is sustained at high levels for over 2 h. In contrast, different patterns can be observed in the a PC12 cell line where EGF-stimulated ERK activation is transient, with inactivation initiated within 5 min and nearly complete within 15-30 min, whereas this MAPK displays prolonged activation for several hours on stimulation with NGF [76]. It is believed that different patterns of ERK activation elicited by EGF and NGF underlie their differential effects to drive either cellular proliferation of differentiation, respectively [77]. Using PC12 cells as a model system to identify key phosphatases suppressing ERK activation, biochemical studies revealed that early rapid inactivation of these MAPKs reflects, in part, threonine dephosphorylation by the serine/threonine protein phosphatase PP2A [76].

In addition to threonine dephosphorylation, these studies also indicated that tyrosine-specific protein phosphatases (PTPs) also contribute to ERK inactivation [76]. Currently, 50 or more PTPs have been characterized [78-80], and although the PC12 cell PTPs were not identified molecularly [76], recent studies in other cell types have identified a possible role for three related PTP gene family members [81-84]. Notwithstanding the importance of these early reports on PP2A and tyrosine-specific PTPs inactivating ERKs, little is known about their general importance in terminating MAPK signaling, of the molecular mechanisms that may control phosphatase catalytic activity, or of their specificity for inactivating different MAPK isoforms.

In contrast to these protein phosphatase classes, there has been significant and rapid progress in our understanding of the role played by a subclass of PTP that possess activity for dephosphorylating both phosphotyrosine and phosphothreonine residues, known as the dual specificity phosphatases (DSPs).

The first mammalian DSP was identified as the mouse immediate early gene 3CH134 or its human orthologue CL100, which is induced rapidly after exposure to growth factors, heat shock, or oxidative stress [85-87]. Recombinant CL100/3CH134 was shown to dephosphorylate threonine and tyrosine residues of ERK, which was paralleled by its inactivation. These studies showed that CL100/3CH134 was specific for dephosphorylation of ERK when compared to a number of other unrelated phosphoproteins [76]. A correlation between 3CH134 levels and ERK inactivation was also found in mammalian cells, leading to its renaming as MAPK phosphatase-1 (MKP-1) [88]. Despite this important early work, the relevance of MKP-1 in ERK inactivation remains to be elucidated. Firstly, ERK activity is apparently normal after deletion of the MKP-1 gene in mice [89]. Secondly, it has also become evident that MKP-1 is at least as effective in inactivating JNK and p38 when compared to the ERKs [90-91]. Thirdly, newly identified members of the DSP gene family appear highly selective for ERK and may represent the true physiological regulators of this MAPK isoform. Since the initial cloning of MKP-1, eight additional mammalian DSP gene family members have been identified and characterized, which include MKP-2, MKP-3, MKP-4, MKP-5, MKP-X, PAC1, M3/6 and B59. These DSPs all appear to be effective in mediating inactivation of MAPKs.

The following model for MAPK inactivation by DSP is suggested (Figure 5). Stimulation by growth factors, cytokines, cellular stresses or some active oncogenes leads to rapid transcription of one or a subset of DSP genes. Increased DSP transcription may reflect activation of specific MAPK, although alternative pathways are not excluded. After translation of the DSP mRNA into protein, the catalytically inactive DSP translocates to a specific subcellular compartment within either the nucleus or the cytosol. Upon encountering its target MAPK, the DSP binds tightly through its amino terminus, which in turn triggers activation of the phosphatase catalytic domain. If the bound MAPK is already activated, then this will result in its rapid inactivation. Conversely, if the MAPK is not

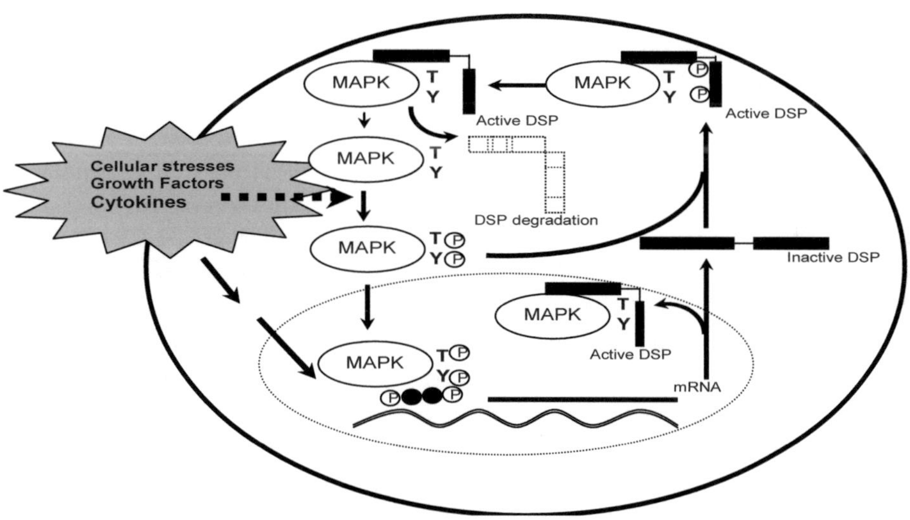

Figure 5. Cell exposure to growth factors, cytokines and cell stresses leads to induction of a subset of DSP genes. Increased expression is likely to reflect activation of transcription factors (black circles) via both MAPK-dependent and independent pathways. Newly synthesized DSPs translocate to specific subcellular compartments as dictated by anchorage and/or localization motifs not yet identified. Specific binding to target MAPKs through regions within the DSP amino terminus then triggers activation of the phosphatase catalytic domain. Bound MAPKs are in turn inactivated by dephosphorylation on threonine and tyrosine residues localized within the "activation loop" motif of TxY. Inactive MAPKs then dissociate, leaving the DSP free to bind and inactivate another MAPK molecule. In the absence of continued DSP gene transcription and protein synthesis, rapid degradation may limit their duration of activity in cells (Camps et al., 1999).

active, then its tight interaction with an active DSP is expected to block any possibility of kinase activation by a subsequent stimulus. MAPKs that fail to bind the DSP within its amino terminus remain active or susceptible to activation after extracellular stimulation. Depending on their cellular localization, these regulatory effects allow for selected inhibition of MAPK activities in specific subcellular compartments. Some DSPs have been shown to possess short half-lives [76], suggesting that in the absence of continued gene transcription and protein synthesis, their rapid turnover limits their duration of action in cells. Overall, tight control of DSP gene induction, combined with their differential binding and catalytic activation by a specific repertoire of MAPKs, provides a sophisticated mechanism for rapid targeted inactivation of selected MAPK activities.

12. MAP kinase phosphatase-1 (MKP-1): A mediator of the beneficial effects of glucocorticoids during ischemia/reperfusion-induced stress in the heart

It is noteworthy that many genes that are positively regulated at post-transcriptional level by p38-MAPK, are negatively regulated at the same level by glucocorticoids. Lasa and co-workers investigated the effects of GCs on the p38-MAPK pathway and have shown that dexamethasone destabilized cyclooxygenase-2 (COX-2) mRNA by inhibiting the function, but not the expression of p38-MAPK [92]. The inhibition of p38-MAPK was then shown to be mediated by MKP-1. We and others have also demonstrated that dexamethasone induces the expression of MKP-1 which potently inactivated p38-MAPK [93-94].

Wu and Bennet (2005) demonstrated that MKP-1 promotes cell survival in fibroblasts through the attenuation of stress responsive MAPK-mediated apoptosis [95]. Upregulation of MKP-1 has also been shown to be associated with cardioprotection by long-chain polyunsaturated fatty acids [93]. It has also been reported that transgenic mice overexpressing MKP-1 were protected, whereas knock-out mice show greater injury after ischemia/reperfusion [96]. The exact mechanism of the beneficial effects of glucocorticoids on the heart during ischemia/reperfusion-induced stress still remain to be established. In view of the significant contribution of apoptosis, necrosis and autophagy during ischemia/reperfusion-induced stress, it is expected that GC-induced cardioprotection to be associated with reduced apoptosis and necrosis. Indeed, Fan and co-workers have demonstrated that dexamethasone, administered intraperitoneally or added directly to the perfusate, significantly improved post-ischemic functional recovery and reduced infarct size compared to untreated controls [94]. These were associated with associated with upregulation of MKP-1 protein expression [94]. Furthermore, it was also shown by us that upregulation of MKP-1 during simulated ischemia/reperfusion is associated with an attenuation of apoptosis in neonatal cardiomyocytes [93].

13. Conclusions

It has been suggested that upregulation of MKP-1 during ischemia/reperfusion-induced stress attenuates myocardial injury [93,94]. MKP-1, found predominantly in the nucleus, is a dual specific phosphatase which dephosphorylates phosphotyrosine and phosphothreonine-containing protein kinases such as the MAPKs. MAPKs are known to be involved in intracellular signalling pathways that regulate gene expression in response to a variety of extracellular signals. MAPKs are activated during ischemia/reperfusion-induced stress in the heart. It was also demonstrated that glucocorticoids act via MKP-1 induction and subsequent p38-MAPK inhibition to induce cardioprotection during ischemia/reperfusion-induced stress [94].

MAPKs have been found to be involved in autophagic, apoptotic and necrotic cell death during stress responses of the heart [97-102]. Autophagy is foremost a survival mechanism which is activated in cells subjected to nutrient or growth factor deprivation. However, when the cellular stress continues, cell death may occur via autophagy, or becomes associated with features of apoptotic or necrotic cell death [103]. Apoptosis is essential for removal of specifically targeted cells, through the process of apoptotic body formation and phagocytosis [104]. Necrosis is a pathological cellular response requiring no ATP. Necrotic cells are morphologically characterized by disrupted membranes, cytoplasm and mitochondrial swelling, disintegration of organelles and complete cell lysis [105]. Cell death following ischemia/reperfusion-induced stress is thought to manifest in morphological features indicative for all three, apoptotic, necrotic and autophagic cell death [106].

MKP-1 has been shown to be involved in the regulation of apoptosis [107] and it was also very recently demonstrated that MKP-1 may lead to autophagy induction in cancer cells [108]. We have recently demonstrated that inhibition of MKP-1 and subsequent increased p38-MAPK phosphorylation during ischemia/reperfusion-induced stress is associated with attenuated autophagy and increased apoptosis and necrosis in the heart (unpublished data). We thus propose the following mechanism of GC-induced protection in the heart: During ischemia/reperfusion-induced stress in the heart, p38 MAPK is activated, GCs sustain/upregulate autophagy via an increase in MKP-1 and subsequent dephosphorylation of p38 MAPK which ultimately protects the heart from apoptosis and necrosis, driven by the effects of autophagy on the metabolic balance sheet of the heart.

Author details

Anna-Mart Engelbrecht* and Benjamin Loos
Dept of Physiological Sciences, Stellenbosch University, Stellenbosch, South Africa

14. References

[1] Dallman MF, Strack AM, Akana SF, Bradbury MJ, Hanson ES, Scribner KA (1993) Feast and famine: critical role of glucocorticoids with insulin in daily energy flow. Fron Neuroendocrinol 14: 303-347.

---

* Corresponding Author

[2] Hammond GL, Smith CL, Paterson NAM, Sibbald WJ (1990) A role for corticosteroid-globulin in delivery of cortisol to activated neutrophils. J Clin Endocrinol Metab 71: 34-39.

[3] Buttgereit F, Scheffod A (2002) Rapid glucocorticoid effects on immune cells. Steroids 6: 529-534.

[4] Stellato C (2004) Port-transcriptional and nongenomic effects of glucocorticoids. Proc Am Thorac Soc 1: 255-263.

[5] Limbourg FP, Liao JK (2003) Nontranscriptional actions of the glucocorticoid receptor. J Mol Med 81: 168-174.

[6] Wehling M (1997) Specific, nongenomic actions of steroid hormones. Annu Rev Physiol 59: 365-393.

[7] Ito K, Chung KF, Adcock IM (2006) Update on glucocorticoid action and resistance. J Allergy Clin Immunol 117: 522-543.

[8] Clark AR, Dean JL, Saklatvala J (2003) Post-transcriptional regulation of gene expression by mitogen-activated protein kinase p38. FEBS Letters 546: 37-44.

[9] Sapolsky RM, Romero LM, Munck AU (2000) How do glucocorticoids influence stress responses? Integrating permissive, suppressive, stimulatory, and preparative actions. Endocr Rev 21: 55-89.

[10] Libby P, Maroko PR, Bloor CM, Sobel BE, Braunwald E (1973) Reduction of experimental myocardial infarct size by corticosteroid administration. J Clin Invest 52: 599-607.

[11] Valen G, et al (2000) Glucocorticoid pre-treatment protects cardiac function and induces cardiac heat shock protein 72. Am J Physiol Heart Circ Physiol 279: H836-H843.

[12] Varga E, et al (2004) Inhibition of ischemia/reperfusion-induced damage by dexamethasone in isolated working rat hearts: the role of cytochrome c release. Life Sci 75: 2411-2423.

[13] Skyschally A, et al (2004) Glucocorticoid treatment prevents progressive myocardial dysfunction resulting from experimental coronary microembolization. Circulation 109: 2337-2342.

[14] Giugliano GR, Giugliano RP, Gibson CM, Kuntz RE (2003) Meta-analysis of corticosteroid treatment in acute myocardial infarction. Am J Cardiol 91: 1055-1059.

[15] Dennis SC, Gevers W & Opie LH (1991) Protons in ischemia: where do they come from: where do they go to? J Mol Cell Cardiol 23: 1077-1086.

[16] Zong WX & Thompson SB (2006) Necrotic death as a cell fate. Genes Dev 20: 1-15.

[17] Murry CE, Jennings RB & Reimer KA (1986) Preconditioning with ischemia: a delay of lethal cell injury in ischemic myocardium. Circulation 74: 1124-1136.

[18] Nishida K, Kyoi S, Yamaguchi O, Sadoshima J & Otsu K (2009) The role of autophagy in the heart. Cell Death Differ 16: 31-38.

[19] Olivetti G, Abbi R, Quaini F, Kajstura J, Cheng W, Nitahara JA, Quaini E, Di Loreto C, Beltrami CA, Krajewski S, Reed JC & Anversa P (1997) Apoptosis in the failing human heart. N Engl J Med 336: 1131-1141.

[20] De Duve C & Wattiaux R (1966) Functions of Lysosomes. Ann Rev Physiol 28: 435-92.

[21] Mizushima N, Levine B, Cuervo AM, Klionsky DJ (2008) Autophagy fights disease through cellular self-digestion. Nature 451(7182):1069-75.
[22] Baba M, Takeshige G, Baba N and Ohsumi Y (1994) Ultrastructural analysis of the autophagic process in yeast: Detection of autophagosomes and their characterization. J Cell Biol 6:903-13.
[23] Dice FJ (2007) Chaperone-Mediated Autophagy. Autophagy 4:295-9.
[24] He C, Klionskly DJ (2009) Regulation mechanisms and signaling pathways in autophagy. Annu Rev Genet 43:67-93.
[25] Cuervo AM (2010) The plasma membrane brings autophagosomes to life. Nat.Cell Biol12: 735-737.
[26] Cuervo AM (2004) Autophagy: Many paths to the same end. Mol Cell Biochem 263:55-72.
[27] Yorimitsu T and Klionsky DJ (2005) Autophagy: molecular machinery for self-eating. Cell Death Differ 12:1542-1552.
[28] Fass E, Amar N and Elazar Z (2007). Identification of essential residues for the c-terminal cleavage of mammalian LC3. Autophagy 3:1:48-50.
[29] Scherz-Shouval R, Shvets E, Elazar Z (2007) Oxidation as a post-translational modification that regulates autophagy. Autophagy 4:371-3.
[30] Sybers HD, Ingwall J, DeLuca M (1978) Autophagy in cardiac myocytes. Recent Adv Stud Cardiac Struct Metab 12:453-463.
[31] Hamacher-Brady A, Brady NR, Gottlieb RA (2006) Enhancing macroautophagy protects against ischemia/reperfusion injury in cardiac myocytes. J Biol Chem 281: 29776-29787.
[32] Loos B, Engelbrecht AM (2009). Cell death: a dynamic response concept. Autophagy 5(5):1–14.
[33] Loos, B; Genade, S.; Ellis, B.; Lochner, A.; Engelbrecht, A. M (2011). At the core of survival: Autophagy delays the onset of both apoptotic and necrotic cell death in a model of ischemic cell injury. Exp Cell Res 317: 1437-1453.
[34] Matsui Y, Takagi H, Qu X, Abdellativ M, Sakoda H, Asano T (2007) Distinct roles of autophagy in the heart during ischemia and reperfusion: roles of AMP-activated protein kinase and beclin 1 in mediating autophagy. Circ Res100: 914-922.
[35] Dosenko VE, Nagibin VS, Tumanovska LV and Moibenko AA (2006) Protective effect of autophagy in anoxia-reoxygenation of isolated cardiomyocytes? Autophagy 2(4): 305-306.
[36] Yue Z, Jin S, Yang C, Levine AG, Heintz N (2003). Beclin 1, an autophagy gene essential for early embryonic development, is a haploinsufficient tumor suppressor. Proc Natl Acad Sci USA; 100: 15077-15082.
[37] Nakai A, Yamaguchi O, Takeda T, Higuchi Y, Hikoso S, Taniike M (2007) The role of autophagy in cardiomyocytes in the basal state and in response to hemodynamic stress. Nat Med 13: 619-624.
[38] Gustafsson ÅB, Gottlieb RA (2009). Autophagy in ischemic heart disease. Circ Res 104:150-158.
[39] Lam A, Lopaschuk GD (2007) Anti-anginal effects of partial fatty acid oxidation inhibitors. Curr Opin Pharmacol 7:179-185.

[40] Altarejos JY, Taniguchi M, Clanacham AS, Lopaschuk GD (2005). Myocardial ischemia differentially regulates LKB1 and an alternate 5'-AMP-activated protein kinase kinase. J Biol Chem 280:183-190.
[41] Jafri MS, Dudycha SJ, O'Rourke B (2001). Cellular energy metabolism: models of cellular respiration. Annu Rev Biomed Eng 3:57–81.
[42] Takagi H, Matsui Y, Sadoshima J (2007). The role of autophagy in mediating cell survival and death during ischemia and reperfusion in the heart. Antioxid Redox Signal 9:1373-1381.
[43] Grover GJ, Atwal KS, Sleph PG, Wang FL, Monshizadegan H, Monticello T (2004) Excessive ATP hydrolysis in ischemic myocardium by mitochondrial F1F0 ATPase: effect of selective pharmacological inhibition of mitochondrial ATPase hydrolase activity. Am J Physiol Heart Circ Physiol 287: 1747-1755.
[44] Kunapuli S, Rosanio S, Schwarz ER (2006) "How do cardiomyocytes die?" Apoptosis and autophagic cell death in cardiac myocytes. J Card Fail 12:381-391.
[45] Leist M, Single B, Castoldi AF, Kuhnle S, Nicotera P (1997) Intracellular adenosine triphosphase (ATP) concentration: A switch in the decision between apoptosis and necrosis. J Exp Med 185: 1481-6.
[46] Tatsumi T, Shiraishi J, Keira N, Akashi K, Mano A, Yamanaka S (2003) Intracellular ATP is required for mitochondrial apoptotic pathways in isolated hypoxic rat cardiac myocytes. Cardiovasc Res 59: 428-40.
[47] Singh R and Cuervo AM (2011). Autophagy in the cellular energetic balance. Cell Metabolism 13: 495-504
[48] Mizushima N and Klionsky DJ (2007) Protein turnover via autophagy: implications for metabolism. Annu Rev Nutr 27:19-40.
[49] Singh R , Kaushik S, Wang Y, Xiang Y, Novak I, Komatsu M, Tanaka K, Cuervo AM and Czaja MJ (2009) Autophagy regulates lipid metabolism. Nature 458: 1131-1135.
[50] Nemchenko A, Chiong M, Turer A, Lavandero S, Hill JA (2011). Autophagy as therapeutic target in cardiovascular disease. JMCC 51: 584-593.
[51] Juhász G, Csikós G, Sinka R, Erdélyi M, Sass M (2003) The Drosophila homolog of Aut1 is essential for autophagy and development. FEBS Lett 543: 154-8.
[52] Levine B and Klionsky DJ (2004). Development by self-digestion: molecular mechanisms and biological functions of autophagy. Developmental Cell 6: 463-477.
[53] Martin DN, Balgley B, Dutta S, Chen J, Rudnick P, Cranford J, Kantartzis S, DeVoe DL, Lee C, Baehrecke EH (2007) Proteomic analysis of steroid-triggered autophagic programmed cell death during Drosophila development. Cell Death Differ 14: 916-23.
[54] Kuma A, Hatano M, Matsui M, Yamamoto A, Nakaya H, Yoshimori T, Ohsumi Y, Tokuhisa T, Mizushima N (2004) The role of autophagy during the early neonatal starvation period. Nature 432: 1032-6.
[55] Yue Z, Jin S, Yang C, Levine AG, Heintz N (2003). Beclin 1, an autophagy gene essential for early embryonic development, is a haploinsufficient tumor suppressor. Proc Natl Acad Sci USA 100: 15077-15082.
[56] Yu L, Alva A, Su H, Dutt P, Freundt E, Welsh S (2004) Regulation of an ATG7-beclin 1 program of autophagic cell death by caspase-8. Science 304: 1500-1502.

[57] Shimizu S, Kanaseki T, Mizushima N, Mizuta T, Arakawa-Kobayashi S, Thompson CB and Tsujimoto Y (2004) Role of Bcl-2 family proteins in a non-apoptotic programmed cell death dependent on autophagy genes. Nature Cell Biology 6: 1221 – 1228.

[58] Kinch G, Hoffman KL, Rodrigues EM, Zee MC, Weeks JC (2003) Steroid-triggered programmed cell death of a motorneuron is autophagic and involves structural changes in mitochondria. J Comp Neurol 17: 384-403.

[59] Khamzina L, Veilleux A, Bergeron S, Marette A (2005). Increased activation of the mammalian target of rapamycin pathway in liver and skeletal muscle of obese rats: possible involvement in obesity-linked insulin resistance. Endocrinology 146:1473-1481.

[60] Hadoke PWF, Iqbal J, Walker BR (2009). Therapeutic manipulation of glucocorticoid metabolism in cardiovascular disease. Brit J Pharmacol 156: 689-712.

[61] Laane E, Tamm KP, Buentke E, Ito K, Khahariza P, Oscarsson J, Corcoran M, Bkörklund AC, Hultenby K, Lundin J, Heyman M, Söderhäll S, Mazur J, Porwit A, Pandolfi PP, Zhivotovsky B, Panaretakis T and Grandér D (2009). Cell death induced by dexamethasone in lymphoid leukemia is mediated through initiation of autophagy. Cell Death Differ 16: 1018-1029.

[62] Cadwell K, Liu JY, Brown SL, Miyoshi H, Loh J, Lennerz JK, Kishi C, Kc W, Carrero JA, Hunt S, Stone CD, Brunt EM, Xavier RJ, Sleckman BP, Li E, Mizushima N, Stappenbeck TS, Virgin HW (2008) A key role for autophagy and the autophagy gene Atg16 in mouse and human intestinal Paneth cells. Nature 13(456): 259-63.

[63] Deretic V (2009) Links between autophagy, innate immunity, inflammation and Chron's disease. Dig Dis 27:246-251.

[64] Begum N, Ragolia L, Rienzie J, McCarthy M & Duddy N (1989) Regulation of mitogen-activated protein kinase phosphatase-1 induction by insulin in vascular smooth muscle cells. Evaluation of the role of the nitric oxide signalling pathway and potential defects in hypertension. J Biol Chem 273: 25164-25170.

[65] Cowan KJ & Storey (2003) Mitogen-activated protein kinases: new signalling pathways functioning in cellular responses to environmental stress. J Exp Biol 206: 1107-1115.

[66] Marczin N, El-Habashi N, Hoare GS, Bundy RE & Yacoub M (2003) Antioxidants in myocardial ischemia-reperfusion injury: therapeutic potential and basic mechanisms. Arch Biochem Biophys 420: 222-236.

[67] Junttila MR, Li SP, Wetermarck J (2008) Phosphatase-mediated crosstalk between MAPK signalling pathways in the regulation of cell survival. Faseb J 22: 954-965.

[68] Weston CR & Davis RJ (2007) The JNK signal transduction pathway. Curr Opin Cell Biol 19: 142-149.

[69] Mackay K, Mochly-Rosen D (2001) Arachidonic acid protects neonatal rat cardiac myocytes form ischaemic injury through ε protein kinase C. Cardiovasc Res 50: 65-74.

[70] Saurin AT, Martin JC, Heads RJ, Foley C, Mockridge JW, Wright MJ, Wang Y, Marber S (2000) The role of differential activation of p38 mitogen activated protein kinases in preconditioned ventricular myocytes. Faseb J 14: 2237-2246.

[71] Barancik M, Htun P, Strohm C, Killian S, Schaper W (2000) Inhibition of the cardiac p38-MAPK pathway by SB20350 delays ischemic cell death. J Cardiovasc Pharmacol 35: 474-483.

[72] Ma XL, Kumar S, Gao F, Louden CS, Lopez BL, Christopher TA, Wang C, Lee JC, Feuerstein GZ, Yue TL (1999) Inhibition of p38 mitogen-activated protein kinase decreases cardiomyocyte apoptosis and improves cardiac function after myocardial ischemia and reperfusion. Circulation 99: 1685-1691.
[73] Yue TL, Wang C, Gu J-L, Ma XL, Kumar S, Lee JC, Feuerstein GZ, Thomas H, Maleeff B, Ohlstein EH (2000) Inhibition of extracellular signal-regulated kinase enhances ischemia/reoxygenation-induced apoptosis in cultured cardiac myocytes and exaggerates reperfusion injury in isolated perfused hearts. Circ Res 86: 692-699.
[74] Zechner D, Craig R, Hanford HS, McDonough PM, Sabbadini RA, Glembotski CC (1998) MKK6 activates myocardial cell NF-kappaB and inhibits apoptosis in a p38 mitogen-activated protein kinase-dependent manner. J Biol Chem 273: 8232-8239.
[75] Wang X, Martindale JL, Liu Y, Holbrook NJ (1998) The cellular response to oxidative stress: influences of mitogen-activated protein kinase signalling pathways on cell survival. Biochem J 333: 291-300.
[76] Alessi DR, Gomez N, Moorhead G, Lewis T, Keyse SM, Cohen P (1995) Inactivation of p42 MAPK kinase by protein phosphatase 2A and a protein tyrosine phosphatase, but not CL 100, in various cell lines. Curr Biol 5: 283-295.
[77] Marshall CJ (1995) Specificity of receptor tyrosine kinase signalling: transient versus sustained extracellular signal-regulated kinase activation. Cell 80: 179-185.
[78] Neel BG, Tonks NK (1997) Protein tyrosine phosphatases in signal transduction. Curr Opin Cell Biol 9: 193-204.
[79] Hooft van Huijsduijnen R (1998) Protein tyrosine phosphatases: counting trees in the forest. Gene 225: 1-8.
[80] Denu JM, Dixon JE (1998) Protein tyrosine phosphatases: mechanisms of catalysis and regulation. Curr Opin Chem Biol 2: 663-641.
[81] Wurgler-Murphy SM, Maeda T, Witten EA, Saito H (1997) Regulation of the Saccharomyces cerevisiae HOG1 mitogen activated protein kinase by PTP2 and PTP3 protein tyrosine phosphatases. Mol Cell Biol 15: 1289-1297.
[82] Shiozaki K, Russel P (1995) Cell-cycle control linked to extracellular environment by MAP kinase pathway in fission yeast. Nature 378: 739-743.
[83] Millar JB, Buck V, Wilkinson MG (1995) Pyp1 and Pyp2 PTPases dephosphorylated an osmosensing MAP kinase controlling cell size at division in fission yeast. Genes Dev 9: 2117-2130.
[84] Zhan X-L, Deschenes RJ, Guan KL (1997) Differential regulation of FUS3 MAP kinase by tyrosine-specific phosphatases PTP2/PTP3 and dual-specificity phosphatase MSG5 in Saccharomyces cervisiae. Genes Dev 11: 1690-1702.
[85] Keyse SM & Emslie EA (1992) Oxidatives stress and heat shock induce a human gene encoding a protein-tyrosine phosphatase. Nature 359: 644-646.
[86] Charles CH, Sun H, Lau LF, Tonks NK (1993) MKP-1, an immediate early gene product is a dual specificity phosphatase that dephosphorylates MAP kinases in vivo. Cell 75(3): 487-493.
[87] Noguchi T, Metz R, Chen L, Mattei MG, Carasco D, Bravo R (1993) Structure, mapping and expression of erp, a growth factor-inducible gene encoding a nontransmembrane

protein tyrosine phosphatase, and effect of ERP on cell growth. Mol Cell Biol 13: 5195-5205.
[88] Sun H, Charles CH, Lau LF, Tonks NK (1993) MKP-1 (3Ch134), an immediate early gene product, is a dual specificity phosphatase that dephosphorylates MAP kinase in vivo. Cell 75: 487-493.
[89] Dorfman K, Carrasco D, Gruda M, Ryan C, Lira SA, Bravo R (1996) Disruption of the erp/mkp-1 gene does not affect mouse development: normal MAP kinase activity in ERP/MKP-1-deficient fibroblasts. Oncogene 13: 925-931.
[90] Chu Y, Solski PA, Khosravi-Far R, Der CJ, Kelly K (1996) the mitogen-activated protein kinase phosphatases PAC1, MKP-1 and MKP-2 have unique substrate specificities and reduced activity in vivo towards ERK2 sevenmaker mutation. J Biol Chem 271: 6497-6501.
[91] Franklin CC, Kraft AS (1997) Conditional expression of the mitogen-activated protein kinase (MAPK) phosphatase MKP-1 preferentially inhibits p38 MAPK and stress-activated protein kinase in U937 cells. J Biol Chem 272: 16917-16923.
[92] Lasa M, Abraham SM, Boucheron C, Saklatvala J, Clark AR (2002) Dexamethasone causes sustained expression of mitogen-activated protein kinase (MAPK) phosphatase 1 and phosphatase-mediated inhibition of MAPK p38. Mol Cel Biol 22: 7802-7811.
[93] Engelbrecht A-M, Engelbrecht P, Genade S, Niesler C, Page C, Smuts M, Lochner A (2005) Long-chain polyunsaturated fatty acids protect the heart against ischemia/reperfusion-induced injury via a MAPK dependent pathway. J Mol Cell Cardiol 39: 940-954.
[94] Fan WJ, Genade S, Genis A, Huisamen B, Lochner A (2009) Dexamethasone-induced cardioprotection: a role for the phosphatase MKP-1? Life Sci 84: 838-846.
[95] Wu JJ & Bennett AM (2005) Essential role for mitogen-activated protein (MAP) kinase phosphatase-1 in stress-responsive MAPK and cell survival signalling. J Biol Chem 280: 16461-16466.
[96] Kaiser RA, Bueno OF, Lips DJ, Doevendans PA, Jones F, Kimball TF, Molkentin JD (2004) Targeted inhibition of p38 mitogen-activated protein kinase antagonizes cardiac injury and cell death following ischemia-reperfusion in vivo. J Biol Chem 279: 15524-1530.
[97] Lee TH, Huang Q, Oikemus S, Shank J, Ventura JJ, Cusson N, Vaillancourt RR, Su B, Davis RJ, Kelliher MA (2003) The death domain kinase RIP1 is essential for tumor necrosis factor alpha signalling to p38 mitogen-activated protein kinase. Mol Cell Biol 23: 8377-8385.
[98] Khan TA, Bianchi C, Ruel M, Voisine P, Sellke FW (2004) Mitogen-activate protein kinase pathways and cardiac surgery. J Thorac Cardiovasc Surg 127: 806-811.
[99] Lee TH, Cusson N, Kelliher MA (2004) The kinase activity of Rip1 is not required for tumor necrosis factor alpha-induced IkappaB kinase or p38 MAP kinase activation or for ubiquitination of Rip1 by Traf2. J Biol Chem 279: 33185-33191.
[100] Codongo P & Meijer AJ (2005) Autophagy and signalling: Their role in cell survival and cell death. Cell Death Differ 12(2): 1509-1518.

[101] Park KJ, Lee SH, Lee CH, Jang JY, Chung J, Kwon MH, Kim YS (2009) Upregulation of beclin-1 expression and phosphorylation of Bcl-2 and p53 are involved in the JNK-mediated autophagic cell death. Biochem Biophys Res Commun 382: 762-729.

[102] Yang LY, Wu KH, Chiu WT, Wang SH & Shih CM (2009) The cadmium-induced death of mesangial cells results in nephrotoxicity. Autophagy 5: 571-572.

[103] Maiuri MC, Zalckvar E, Kimchi A, Kroemer G (2007) Self-eating and self-killing: crosstalk between autophagy and apoptosis. Nat Rev Mol Cell Biol 8: 741-752.

[104] Peter C, Waibel M, Radu CG, Yang LV, Witte ON, Schulze-Osthoff K, Wesselborg S, Lauber K (2008) Migration to apoptotic "find-me" signals is mediated via the phagocyte receptor G2A. J Biol Chem 283: 5296-5305.

[105] Zong WX & Thompson CB (2006) Necrotic death as a cell fate. Genes Dev 20: 1-15.

[106] Murphy E & Steenbergen C (2008) Mechanisms underlying acute protection from cardiac ischemia-reperfusion injury. Physiol Rev 88: 581-609.

[107] Morisco C, Marrone C, Trimarco V, Crispo S, Monti MG, Sadoshima J, Trimarco B (2007) Insulin resistance affects the cytoprotective effect of insulin in cardiomyocytes through an impairment of MAPK phosphatase-1 expression. Cardiovasc Res 76: 453-464.

[108] Lu HH, Kao SY, Liu TY, Liu ST, Huang WP, Chang KW, Lin SC (2010) Areca nut extract induced oxidative stress and upregulated hypoxia inducing factor leading to autophagy in oral cancer cells. Autophagy 6: 725-737.

Chapter 6

Glucocorticoids and the Intestinal Environment

Hümeyra Ünsal and Muharrem Balkaya

Additional information is available at the end of the chapter

http://dx.doi.org/10.5772/51977

1. Introduction

For thousands, perhaps millions of years, human have marveled to understand how the body is formed and function, how it maintains its wholeness and healthy state, and how disordered states occur. In frame of holistic philosophy of ancient eastern cultures, a person had been accepted as physical, emotional, mental, and spiritual ones. In this concept, the balance of the body, mind and spirit were accepted as the healthy state of an individual [1,2]. The ancient Greeks defended the concept of the four humors doctrine; blood, black bile, yellow bile, and phlegm. *Ad modum* this doctrine these four humors in a healthy person were believed to be balanced, and the reason why a person fell ill was due to the fact that these fluids were disturbed [3,4]. With the separation of medicine from superstition, magic and religion by famous Greek physician Hippocrates in around 5th century B.C., more realistic and relevant approaches could be developed to better understanding the life, structures of living creatures and their healthy and diseased conditions. These and the time-dependent innovative developments in technology and science throughout the following centuries led to more concrete observations, mainly on animals. Gathered evidences and additive knowledge base from these observations mankind led mankind to make realistic definitions on the subjects "the structure, integrity and functions" of the animal and human body. In 19th century Louis Pasteur, a French chemist and microbiologist, stated the germ theory of diseases. He believed that micro-organisms (bacteria) infect animals and humans, thus they cause diseases [5]. At the same times, a French Physiologist Claude Bernard tried to understand how living creatures maintain their integrity, and how it is regulated, and defeated. He discriminated the internal environment from the external environment and was in opinion that living creatures maintain their internal milieu relatively constant under continuously changing environmental conditions. Claude Bernard [6] attributed also an important role to nervous system in the maintenance of internal environment in physiological ranges in human and animal organisms and remarked the substantial differences between animals and plants in this respect. Since that time, the interest of the researchers in different fields worldwide is mainly focused on possible regulation mechanisms of various living species. Thus, it can be said that the philosophical roots of the concept "stress" and "stress physiology" is going back to the early observations that living creatures are exposed continuously to the effects of various environmental challenges against which they have to defend their integrity, and following statement from Claude Bernard that living creatures strive to maintain their internal environments relatively constant *via* various homeokinetic mechanisms even if their environmental conditions are changing, thereby keep their normal physiological functioning and prerequisite for a free, independent live or shortly *'la fixité du miliéu interieur est la condition d'une vie libre et indépendante'* as defined by him *"Il y a pour l'animal deux milieux: un milieu extérieur dans lequel est placé l'organisme, et un milieu intérieur dans lequel vivent les éléments des tissus"*. However, Hans Selye, one of the Pioneers and founders of stress from 1930's, was the first who introduced the term "stress" as the real or perceived physical or psychological events which are threaten the homeokinesis in medical terminology. *Ad modum* Selye the stress is somewhat like living, not so easy to define, although there is no doubt about its presence [7]. The environmental challenges affecting a living creature, thus causing stress, can vary from physical, to chemical and bio-psycho-social factors, while all the reactants, their contra- and/or co-players within the living systems are of chemical nature at the last instance; intracellular or intra-bodily signaling elements as either hormones including glucocorticoids and catecholamines or neurotransmitters, cytokines and chemokines, etc., or a group or all of them functioning simultaneously within the body for the same purposes.

Stress and the glucocorticoids are associated or interweaving concepts with each other. Indeed, to physiologists the term "stress" has come to mean any event that elicits increased cortisol secretion [8]. However, as it is well known, glucocorticoids are not only mediators of the stress responses; they take a part in peripheral components of stress responses. The stress response is mediated by the stress system which is composed of two components; central nervous system and the peripheral part. The central, greatly interconnected effectors of this system include the hypothalamic hormones arginine vasopressin, corticotropin-releasing hormone/factor (CRH/CRF) and pro-opiomelanocortin-derived peptides, and the locus ceruleus and autonomic norepinephrine centers in the brainstem. The peripheral components of the stress system include (*a*) the peripheral limbs of the hypothalamic-pituitary-adrenal (HPA) axis; (*b*) the efferent sympathetic-adrenomedullary system, and (*c*) components of the parasympathetic system [9-11]. There are also bidirectional positive feedback regulation between the CRF secreted paraventricular nucleus of hypothalamus and central noradrenergic system [9,11,12].

Stressors activate different physiological processes. The first classical response is the secretion of adrenalin and noradrenalin hormones from the adrenal medulla *via* activation of sympathetic nervous system. This response is called "fight or flight syndrome", because adrenaline and noradrenalin increase the respiratory rate, the heartbeat, the concentration of glucose in circulating blood and the blood flow to the skeletal muscles. This fast response is primarily related to survival. Stressors also activate the HPA axis. The activation of this axis begins with the stimulation of parvocelular neurons of hypothalamus and secretion of CRH. CRH stimulates the secretion of adrenocorticotrophic hormone (ACTH) from the adenohypophsis and the ACTH acts on cortex of adrenal glands and stimulates the release of glucocorticoid hormones. GC hormones (corticosterone in rodents and cortisol in humans), which are the ultimate product of HPA axis activation, act on multiple bodily systems to maintain homeokinesis. They stimulate protein catabolism, gluconeogenesis and release of glycerol and fatty acids into the blood, maintain the vasoconstructive effect of norepinephrine, inhibit glucose uptake and oxidation by many body cells except the brain (insulin antagonism) and also inhibit inflammation and specific immune response [8-11].

The secretion of ACTH, and therefore of cortisol or corticosterone, is stimulated by several hormones and molecules in addition to hypothalamic CRH. Depending on the stressor, substances such as vasopressin, epinephrine, angiotensin II, various cytokines (tumor necrosis factor (TNF)-α, interleukin (IL)-1, and IL-6), and lipid mediators of inflammation affect the hypothalamic, pituitary, and/or adrenal components of the HPA axis and potentiate its activity. Glucocorticoids play an important role in the regulation of basal activity of the HPA axis, as well as in the termination of the stress response by acting at extra-hypothalamic centers, the hypothalamus, and the pituitary gland. The negative feedback of glucocorticoids on the secretion of CRH and ACTH serves to limit the duration of the total tissue exposure of the organism to glucocorticoids, thus minimizing the catabolic, lipogenic, anti-reproductive, and immunosuppressive effects of these hormones [8,10,11].

The activation of the HPA is a longer-term adjustment by the humans or animals to the changes in their micro- or surrounding environments. Selye [7] called it as the 'general adaptation syndrome' (GAS). The process of adaptation, also known as "allostasis" (literally "maintaining stability, through change"), supports the homeokinesis [13]. In acute stress, the activation of both sympathetic system and HPA axis are essential for survival of individual and they help to re-establish or maintain homeokinesis through adaptation. However, in chronic periods, prolonged or repeated activation of stress systems can result in cumulative biological changes (known as allostatic load) and can alter adaptive mechanism. If the ability of the organisms to maintain their integrity is poor or not strong enough to compensate the effects of environmental challenges, they can also harm the living creatures *via* various mechanisms. Excessive or inappropriate, inadequate adaptive responses to stress may play a causal role in development of certain diseases [10,11,14,15]. Indeed, depending on the stressors and their severity as well as the capability of living creatures to respond them, the reactions of living creatures to the stressors can be systematic, also reflecting itself throughout the whole body, or mainly local or regional, reflecting self at the organel/celluler/organ or system levels [11,14]. Similarly, the application of glucocorticoids for a long time can also cause events with serious consequences [16].

The gastrointestinal tract and the immune system are particularly responsive to different stressors. This system has many cellular targets for the stress mediators such as catecholamines, glucocorticoids and CRF [17-19]. The association between stress and various gastrointestinal diseases, including functional bowel disorders, inflammatory bowel disease (IBD), peptic ulcer disease and gastroeosophageal reflux disease, is being actively investigated [15,17]. However, there is a parodox that the chronic stress plays a role in inflammatory bowel disease while the glucocorticoid therapy is widely used to cure the same disease.

Gastrointestinal system (GIS) is the biggest surface area (~200 m^2) of the body that is binding the organism to the external environment. This system is continuously exposed to various antigens from consumed foods and resident bacteria and also from potentially harmful pathogens, such as viruses, bacteria, fungi or parasites. Besides digestion and absorption processes, it forms a barrier between the internal and external environments [20]. Intestinal barrier is composed of various components such as tight junction conformation between the intestinal epithelial cells, mucosal immune system, mucin secretion, and intestinal microbiota. The barrier function is quite critical process because of the barrier should confirm the hyporesponsiveness or tolerance towards commensal bacteria while maintaining the ability to fight pathogenic microorganisms. The breakdown of this critical balance usually results in inflammation-associated damages. Gastrointestinal system is rather complex system, which has own nervous and endocrine system. The enteric nervous system is connected bidirectionally to the brain by parasympathetic and sympathetic pathways forming the brain–gut axis. The description of stress-induced alterations in this axis is thought to be important for the solving problems of many stress-related gastrointestinal disorders [17,20]. A number of paracine acting endocrine cells have important functions for the regulation of digestion processes. These hormones exist in both central nervous system and gastrointestinal plexus neurons where they function as neurotransmitters or neuromodulators [8]. Recent findings suggest that glucocorticoid hormones may also be synthesized from extra-adrenal tissues such as brain, skin, vascular endothelium and intestine. These tissues express steroidogenic enzymes and were claimed to be potential extra-adrenal sources of glucocorticoids [21]. It is emphasized that intestinal glucocorticoid synthesis might be of potential importance in regulation of mucosal immune responses and information of inflammatory bowel disease [22].

Gastrointestinal system hosts also a large number of microorganisms. They all together are called as gastrointestinal microbiota, and form the great part of the system. The microbiota–host interactions play an active role in many physiologic and pathophysiologic processes of the host [19,23,24]. While gastrointestinal microbiota could affect the stress response [25] and intestinal structure and functions of the host [23,24], stress hormones of the host organism such as the catecholamines can also alter directly growth, motility, biofilm formation and/or virulence of pathogens and commensal bacteria [19,26,27] or they may affect their microbiota indirectly by changing the intestinal environment [20].

The effects of stress on important physiological functions of the gut include; motility, secretion and absorption, visceral sensitivity, mucosal integrity, permeability, immune system, blood flow, microbiota and microbiota-host interactions [17,20]. Some stress-related alterations in gut physiology also can be induced by exogenous glucocorticoids [28-30]. However; recent findings using central and peripheral CRF administration showed that CRF and their receptor subtypes (CRF1 and CRF2) are playing important roles in many stress-related alterations of the gut. The stress-related alterations including intestinal permeability, mast cell activity [20], goblet cell and mucin formation [31], and motility alterations [32] can be mimicked by the CRF agonists and inhibited by CRF receptor antagonists. Therefore; CRF have been suggested as a target to treat stress-induced functional gastrointestinal disorders.

In this chapter, the effects of stress and stress-related hormones, especially glucocorticoids on the components of intestinal environment suc as intestinal epithelium, mucin formation, mucosal immune system, intestinal microbiota and microbiota-host interactions, and also the role of corticosteroids and stress in bacterial colonization and intestinal diseases were reviewed.

2. Stress models for gastrointestinal studies

A great number of animal models of stress (acute/chronic, early life/adult, physical/ psychological or both physical and psychological) have been described for studying the effects of stress on gastrointestinal functions. For this purpose, rather naturally (Wistar-Kyoto rats) or genetically modified stress susceptible animals were also used. As denoted by Soderholm and Perdue [20], stress models that psychological effects are more powerful than the physical effects are preferred for mimicking the effects of the life and environmental stress on several pathologies. However, the kind and duration of stressors and other factors including genetic or perinatal environment, etc. might be a key factor in the evaluation of the stress effects on specific gastrointestinal functions such as stress-induced visceral hyperalgesia. Depending on the characteristics of the stressors and the time-course of their effects, alterations caused by stress can be immediate, delayed, transient or sustained or never be seen [33,34]. For example, the small intestinal transit was significantly inhibited by restraint stress, but not by footshock stress although plasma corticosterone levels were significantly elevated to the same extent by restraint stress and foot-shock stress [33].

Williams et al [35] reported that acute mild restraint (wrap restraint) elevated plasma levels of adrenocorticotropic hormone and beta-endorphin, and caused analgesia. Gastric ulcer did not form, gastric emptying was not affected, however, small intestinal transit was inhibited, and large intestinal transit was stimulated by wrap restraint stress, and there was an associated increase in fecal excretion. Because of neither adrenalectomy nor hypophysectomy have prevented the response of the intestine to stress, they suggested that adrenal or pituitary-derived factors are not responsible for mediating the effects of stress on the gut.

Restraint stress is most widely used as an acute stress model. Restraining can be supplied with restraint devices or by wrap restraint for times varying from 30 min to 4 hours. This model could be modified with a cold environment (cold restraint stress) or water immersion (water immersion restraint stress) for creating both physical and psychological stress [20]. Cold enhanced the changes in rat intestine caused by restraining. However, plasma corticosterone levels increased in both restraint and cold restraint stressed rats in same extent compared with fasted unstressed rats. Fasting corticosterone levels also increased compared with the fed rats [36].

The acute (one time) and chronic (1 hour/day for 10 consecutive days) models of water avoidance stress are also preferred potent psychological models in determination of stress-induced gastrointestinal functions. These models result in elevations of ACTH and corticosterone within 30 min [37], and induce enlargement of the adrenal glands [38]. Recently, Vicario et al [39,40] reported that crowding stress (8 rats/cage) or sham-crowding (2 rats/cage) for up to 15 consecutive days triggers reversible inflammation, mast cell-mediated barrier dysfunctions, persistent epithelial dysfunction, and colonic hyperalgesia. Crowding-stressed rats showed higher plasma corticosterone levels than sham-stressed animals from day 1 and up to day 15. After 15 days of crowding stress, corticosterone levels decreased %38 (slightly adaptation), but HPA reactivity to incoming stressors was preserved. Crowding stress, differently from the stress models induced in laboratory, is actualized in natural environment of animals and may reflect life stress well for humans. Thus, this model has been also suggested as a suitable animal model to unravel the complex pathophysiology underlying to common human intestinal stress-related disorders, such as IBS.

Early life stress models such as maternal deprivation of pups from the dams have also been widely used [31,41,43,44], because stressful events in the early period of life (in the form of abuse, neglect or loss of the primary caregiver) have been shown to modify adult immune and gastrointestinal tract functions [12].

3. Intestine and its microenvironment

The gastrointestinal system is a tubular organ and the part 'intestine' extends downwards from the pyloric sphincter. With its many loops and coils, small and large intestines fill much of the abdominal cavity. Microscopically, both the small and large intestine are composed of four distinct layers; the mucosa covering the internal site of the tube, the submucosa, the muscularis externa and the serosa. The mucosa consists of layer of epithelia, loose connective tissue layer (lamina propia) containing blood vessels, lymphatics, and some lymphoid tissue, and muscularis mucosa. They both have different types of cells as building blocks; however, some of them are especially important in relation to luminal challenges *via* different agents including undigested or partly digested dietary proteins, gut microbiota and its metabolites. Located among the enterocytes are goblet cells secreting mucin which *per se* build a barrier; scattered enteroendocrine cells with paracrine and endocrine actions; Paneth cells characterized by their granules containing lysozyme, tumor necrosis factor-α and defensins have antibacterial roles; M cells with their well-known roles in antigen sampling and transportation; and the intestinal subepithelial myofibroblasts located in proximity to the mucosal epithelium and produce growth factors including hepatocyte growth factor promoting the proliferation of the intestinal epithelial stem cells, thus responsible for regeneration and maintaining of the integrity of the intestinal mucosa; and dendritic cells (DCs) highly specialized for antigen presentation which can capture non-self proteins and recognize microbial products [45-55].

Intestinal epithelial cells continuously contact with two different environments; first, luminal environment, which include intestinal secretions, food antigens, commensal bacteria, and also noxious or pathogenic materials, and second, the interstitial fluid surrounding the cells at the basolateral side. The single layer intestinal epithelium along the small and large intestine has a number of physiologic functions; it forms a barrier between the external (luminal) and internal environments besides its digestive and absorptive functions, and this epithelial barrier limits the space for bacterial growth. The ability of the epithelium to control uptake of molecules into the body is denoted as the intestinal barrier function [20,56,57]. The characteristics of intestinal epithelium for participation to the barrier function include; tight junction adherence between the epithelial cells, fluid and mucin secretions, secretions of numerous antimicrobial peptides, transepithelial transport of secretory IgA and the antigen presenting cell activity. However, intestinal epithelium is not only component of the intestinal barrier. Mucosal immune system, microbiota and microbiota-host interactions exist in major components of intestinal barrier [23,24]. All these components of intestinal barrier are controlled by the mediators of neuro-endocrine-immune network, and stress and stress mediators have significant impact on these components and regulatory network [20,24].

4. The effects of stress and glucocorticoids on intestinal barrier function

Intestinal mucosal epithelium is very sensitive against different types of stress because of the half-time of mucosal epithelia which may be as short as one and half day in certain parts. In other words, compared to many other tissues in the human and animal body, it is not well differentiated and very fragile [8,57]. The effects of acute or chronic stress on intestinal barrier function or intestinal permeability does not appear very different from each other in animal models of stress. However, the duration and repetition of stressors may influence severity, and the alterations may be temporary or permanent [34,58]. Generally, intestinal ion secretion [40,59], macromolecular permeability [60,61], inflammation [40,59], visceral hypersensivity and colonic motility increased [40], while gastric motility decreased in various animal models of stress [62-64]. These stress responses have been also described in IBD patients and involve dysregulation of HPA axis [12,15,17]. They are mediated by stress-related neuropeptides such as CRF, neural mechanisms and mast cells [18,20,65]. Various stress factors including heat, nutritional alterations, overcrowding, physical restraints and transporting also destroy the microbial balance and their microenvironment in the gut [66,67]. When the stressful events cause a decrease in beneficial bacteria, they generally increase the pathogenic species within the gut microenvironment [67-69]. In following sections, the effects of stress mediators on each component of barrier were discussed in details.

5. The physical barrier of epithelium

Cell-cell and cell–basement membrane interactions of intestinal epithelial cells control the transcellular and paracellular transports of luminal macromolecules and prevent bacteria from translocating into the subepithelial layer. Tight junctions (TJ) are primary physical components of intestinal barrier, located at the most apical part of lateral membranes of epithelial cells and restrict paracellular passage. The breakdown of tight junctions during bacterial infections results in gut barrier failure, often termed "leaky gut" [20,23]. Proteins that constitute the TJ complex include transmembrane proteins such as occludin, claudin, junction adhesion molecules and intracytoplasmic proteins zonula occludens 1 and 2 (ZO1-ZO2) and members of the membrane-associated guanylate kinase (MAGUK) protein family [70]. Tight junctions are highly dynamic structures, and their permeability is regulated by several physiological and pathophysiological conditions. Signals from intestinal microbiota may promote integrity of the epithelial barrier and have been shown to regulate tight junctions and protect intestinal epithelial cells (IECs) from injury by controlling the rate of IEC proliferation and inducing cytoprotective proteins [23]. Inflammatory cytokines can disrupt tight junctions and impair gut barrier integrity. Treating epithelial monolayers with TNF-α or IL-1b increased the permeability of tight junctions by stimulating transcription and activation of myosin light chain kinase (MLCK) [71-73]. The acute partial wrap restraint stress increased colonic permeability and rectal hypersensitivity *via* epithelial cell cytoskeleton contraction through myosin light chain kinase activation [74]. Acute immobilization stress also induced an increase in TJ permeability in the rat terminal ileum. These changes were mainly due to irregularly distribution of TJ transmembrane protein occludin and of the plaque protein ZO-1 which were seen after 2 hours from the stress induction and returned to a normal pattern within 24 hours [70]. Mazzon and Cuzzocrea [75] also suggested that TNF-α has active roles in the increase of tight junction permeability during acute restraint stress. They demonstrated *in vivo* in a TNF-α R1 knock-out mouse (TNF-α R1KO) model of restraint stress that the inhibition of TNF-α attenuates the development of TJ alteration in the ileum. Restraint stress caused the increase of heat shock protein-70 expression and associated decrease in the expression of type 1 (ZO-1) protein in the colonic epithelium of mice. These stress-induced changes can be inhibited by the glucocorticoid receptor antagonist mifepristone [76]. However, Boivin et al. [77] reported that glucocorticoids enhanced epithelial barrier function by suppressing transcription of myosin light chain kinase. Bacterial pathogens target tight junctions and breach epithelial integrity to promote colonization, obtain nutrients and access the underlying tissues [23]. So, alterations in gastrointestinal microbiota induced by several stressors or exogenous glucocorticoids might be an important threat for the barrier disruption.

6. Fluid and ion secretion

Due to their diluting and flushing effects, fluid and ion secretion of epithelial cells is another protective mechanism contributing to the barrier function [20]. In humans, the jejunal net water and sodium chloride absorption decreased during both psychological (induced by dichotomous listening) [78] and physical stress (induced by cold pain) [79], and also ion absorption is changed toward secretion in psychological form [78]. Both acute and chronic stress inductions increased short circuit current (an *in vitro* technique used for measuring the secretory response of intestines) in several parts of rodent intestines [36,41,59,80]. In addition, the peripheral non-selective CRF antagonists astressin or α-helical CRF9-41 abolished stress- induced alterations [41,80,81]. Intraperitoneal injection of a newly developed selective CRF(1) peptide agonist cortagine also induced an increase in defecation and watery diarrhea in mice and rats [82]. The effects of mineralocorticoids and glucocorticoids on intestinal water and ion movements are well known. Methylprednisolone for 3 days increased Na^+K^+adenosinetriphosphatase activity and Na^+ absorption [83]; it also increased guanylate cyclase activity and Cl^- secretion in the jejunum and ileum 6 h after administration [84,85]. However, there is no direct information about the increase of water and ion secretion related with increased glucocorticoid secretions in different stressful conditions.

7. Intestinal permeability and mast cell functions

An increase in intestinal permeability was reported in animals [61,86] and humans [87] submitted to acute or chronic stress, and in IBD and IBS patients [88,89]. Increase of intestinal permeability or macromolecular permeability also involves mucosal inflammation, mucosal damage, and mast cell hyperactivity. The barrier properties of the intestinal epithelium are usually studied by assessing the permeability to various probe/marker molecules (such as horseradishperoxidase, ^{51}Cr-EDTA, mannitol) *in vivo* or *in vitro* with intestinal segments mounted in Ussing-type chambers [20]. Bagchi et al [90] investigated the effects of acute (90 minute by water immersion) and chronic (15 min/day for 15 consecutive days by water immersion) stress on the production of reactive oxygen species (ROS) and oxidative tissue damage in gastric and intestinal mucosa. Both acute and chronic stress increased ROS production, lipid peroxidation and DNA fragmentation in both gastric and intestinal mucosa, but acute stress produced greater injury when compared to chronic stress. Colonic myeloperoxidase, mucosal mast cell activity and colonic permeability increased (as assessed with macroscopic damage and bacterial translocation to mesenteric lymph nodes, liver and spleen) at 12 weeks-period in maternally deprived rat pups induced by separation from their mothers on 2-14 days period for 3 hours a day [91]. Besides, the responses of maternally deprived rats to the TNBS-induced colitis were more prominent compared with the control rats. Both acute and chronic cold stress could cause oxidative stress of duodenum and a change in iNOS, which was related to the intestinal damage process in broiler chicks [92]. There are also evidences about the bacterial production of iNOS [93]. Boudry et al [58] suggested that both apoptosis in the crypts and an immature epithelium covering the villus surface can be responsible for a barrier defect in rats submitted to WAS (1 h/day) for 5 or 10 days. Morphologic [39,94] and enzymatic alterations [40] in mitochondria of the intestinal epithelium can also participate to promotion of intestinal dysfunctions in stress-induced animals.

Mast cell activity of gastrointestinal mucosa has altered in both acute and chronic stress models. They contain inflammatory and immunmodulating mediators such as prostaglandins, histamine and serotonin that directly alter epithelial transport properties [80] and nerve and muscle functions [95]. So it has a pivotal role in visceral hypersensivity [34], intestinal inflammation, intestinal mucin secretion [96] and epithelial barrier disruption [20,61]. Castagliuolo et al. [96] found that mast cells are essential for the colonic mucin and prostaglandin secretions in immobilization stressed mice, because of these secretions were absent in mast-cell deficient animals. Even, reconstitution of bone marrow with mast cells reversed that response to normal stress values [96]. Mast cell-deficient rats (Ws/Ws) and their normal mast cell-containing littermates (1/1) were submitted to water avoidance (1 h/day) or sham stress for 5 consecutive days. Stress increased baseline jejunal epithelial ion secretion, ionic permeability, macromolecular permeability [61,94], and the number and proportion of mucosal mast cells [94] in 1/1 rats but not in Ws/Ws rats, compared with non-stressed controls. Morphological, inflammatory and permeability changes were not seen in ileum and colon of mast cell-deficient rats in a chronic stress model [42]. Kim et al [97] reported that acute stress increased mast cell number and mucosal proteinase-activated receptor-2 (PAR2) expression (G-protein coupled receptor which can be activated by mast cell tryptase and modulate gastrointestinal functions) in the rat colon. Because of CRF-antagonist astressin inhibited these alterations, they suggested that CRF can be mediator of these events. Dexamethasone treatment improves PAR-2 agonist-induced visceral hypersensitivity, but does not prevent PAR-2 agonist-induced increase in colonic permeability in rats. This effect is coupled with a reduction of colonic mast cell numbers and RMCP-II contents [98]. Chronic stressful stimulus also caused greatest numbers of degranulated mast cells [99] and mast cell hyperplasia in the intestine of rats [100]. In our unpublished study, we found that while acute cold swimming stress (swimming in 18 ^{0}C water, for 15 min) increased the mucosal mast cell numbers in ileum, dexamethasone decreased their numbers significantly. It has been reported that mast cell numbers and their protease II activity were decreased in different dexamethasone treatments [98,101,102]. Wrap restraining stress in rats for 2 hours increased histamine content in colonic mast cells without degranulation, and this was found to be mediated by interleukin I and CRF [103]. Santos et al [80] reported that CRH, when injected intraperitoneally, mimicked the effects of acute restraint stress on colon epithelium such as increased colonic ion secretion, macromolecular permeability *via* cholinergic and adrenergic nerves and mast cells. Because CRH-induced alterations in colon epithelium inhibited by CRH-antagonist, adrenergic, nicotinic and muscarinic receptor antagonists and mast cell stabilizing agent doxantrazole, but not by aminoglutethimide (mineralcorticoid and glucocorticoid synthesis blocker, they suggested that steroids have no role in CRH-induced colonic pathology. They also denoted that stimulatory effects of CRH on mast cells can be mediated by direct or indirect neural pathways. Also in humans, CRH mediates transcellular uptake of HRP in colonic mucosal biopsy samples *via* CRH receptor subtypes R1 and R2 on subepithelial mast cells [104].

8. Mucin – Physicochemical barrier

Mucin secretion is also a major component of intestinal barrier which protects the mucosa by forming a coating layer over the epithelium against bacterial penetration. In addition to providing a biophysical barrier, mucus forms a matrix that allows the retention of high concentrations of specific and nonspecific antimicrobial molecules, such as secretory IgA and defensins in close proximity to the epithelial surface [23,105,106]. The secreted mucus forms two layers, a thinner inner layer that is accepted to be sterile and difficult to dislodge and an outer layer that is not sterile and is more easily removed. Mainly MUC2 type mucin is synthesized from goblet cells in small and large intestines. Epithelial cells and Paneth cells secrete antimicrobial peptides that help preventing of bacteria to penetrate the inner mucus layer. Both the physicochemical structure and thickness of mucin coating show differences through the gastrointestinal canal. It was suggested that mucus thickness is increased and the increase was correlated with luminal bacterial concentrations of related parts of gastrointestinal canal. The inner layer is ~15–30 μm and the outer layer is 100–400 μm in small intestine and it is thickest in ileum because there are approximately 10^5–10^7 bacteria per gram of faeces in the lumen. Otherwise, the inner layer of ~100 μm and a thick outer layer of ~700 μm in large intestine where 10^{10}–10^{12} bacteria per gram of luminal content resides [106]. Mucin is not only a barrier against the bacteria but also nutritional source for bacteria. In addition, bacteria capable of colonizing mucus can avoid rapid expulsion *via* peristalsis of the intestine and take an advantage for transmitting their signaling pathway to the host [107]. Microbiota can stimulate mucin secretion *via* bacterial products and increase MUC2 expression *via* activation of TLRs and NOD-like receptors or other signaling pathways at transcriptional level. Mucin secretion is also influenced by hormones, inflammatory mediators, several signaling peptides, growth factors and infectious bacteria [106,107]. Castagliuolo et al. [108] reported that acute stress caused a depletion of goblet cells and an increase of mucin secretion related with decrease of mucin containing goblet cell numbers *via* an increase of CRF secretion [20]. They proposed that although rapid mucin release during acute stress would increase the barrier properties and provide a degree of protection against invasion of a leaky epithelium, goblet cell depletion would be deleterious in a longer time period because of the reduced capacity to respond to ongoing or new threats. A 10-day chronic stress model was resulted in barrier dysfunction in the ileum and colon (increased macromolecular permeability and depletion of mucus) and ultrastructural changes in epithelial cells (enlarged mitochondria and presence of autophagosomes) associated with bacterial adhesion and their penetration into enterocytes [42]. Studies revealed that CRF signaling can activate mucin secretion because goblet cells have CRF1 receptors and stress and peripheral injection of CRF induces mucus depletion in rat distal colon [18]. On the other hand, maternal separation stress increased mucus secretion and thus caused an elevation in the number of mucosal goblet cells in rats [109]. In our unpublished study, both acute cold swimming stress and dexamethasone injection increased the goblet cell counts in the ileum within six hours, but the effects of dexamethasone were more prominent than the swimming stress. Further, while the effect of the dexamethasone on goblet cells maintained in 24 hours period that of swimming stress was disappeared [Ünsal et al., unpublished data]. Finnie et al. [110] reported that exogenous prednisolone and hydrocortisone also increased the mucin secretion significantly in left slightly and in right uninvolved colonic biopsies of patients with ulcerative colitis. They suggested that therapeutic effects of corticosteroids in ulcerative colitis may be related partly with their stimulatory effects on mucin synthesis.

As partly mentioned above, most stress-induced gastrointestinal (GI) dysfunctions can be induced by peripheral CRF agonists and prevented by CRF receptor antagonists [18]. In a review article Larauche et al [18] reported about "CRF signaling" and emphasized that peripheral injection of CRF or urocortin stimulates colonic transit, motility, Fos expression in myenteric neurons, and defecation through activation of CRF1 receptors, whereas it decreases ileal contractility *via* CRF2 receptors. Additionally, intraperitoneal administration of CRF induces colonic mast cells degranulation *via* both CRF1 and CRF2 receptors and increases ion secretion and mucosal permeability to macromolecules, which can in turn promote intestinal inflammation and alters visceral sensitivity. Furthermore, CRF peptides can reproduce secretomotor and mucosal alterations *in vitro*. Although there are a lot of events that CRF is primary mediator in stress-induced alterations of GIS in animals and humans [17,18,32,80-82,111], similar reports for the glucocorticoids are limited [28-30]. Meddings and Swain [28] reported that stress-induced increases in gastrointestinal epithelial permeability seemed to be mediated by adrenal corticosteroids and disappeared after adrenalectomy or pharmacologic blockade of glucocorticoid receptors. Besides, dexamethasone treatment of control animals increased gastrointestinal permeability and mimicked the effects of stress. Spitz et al. [29,30] evaluated the effects of dexamethasone on intestinal barrier functions in various conditions such as starvation and after bacterial contamination. They found that starvation significantly impairs secretory IgA, promotes bacterial adherence to the mucosa and increases intestinal permeability to f-MLP in rats given 0.8 mg/kg dexamethasone intraperitoneally. These effects are significantly attenuated by the feeding of rat chow [30]. In other study, they also found out that dexamethasone administration increased intestinal permeability and bacterial adherence to the mucosa [29]. However, antibiotic decontamination of the intestine completely abrogated the intestinal permeability defects observed in this model. Basing these findings they concluded that bacterial-mucosal cell interactions may be responsible for alterations in intestinal permeability after dexamethasone administration.

9. Intestinal immune system

Intestinal homeokinesis depends on complex interactions between the microbiota, the intestinal epithelium and the host immune system. Innate and acquired immune cells of the intestine have critical roles in barrier function because of they should tolerate the antigens belonging to the food and commensal microbiota as well as they should protect the body against pathogen microorganisms [20,57]. Systemic nonresponsiveness to antigens that are introduced orally is a phenomenon known as "oral tolerance". Oral tolerance is typically characterized by the suppression of the systemic T helper 1 (Thl) response to antigens and elevated levels of IL-I0, TGF-β and antigen-specific sIgA at the mucosal surface. The T helper 2 (Th2) response also promotes the induction of tolerance in the gut. Production of IL-4 and IL- 5 during Th2 response acts synergistically to enhance IgA production. These cytokines also act further to inhibit the Thl response [57]. The cells of the innate immunity discriminate potentially pathogenic microbes from harmless antigens through pattern recognition receptors (PRR). Toll-like receptors (TLRs) are a family of pathogen-recognition receptors of the innate immune system. TLRs are present on a variety of cell types such as intestinal epithelium, monocytes, and dendritic cells. They recognize conserved molecular motifs on microorganisms called pathogen associated molecular patterns (PAMPS). TLRs are activated by various components of microorganisms, e.g. TLR4 binds lipopolysaccharide (LPS) in gram-negative bacteria. Besides, TLR5 binds to flagellin, TLR2/6 binds to fungal zymosan and TLR7 binds single stranded RNA (ssRNA) from viruses. Activation of the TLRs by either pathogenic ligands or host factors results in downstream activation or inhibition of pathways involved in inflammation. Toll-like receptor activation by commensal bacteria plays an essential role in maintaining colonic homeostasis and controlling tolerance in the gut [57,112,113,114]. However, inappropriate activation of their signaling pathways may lead to deleterious inflammation and tissue injury. TLRs have been implicated in the pathogenesis of many GI disorders [57,114]. Although intestinal immune system is thought to have a critical role in stress-induced alterations of GIS functions, the studies about this situation are limited as this also the case for other functions of GIS such as motility, secretion and permeability [18,115,116]. McKernan et al. [116] investigated for the first time the regulation of TLR expression in the colonic mucosa in two distinct chronic stress models; Wistar-Kyoto (WKY) rats and maternally separated rats where Sprague Dawley rats were used as controls. Significant increases are seen in the mRNA levels of TLR3, 4 and 5 in both the distal and proximal colonic mucosa of MS rats compared with controls. No significant differences were noted for TLR 2, 7, 9 and 10 while TLR 6 could not be detected in any samples in both rat strains. The WKY strain showed increased levels of mRNA expression of TLR3, 4, 5, 7, 8, 9 and 10 both in the distal and proximal colonic mucosa compared to the control animals of Sprague-Dawley strain. No significant differences in expression were found for TLR2 in all samples of both strains. These authors suggested that the up-regulation of TLR 4 and 5 may indicate increases in cytokine production in response to the increases in sensitivity to gut bacteria. In addition, they suggested that the observed differences in TLR expression activity between MS and WKY rats might be related with their different neuroendocrine responses or microbiota. In spleens isolated from mice subjected to chronic 12-hour daily physical restraint for two days, TLR-4 expression significantly increased, T helper 1 (Th1) cytokine IFN-γ and IL-2 levels were found to be decreased, but Th2 cytokine and IL-4 increased. They suggested that stress modulates the immune system through a TLR4-dependent mechanism, because TLR4-deficient mice are resistant to stress-induced lymphocyte reduction and the restraint stress significantly inhibits changes of Th1 and Th2 cytokines in TLR4-deficient mice compared with the wild type mice [117]. Repeated social defeat stress (SDR) has been shown to increase the expression of TLR2 and TLR4 [118] and can activate dendritic cells for enhanced cytokine secretion in response to TLR specific stimuli. Besides, glucocorticoid resistance was determined in CD11+ dendritic cells isolated from spleens of SDR mice, whereas under baseline conditions DCs are highly sensitive to glucocorticoids [119]. Glucocorticoids and catecholamines appear to be able to regulate the expression of certain TLRs [116]. Toll-like receptor agonist-induced cytokine (IL1b, IL6, IL8 and TNF-α) release was markedly enhanced in stimulated whole blood samples from IBS patients compared with healthy controls. Plasma levels of cortisol, IL-6 and IL-8 were also significantly increased in IBS patients [120].

Chronic stress (induced by water avoidance stress for 1 hour/day for 10 consecutive days) induced the infiltration of neutrophils and mononuclear cells, and increased myeloperoxidase (MPO) activity in ileum and colon mucosa, but these changes were not shown in mast cell deficient rats [42]. Similary, jejunal inflammatory cells such as neutrophils, eosinophils and mononuclear cells and expression of IL-4 (TH2 type cytokine) increased, while interferon–γ (IFN- γ) (TH1 type cytokine) decreased in same chronic stress model of rats. Treatment of stressed rats with an antagonist to CRH eliminated the manifestations of intestinal hypersensitivity [121].

Velin et al [122] evaluated the M cell-containing follicle associated epithelium (specialized in antigen uptake) in acute and chronic stress conditions. Acute stress increased horseradish peroxidase (HRP) flux in villus as well as in follicle-associated epithelium (FAE), and chronic stress increased *E. coli* passage in follicle-associated epithelium whereas there was no significant increase in villus epithelium. In patients with Crohn's disease (CD), transmucosal uptake of non-pathogenic *E. coli* across the FAE increased in ileum, despite unchanged macromolecular permeability, but these changes were not observed in patients with ulcerative colitis [123]. Recently, Keita [124] showed that application of CRF agonist increased HRP and *E. coli* passage, stress-induced increases in uptake across FAE of HRP, and *E. coli* were reduced by CRF antagonist, mast cell stabilizer and atropine. Chronic restraint stress increases eosinophils expressing CRF in the jejunum, which participate to the recruitment of mast cells and epithelial barrier dysfunction [125]. The influence of CRF signaling on intestinal mast cell activity is detailed above. However, the information about their effects on other immune components of intestine (such as intestinal epithelial cells, TLR expression or intraepithelial lymphocytes) is limited. Larauche et al [82] reported that treatment of mice with CRF-1 agonist cortagine exhibits a dose-related interferon-γ (IFNγ) response indicating T cell and/or natural killer (NK) cell activation, which is followed by tight junction deregulation and dose dependent apoptotic loss of different cell populations in ileum.

IECs participate in initiating adaptive immune responses in the gut by transporting luminal antigens to underlying immune cells for presentation by professional antigen presenting cells or can present antigen themselves [57]. intraepithelial lymphocyte (IEL) and paneth cells (specialized IEC located at the base of intestinal crypts in small intestine) do also synthesis the antimicrobial peptides such as lysozymes, alpha defensins, cathelicidins, lipocalins, and C-type lectins such as RegIIIγ [126]. Production of RegIIIg [127] and alpha-defensins [128] as well as that of secretory IgA [129] are induced by commensal bacteria. Nutritional and infection stress affected the secretory activity of Paneth cells in human [130]. In women, acute cold stress induced the release of α-defensin in the jejunum [131]. Evidences suggested that dysfunction of Paneth cells and impaired defensin secretion may contribute to IBD susceptibility [57,105].

Corticosteroids and catecholamines are well recognized and accepted powerful regulators and players of the body in its response to environmental challenges including biological factors of stress. Stress or corticosteroid applications are known to have also profound effects on intestinal wall structure and functioning. Intestinal submucosa is the place where lymphocytes, eosinophils and mast cells reside in men and animals under normal conditions. Jarillo-Luna et al. [115] investigated the effects of chronic restraint stress in mice submitted to different procedures (adrenalectomy, chemical sympathectomy, and treatment with a glucocorticoid antagonist (RU486), dexamethasone, and epinephrine) on intraepithelial lymphocyte (IEL) numbers. They found that chronic restraint-stress reduced the IEL population in the small intestine and adrenal catecholamines and glucocorticoids are essential in preserving IEL population because adrenalectomy, treatment with RU-486 and chemical sympathectomy decreased the number of γδ, CD4+ and CD8+ T cells in non-stressed groups. They also found that adrenalectomy did not buffered the stress-induced reduction in CD8 lympocytes, but glucocorticoid receptor antagonist RU-486 buffered stress-induced decrease in γδ and CD8+, but not in CD4+ T cells. Besides, low and high doses of dexamethasone (5 and 50 mg/kg BW) significantly reduced the number of γδ and CD8+ T cells, and epinefrin (0.1-0.5 mg/kg) reduced the number of γδ, CD4+ and CD8+ T cells in intact mice. Also many other studies reported that both stress-related endogen rises of glucocorticoids [115,132-134] and exogenous glucocorticoid administrations [135,136] induce decreases in intraepithelial lymphocytes and/or those in ileal Peyer patches. Pretreatment with glucocorticoid receptor antagonist mifepristone significantly reduced apoptosis in both T- and B-cell populations in intraepithelial lymphocytes after the burn injury [133]. Experimental studies also suggested that single or repeated parenteral applications of cortisone cause a decrease in eosinophil concentration in all parts of examined gastrointestinal wall from stomach up to colon [137,138]. Immunosuppressive effects of glucocorticoids are explained mainly by an increase of apoptosis and a decrease of cytokine production. Corticosterone impaired the maturation of DCs and cytokine production and reduced the ability of DCs to prime naive CD8+ T cells *in vivo*; there was no reduction in surface TLR4 expression in CORT-treated DCs [139]. However, McEwen et al. [140] proposed that although glucocorticoids are mainly known with and used widely for their immunsuppressive aspects, adrenal steroids play also different roles as important modulators of the immune system. Pharmacological as well as physiological changes in glucocorticoids result in a decrease in lymphocyte, monocyte and eosinophil numbers and an increase in neutrophil numbers in the blood of men and rodents. These changes are not related with the glucocorticoid-induced leukocyte deaths. The nonspecific stress and glucocorticoid administration cause redistribution of leukocytes from peripheral blood into various tissues and organs, such as bone marrow, spleen and lymph nodes [140-142].

10. Intestinal microbiota

One of the important groups of the environmental biological stressors belongs to the microbiota, and it is associated with every multicellular organism on earth. It is estimated that in humans and many animals reside at least 10^{14} microorganisms, making approximately 1.5 kg biomass, in various parts of the body, most abundant of them residing the distal part of the gut in humans and animals with exception of ruminants [143-146]. These parts of the body lined by the skin or mucous membranes and all are in direct contact with the environment. Although the microorganisms are preferable grouped as pathogenic, while they harm the multicellular organisms, and saprophytic, while they seemingly do not harm their hosts instead they build symbiotic relationships, but possibly this depends only on the balance or imbalance among numerous groups of microorganisms constituting the microbiota in a definite part of the body and between the microbiota and its host, in general.

The first days, weeks, months or years, the time spent in mothers' womb or in egg-shall of the metazoan life is the only time which they are free of microbes. The delivery into the outside exposes them to an enormous range of microbes from diverse environments. This is the first encounters with life forms with different morphology and functions. The studies have shown that within a short time following delivery, the microrganisms are present on the skin and mucosal surfaces of the body. With time, a dense, complex gastrointestinal microbiota develops [147,148]. Due to the unique properties of microorganisms including their small size, metabolic versatility and genetic plasticity, microorganisms can tolerate and easily adapt to unfavorable and immense variety of continuously changing environmental conditions [149]. However, although a wide variety of microorganisms were exposed to representative individuals from start up throughout the life periods, only a limited numbers of species are able to colonize permanently in available body surfaces of man and animals. The microorganisms display a tissue tropism; e.g., they colonize predominantly only certain body sites. Consequently, each side is inhabited by only certain species of microorganisms. The microorganisms found at a particular body site constitute what is known as the indigenous or normal microbiota of this site, wherein the term 'indigenous' include all of viruses, protozoa, archae, and fungi [150,151]. The GIT is inhabited with 10^{13}–10^{14} microorganisms, approximately 500 to over 1000 different species and more than 7000 strains. Their counts exceed ten times the numbers of somatic cells of their hosts [144,151-154].

The very complex and diverse gastro-intestinal microbiota differs from species to species, in dependence of nutritional habits with some geographic motives. Besides, it varies from one segment to another and varies over time in the same individual, because the environment of the GIT varies considerable along its length and with the lifetime of an individual [144]. Thus, the composition and intensity of the microbiota of a newborn is quite different from those of an adult which are in turn quite different from that of an elderly individual [155,156]. Colonization begins at birth with facultative bacteria and the colonization of anaerobic bacteria which are composed of more than %90 of GIS microbiota develops later. In humans, the microbiota has a stable adult-like signature by 1 year of age [113,154]. Similarly, the composition and intensity of the microbiota varies along the gastrointestinal tract where they are attached to the mucosa or are present in the contents. In stomach and duodenum of humans, microorganism numbers is 10^3CFU/ml and include more lactobacilli, streptococci and yeasts species. In jejunum (10^4CFU/ml) and ileum ($10^{7\text{-}8}$ CFU/ml) *Lactobacillus, Bacteroides, Enterobacteriaceae,* Streptococci, *Bifidobacterium and Fusobacteria species* are more existent. The highest numbers of bacteria ($10^{11\text{-}12}$ CFU/ml) displaying enormous diversity are found in colon, predominant species being *Bacteroides, Fusobacterium, Eubacterium,Peptococcus, Peptostreptococcus, Veillonella, Bifidobacterium, Escherichia, Clostridium, Lactobacillus* and others [147,154]. Although only 40-45% part of GI microbiota could be growth with classical microbial culture tecniques, recently developed moleculer techniques allow the definition of non-culturable members of microbiota. The vast majority of microorganisms belong to the phyla of *Firmicutes, Bacteroidetes, Actinobacteria,* and *Proteobacteria* while *Fusobacteria, Verrucomicrobia and TM7* are represent in relatively lower numbers [144,145,157,158]. There are also some fungi and *Archaea* present in the gastrointestinal tract [144,159,160], but they comprise less than 1% of total inhabitants. The majority of the intestinal bacteria are composed of gram-negative anaerobes [143].

With the acquisition and establishment in the intestinal lumina with various microbial populations bidirectional interactions between microbiota and host organism starts [161,162]. There are symbiotic relationships between the host and its GI microbiota in steady-state conditions. The gastrointestinal tract serves a natural habitat for a dynamic microbial community of different origins while the microbiota is very essential for both gastrointestinal integrity [163] and general health of host organisms [113]. Comparison between the conventional and germ-free animals has allowed obtaining information about the effects of microbiota on morphologic, functional and metabolic characteristics of host organisms [23,113,154,160]. Germ free animals have enlarged cecum [164], they have thinner gut wall, smaller total surface area and more cubic epithelium than the columnar, increased enterochromaffin cell area and smaller Peyer's patches, and intestinal epithelium has slower turnover rate compared with the conventional animals [160,165]. The materiality of the gut microbiota also for many gut functions such as motility, immune and barrier functions are reviewed by several authors [23,113].

Complex association between the host and its microbiota collectively extends the processing indigestible parts of food to the benefits of the host organisms *via* metabolic capacities which are not coded in host genomes like mammalian and avian species [166-168]. They digest the unusable parts of the diets; metabolites reach to the intestinal lumina within various secretions and desquamated cells of their hosts for growth and proliferation. At the same time, they also supply the host organisms with a considerable amount of nutrients, which makes this ecosystem an invaluable, essential metabolic organ, which contributes significantly to the homeokinesis of the host organisms [23,113,152,169]. They produce substances including vitamins, volatile or short-chain fatty acids (SCFAs) and polyamines which are absorbed throughout the intestinal wall and used directly by intestinal epithelial cells or other cells of the body [170,171]. SCFA profoundly influence gut barrier functions, host immunity, epithelial proliferation and bacterial pathogenesis [172]. Zheng et al. [171] showed extensive gut microbiota modulation of host systemic metabolism involving short-chain fatty acids, tryptophan and tyrosine metabolism, and possibly a compensatory mechanism of indole-melatonin production. All these metabolites have also many regulatory functions in host organisms. Tryptophan and tyrosine are precursors of neurotransmitters acting directly at the central nervous system level [113]. Thus, the gut microbiota enhances the host's metabolic capacity for processing nutrients and modulates the activities of multiple pathways in a variety of organ systems, including the brain.

Microbiota acts as a luminal barrier against incoming pathogens; this phenomenon has been described as colonization resistance [23,154]. Beneficial and pathogen microorganism compete with each other for the attachment sites and for nutrients, so microbiota and their products can prevent pathogen colonization directly. On the other hand, microbiota acts on barrier functions also indirectly by stimulating mucosal immune system [172]. The abundant antigenic stimulus supplied by microbiota and their products are essential for the stimulation of immune system cells locally and systemically [173-175]. In germ-free animals, besides the poor developed Peyer's patches, altered compositions of CD4+ T cells and IgA-producing B cells in the lamina propria [165], TH 17 cells, which is a subset of the T cells and contribute to resistance against colonization by pathogens were virtually absent in germ free animals [176,177]. Chow and Mazmanian [177] denoted that although Th17 cells are essential for immunity, they have also been implicated in the pathogenesis of many autoimmune diseases, including IBD, arthritis, psoriasis, and experimental autoimmune encephalomyelitis (EAE).

The gut microbiota has recently been identified as the main source of highest biological variability confined in an individual [178]. Because the metazoan life-forms and the inhabitation of their gastrointestinal tract with microorganisms evolved together, there are close links between any host or its epi-genome and its very complex diverse gastrointestinal microbiota with their multitude genomes. It is estimated that this microbial community has 70–140 times more total genes than the human host. These functional inter-relationships between host and microbiota or two different genomes determine the health or disease state of the metazoan hosts and the balance among different microorganism populations [113,172,179]. It is well accepted that the intestinal microbiota involves in metabolome of the host, thus promotes actively fat accumulation and weight gain and sustains indirectly a low-grade systemic inflammation especially when imbalanced, and consequently, enhances the risk for complex, multifactorial diseases such as insulin resistance, diabetes, obesity and cardiovascular diseases. The search of global obesity epidemic led to the growing evidences about the possible roles of intestinal microbiota in these respects [180,181,182]. Claus et al. [170] has noted that the colonization of the gut microbiota was associated with a rapid increase in body weights of animals up to 4% within 5 days of colonization. Findings of various studies also revealed that gut microbiota profile of obese and diabetic individuals differ by phylum level both in its quantity and quality from that of lean and nonobese individuals [182,183]. Recent evidences exhibit that the composition of the gut microbiome may influence body weight of the host by various mechanisms including enhancing the ability of intestines to extract energy from food [184], regulating fat storage in tissues [185] and affecting satiety by modulating the levels of local hormones that regulate satiety and by direct effects in central nervous system [186].

There is a growing appreciation of the critical roles played by the commensal microbiota, both in general well-being of the hosts and in the specific functioning of the brain–gut axis [113]. Bidirectional communications of brain–gut–enteric microbiota axis simply actualized by through signals from the brain can influence the motor, sensory, and secretory modalities of the gastrointestinal tract and conversely, visceral messages from the gastrointestinal tract can influence brain functions [187]. Sudo and colleagues [25] showed that gut microbiota effect the stress responses of host organisms. They compared the response of the HPA axis to stress in GF, specific pathogen free (SPF) and gnotobiotic mice that were mono-associated with a single bacterium. Restraint stress caused an exaggerated ACTH and corticosterone elevation in GF rather than SPF mice. This hyper-response of the HPA axis was reversed by mono-association with *Bifidobacterium infantis*. They also showed in following experiments that the levels of brain-derived nerve factor (BDNF), norepinephrine and 5- 5-hydroxytryptamine (5-HT) in the cortex and hippocampus were significantly lower in GF mice than in SPF mice [188]. Improvements of stress-related symptoms by probiotic administration also support the possible regulatory effects of microbiota on HPA axis and brain functions [44,189]. Gareau et al [44] reported that probiotic treatments improved colonic dysfunction and corrected the higher corticosterone levels in stressed rats induced by maternal seperation. L. rhamnosus (JB-1) reduced stress-induced corticosterone and anxiety- and depression-related behavior in mice. In different region of brain, this therapy also altered GABA receptor expression implicated in the pathogenesis of anxiety and depression, which are highly comorbid with functional bowel disorders. Due to the neurochemical and behavioral effects were not found in vagotomized mice, they suggested that vagus could be a major modulatory constitutive communication pathway between the bacteria exposed to the gut and the brain [189]. The roles of probiotics and gut microbiota in modulation of visceral and even somatic pain perception and their possible roles in alterations of mood and behavior were reviewed by Forsythe et al. [190] and Grenham et al. [113].

As mentioned above, intestinal dysbiosis can adversely influence gut physiology both by direct effects to the surrounding gut wall and by leading to inappropriate brain–gut axis signaling and associated consequences for CNS functions and disease states. Stress at the level of the CNS can also impact on gut functions and lead to perturbations of the microbiota [113].

11. Stress and intestinal microbiota

Intestinal microbiota have once been seen as potential treat for the host organisms, but recently accepted as an integral part of metazoan life and even as an organ with a huge variety of building blocks which mainly cooperate with each other and with the host for maintaining the health and survival [113,144]. However, various stress factors such as heat, cold, nutritional alterations, overcrowding, physical restraints and transporting or fouled or contaminated foods can destroy the microbial balance in the gastrointestinal system [66,67,191-195] and alter their relationships with each other and with their hosts. Stressful stimuli can affect gastrointestinal microbiota directly, for example *via* limited availability of food ingredients or direct actions of stress mediators such as adrenaline or noradrenaline on microbiota [27,196], and indirectly *via* altering the intestinal environment of bacteria such as intestinal secretion, motility, permeability and immune functions as reviewed above.

The effects of several stressors and stress mediators on intestinal microbiota were given in Table 1. Bailey et al [197] induced social disruption stress (SDR) in mice to determine whether the microbiome contributes to stressor-induced immune enhancements. They analyzed bacterial populations in the cecum with using bacterial tag-encoded FLX amplicon pyrosequencing (bTEFAP) and found that microbiota significantly changed immediately after stressor exposure as summarized in Table 1, and stress also increased circulating levels of IL-6 and MCP-1, which were significantly correlated with stressor-induced changes to three bacterial genera (i.e., *Coprococcus, Pseudobutyrivibrio,* and *Dorea spp*). However in antibiotic treated mice, exposure to SDR failed to increase IL-6 and MCP-1. Bailey et al [191] reported that restraint stress also significantly change the composition of the intestinal microbiota in mice and disruption of the microbiota increased susceptibility to murine enteric pathogen *Citrobacter rodentium* which can be associated with reduced competitive exclusion of commensal bacteria and increased tumor necrosis factor alpha (TNF-α) gene expression in colonic tissue. Reduction in bifidobacteria and lactobacilli numbers in fecal samples of infant monkeys whose mother had been exposed to stress in either early or late pregnancy period showed that maternal pregnancy conditions affect infant health and can enhance susceptibility to infection [68]. Similarly, early life stress induced by maternal separation altered fecal microbiota with concomitant increases in corticosterone and also visceral hypersensitivity and systemic immune response to *in vitro* lipopolysaccharide challenges in rats [198]. Knowles et al [199] reported that non-extreme 'every day' stress events such as exam stress can affect the integrity of the indigenous gastrointestinal microflora of humans but these changes are not supported by cortisol responses. Maternal separation of rhesus macaques also caused to decrease of lactobacilli at 3th days post-separation but significant differences in the cortisol responses did not predict the magnitude of the reduction of lactobacilli numbers. These authors suggested that more than one neuro-hormone can modulate microbiota changes.

Because of their immune-suppressive or stress-mediating effects, some studies have been focused on the effects of glucocorticoids on intestinal microbiota. These studies showed that exogenous glucocorticoid applications to the host organisms are also able to cause changes in gastrointestinal microbiota. We [200,Ünsal et al., unpublished study] and others [29,30,201] demonstrated that exogenous glucocorticoid administrations can also affect gut microbiota by enhancing total aerobe and gram negative enteric bacteria and their translocation to extraintestinal tissues [201]. We compared the effects of different doses of dexamethasone on ileal microbiota and found, in contrast to well-known stress effects, that 5mg/kg dexamethasone injection also increased the numbers of total anaerobe and lactobacilli in ileal content of rats [200]. However, their number did not change in lower doses of dexamethasone. Also in our unpublished study acute cold swimming stress decreased the numbers of lactobacilli, while dexamethasone in dose of 5 mg/kg increased total aerobe, gram-negative enteric bacteria and lactobacilli. Thus, the evidences available suggest that several stressors reduce the number of lactobacilli, while on the contrary, they increases growth, epithelial adherence and mucosal uptake of Gram-negative pathogens. Lactobacilli may possible be defined as stress indicator bacteria of the gut microbiota which is sensible to the effects of various stressors, in general. Although it is known that exogenous glucocorticoids increase the counts of gram negative enteric bacteria [29,30,201], no other information about their effects on the lactobacilli in the gut could be found.

The roles of stress and stress-related hormones in the pathogenesis of infectious diseases are beyond any argument. Microbial endocrinology is a new research area which appeared from the demand how stress influence the bacterial infections, how neuro-endocrine-immune secretions of host organisms influence their harboring microbiota and how infectious microbes can actively use the neurohormonal products of the stress to their own advantages [202,203]. Recently, several *in vitro* studies have focused on direct effects of stress hormones on bacterial growth and their virulence in an effort to explore and understand the interactions of so-called stress hormones and infections. These studies gathered the evidence that catecholamines stimulate the growth of a wide variety of gram-negative bacterial species, including those of medical importance [27,196,204-209]. Furthermore, catecholamines were also found to be able to induce *E.coli* to produce a heat-stable autoinducer of growth [19,27,204,210] as well as for adhesion required K99 pilus and shigella-like toxins I and II, which may have important roles in its pathogenic activity [210].

The effects of norepinephrine and its receptor antagonists on mucosal bacterial adherence were also determined in sheets obtained from different parts of the gut, mounted in Ussing chamber. Norepinephrine increased the adherence of enterohemorrhagic *Escherichia coli* O157:H7 (EHEC) to colonic epithelium through interactions with α-2 adrenergic receptors [211-213] and it increased the internalization of enterohemorrhagic E. coli O157:H7 (EHEC) and S. enterica serovar Choleraesuis in jejunal mucosa containing Peyer's patch follicles [214,215]. Parallel studies related to the direct actions of other stress mediators such as cortisol or CRF on bacterial growth could not be found. However, Kakuno et al. [216] suggested that hydrocortisone enhance intracellular colonizations of E. coli and Schreiber and Brown [217] reported that ACTH increased EHEC adherence to the porcine colonic mucosa.

Many factors participate in the pathology of inflammatory bowel disease (IBD) such as genetic and immune status of host organism, the gut microbiota, and environmental triggers [218]. Some scientific events support that the enteric microbiota is involved in abnormal inflammatory responses observed in diverse animal models for inflammatory bowel disease [219,220]. These events reviewed by the authors [219,220] are arranged as the reduction or absence of intestinal inflammation in animal models of colitis in antibiotic-treated or germ-free animals; colitis formation with some bacterial inoculations to germ free rats or not to formation with other bacterial species; and beneficial effects of probiotics and prebiotics in IBD patients or animal models of IBD. However, although microbiota has been thought to play an active role in etiopathogenesis of inflammatory bowel disease, it is not clear whether they are cause or outcome. In other words, whether alterations in intestinal microenvironment of microbiota such as mucin secretion, immune modifications and epithelial dysfunctions cause to changes in commensal microbiota or microbial alterations cause to inflammatory responses of intestinal mucosa in stressful conditions is not clear yet [221].

Although the reports in microbiome composition of IBD-patients or models show differences, changes in microbiota composition are characterized more likely by decreases in lactobacilli and bifidobacteria, and increases or unchange in aerobe and facultative anaerobic bacteria [222]. Molecular analysis of the microbiota of IBD patients have shown that temporal stability and diversity of the gut microbiota composition in IBD patients decreased compared to non-IBD controls [223], and commensal bacteria, particularly members of the phyla *Firmicutes* and *Bacteroidetes* decreased and *Proteobacteria* and *Actinobacteria* increased [224]. These changes look alike to those that seen following effects of stress on intestinal microbiota.

Stress and/or Stress Mediators	Microbiota	Method	References
Social disruption stress (SDR) in mice (total of 6, two-hour cycles of SDR)	Decrease in *Bacteroides* spp., tended to decrease in *Lactobacillus* spp., tended to increase in *Clostridium* spp. and changes in *Coprococcus, Pseudobutyrivibrio*, and *Dorea spp. in cecal content*	(bTEFAP)	197
Restraint stress for 7 days in mice (between 18.00- 08.00 h)	Overgrowth of facultatively anaerobic microbiota, reduction in family *Porphyromonadaceae,and genus Tannerella,*reducing microbial richness and diversity in the ceca	both culture technique and bTEFAP	191
Prenatal stress induced by acoustical startle paradigm for 6 weeks in early or late pregnancy in Rhesus Monkey	prenatal stress reduced the overall numbers of bifidobacteria and lactobacilli in fecal cultures of infants	culture technique	68
Maternal separation in rhesus macaques *(Macaca mulatta)*	Decrease of lactobacilli in fecal samples at 3th days postseparation, not correlated with cortisol responses	culture technique	26
Academic stress in undergraduate students	Reduction in fecal lactic acid bacteria, unsignificantly cortisol enhancement	culture technique	199
Food, water and bedding deprivation in mice	Decrease in lactobacilli in stomach, increase of coliforms in jejunum, ileum and cecum, reduction in fusiform-shaped bacteria associated with mucosal epithelium of cecum and colon	culture technique	192
Dexemethasone (0.8 mg/kg) Dexamethosone (0.8 mg/kg)+ starvation for 48 h in Fischer rat	impairs secretory IgA, promotes bacterial adherence to the mucosa, increase of intestinal permeability		29,30,225

Stress and/or Stress Mediators	Microbiota	Method	References
Dexamethasone 5 mg/kg in rats	Increase of total aerobe bacteria and lactobacilli in ileum	culture technique	200, Ünsal et al., unpublished study
Methylprednisolone (3 mg/kg) in rats subjected to temporary liver inflow occlusion	Increase of intestinal *Klebsiella spp* and *Proteus spp* and of translocation to multiple organs.	culture technique	201
Pregnant rats were treated with either cortisone acetate or normal saline on days 18-21 of gestation	Total bacteria and gram-negatives found in association with the mucosa were significantly lower in pups prenatally treated with steroids.	culture technique	226
Norepinephrine action on porcine or murine cecum/ colon/jejunum explants	Increases cecal-colonic adherence of E. coli O157:H7; changes Salmonella and E. coli uptake into Peyer's patches		211-215
ACTH action on explants of porcine distal colonic mucosa	Increases adherence of E. coli O157:H7 to colonic mucosa		217

Table 1. The effects of some different type stressors and/or stress mediators on intestinal microbiota

12. Nutritional stress

Nutrition and nutrients of metazoans play very important multifunctional key roles both for metazoan host and for its gastrointestinal microbiota. They are essential not only in colonization, growth and survival of the microbiota in intestinal system but also in maintaining the balance among different species and their localization within its lumina [67,192,227,228]. Nutrition plays an important role as stressor for host organisms and their gastrointestinal tract *via* three mechanisms. Firstly, foods supply nutrients for intestinal microbiota and also serve as carriers of various microorganisms into gastrointestinal tract which may under circumstances lead to imbalances among different species; secondly, nutritional deficiencies or imbalances are perceived from the organisms as stressors setting them to the state of well-known alarm reaction of stress; and thirdly, certain food ingredients in their undigested forms as foreign substances accepted as non-self from organisms and stimulate a stress situation. In cases of carrying the microorganisms into gastrointestinal tract or acting as antigens, the foreign treats come into direct contact with the wall of gastrointestinal tract. A great part of microorganisms stay in gastrointestinal canal for a short time period, while others colonize its lumina permanently and their genera can be life-long present there, mostly in a symbiotic relationship with the host organisms.

Dietary ingredients, which are not digestible for the host organisms or which are digestible but escape from the intestinal digestion can be utilized as substrate for growth from microbiota colonized in the following sections of the gut [229,230]. All microorganisms residing in gastrointestinal tract needs the nutrients that necessary for their growth and proliferation are continuously supplied *via* foods of their hosts and from host organisms in secretions of digestive organs including saliva, gastric juice, pancreatic, hepatic (bile) and intestinal wall secretions and desquamated epithelial structures. The composition and amount of the food, even the compositions of these secrets may undergo substantial changes. This is why the hosts' balanced nutrition and physiological state exerts a strong controlling effect on its microbiota [160,181,192,231-237]. Thus, any nutritional deficiency or imbalance of their hosts serve the most important challenge for the growth, survival and balance of different microbial species within the intestinal lumina.

Malnutritions in different nature or nutritional imbalances had always been and are still very widespread health problems of men and animals worldwide and frequently seen in infants and elderly, and those subjects having malignancies, getting chemotherapy and/or radiotherapy or infected with human immunodeficiency virus. Very common forms of malnutrition are protein, calorie and protein calorie deficiencies which almost always are complicated with deficiencies of other nutrients, especially that of minerals and vitamins [238]. As mentioned above, deficiencies of calories, proteins, minerals or vitamins in hosts' food can influence the indigenous microbiota both directly *via* the restricted availability of the metabolites and their indigestible parts for hosts and indirectly by inducing a stress response within the host organism and affecting the compositions of gastrointestinal morphology and secretions as well as by impairing the general and local immune responses and neuro-endocrine-immune network leading to an imbalance between the host organism and its microbiota, in general. These changed milieus offer possibilities to certain new species of the microbiota for adaptation in gastrointestinal tract or cause their dispersion from their localization areas to others. In protein calorie malnutrition, colonic type microbiota known to spread to and proliferate in the upper small intestine which may cause a variety of metabolic disturbances including steatorrhea, vitamin deficiencies, nutrient malabsorbtions, and consequently water leakage into lumina and diarrhea [160,239-241]. Generally, pathogenic microorganisms including Enterobacteriaceae, Pseudomonas, Klebsiella and Candida were increased [240,241]. In such clinical cases of complicated protein and/or calorie malnutrition, pathogenic microorganisms often cause endotoxemia and infection in addition to intestinal disruptions including diarrhea and metabolic diseases [242,243]. Thus, they all affect the composition of the intestinal digesta and its passage time, which in turn may influence the composition of the indigenous intestinal microbiota and their relationships with the intestinal wall [244-246].

Generally, experimental studies use deficiencies or excesses of a definite dietary component or several components, and animals are held under more hygienic, defined conditions throughout the rearing and experimental periods than their counterparts, whereas clinical cases develop spontaneously in man and animals. Thus, they give the possibility to detect the possible effects of a certain dietary component on the behavior of the gastrointestinal microbiota. However, such experimental evidences from studies using deficiencies or imbalances of definite nutrients in this respect are very sparse. So, an almost protein-free diet disrupted the cecal microbiota, and made mice more susceptible to bacterial translocation than those mice nourished adequately [227,236,247]. The counts of cecal total aerobic bacteria and Gram-negative enteric bacilli were found to be increased time-dependently when CD-1 mice were fed an almost N-free diet for 21 days [236]. The results of another study on adult female Crl:CD-1[CR]BR mice also showed that both the feeding an almost protein-free and 20% fat containing diet for 14 days and starvation for 3 days resulted in an increase in counts of Gram-negative enteric bacilli and a decrease in counts of lactobacilli and strict anaerobes [227]. In certain studies the effects of dietary manipulations combined and/or compared with those of endotoxemia were investigated. So, Deitch et al. [227] studied the effects of starvation and malnutrition alone or in combination with endotoxemia and found that the spread of bacteria from the gut could not be controlled nor translocated bacteria be cleared in protein malnourished mice as effectively as in the controls. However, no association between protein malnutrition and bacterial translocation could be found by Katayama et al. [247]. Instead, these authors determined that the total numbers of Gram-negative enteric bacilli adherent to the mucosa of ileum and cecum were less in protein malnourished rats than in their adequately nourished controls. Further, there was also a significant negative correlation between the duration of protein malnutrition and bacterial adherence to the intestinal mucosa. Only, *E. coli* binding to insoluble ileal mucus was increased in the rats receiving endotoxin. Tannock and Savage [192] reported that the deprivation of food and water and bedding for 48 hours increased the counts of coliform bacteria while they decreased the counts of cecal lactobacilli of CD-1 and C57BL mice strainsIn a preliminary study, we found that feeding an almost protein-free diet to male Wistar rats for 35 days affected especially the total aerobe microorganisms and lactobacilli while total anaerobe and *Enterobacteriaceae* remained relatively unaffected. Compared to controls with balanced nutrition, both dietary qualitative and quantitative protein malnutrition decreased mean lactobacilli counts. Also, the quality and quantity of the dietary protein made a difference in their effects on intestinal microbiota; compared to gelatin-fed animals, lower aerobe and higher lactobacilli counts could be observed in cecal samples of rats given an almost protein-free diet. Furthermore, it could also be shown that the actual immune status (e.g. suppression of neutrophils) of the host can modify the effects of the qualitative and quantitative protein malnutrition on the intestinal microbiota [193].

Human cultural characteristics may also have implications on the compositions of the gastrointestinal microbiota. Living on a high carbohydrate diet caused also the presence of fewer bacteriodes and more enterococci in feces of the people than those living on a Western diet with more fat and animal proteins [231].

After all, the mechanisms *via* which different type of diets or dietary manipulations affect the host and its guest organ 'gut microbiota' are still not exactly cleared. The effects of dietary qualitative and/or quantitative protein malnutrition on regulatory systems in men and animals are well characterized and are the topic of numerous texts. Earlier studies with definite protein malnutrition were summarized by Aschkenasy [248] and suggest that protein malnutrition of different types or amino acid imbalances generally result in increases of adrenalin and glucocorticoid concentrations in man and animals. Torún and Viteri [249] also noted that in protein and/or protein-calorie malnutrition, the concentrations of adrenalin and glucocorticoids are either increased or showed no important change while many other hormones with exceptions of aldosterone and growth hormone decreased significantly. However, such studies have very important drawbacks as they look only one aspect of the regulators such as their concentrations in blood. Generally, the concomitant expression status of the enzymes which interconvert active and inactive forms of a given hormone and their receptors in target tissues or cells are ignored or not evaluated concurrently. A study conducted by Marroqui et al. [250] on mice demonstrated that during a protein malnutrition plasma glucagon concentration increased, but the ability of exogenous glucagon to raise plasma glucose levels were lower in mice given a low protein diet.

13. Conclusion

Since their introduction in the terminology of scientific medicine, the terms environment, stress and microorganisms were probably never been so important in mind of mankind for the development, health and welfare of men and animals. Although the roles of stress and stress-dependent disruptions of the intestinal microbiota both in developments and in promotion of the symptoms of various diseases and disorders including those of gastrointestinal system in men and animals are well accepted, there is still a lack of information about many aspects including which strains play really a role in the etiopathogenesis of a given condition, and which mechanisms are effective in such cases [24,113]. The stress-dependent dysfunctions of HPA axis can manifest itself in different ways. In many cases it may be related to high or low cortisol concentrations in blood whereas in other situations no detectable change of cortisol occurs. Further, the response given by hypothalamus and pituitary gland to the cortisol can be increased or decreased depending on the receptor numbers [10,11,14,15]. While in classic stress response sympathetic nervous system and glucocorticoids thought to be responsible for stress-dependent processes, studies within last two decades suggest that many disordered situations of the gastrointestinal system mediated by CRF. Both CRF-related peptides and CRF receptors are also expressed within the intestine, where they may activate directly the enteric, endocrine, and immune cells and may be involved in intestinal manifestations such as mucosal permeability, secretion, mast cell function, motility, mucin formation, immune function and many disorders of the gut. In other words, the peripheral changes produced by stress can be mimicked by CRF-injection and prevented by CRF-receptor antagonists [18,20,31,32,82]. Therefore, CRF have been suggested as a new target in treating stress induced functional gastrointestinal disorders.

Recently, intestinal microbiota imbalances gain growing interests both as the subject and cause of stress and stress-related diseases which are connected with not only the gastrointestinal system but also all other systems or organs of the metazoan hosts including the adipose tissue [24,113, 179, 184,185]. Basing on experimental and clinical studies, certain phyla and species are currently related with a given specific condition [180,181]. However, all these studies are looking mainly on one side of the iceberg, like for example changes in a specific member of the microbiota in respect to stress stimuli and a specific neurotransmitter in brain, as it also the case in search of the mediating regulatory pathways. Understanding the roles of stress and stress-related microbiotal changes and their mechanisms in the role of various physiopathological conditions would be helpful in improvements of the relationships of the metazoan hosts with their microenvironments including its microbiota and thus, would contribute greatly to the health state of men and animals.

Author details

Hümeyra Ünsal* and Muharrem Balkaya
Adnan Menderes University, Faculty of Veterinary Medicine, Department of Physiology, Işıklı, Aydın, Turkey

14. References

[1] Adams JD, Jr Garcia C (2005) Spirit, Mind and Body in Chumash Healing. Evid. based. complement. alternat. med. 2: 459-463.
[2] Yang Y (2009) Chinese Herbal Medicines. Comparisons and Characteristics. 2nd Editions. China. Churchill Livingstone Elsevier, pp
[3] Fornaro M, Clementi N, Fornaro P (2009) Medicine and Psychiatry in Western Culture: Ancient Greek Myths and Modern Prejudices. Ann. gen. psychiatry 8: 21.
[4] Yapijakis C (2009) Hippocrates of Kos, the Father of Clinical Medicine, and Asclepiades of Bithynia, the Father of Molecular Medicine. In vivo: 507-514.
[5] Kelly K. The History of Medicine. Medicine Becomes a Science: 1840-1999. Facts on File Inc.
[6] Bernard C. (1865). Introduction à l'étude de la médecineexpérimentale. Available: http://classiques.uqac.ca/classiques/bernard_claude/intro_etude_medecine_exp/intro_medecine_exper.pdf
[7] Selye H (1936) A Syndrome Produced by Diverse Nocuous Agents. Nature. 138: 32.
[8] Vander Sherman and Luciano's Human Physiology: The Mechanisms of Body Function. 8th Edition. The McGraw-Hill Companies, pp. 728-732
[9] Chrousos GP, Gold PW (1992) The Concepts of Stress and Stress System Disorders. Overview of Physical and Behavioral Homeostasis. JAMA. 267: 1244-1252.
[10] Charmandari E, Tsigos C, Chrousos G (2005) Endocrinology of the Stress Response. Annu. rev. physiol. 67: 259-84.
[11] Chrousos GP (2009) Stress and Disorders of Stress Systems. Nature rev. endoc. 5: 374-381.
[12] Mayer EA, Naliboff BD, Chang L, Coutinho SV (2001) Stress and Irritable Bowel Syndrome. Am. j. physiol. gastrointest. liver physiol. 280: G519-G524.

* Corresponding Author

[13] Goymann W, Wingfield JC (2004) Allostatic Load, Social Status and Stress Hormones: The Costs of Social Status Matter. Anim. beh. 67: 591-602.

[14] McEwen BS (2000) Allostasis, Allostatic Load, and the Aging Nervous System: Role of Excitatory Amino Acids and Excitotoxicity. Neurochem. res. 25: 1219-1231.

[15] Mayer EA (2000) The Neurobiology of Stress and Gastrointestinal Disease. *Gut.* 47: 861-869.

[16] Papadimitriou A, Priftis KN (2009) Regulation of the Hypothalamic-Pituitary-Adrenal Axis. Neuroimmunomodulation. 16: 265-271.

[17] Bhatia V, Tandon RK (2005) Stress and the Gastrointestinal Tract. J. gastroenterol. hepatol. 20: 332-339.

[18] Larauche M, Kiank C, Tache Y (2009) Corticotropin Releasing Factor Signaling in Colon and Ileum: Regulation by Stress and Pathophysiological Implications. J. physiol. pharmacol. 60 (Suppl 7): 33-46.

[19] Lyte M, Vulchanova L, Brown DR (2011) Stress at the Intestinal Surface: Catecholamines and Mucosa-Bacteria Interactions. Cell tissue res. 343: 23-32.

[20] Söderholm JD, Perdue MH (2001) Stress and Gastrointestinal Tract. II. Stress and Intestinal Barrier Function. Am. j. physiol. gastrointest. liver physiol. 280: G7-G13.

[21] Davies E, MacKenzie SM (2003) Extra-Adrenal Production of Corticosteroids. Clin. Exp. pharmacol. physiol. 30: 437-445.

[22] Noti M, Sidler D, Brunner T (2009) Extra-Adrenal Glucocorticoid Synthesis in the Intestinal Epithelium: More than a Drop in the Ocean? Semin. immunopathol. 31: 237-248.

[23] Ashida H, Ogawa M, Kim M, Mimuro H, Sasakawa C (2011) Bacteria and Host Interactions in the Gut Epithelial Barrier. Nat. chem. biol. 8: 36-45.

[24] Sekirov I, Russell SL, Antunes LC, Finlay BB (2010) Gut Microbiota in Health and Disease. Physiol. rev. 90: 859-904.

[25] Sudo N, Chida Y, Aiba Y, Sonoda J, Oyama N, Yu XN, Kubo C, Koga Y (2004) Postnatal Microbial Colonization Programs the Hypothalamic-Pituitary-Adrenal System for Stress Response in Mice. J. physiol. 558: 263-275.

[26] Bailey MT, Coe CL (1999) Maternal Separation Disrupts the Integrity of the Intestinal Microflora in Infant Rhesus Monkeys. Dev psychobiol. 35:146-155.

[27] Freestone PP, Haigh RD, Williams PH, Lyte M (1999) Stimulation of Bacterial Growth by Heat-Stable Norepinophrine-Induced Autoinducers. FEMS microbial. letters. 172: 53-60.

[28] Meddings JB, Swain MG (2000) Environmental Stress-Induced Gastrointestinal Permeability is Mediated by Endogenous Glucocorticoids in the Rat. Gastroenterology. 119: 1019-1028.

[29] Spitz J, Hecht G, Taveras M, Aoys E, Alverdy J (1994) The Effect of Dexamethasone Administration on Rat Intestinal Permeability: The Role of Bacterial Adherence. Gastroenterology. 106: 35-41.

[30] Spitz JC, Ghandi S, Taveras M, Aoys E, Alverdy JC (1996) Characteristics of the Intestinal Epithelial Barrier During Dietary Manipulation and Glucocorticoid Stress. Crit. care med. 24: 635-641.

[31] Estienne M, Claustre J, Clain-Gardechaux G, Paquet A, Taché Y, Fioramonti J, Plaisancié P. (2010) Maternal Deprivation Alters Epithelial Secretory Cell Lineages in Rat Duodenum: Role of CRF-Related Peptides. Gut. 59: 744-751.

[32] Taché Y, Martinez V, Million M, Wang L (2001) Stress and the Gastrointestinal Tract III. Stress-Related Alterations of Gut Motor Function: Role of Brain Corticotropin-Releasing Factor Receptors. Am. j. physiol. gastrointest. liver physiol. 280: G173-G177.

[33] Tsukada F, Sugawara M, Kohno H, Ohkubo Y (2001) Evaluation of the Effects of Restraint and Footshock Stress on Small Intestinal Motility by an Improved Method Using a Radionuclide, 51 Cr, in the Rat. Biol. pharm. bull. 24:488-90.

[34] Bradesi S, Schwetz I, Ennes HS, Lamy CM, Ohning G, Fanselow M, Pothoulakis C, McRoberts JA, Mayer EA (2005) Repeated Exposure to Water Avoidance Stress in Rats: A New Model for Sustained Visceral Hyperalgesia. Am. j. physiol. gastrointest. liver physiol. 289: G42–G53.

[35] Williams CL, Villar RG, Peterson JM, Burks TF (1988) Stress-Induced Changes in Intestinal Transit in the Rat: A Model for Iirritable Bowel Syndrome. Gastroenterology. 94: 611-621.

[36] Saunders PR, Kosecka U, McKay DM, Perdue MH (1994) Acute Stressors Stimulate Ion Secretion and Increase Epithelial Permeability in Rat Intestine. Am. j. physiol. 267: G794-G799.

[37] Million M, Taché Y, Anton P (1999) Susceptibility of Lewis and Fischer Rats to Stress-Induced Worsening of TNB-Colitis: Protective Role of Brain CRF. Am. j. physiol. 276: G1027-G1036.

[38] Söderholm JD, Streutker C, Yang PC, Paterson C, Singh PK, McKay DM, Sherman PM, Croitoru K, Perdue MH (2004) Increased Epithelial Uptake of Protein Antigens in the İleum of Crohn's Disease Mediated by Tumour Necrosis Factor Alpha. Gut. 53: 1817-1824.

[39] Vicario M., Guilarte M, Alonso C, Yang PC, Martínez C, Ramos L, Lobo B, González A, Guilà M, Pigrau M, Saperas E, Azpiroz F, Santos J (2010) Chronological Assessment of Mast Cell-Mediated Gut Dysfunction and Mucosal Inflammation in a Rat Model of Chronic Psychosocial Stress. Brain behav. immun. 24: 1166-1175.

[40] Vicario M, Alonso C, Guilarte M, Serra J, Martínez C, González-Castro AM, Lobo B, Antolín M, Andreu AL, García-Arumí E, Casellas M, Saperas E, Malagelada JR, Azpiroz F, Santos J (2012) Chronic Psychosocial Stress Induces Reversible Mitochondrial Damage and Corticotropin-Releasing Factor Receptor Type-1 Upregulation in the Rat Intestine and IBS-like Gut Dysfunction. Psychoneuroendocrinology 37: 65-77.

[41] Söderholm JD, Yates DA, Gareau MG, Yang PC, MacQueen G, Perdue MH (2002) Neonatal Maternal Separation Predisposes Adult Rats to Colonic Barrier Dysfunction in Response to Mild Stress. Am. j. physiol. gastrointest. liver physiol. 283: G1257-G1263.

[42] Söderholm JD, Yang PC, Ceponis P, VohraA, Riddell R, Sherman PM, Perdue MH (2002) Chronic Stress Induces Mast Cell-Dependent Bacterial Adherence and Initiates Mucosal Inflammation in Rat Intestine. Gastroenterology. 123: 1099-1108.

[43] Gareau MG, Jury J, Yang PC, MacQueen G, Perdue MH (2006) Neonatal Maternal Separation Causes Colonic Dysfunction in Rat Pups Including Impaired Host Resistance. *Pediatr. res.* 59: 83-88.

[44] Gareau MG, Jury J, Perdue MH (2007) Neonatal Maternal Separation of Rat Pups Results in Abnormal Cholinergic Regulation of Epithelial Permeability. Am. j. physiol. gastrointest. liver physiol. 293: G198-G203.

[45] Iwasaki A, Kelsall BL (1999) Mucosal Dendritic Cells: Their Specialized Role in Initiating T Cell Responses. Am. j. physiol. gastroenterol. liver physiol. 276: G1074-G1078.

[46] Powell DW, Mifflin RC, Valentich JD, Crowe SE, Saada JI, West AB. (1999) Myofibroblasts. I. Paracrine Cells Important in Health and Disease. Am j. physiol. 277: C1-C9.

[47] Powell DW, Mifflin RC, Valentich JD, Crowe SE, Saada JI, West AB. (1999) Myofibroblasts. II. Intestinal Subepithelial Myofibroblasts. Am. j. physiol. 277: C183-C201.

[48] Stagg AJ, Hart AL, Knight SC, Kamm MA (2003) The Dendritic Cell: Its Role in Intestinal Inflammation and Relationship with Gut Bacteria. Gut. 52: 1522-1529.

[49] Catron DM, Itano AA, Pape KA, Mueller DL, Jenkins MK (2004) Visualizing the First 50 Hr of the Primary Immune Response to a Soluble Antigen. Immunity. 21: 341-347.

[50] Macpherson AJ, Uhr T (2004) Induction of Protective IgA by Intestinal Dendritic Cells Carrying Commensal Bacteria. Science. 303: 1662-1665.

[51] Saada JI, Barrera CA, Reyes VE, Adegboyega PA, Suarez G, Tamerisa RA, Pang KF, Bland DA, Mifflin RC, DI Mari JF, Powell DW (2004) Intestinal Myofibroblasts and Immune Tolerance. Ann. n. y. acad sci. 1029: 379-381.

[52] Niess JH, Reinecker HC (2005) Lamina Propria Dendritic Cells in the Physiology and Pathology of the Gastrointestinal Tract. Curr. opin. gastroenterol. 21: 687-691.

[53] Leon F, Symythies LE, Smith PD, Kelsall BL (2006) Involvement of Dendritic Cells in the Pathogenesis of Inflammatory Bowel Diseases. Adv. exp. med. biol. 579: 117-132.

[54] Inman CF, Singha, Lewis M, Bradley B, Stokes C, Bailey M (2010) Dendritic Cells Interact with CD4 T Cells in Intestinal Mucosa. J. leukocyte biol. 88: 571-578.

[55] Manicassamy S, Reizis B, Ravindran R, Nakaya H, Salazar-Gonzalez RM, Wang YC, Pulendran B (2010) Activation of Beta-Catenin in Dendritic Cells Regulates Immunity Versus Tolerance in the Intestine. Science. 329: 849-853.

[56] Perdue MH (1999) Mucosal Immunity and Inflammation III. The Mucosal Antigen Barrier: Cross Talk with Mucosal Cytokines Am. j. physiol. gastrointest. liver physiol. 277: G1-G5.

[57] Mason KL, Huffnagle GB, Noverr MC, Kao JY (2008) Overview of Gut Immunology. In: Huffnagle GB, Noverr MC, editors. GI Microbiota and Regulation of the Immune

System: Advances in Experimental Medicine and Biology Vol 635. Landes Bioscience Springer Science+Business Media. pp: 1-10.

[58] Boudry G, Jury J, Yang PC, Perdue MH (2007) Chronic Psychological Stress Alters Epithelial Cell Turn-Over in Rat Ileum. Am. j. physiol. gastrointest. liver physiol. 292: G1228-G1232.

[59] Cameron HL, Perdue MH (2005) Stress Impairs Murine İntestinal Barrier Function: Improvement by Glucagon-Like Peptide-2. J. pharmacol. exp. ther. 314: 214-220.

[60] Kiliaan AJ, Saunders PR, Bijlsma PB, Berin MC, Taminiau JA, Groot JA, Perdue MH. (1998) Stress Stimulates Transepithelial Macromolecular Uptake in Rat Jejunum. Am. j. physiol. gastrointest. liver. physiol. 275: G1037-G1044.

[61] Santos J, Benjamin M, Yang PC, Prior T, Perdue MH (2000) Chronic Stress Impairs Rat Growth and Jejunal Epithelial Barrier Function: Role of Mast Cells. *Am. j. physiol. gastrointest. liver physiol.* 278: G847-G854.

[62] Hung CR. (1998) Low Susceptibility of Stress Ulcer in Diabetic Rats: Role of Cholinergic Gastric Motility. Chin. j. physiol. 41: 151-159.

[63] Babygirija R, Zheng J, Bülbül M, Ludwig K, Takahashi T (2010) Beneficial Effects of Social Attachment to Overcome Daily Stress. Brain res.1352: 43-49.

[64] Zheng J, Babygirija R, Bülbül M, Cerjak D, Ludwig K, Takahashi T (2010) Hypothalamic Oxytocin Mediates Adaptation Mechanism Against Chronic Stress in Rats. Am. j. physiol. gastrointest. liver physiol. 299: G946-G953.

[65] Wallon C, Söderholm JD (2009) Corticotropin-Releasing Hormone and Mast Cells in the Regulation of Mucosal Barrier Function in the Human Colon. Ann. n. y. acad. sci. 1165: 206-210.

[66] Suzuki K, Harasawa R, Yoshitake Y, Mitsuoka T (1983) Effects of Crowding and Heat Stress on Intestinal flora, Body Weight Gain, and Feed Efficiency of Growing Rats and Chicks. Jpn. j. vet. sci. 45:331-338.

[67] Tannock GW (1997) Modification of the Normal Microbiota by Diet, Stress, Antimicrobial Agents, and Probiotics. In: Mackie RI, White BA, Isaacson RE, editors. Gastrointestinal Microbiology. New York. Chapman & Hall, pp 434-466.

[68] Bailey MT, Lubach GR, Coe CL (2004) Prenatal Stress Alters Bacterial Colonization of the Gut in Infant Monkeys. J. pediatr. gastroenterol. nutr. 38: 414-421.

[69] Lutgendorff F, Akkermans LM, Söderholm JD (2008) The Role of Microbiota and Probiotics in Stress-Induced Gastro-Intestinal Damage. Curr. mol. med. 8(4): 282-298.

[70] Mazzon E, Sturniolo GC, Puzzolo D, Frisina N, Fries W (2002) Effect of Stress on the Paracellular Barrier in the Rat Ileum. Gut. 51: 507-513.

[71] Wang F, Graham WV, Wang Y, Witkowski ED, Schwarz BT, Turner JR (2005) Interferon-Gamma and Tumor Necrosis Factor-Alpha Synergize to Induce Intestinal Epithelial Barrier Dysfunction by Up-regulating Myosin Light Chain Kinase Expression. Am. j.pathol. 166: 409-419.

[72] Graham WV, Wang F, Clayburgh DR, Cheng JX, Yoon B, Wang Y, Lin A, Turner JR. (2006) Tumor Necrosis Factor-Induced Long Myosin Light Chain Kinase Transcription

is Regulated by Differentiation-Dependent Signaling Events. Characterization of the Human Long Myosin Light Chain Kinase Promoter. J. biol. chem. 281: 26205-26215.
[73] Al-Sadi R, Ye D, Dokladny K, Ma TY (2008) Mechanism of IL-1 Beta-Induced Increase in Intestinal Epithelial Tight Junction Permeability. J. immunol. 180: 5653-5661.
[74] Ait-Belgnaoui A, Bradesi S, Fioramonti J, Theodorou V, Bueno L (2005) Acute Stress-Induced Hypersensitivity to Colonic Distension Depends upon Increase in Paracellular Permeability: Role of Myosin Light Chain Kinase. Pain. 113: 141-147.
[75] Mazzon E, Cuzzocrea S (2008) Role of TNF-Alpha in Ileum Tight Junction Alteration in Mouse Model of Restraint Stress. Am. j. physiol. gastrointest. liver physiol. 294: G1268-G1280.
[76] Matsuo K, Zhang X, Ono Y, Nagatomi R (2009) Acute Stress-Induced Colonic Tissue HSP70 Expression Requires Commensal Bacterial Components and Intrinsic Glucocorticoid. Brain behav. immune. 23: 108-115.
[77] Boivin MA, Ye D, Kennedy JC, Al-Sadi R, Shepela C, Ma TY (2007) Mechanism of Glucocorticoid Regulation of the Intestinal Tight Junction Barrier. Am. j physiol. gastrointest. liver physiol. 292: G590-G598.
[78] Barclay GR, Turnberg LA (1987) Effect of Psychological Stress on Salt and Water Transport in the Human Jejunum. Gastroenterology. 93: 91-97.
[79] Barclay GR, Turnberg LA (1988) Effect of Cold-Induced Pain on Salt and Water Transport in the Human Jejunum. Gastroenterology. 94: 994-998.
[80] Santos J, Saunders PR, Hanssen NP, Yang PC, Yates D, Groot JA, Perdue MH (1999) Corticotropin-Releasing Hormone Mimics Stress-Induced Colonic Epithelial Pathophysiology in the Rat Am. j. physiol. 277: G391-G399.
[81] Saunders PR, Santos J, Hanssen NP, Yates D, Groot JA, Perdue MH (2002) Physical and Psychological Stress in Rats Enhances Colonic Epithelial Permeability via Peripheral CRH. Dig. dis. sci. 47: 208-215.
[82] Larauche M, Gourcerol G, Wang L, Pambukchian K, Brunnhuber S, Adelson DW, Rivier J, Million M, Taché Y (2009) A Cortagine CRF1 Agonist, Induces Stresslike Alterations of Colonic Function and Visceral Hypersensitivity in Rodents Primarily Through Peripheral Pathways. Am. j. physiol. gastrointest. liver physiol. 297: G215-G227.
[83] Charney AN, Kinsey MD, Myers L, Gainnella RA, Gots RE (1975) Na+-K+-Activated Adenosine Triphosphatase and Intestinal Electrolyte Transport. Effect of Adrenal Steroids. J. clin invest. 56: 653-660.
[84] Marnane WG, Tai YH, Decker RA, Boedeker EC, Charney AN, Donowitz M (1981) Methylprednisolone Stimulation of Guanylate Cyclase Activity in Rat Small Intestinal Mucosa: Possible Role in Electrolyte Transport. Gastroenterology.81: 90-100.
[85] Tai YH, Decker RA, Marnane WG, Charney AN, Donowitz M (1981) Effects of Methylprednisolone on Electrolyte Transport by In Vitro Rat Ileum. Am. j. physiol. 240: G365-G370.

[86] Yates DA, Santos J, Söderholm JD, Perdue MH (2001) Adaptation of stress-induced mucosal pathophysiology in rat colon involves opioid pathways. Am. j. physiol. gastrointest. liver physiol. 281: G124-G128.

[87] Santos J, Saperas E, Nogueiras C, Mourelle M, Antoli'n M, Cadahia A, Malagelada JR (1998) Release of Mast Cell Mediators into the Jejunum by Cold Pain Stress in Humans. Gastroenterology 114: 640-648.

[88] Gerova VA, Stoynov SG, Katsarov DS, Svinarov DA (2011) Increased Intestinal Permeability in Inflammatory Bowel Diseases Assessed by Iohexol Test. World j. gastroenterol. 17: 2211-2215.

[89] Gecse K, Róka R, Séra T, Rosztóczy A, Annaházi A, Izbéki F, Nagy F, Molnár T, Szepes Z, Pávics L, Bueno L, Wittmann T (2012) Leaky Gut in Patients with Diarrhea-Predominant Irritable Bowel Syndrome and Inactive Ulcerative Colitis. Digestion. 85: 40-46.

[90] Bagchi D, Carryl OR, Tran MX, Bagchi M, Garg A, Milnes MM, Williams CB, Balmoori J, Bagchi DJ, Mitra S, Stohs SJ (1999) Acute and Chronic Stress-Induced Oxidative Gastrointestinal Mucosal Injury in Rats and Protection by Bismuth Subsalicylate. Mol. cell biochem. 196: 109-116.

[91] Barreau F, Ferrier L, Fioramonti J, Bueno L (2004) Neonatal Maternal Deprivation Triggers Long Term Alterations in Colonic Epithelial Barrier and Mucosal Immunity in Rats. Gut. 53: 501-506.

[92] Zhang ZW, Lv ZH, Li JL, Li S, Xu SW, Wang XL (2011) Effects of Cold Stress on Nitric Oxide in Duodenum of Chicks. Poult. sci. 90: 1555-1561.

[93] Witthöft T, Eckmann L, Kim JM, Kagnoff MF (1998) Enteroinvasive Bacteria Directly Activate Expression of INOS and NO Production in Human Colon Epithelial Cells. Am. j. physiol. 275: G564-G571.

[94] Santos J, Yang PC, Soderholm JD, Benjamin M, Perdue MH (2001) Role of Mast Cells in Chronic Stress Induced Colonic Epithelial Barrier Dysfunction in the Rat. Gut 48: 630-636.

[95] Perdue MH, McKay DM (1994) Integrative Immunophysiology in the Intestinal Mucosa. Am. j. physiol. 267: G151-G165.

[96] Castagliuolo I, Wershil BK, Karalis K, Pasha A, Nikulasson ST, Pothoulakis C (1998) Colonic Mucin Release in Response to Immobilization Stress is Mast Cell Dependent. *Am. j. physiol. gastrointest. liver physiol.* 274: G1094-G1100.

[97] Kim DH, Cho YJ, Kim JH, Kim YB, Lee KJ (2010) Stress-Induced Alterations in Mast Cell Numbers and Proteinase-Activated Receptor-2 Expression of the Colon: Role of Corticotrophin-Releasing Factor. J. korean med. sci. 25: 1330-1335.

[98] Róka R, Ait-Belgnaoui A, Salvador-Cartier C, Garcia-Villar R, Fioramonti J, Eutamène H, Bueno L (2007) Dexamethasone Prevents Visceral Hyperalgesia but not Colonic Permeability Increase Induced by Luminal Protease-Activated Receptor-2 Agonist in Rats. Gut. 56: 1072-1078.

[99] Wilson LM, Baldwin AL (1999) Environmental Stress Causes Mast Cell Degranulation, Endothelial and Epithelial Changes, and Edema in the Rat Intestinal Mucosa. Microcirculation. 6: 189-198.

[100] Jorge E, Fernández JA, Torres R, Vergara P, Martin MT (2010) Functional Changes Induced by Psychological Stress are not Enough to Cause Intestinal Inflammation in Sprague-Dawley Rats. Neurogastroenterol. motil. 22: e241-e250.

[101] Godot V, Garcia G, Capel F, Arock M, Durant-Gasselin I, Asselin-Labat ML, Emilie D, Humbert M (2006) Dexamethasone and IL-10 Stimulate Glucocorticoid-Induced Leucine Zipper Synthesis by Human Mast Cells. Allergy 61: 886-890.

[102] Rijnierse A, Koster AS, Nijkamp FP, Kraneveld AD (2006) TNF-Alpha is Crucial for the Development of Mast Cell-Dependent Colitis in Mice. Am. j. physiol. gastrointest. liver physiol. 291: G969-G976.

[103] Eutamene H, Theodorou V, Fioramonti J, Bueno L (2003) Acute Stress Modulates the Histamine Content of Mast Cells in the Gastrointestinal Tract Through Interleukin-1 and Corticotropin-Releasing Factor Release in Rats. J. physiol. 553: 959-966.

[104] Wallon C, Yang PC, Keita AV, Ericson AC, McKay DM, Sherman PM, Perdue MH, Söderholm JD (2008) Corticotropin-Releasing Hormone (CRH) Regulates Macromolecular Permeability via Mast Cells in Normal Human Colonic Biopsies In Vitro. Gut. 57: 50-58.

[105] Maloy KJ, Powrie F (2011) Intestinal Homeostasis and Its Breakdown in Inflammatory Bowel Disease. Nature. 474: 298-306.

[106] McGuckin MA, Lindén SK, Sutton P, Florin TH. (2011) Mucin Dynamics and Enteric Pathogens. Nat. rev microbiol. 9: 265-278.

[107] Dharmani P, Srivastava V, Kissoon-Singh V, Chadee K (2009) Role of Intestinal Mucins in Innate Host Defense Mechanisms Against Pathogens. J. innate immun. 1: 123-135.

[108] Castagliuolo I, Lamont JT, Qiu B, Fleming SM, Bhaskar KR, Nikulasson ST, Kornetsky C, Pothoulakis C (1996) Acute Stress Causes Mucin Release From Rat Colon: Role of Corticotropin Releasing Factor and Mast Cells. Am. j. phyiol. 271: G884-G892.

[109] O'Malley D, Julio-Pieper M, Gibney SM, Dinan TG, Cryan JF (2010) Distinct Alterations in Colonic Morphology and Physiology in Two Rat Models of Enhanced Stress-Induced Anxiety and Depression-like Behaviour. Stress. 13(2): 114-122.

[110] Finnie IA, Campbell BJ, Taylor BA, Milton JD, Sadek SK, Yu LG, Rhodes JM (1996) Stimulation of Colonic Mucin Synthesis by Corticosteroids and Nicotine. Clin. sci. (Lond) 91: 359-364.

[111] Tsukamoto K, Nakade Y, Mantyh C, Ludwig K, Pappas TN, Takahashi T (2006) Peripherally Administered CRF Stimulates Colonic Motility via Central CRF Receptors and Vagal Pathways in Conscious Rats. Am. j. physiol. regul. integr. comp. physiol. 290: R1537-R1541.

[112] Michelsen KS, Arditi M (2007) Toll-like Receptors and Innate Immunity in Gut Homeostasis and Pathology. Curr. opin. hematol. 14: 48-54.

[113] Grenham S, Clarke G, Cryan JF, Dinan TG (2011) Brain-Gut-Microbe Communication in Health and Disease. Front. physiol. 2: 1-14.

[114] Shibolet O, Podolsky DK (2007) TLRs in the Gut. IV. Negative Regulation of Toll-like Receptors and Intestinal Homeostasis: Addition by Subtraction. Am. j. physiol. gastrointest. liver physiol. 292: G1469-G1473.

[115] Jarillo-Luna A, Rivera-Aguilar V, Martìnez-Carrillo BE, Barbosa-Cabrera E, Garfias HR, Campos-Rodrĺguez R (2008) Effect of Restraint Stress on the Population of Intestinal Intraepithelial Lymphocytes in Mice. Brain behav. immun. 22: 265-275.

[116] McKernan DP, Nolan A, Brint EK, O'Mahony SM, Hyland NP, Cryan JF, Dinan TG (2009) Toll-Like Receptor mRNA Expression is Selectively Increased in the Colonic Mucosa of Two Animal Models Relevant to Irritable Bowel Syndrome. PLoS ONE 4(12): e8226. Available: http://www.plosone.org/article/info%3adoi%2fF10.1371%2Fjournal.pone.0008226.

[117] Zhang Y, Woodruff M, Zhang Y, Miao J, Hanley G, Stuart C, Zeng X, Sprabhajar S, Moorman J, Zhao B, Yin D (2008) Toll-like Receptor 4 Mediates Chronic Restraint Stress-Induced Immune Suppression. *J. neuroimmunol.* 194:115–122.

[118] Bailey MT, Engler H, Powell ND, Padgett DA, Sheridan JF (2007) Repeated Social Defeat Increases the Bactericidal Activity of Splenic Macrophages Through a Toll-like Receptor-Dependent Pathway. Am. j. physiol. regul. integr. comp. physiol. 293: R1180-R1190.

[119] Powell ND, Bailey MT, Mays JW, Stiner-Jones LM, Hanke ML, Padgett DA, Sheridan JF (2009) Repeated Social Defeat Activates Dendritic Cells and Enhances Toll-like Receptor Dependent Cytokine Secretion. *Brain behav. immun.* 23: 225-231.

[120] McKernan DP, Gaszner G, Quigley EM, Cryan JF, Dinan TG (2011) Altered Peripheral Toll-like Receptor Responses in the Irritable Bowel Syndrome. Aliment. pharmacol. ther. 33: 1045-1052.

[121] Yang PC, Jury J, Söderholm JD, Sherman PM, Mckay DM, Perdue MH (2006) Chronic Psychological Stress in Rats Induces Intestinal Sensitization to Luminal Antigens. Am. j. pathol. 168: 104-114.

[122] Velin AK, Ericson AC, Braaf Y, Wallon C, Söderholm JD (2004) Increased Antigen and Bacterial Uptake in Follicle Associated Epithelium Induced by Chronic Psychological Stress in Rats. Gut. 53: 494-500.

[123] Keita AV, Salim SY, Jiang T, Yang PC, Franzén L, Söderkvist P, Magnusson KE, Söderholm JD (2008) Increased Uptake of Non-pathogenic E. Coli via the Follicle-Associated Epithelium in Longstanding Ileal Crohn's Disease. J. pathol. 215: 135-144.

[124] Keita AV, Söderholm JD, Ericson AC (2010) Stress-Induced Barrier Disruption of Rat Follicle-Associated Epithelium Involves Corticotropin-Releasing Hormone, Acetylcholine, Substance P, and Mast Cells. Neurogastroenterol. motil. 22: 770-778.

[125] Zheng PY, Feng BS, Oluwole C, Struiksma S, Chen X, Li P, Tang SG, Yang PC (2009) Psychological Stress Induces Eosinophils to Produce Corticotrophin Releasing Hormone in the Intestine. Gut. 58:1473-1479.

[126] Koslowski M J, Beisner J, Stange EF, Wehkamp J (2010) Innate Antimicrobial Host Defense in Small Intestinal Crohn's Disease. Int. j. med. microbiol. 300: 34-40.

[127] Cash HL, Whitham CV, Behrendt CL, Hooper LV (2006) Symbiotic Bacteria Direct Expression of an Intestinal Bactericidal Lectin. Science. 313: 1126-1130.

[128] Ayabe T, Satchell DP, Wilson CL, Parks WC, Selsted ME, Ouellette AJ (2000) Secretion of Microbicidal Alpha-Defensins by Intestinal Paneth Cells in Response to Bacteria. Nat. immunol. 1: 99-100.

[129] Macpherson AJ, Slack E (2007) The Functional Interactions of Commensal Bacteria with Intestinal Secretory IgA. Curr. opin. gastroenterol. 23: 673-8.

[130] Kelly P, Feakins R, Domizio P, Murphy J, Bevins C, Wilson J, McPhail P, Poulsom R, Dhaliwal W (2004) Paneth Cell Granule Depletion in Human Small Intestine under Infective and Nutritional Stress. Clin. exp. immunol. 135: 303-309.

[131] Alonso C, Guilarte M, Vicario M, Ramos L, Ramadan Z, Antolín M, Martínez C, Rezzi S, Saperas E, Kochhar S, Santos J, Malagelada JR (2008) Maladaptive Intestinal Epithelial Responses to Life Stress may Predispose Healthy Women to Gut Mucosal Inflammation. Gastroenterology. 135: 163-172.

[132] Murosaki S, Inagaki-Ohara K, Kusaka H, Ikeda H, Yoshikai Y (1997) Apoptosis of Intestinal Intraepithelial Lymphocytes Induced by Exogenous and Endogenous Glucocorticoids. Microbiol. immunol. 41: 139-148.

[133] Fukuzuka K, Edwards CK 3rd, Clare-Salzer M, Copeland EM 3rd, Moldawer LL, Mozingo DW (2000) Glucocorticoid and Fas Ligand Induced Mucosal Lymphocyte Apoptosis After Burn Injury. J. trauma. 49: 710-716.

[134] Reber SO, Peters S, Slattery DA, Hofmann C, Schölmerich J, Neumann ID, Obermeier F (2011) Mucosal Immunosuppression and Epithelial Barrier Defects are Key Events in Murine Psychosocial Stress-Induced Colitis. Brain behav. immun. 25: 1153-1161.

[135] Motyka B, Bhogal HS, Reynolds JD (1995) Apoptosis of Ileal Peyer's Patch B Cells is Increased by Glucocorticoids or Anti-immunoglobulin Antibodies. Eur. j. immunol. 25: 1865-1871.

[136] Ruiz-Santana S, Lopez A, Torres S, Rey A, Losada A, Latasa L, Manzano JL, Diaz-Chico BN, (2001) Prevention of Dexamethasone Induced Lymphocytic Apoptosis in the Intestine and in Peyer Patches by Enteral Nutrition. J. parenter. enteral nutr. 25: 338-345.

[137] Vaughn J (1961) Experimental Eosinophilia: Local Tissue Reactions to Ascaris Extracts. J. allergy. 32: 501-513.

[138] Browaeys J, Wallon D (1958) Éosinophilies tissulaires du rat a l'état normal et dans les éosinopénies sanguine. Le sang 29: 686-695.

[139] Elftman MD, Norbury CC, Bonneau RH, Truckenmiller ME (2007) Corticosterone Impairs Dendritic Cell Maturation and Function. Immunology. 122: 279-290.

[140] McEwen BS, Biron CA, Brunson KW, Bulloch K, Chambers WH, Dhabhar FS, Goldfarb RH, Kitson RP, Miller AH, Spencer RL, Weiss JM (1997) The Role of Adrenocorticoids

as Modulators of Immune Function in Health and Disease: Neural, Endocrine and Immune Interactions. Brain res. rev. 23: 79-133.

[141] Toft P, Lillevang ST, Tønnesen E, Svendsen P, Höhndorf K (1993) Redistribution of Lymphocytes Following E. Coli Sepsis. Scand. j. immunol. 38: 541-545.

[142] Toft P, Svendsen P, Tønnesen E, Rasmussen JW, Christensen NJ (1993) Redistribution of Lymphocytes after Major Surgical Stress. Acta anaesthesiol. scand. 37: 245-249.

[143] Tlaskalová-Hogenová H, Stepánková R, Hudcovic T, Tucková L, Cukrowska B, Lodinová-Zádníková R, Kozáková H, Rossmann P, Bártová J, Sokol D, Funda DP, Borovská D, Reháková Z, Sinkora J, Hofman J, Drastich P, Kokesová A (2004) Commensal Bacteria (Normal Microflora), Mucosal Immunity and Chronic Inflammatory and Autoimmune Diseases. Immunol. lett. 93: 97-108.

[144] Eckburg PB, Bik EM, Bernstein CN, Purdom E, Dethlefsen L, Sergent M, Gill SR, Nelson KE, Relman DA (2005) Diversity of Human Intestinal Microbial Flora. Science. 308: 1635-1638.

[145] Ley RE, Peterson DA, Gordon JI (2006) Ecological and Evolutionary Forces Shaping Microbial Diversity in the Human Intestine. Cell. 124: 837-848.

[146] O'Hara AM, Shanahan EM (2006) The gut flora as a forgotten organ. EMBO rep. 7: 688-693.

[147] Holzapfel WH, Haberer P, Snel J, Schillinger U, Jos HJ, Huis in't Veld. (1998) Overview of Gut Flora and Probiotics. Int. j. food microbiol. 41: 85-101.

[148] Mackie RI, Sghir A, Gaskins HR (1999) Developmental Microbial Ecology of the Neonatal Gastrointestinal Tract. Am. j. clin. nutr. 69(suppl.): 1035-1045.

[149] Guerrero R, Berlenga M (2006) Life's Unity and Flexibility: The Ecological Link. Int. microbiol. 9: 225-235.

[150] Savage DC (1999) Mucosal Microbiota. In: Ogra PL, Mestecky J, Lamm ME, Strober W, Bienenstock J, McGhee J, editors. Mucosal immunology. New York: Academic Press. 19-30 pp.

[151] Gill SR, Pop M, Deboy RT, Eckburg PB, Turnbaugh PJ, Samuel BS, Gordon JI, Relman DA, Fraser-Liggett CM, Nelson KE (2006) Meta Genomic Analysis of the Human Distal Gut Microbiome. Science. 312:1355-1359.

[152] Hooper LV, Gordon JI (2001) Commensal Host-Bacterial Relationships in the Gut. Science. 292: 1115-1118.

[153] Turnbaugh PJ, Ley RE, Hamady M, Fraser-Liggett CM, Knight R, Gordon JI (2007) The Human Microbiome Project. Nature. 449: 804-810.

[154] Berg RD (1996) The Indigenous Gastrointestinal Microflora. Trends microbial. 4: 430-435.

[155] Claesson MJ, Cusack S, O'Sullivan O, Greene-Diniz R, DeWeerd H, Flannery E, Marchesi R, Falush D, Dinan T, Fitzgerald G, Stanton C, VanSinderen D, O'Connor M, Harnedy N, O'Connor K, Henry C, O'Mahony D, Fitzgerald AP, Shanahan F, Twomey C, Hill C, Ross RP, O'Toole PW (2011) Composition, Variability, and Temporal Stability of the Intestinal Microbiota of the Elderly. Proc. natl. acad. sci. 108(S1): 4586-4591.

[156] Palmer C, Bik EM, DiGiulio DB, Relman DA, Brown PO (2007) Development of the Human Infant Intestinal Microbiota. PLoS Biol 5(7): e177. doi: 10.1371/journal.pbio.0050177.

[157] Andersson AF, Linberg M, Jakobsson H, Bäkhed F, Nyrén P, Engstrand L (2008) Comparative Analysis of Human Gut Microbiota by Barcoded Pyrosequencing. PLoS One. 3(7): Article ID e2836.

[158] Frank DN, Pace NR (2008) Gastrointestinal Microbiology Enters the Metagenomics Era. Curr. opin. gastroent. 24: 4-10.

[159] Miller TL, Wolin MJ (1983) Stability of Methanobrevibacter Smithii Populations in the Microbial Flora Excreted from the Human Large Bowel. Appl. environ. microbiol. 45: 317-318.

[160] Simon GL, Gorbach SL (1984) Intestinal Flora in Health and Disease. Gastroenterology 86: 174-193.

[161] Dubos R, Schaedler RW, Costello R, Hoet P (1965) Indigenous, Normal, and Autochthonous Flora of the Gastrointestinal Tract. J. exp. med. 122: 67-76.

[162] Khoury KA, Floch MH, Hersh T (1969) Small Intestinal Mucosal Cell Proliferation and Bacterial Flora in the Conventionalization of the Germfree Mouse. J. exp. med. 130: 659-670.

[163] Guarner F, Malagelada JR (2003) Gut Flora in Health and Disease. Lancet 361: 512-519.

[164] Wotsmann BS, Kardoss EB, Knight PL (1968) Cecal Enlargement, Cardiac Output and O_2 Consumption in Germfree Rats. Proc. soc. exp. biol. med. 128: 137-140.

[165] Hooper, LV, Macpherson, AJ (2010) Immune Adaptations that Maintain Homeostasis with the Intestinal Microbiota. Nat. rev. immunol. 10: 159-169.

[166] Gilmore MS, Ferretti JJ (2003) Microbiology. The Thin Line Between Gut Commensal and Pathogen. Science. 299: 1999-2002.

[167] Tannock GW (2005) New Perceptions of the Gut Microbiota: Implications for Future Research. Gastroenterol. clin. north am. 34: 361-382.

[168] Martin FP, Sprenger N, Montoliu I, Rezzi S, Kochhar S, Nicholson JK (2010) Dietary Modulation of Gut Functional Ecology Studied by Fecal Metabonomics. J. proteome res. 9: 5284-5295.

[169] Heath P, Claus SP (2011) Assessing hepatic metabolic changes during progressive colonization of germ-free mouse by 1H NMR spectroscopy. J. vis exp. (58) pii: 3642. doi: 10.3791/3642.

[170] Claus SP, Tsang TM, Wang Y, Cloarec O, Skordi E, Martin FP, Rezzi S, Ross A, Kochhar S, Holmes E, Nicholson JK (2008) Systemic Multicompartmental Effects of the Gut Microbiome on Mouse Metabolic Phenotypes. Mol. syst. biol. 4: 219.

[171] Zheng X, Xie G, Zhao A, Zhao L, Yao C, Chiu NH, Zhou Z, Bao Y, Jia W, Nicholson JK, Jia W (2011) The Footprints of Gut Microbial-Mammalian Co-metabolism. J. proteome res. 10: 5512-5522.

[172] Keeney KM, Finlay BB (2011) Enteric Pathogen Exploitation of the Microbiota-Generated Nutrient Environment of the Gut. Curr. opin. microbiol. 14: 92-98.

[173] Bouskra D, Brezillon C, Berard M, Werts C, Varona R, Boneca IG, Eberl G (2008) Lymphoid Tissue Genesis Induced by Commensals Through NOD1 Regulates Intestinal Homeostasis. Nature. 456: 507- 510.

[174] Macpherson AJ, Harris NL (2004) Interactions Between Commensal Intestinal Bacteria and the Immune System. Nat. rev. immunol. 4: 478-485.

[175] Vijay-Kumar M, Aitken JD, Carvalho FA, Cullender TC, Mwangi S, Srinivasan S, Sitaraman SV, Knight R, Ley RE, Gewirtz AT (2010) Metabolic Syndrome and Altered Gut Microbiota in Mice Lacking Toll-like Receptor 5. Science. 328: 228-231.

[176] Atarashi K, Nishimura J, Shima T, Umesaki Y, Yamamoto M, Onoue M, Yagita H, Ishii N, Evans R, Honda K, et al (2008). ATP Drives Lamina Propria T(H)17 Cell Differentiation. Nature. 455: 808-812.

[177] Chow J, Mazmanian SK (2009) Getting the Bugs out of the Immune System: Do Bacterial Microbiota "Fix" Intestinal T Cell Responses? Cell host microbe. 5: 8-12.

[178] Fetissov and Déchelotte (2011) The New Link Between Gut-Brain Axis and Neuropsychiatric Disorders. Curr. opin. clin. nutr. metab. care. 14: 477-482.

[179] Hooper LV, Wong MH, Thelin A, Hansson L, Falk PG, Gordon JI (2001) Molecular Analysis of Commensal Host-Microbial Relationships in the Intestine. Science 2: 881-884.

[180] Mozeš S, Bujňáková D, Šefčiková Z, Kmet' V (2008) Developmental Changes of Gut Microflora and Enzyme Activity in Rat Pups Exposed to Fat-Rich Diet. Obesity 16: 2610-2615.

[181] Turnbaugh PJ, Hamady M, Yatsunenko T, Cantarel BL, Duncan A, Ley RE, Sogin ML, Jones WJ, Roe BA, Affourtit JP, Egholm M, Henrissat B, Heath AC, Knight R, Gordon JI (2009) A Core Gut Microbiome in Obese and Lean Twins. Nature. 457: 480-484.

[182] Šefčiková Z, KmeŤ V, Bujňáková D, Raček L', Mozeš Š (2010) Development of Gut Microflora in Obese and Lean Rats. Folia microbiol. 55: 373-375.

[183] Manco M, Putignani L, Bottazzo GF (2010) Gut Microbiota, Lipopolysaccharides, and Innate Immunity in the Pathogenesis of Obesity and Cardiovascular Risk. Endocr. rev. 31: 817-844.

[184] Turnbaugh P, Ley RE, Mahowald MA, Magrini V, Mardis ER, Gordon JI (2006) An Obesity-Associated Gut Microbiome with Increased Capacity for Energy Harvest. Nature 444: 1027-1031.

[185] Bäckhed F, Ding H, Wang T, Hooper LV, Koh GY, Nagy A, Semenkovich CF, Gordon JI (2004) The Gut Microbiota as An Environmental Factor that Regulates Fat Storage. Proc. natl. acad. sci. 2: 15718-15723.

[186] Prins A (2011) The Brain-Gut Interaction: The Conversation and the Implications. S. afr. j. clin. nutr. 24: 8-14.

[187] O'Mahony SM, Hyland NP, Dinan TG, Cryan JF. (2011) Maternal Separation as A Model of Brain-Gut Axis Dysfunction. Psychopharmacology 214: 71-88.

[188] Sudo N (2006) Stress and Gut Microbiota: Does Postnatal Microbial Colonization Programs the Hypothalamic-Pituitary-Adrenal System for Stress Response? International Congress Series 1287: 350-354.

[189] Bravo JA, Forsythe P, Chew MV, Escaravage E, Savignac HM, Dinan TG, Bienenstock J, Cryan JF (2011) Ingestion of Lactobacillus Strain Regulates Emotional Behavior and Central GABA Receptor Expression in a Mouse Via the Vagus Nerve. Proc. natl. acad. sci. 108: 16050-16055.

[190] Forsythe P, Sudo N, Dinan T, Taylor VH, Bienenstock J (2010) Mood and Gut Feelings. Brain behav. immun. 24(1): 9-16.

[191] Bailey MT, Dowd SE, Parry NM, Galley JD, Schauer DB, Lyte M (2010) Stressor Exposure Disrupts Commensal Microbial Populations in the Intestines and Leads to Increased Colonization by Citrobacter Rodentium. Infect. immun. 78: 1509-1519.

[192] Tannock GW, Savage DC (1974) Influences of Dietary and Environmental Stress on Microbial Populations in the Murine Gastrointestinal Tract. Infect, immun. 9: 591-598.

[193] Bıyık H. Balkaya M, Ünsal H, Ünsal C. (2005) The Effects of Qualitative and Quantitative Protein Malnutrition on Cecal Microbiota in Wistar Rats with or without Neutrophil Suppression. Turk. j. vet. anim. sci. 29: 767-773.

[194] Ünsal H, Balkaya M, Bıyık H, Ünsal C, Basbulbul G, Poyrazoglu E, Kozacı LD (2009) Time-dependent Effects of Dietary Qualitative and Quantitative Protein Malnutrition on Some Members of the Cecal Microbiota in Male Wistar Rats. Microb. ecol. health dis. 21: 44-449.

[195] Ünsal H, Çötelioglu Ü. (2007) The Effects of Food Restriction on Some Biochemical Parameters and Certain Bacterial Groups in the Cecum in Sprague Dawley Rats. Microb. ecol. health dis. 19: 17-24.

[196] Lyte M, Ernst S (1992) Catecholamine Induced Growth of Gram Negative Bacteria. Life sci. 50: 302-312.

[197] Bailey MT, Dowd SE, Galley JD, Hufnagle AR, Allen RG, Lyte M (2011) Exposure to a Social Stressor Alters the Structure of the Intestinal Microbiota: Implications for Stressor-Induced Immunomodulation. Brain behave. immun. 25: 397-407.

[198] O'Mahony SM, Marchesi JR, Scully P, Codling C, Ceolho AM, Quigley EM, Cryan JF, Dinan TG (2009) Early Life Stress Alters Behavior, Immunity, and Microbiota in Rats: Implications for Irritable Bowel Syndrome and Psychiatric Illnesses. *Biol. psychiatr.* 65: 263-267.

[199] Knowles SR, Nelson EA, Palombo EA (2008) Investigating the Role of Perceived Stress on Bacterial Flora Activity and Salivary Cortisol Secretion: A Possible Mechanism Underlying Susceptibility to Illness. Biol. psychol. 77: 132-137.

[200] Ünsal H, Balkaya M, Ünsal C, Bıyık H, Başbülbül G, Poyrazoğlu E (2008). The Short-term Effects of Different Doses of Dexamethasone on the Numbers of Some Bacteria in the Ileum. Dig. dis. sci. 53, 1842-1845.

[201] Kirimlioglu V, Kirimlioglu H, Yilmaz S, Piskin T, Tekerekoglu S, Bayindir Y (2006) Effect of Steroid on Mitochondrial Oxidative Stress Enzymes, Intestinal Microflora, and

Bacterial Translocation in Rats Subjected to Temporary Liver Inflow Occlusion. Transplant. proc. 38: 378-381.

[202] Lyte M (1993) The Role of Microbial Endocrinology in Infectious Disease. J. endocrinol. 137: 343-345.

[203] Freestone PP, Sandrini SM, Haigh RD, Lyte M (2008) Microbial Endocrinology: How Stress Influences Susceptibility to Infection. Trends microbiol. 16: 55-64.

[204] Freestone PP, Lyte M, Neal CP, Maggs AF, Haigh RD,Williams PH (2000) The Mammalian Neuroendocrine Hormone Norepinephrine Supplies Iron for Bacterial Growth in the Presence of Transferrin or Lactoferrin. J. bacteriol. 182: 6091-6098.

[205] Kinney KS, Austin CE, Morton DS, Sonnenfeld G (1999) Catecholamine Enhancement of Aeromonas Hydrophila Growth. Microb. pathol. 26: 85-91.

[206] Kinney KS, Austin CE, Morton DS, Sonnenfeld G (2000) Norepinephrine as a Growth Stimulating Factor in Bacteria-Mechanistic Studies. Life sci. 67: 3075-3085.

[207] Neal CP, Freestone PP, Maggs AF, Haigh RD, Williams PH, Lyte M (2001) Catecholamine Inotropes as Growth Factors for Staphylococcus Epidermidis and Other Coagulase-Negative Staphylococci. FEMS microbiol. lett. 194: 163-169.

[208] Belay T, Sonnenfeld G (2002) Differential Effects of Catecholamines on In Vitro Growth of Pathogenic Bacteria. Life sci. 71: 447-456.

[209] Belay T, Aviles H, Vance M, Fountain K, Sonnenfeld G (2003) Catecholamines and in vitro Growth of Pathogenic Bacteria: Enhancement of Growth Varies Greatly Among Bacterial Species. Life sci 73: 1527-1535.

[210] Lyte M, Arulanandam BP, Frank CD (1996) Production of Shigela-Like Toxins by Escherichia Coli O157:H7 can be Influenced by the Neuroendocrine Hormone Norepinephrine. J. lab. Clin. Med. 128: 392-398.

[211] Green BT, Lyte M, Chen C, Xie Y, Casey MA, Kulkarni-Narla A, Vulchanova L, Brown DR (2004) Adrenergic Modulation of Escherichia Coli O157:H7 Adherence to the Colonic Mucosa. Am. j. physiol. gastrointest. liver physiol. 287: G1238-G1246.

[212] Chen C, Brown DR, Xie Y, Green BT, Lyte M (2003) Catecholamines Modulate Escherichia Coli O157:H7 Adherence to Murine Cecal Mucosa. Shock. 20: 183-188.

[213] Chen C, Lyte M, Stevens MP, Vulchanova L, Brown DR (2006) Mucosally-Directed Adrenergic Nerves and Sympathomimetic Drugs Enhance Non-Intimate Adherence of Escherichia Coli O157:H7 to Porcine Cecum and Colon. Eur. j. pharmacol. 539: 116-124.

[214] Green BT, Lyte M, Kulkarni-Narla A, Brown DR (2003) Neuromodulation of Enteropathogen Internalization in Peyer's Patches from Porcine Jejunum. J. neuroimmunol. 141: 74-82.

[215] Brown DR, Price LD (2008) Catecholamines and Sympathomimetic Drugs Decrease Early Salmonella Typhimurium Uptake into Porcine Peyer's Patches. FEMS immunol. med. microbiol. 52: 29-35.

[216] Kakuno Y, Honda M, Takakura K (1997) Colonization Types of Escherichia Coli in Experimental Urinary Tract Infection in Compromised Mice Treated with Hydrocortisone. Kansenshogaku zasshi. 71: 652-658.

[217] Schreiber KL, Brown DR (2005) Adrenocorticotrophic Hormone Modulates Escherichia Coli O157: H7 Adherence to Porcine Colonic Mucosa. Stress. 8: 185-190.

[218] Sands BE (2007) Inflammatory Bowel Disease: Past, Present, and Future. J. gastroenterol. 42(1): 16-25.

[219] Foligné B, Nutten S, Steidler L, Dennin V, Goudercourt D, Mercenier A, Pot B. (2006) Recommendations for Improved Use of The Murine TNBS-Induced Colitis Model in Evaluating Anti-İnflammatory Properties of Lactic Acid Bacteria: Technical and Microbiological Aspects. Dig. dis. sci. 51: 390-400.

[220] Tamboli CP, Neut C, Desreumaux P, Colombel JF (2004) Dysbiosis in Inflammatory Bowel Disease Gut. 53: 1-4.

[221] Thomas LV, Ockhuizen T (2012) New Insights into the Impact of the Intestinal Microbiota on Health and Disease: A Symposium Report. Br. j. nutr. 107: (Suppl 1): 1-13.

[222] Steidler L (2001) Microbiological and Immunological Strategies for Treatment of Inflammatory Bowel Disease. Microbes infect. 3: 1157-1166.

[223] Scanlan PD, Shanahan F, O'Mahony C, Marchesi JR (2006) Culture-Independent Analyses of Temporal Variation of The Dominant Fecal Microbiota and Targeted Bacterial Subgroups in Crohn's Disease. J. clin. microbiol. 44: 3980-3988.

[224] Frank DN, St Amand AL, Feldman RA, Boedeker EC, Harpaz N, Pace NR (2007) Molecular-Phylogenetic Characterization of Microbial Community Imbalances in Human Inflammatory Bowel Diseases. Proc. natl. acad. sci. 104: 13780-13785.

[225] Alverdy J, Aoys E (1991) The Effect of Glucocorticoid Administration on Bacterial Translocation. Ann. surg. 214:719-723.

[226] Schiffrin EJ, Carter EA, Walker WA, Frieberg E, Benjamin J, Israel EJ (1993) Influence of Prenatal Corticosteroids on Bacterial Colonization in the Newborn Rat. J. Pediatr. Gastroenterol. nutr. 17: 271-275.

[227] Deitch EA, Winterton J, Berg R (1987) Effect of Starvation, Malnutrition and Trauma on the Gastrointestinal Tract Flora and Bacterial Translocation. Arch. Surg. 122: 1019-1024.

[228] Gorbach SL, Goldin BR (1992) Nutrition and the Gastrointestinal Microflora. Nutr. rev. 50: 378-81.

[229] Saunders DR, Wiggins HS (1981) Conservation of Mannitol, Lactulose, and Raffinose by the Human Colon. Am. j. physiol. 241: G397-G402.

[230] Roberfroid MB (2005) Introducing Inulin-Type Fructans. Br. j. nutr. 93(Suppl 1): 13-25.

[231] Drasar BS, Crowther JS, Goddard P, Hawksworth G, Hill MJ, Peach S, Williams RE, Renwick A (1973) The Relation between Diet and The Gut Microflora in Man. Proc. nutr. soc. 32: 49-52.

[232] Gracey M, Suharjono, Sunoto, Stone DE (1973) Microbial Contamination of the Gut: Another Feature of Malnutrition. Am. j. clin. nutr. 26: 1170-1174.

[233] Finegold SM, Attebery HR, Sutter VL. (1974) Effect of Diet on Human Fecal Flora: Comparison of Japanese and American Diets. Am. j. clin. nutr. 27(12): 1456-1469.

[234] Deitch EA, Winterton J, Li M, Berg R (1987) The Gut as a Portal of Entry for Bacteremia. Role of Protein Malnutrition. Ann. surg. 205: 681-692.

[235] Mallett AK, Bearne CA, Young PJ, Rowland IR, Berry C (1988) Influence of Starches of Low Digestibility on the Rat Caecal Microflora. Br. j. nutr. 60: 597-604.

[236] Deitch EA, Ma WJ, Ma L, Berg RD, Specian RD (1990) Protein Malnutrition Predisposes to Inflammatory-Induced Gut-Origin Septic States. Ann. surg. 211: 560-568.

[237] Hinton A Jr, Buhr RJ, Ingram KD (2000) Physical, Chemical, and Microbiological Changes in the Crop of Broiler Chickens Subjected to Incremental Feed Withdrawal. Poult. sci. 79: 212-218.

[238] Munro HN, Crim MC (1988) The Proteins and Amino Acids. In: Shils ME, Young VR editors. Modern nutrition in health and disease. Philadelphia: Lea & Febiger. pp. 1-37.

[239] Viteri FE, Schenider RE (1974) Gastrointestinal Alterations in Protein-Calorie Malnutrition. Med. clin. n. am. 58: 1487-1505.

[240] Heyworth B, Brown J (1975) Jejunal Microflora in Malnourished Gambian Children. Arch. dis. child. 50: 27-33.

[241] Omoike IU, Abiodun PO (1989) Upper Small Intestinal Microflora in Diarrhea and Malnutrition in Nigerian Children. J. pediatr. gastroenterol. Nutr. 9: 314-321.

[242] Jirillo E, Pasquetto N, Marcuccio L, Monno R, De Rinaldis P, Fumarola D. (1975) Endotoxemia Detected by Limulus Assay in Severe Malnourished Children. Plasma Effects on Leucocyte Migration: Preliminary Investigations. G. batteriol. virol. immunol. 68: 174-178.

[243] McCowen KC, Ling PR, Ciccarone A, Mao Y, Chow JC, Bistrian BR, Smith RJ (2001) Sustained Endotoxemia Leads to Marked Down-Regulation of Early Steps in the Insulin-Signaling Cascade. Crit. care med. 29: 839-846.

[244] Schreiber RA, Walker WA (1988) The Gastrointestinal Barrier: Antigen Uptake and Perinatal Immunity. Ann. allergy. 61: 3-12.

[245] Sanderson IR, Walker WA (1993) Uptake and Transport of Macromolecules by the Intestine: Possible Role in Clinical Disorders (an Update). Gastroenterology 104: 622-639.

[246] Stanghellini V, Barbara G, Cremon C, Cogliandro R, Antonucci A, Gabusi V, Frisoni C, De Giorgio R, Grasso V, Serra M, Corinaldesi R (2010) Gut Microbiota and Related Diseases: Clinical Features. Intern. emerg. med. 5 (Suppl 1): 57-63.

[247] Katayama M, Xu D, Specian RD, Deitch EA (1997) Role of Bacterial Adherence and the Mucus Barrier on Bacterial Translocation: Effects of Protein Malnutrition and Endotoxin in Rats. Ann Surg. 225: 317-326.

[248] Aschkenasy A (1957) On the Pathogenesis of Anemias and Leukopenias Induced by Dietary Protein Deficiency. Am. j. clin. nutr. 5: 14-25.

[249] Torun B, Viteri FE (1989) Nutrition and Function, with Emphasis on Physical Activity. In: Nutritional Problems of Children in the Developing World. M. Kretchmer M, Viteri FE, Falkner F, editors.

[250] Marroquí L, Batista TM, Gonzalez A, Vieira E, Rafacho A, Colleta SJ, Taboga SR, Boschero AC, Nadal A, Carneiro EM, Quesada I (2012) Functional and Structural Adaptations in the Pancreatic α-Cell and Changes in Glucagon Signaling During Protein Malnutrition. Endocrinology. 153:1663-1672.

Chapter 7

Molecular Mechanisms Conferring Resistance/Sensitivity to Glucocorticoid-Induced Apoptosis

Ilhem Berrou, Marija Krstic-Demonacos and Constantinos Demonacos

Additional information is available at the end of the chapter

http://dx.doi.org/10.5772/51467

1. Introduction

1.1. Glucocorticoids therapeutic effects

Synthetic glucocorticoids (GCs) as effective anti-inflammatory therapeutics are the most widely prescribed drugs in the clinic for the treatment of various conditions including asthma, ulcerative colitis, rheumatoid arthritis and hay fever [1-4]. Glucocorticoids in some cases exert effective anti-neoplastic effects in cancers of blood origin such as acute lymphocytic leukaemia (ALL) as a result of the ability of these hormones to induce cell death in blood cells [1-3]. Resistance to glucocorticoid mediated cell death remains one of the main reasons for inefficient therapy [1] and usually occurs upon prolonged glucocorticoid treatment [2] compromising significantly the success of therapy [3]. The molecular mechanisms mediating glucocorticoid dependent initiation of programmed cell death have been extensively investigated but there are several aspects of these pathways that have not yet been clearly defined. Since understanding of these mechanisms would be beneficial towards improving the glucocorticoids therapeutic efficacy further research exemplifying resistance to glucocrticoid treatment is necessary.

Glucocorticoids (GCs) exert their anti-inflammatory and immunosuppressive effects through either genomic or non-genomic mechanisms. Non-genomic early effects of glucocorticoids are induced in tissues bearing high concentrations of this hormone by interfering with the physicochemical properties of plasma and mitochondrial membranes [4]. In particular, glucocorticoids intercalate into these membranes altering lipid peroxidation and membrane permeability [5]. In addition, non-genomic effects of glucocorticoids include early suppression of the mitogen-activated protein kinase (MAPK) and hence inflammatory signal transduction cascades such as calcium influx, phagocytosis, neutrophil degranulation and cellular adhesion [6, 7, 8, 9, 10, 11]. The non genomic effects of GCs are very important in delivering short-term therapeutic benefits to asthma and rheumatoid arthritis which are diseases characterized by high inflammatory state [12].

2. Mechanisms of GC-mediated cell death

At the molecular level GCs exert their function by interacting with their intracellular GC receptor (GR), which is a hormone responsive transcription factor that modulates gene expression of its target genes [13]. Glucocorticoids activate the cellular death machinery through transcriptional and non-transcriptional pathways by means of either the extrinsic or intrinsic pathway of apoptosis [3, 14, 15, 16].

The extrinsic pathway is induced upon activation of the membrane death receptors such as the tumour necrosis factor (TNF) receptor superfamily, member 6, Fas-Ligand (Fas-L) [17]. The binding of Fas-L leads to the activation of effector caspases (caspases 3, 6 and 7) via the activation of inducer caspases, particularly caspase 8 [18]. Evidence that glucocorticoids are involved in the regulation of the extrinsic pathway of apoptosis has been provided by observations suggesting that glucocorticoids inhibit the induction of Fas-L (but not Fas) signalling in T-cell hybridomas [19, 20]. On the contrary inhibition of the extrinsic pathway using the caspase 8 inhibitor cytokine response modifier A (crmA) in pre-B leukemic cells treated with glucocorticoids indicated that GR does not initiate apoptosis in these cells through the extrinsic pathway [21, 22]. The involvement of the intrinsic pathway, on the other hand, in the glucocorticoid mediated cell death and in particular the regulation of the balance between pro- and anti-apoptotic members of the bcl-2 family has been shown in hepatocytes, small cell lung cancer, primary ALL lymphoblasts and animal systems [23, 24].

The intrinsic pathway of cell death is stimulated in response to intracellular signals, and involves mitochondria releasing pro-apoptotic molecules, formation of the apoptosome and activation of the effector caspases via the initiator caspase 9 [25]. The balance between pro- and anti-apoptotic members of the B cell leukaemia/ lymphoma 2-like (Bcl-2) family plays a crucial role in the execution of apoptosis by glucocorticoids through the intrinsic pathway [18]. In particular, glucocorticoids regulate the expression of various genes involved in the initiation of apoptosis, including the pro-apoptotic Bcl-2 family member BCL2-like 11 (Bim) [22, 26, 27, 28]. Transactivation of Bim results in the activation of the Bcl-2–associated X protein (Bax) and the Bcl2-antagonist/killer 1 (Bak), which mediate the disruption of mitochondrial membrane potential and the release of cytochrome c into the cytosol [29]. Cytochrome c then binds to its adaptor apoptotic protease activating factor (Apaf-1), thereby activating caspase 9 and several effector caspases [30]. Furthermore, mitochondria mediate the generation of reactive oxygen species (ROS), which may potentially have an add-on effect on glucocorticoid-induced apoptosis [31].

In some cases glucocorticoids induce apoptosis by using both the intrinsic and the extrinsic pathways. This is mediated by the cleaved caspase-8 which subsequently leads to activation of the pro-apoptotic member of the Bcl-2 family, Bcl-2 homology 3 (BH3) interacting domain death agonist (Bid) [32]. The C-terminal truncated Bid (t-Bid) activates caspase 9 and the effector caspases 3, 6 and 7 [33]. The intrinsic and extrinsic pathways through which glucocorticoids induce apoptosis in cells responsive to these hormones are illustrated in Figure 1.

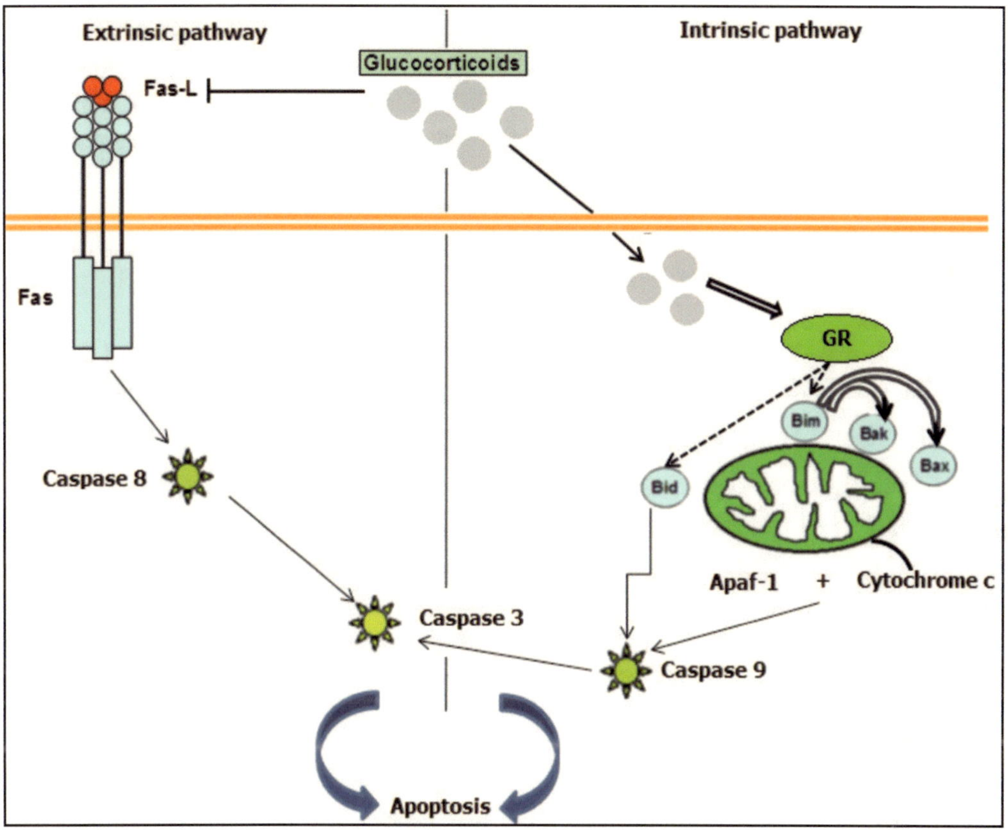

Figure 1. Schematic diagram indicating the extrinsic and intrinsic pathways through which glucocorticoids regulate apoptosis.

Several mechanisms have been proposed to explain the evasion of glucocorticoid mediated apoptosis in resistant cells [34]. These include alterations in the activity of the glucocorticoid receptor [35, 36] either due to changes in GR protein levels, presence of multiple GR variants, or post-translational modifications. GR induces apoptosis by directly modulating the expression of genes involved in cell survival/apoptosis [18, 37], or affecting gene networks involved in stress signalling resulting in an apoptotic stimulus [36, 38].

3. GR transcriptional activity is necessary for its pro-apoptotic function

Glucocorticoid induced apoptosis depends on the presence of adequate amounts of transcriptionally active GR [34, 39, 40, 41, 42]. It has also been shown that the presence of specific GR splicing variants is necessary for the stimulation of GCs dependent apoptosis [3]. Alternative hGR splicing produces two receptor variants called GRα and GRβ, which are highly homologous differing by 50 additional amino acids present in the carboxy terminal region of GRα [43]. GRα is mainly cytoplasmic, and exhibits the typical glucocorticoid receptor function in terms of ligand-dependent transcriptional regulation and as such it is the major functional GR isoform therefore its expression is crucial for cellular sensitivity to GCs [3]. GRβ on the other hand, does not bind ligands, and exerts a dominant negative effect on GRα transcriptional activity [43, 44, 45]. In clinical studies reduced GRα protein levels correlate with resistance to GCs induced apoptosis and disadvantageous prognosis in ALL [3]. Additional indication that GR transcriptional activity is necessary for the initiation of the GCs mediated apoptosis has been provided by the observation that various mutations affecting GR transcriptional activity have been detected in patients exhibiting resistance to glucocorticoids treatment [2, 46]. Furthermore, prolonged glucocorticoid treatment significantly reduces GRα expression [47], whereas GRβ expression is not affected [48].

4. GR dependent regulation of the balance between pro- and anti-apoptotic Bcl-2 family members

B cell leukaemia/ lymphoma 2-like (Bcl-2) family members are categorised into pro- and anti-apoptotic and the balance between the levels of these two types of proteins determines the cellular fate (survival or death) [23]. The involvement of the Bcl-2 family members in the glucocorticoid-induced apoptosis has been shown in cellular and animal studies [49]. For example, the expression of the anti-apoptotic Bcl-2 family member in glucocorticoid-sensitive thymocytes is lower compared to that in glucocorticoid-resistant ones [2], and overexpression of the anti-apoptotic Bcl-2 and B-cell lymphoma-extra large (Bcl-xL) in human ALL prevents glucocorticoids induced apoptosis [50, 51, 52, 53] whereas knock down of the pro-apoptotic member Bim confers resistance to dexamethasone mediated apoptosis [54]. Furthermore, over-expression of the pro-apoptotic Bax [55] and knock down of the myeloid cell leukemia sequence 1 (Mcl-1) sensitises ALL cells to glucocorticoid treatment [56]. We have shown recently that the balance between Mcl-1 and phorbol-12-myristate-13-acetate-induced protein 1 (Noxa) is a determinant of resistance / sensitivity of ALL cells to glucocorticoid-induced apoptosis [57, 58]. Several studies have shown that the pro-apoptotic Bcl-2 family member Bim plays crucial role in the glucocorticoid-induced apoptosis but further investigation is required to define the detailed molecular mechanisms of this process. Up-regulated Bim has been observed in various cell lines upon glucocorticoid treatment including ALL cells [59], primary chronic lymphocytic leukaemia (CLL) cells [27], and some patients with ALL [60]. Moreover knockout of Bim, p53 up-regulated modulator of apoptosis (Puma) or Noxa, or double knockouts of Bax and Bak confer resistance to glucocorticoid-mediated apoptosis in thymocytes [61, 62, 63]. Overall the balance of the levels between pro- and anti-apoptotic Bcl-2 family members has been recognised as a crucial factor in the determination of lymphocytes survival or death and induction of the glucocorticoid dependent programmed cell death.

Gene	Protein	Function	Role in glucocorticoid-induced apoptosis
Bcl2	B-cell Lymphoma 2 (Bcl-2)	Anti-apoptotic	Over-expression of Bcl-2 in human ALL cells prevents glucocorticoids induced apoptosis [41, 64]
BCL-xL	B-cell lymphoma-extra large (Bcl-xL)	Anti-apoptotic	Over-expression of Bcl-xL in human ALL cells prevents glucocorticoids induced apoptosis [23]
BCL2L11	BCL2 Like 11 (Bim)	Pro-apoptotic	Knock down of Bim confers resistance of ALL cells to glucocorticoid-induced apoptosis [65]. Upregulation of Bim sensitizes cells to glucocorticoid-induced apoptosis [27, 66].
Mcl1	Myeloid cell leukemia 1 (Mcl-1)	Anti-apoptotic	Knock down of Mcl-1 sensitises ALL cells to glucocorticoids apoptotic effect [56].
Phorbol-12-myristate-13-acetate-induced protein 1	Phorbol-12-myristate-13-acetate-induced protein 1 (Noxa)	Pro-apoptotic	Noxa regulates the Mcl-1 protein stability and Noxa/Mcl-1 balance determines cell survival or death [57].
p53 up-regulated modulator of apoptosis	p53 upregulated modulator of apoptosis (Puma)	Pro-apoptotic	Puma facilitates glucocorticoid-induced apoptosis of lymphocytes [62, 65].
Bax	Bcl-2–associated X (Bax)	Pro-apoptotic	Bax protein regulates glucocorticoid induced apoptosis in thymocytes [67]. Double knockouts of Bax and Bak confer resistance to glucocorticoid-induced apoptosis in thymocytes [68].
Bak	Bcl-2 homologous antagonist/killer (Bak)	Pro-apoptotic	Double knockouts of Bax and Bak confer resistance to glucocorticoid-mediated apoptosis in thymocytes [68].

Table 1. Pro- and anti-apoptotic Bcl-2 family members implicated in the glucocorticoids induced apoptosis

5. Autophagy

Autophagy is a several steps process leading to cellular degradation of unfolded or aggregated proteins and organelles in response to diverse types of stress such as starvation or metabolic stress and is an essential mechanism contributing to survival, differentiation, development, and homeostasis. Autophagy protects against chronic inflammatory conditions occurring in a variety of pathological situations such as infections, cardiovascular disease, neurodegenaration, inflammatory bowel diseases, aging and cancer [69]. Autophagy has been shown to be involved in prosurvival processes facilitating resistance of cancer cells to chemotherapy as well as under certain conditions in apoptosis [70]. Taking into account the fact that autophagy is prosurvival in addition to reports indicating that inhibitors of autophagy re-sensitise cancer cells to anticancer therapeutics [70, 71] as well as that autophagy is associated with inflammation and resistance to cancer therapy investigators were prompted to study the role of autophagy in the resistance to glucocorticoid induced apoptosis in ALL [72, 73]. These studies have indicated that dexamethasone induces autophagy before the initiation of apoptosis in ALL cells and in actual fact autophagy is a prerequisite for the efficient execution of apoptosis mediated by dexamethasone [72, 73]. More recently the molecular mechanism by which activation of autophagy overturns glucocorticoid resistance has been elucidated [74] signifying the important role of the autophagy inducer beclin-1 and the anti-apoptotic Bcl-2 family member Mcl-1 [74, 75]. Furthermore the inhibition of caspase by selective degradation of catalase and consequent generation of high concentrations of reactive oxygen species might be an alternative mechanism explaining the role of autophagy in dexamethasone induced apoptosis [76].

6. Post-translational modifications

Post-translational modifications of GR are important in regulating its transcriptional activity, protein stability, binding of GR with other transcription factors or co-modulators and subcellular localisation, and for these reasons post-translational modifications are highly relevant to glucocorticoids therapeutic efficacy [77, 78, 79, 80, 81]. GR acetylation is cell type dependent and it is suggested to suppress the receptor's transcriptional activity by reducing its ability to bind to the Glucocorticoid Responsive Elements (GREs) present in its target genes [82], or inhibit the ability of GR to translocate into the nucleus [83]. Regulation of GR transcriptional activity also takes place through ubiquitination and proteasomal degradation of the receptor upon ligand binding [84, 85]. Ubiquitination promotes interaction of GR with E2 conjugating and E3 ligase proteins causing turnover of the receptor and thus down-regulation of its transcriptional activity [85]. In support of these conclusions the proteasome inhibitor MG-132 enhances the transcriptional activity of GR [84]. Ligand-independent sumoylation has been shown to both inhibit [86, 87] as well as to stabilise and potentiate GR transcriptional activity [88]. Three sumoylation sites have been identified within the GR protein conferring GR transcriptional target selectivity [87]. We have recently reported that GR sumoylation is assisted by its phosphorylation at particular sites under certain conditions [89].

GR phosphorylation has been extensively investigated and several different kinases have been identified to induce phosphorylation of the receptor at distinct serine and threonine residues located within the N-terminal AF-1 transactivation domain of the receptor, either in the presence or in the absence of glucocorticoid hormone [90, 91, 92, 93, 94, 95]. S203 residue in human GR is targeted by cyclin/cyclin dependent kinase (CDK) complexes and is located mostly in the cytoplasm thus it is thought to be transcriptionally inactive [89, 95]. GR phosphorylated at S211 is transcriptionally active due to conformational changes which facilitate increased recruitment of the receptor to GRE-containing promoters and is a target for phosphorylation by both cyclin/CDK kinases and MAPK families depending on the cell type [91, 96]. GR phosphorylation at S226 results in inhibition of the GR function, possibly due to increased GR nuclear export and is a result of JNK activation [80, 89, 97, 98]. Finally, phosphorylation of GR at S404 attenuates GR signalling and is due to GSK3 kinase activation [99]. We have recently reported that differential GR phosphorylation in the resistant CEM-C1-15 versus sensitive CEM-C7-14 ALL cells modulates GR transcriptional activity and target selectivity resulting in diverse pro- or anti-apoptotic Bcl-2 family members' gene expression in the two cell lines [58]. In particular we have shown that GR phosphorylation at S211 is predominant in the glucocorticoid-sensitive CEM-C7-14 whereas GR phosphorylation at S226 by c-Jun N-terminal Kinase (JNK) occurs more frequently in the glucocorticoid-resistant CEM-C1-15 cells [58]. These observations lend support to the suggestion that different kinase pathways are responsible for GR phosphorylation in resistant versus sensitive cells to glucocorticoid induced apoptosis, thereby causing GR transcriptional inactivity in the resistant cell lines [58] concomitant Mcl-1 overexpression and hence resistance to GC treatment [56].

Apart from the differential expression of pro- and anti-apoptotic Bcl-2 family members [58] we have recently reported that GR isoforms localised in mitochondria are predominantly phosphorylated at serine 232 compared to serine 246 of the rat GR (corresponding to human GR Ser211 and Ser226 respectively) [96] possibly due to differential conformation of the two phosphoisoforms or diverse interaction patterns with components of the mitochondrial import machinery of the GR phosphorylated at serine 211 versus the GR phosphorylated at serine 226. These observations provide an additional potential explanation for the resistance of the CEM-C1-15 to glucocorticoids induced apoptosis in accord with recent reports indicating differential GR mitochondrial localisation in resistant compared to sensitive ALL cells to glucocorticoid induced apoptosis [93, 94, 95, 97].

7. Mitochondrial GR, glucocorticoids and cellular energy metabolism

Glucocorticoid hormones directly affect mitochondrial membranes inducing loss of mitochondrial transmembrane potential, thereby affecting vital cellular processes mediated by the function of this organelle such as ATP generation via oxidative phosphorylation, regulation of calcium flux and apoptosis [98]. In addition, glucocorticoids exert their effects on mitochondrial biogenesis through the mitochondrial GR [97, 99, 100, 101]. The intracellular trafficking of the glucocorticoid receptor has been shown to play important role in glucocorticoid-induced apoptosis [97, 102]. The glucocorticoid receptor translocates to mitochondria [97, 100, 101, 102], in various cells including rat brain and various other tissues' mitochondria [99], as well as lymphoma cells [97]. GR translocation to the nucleus occurs in both glucocorticoid-sensitive and glucocorticoid-resistant cells, whereas in contrast, GR translocation into mitochondria occurs only in the glucocorticoid-sensitive and not the resistant cells [97, 103]. The mechanisms by which GR translocates to mitochondria and its effects on the regulation of the expression of mitochondrially encoded genes have been partially elucidated [97, 100, 101, 102] and require further investigation. However, it is noteworthy that glucocorticoids modulate mitochondrial biogenesis and mitochondrial energy production pathways by regulating the transcription of the mitochondrial genome [99, 100].

The process of programmed cell death is energy dependent requiring the precise coordination of several biochemical processes including the transcriptional regulation of the expression of genes encoding enzymatic components of the energy production pathways (oxidative phosphorylation (OXPHOS) and glycolysis) [29] and mutations affecting cellular energy production lead to defects in apoptosis and tumourigenesis [104, 105, 106, 107, 108, 109]. In humans the OXPHOS pathway consists of five multi-subunit complexes whose components are encoded by genes located in both the nuclear and the mitochondrial genomes [110] supporting the notion that a transcription factor operating in both subcellular compartments could coordinate the expression of nuclear and mitochondrial genes ensuring appropriate stoichiometry and timely gene expression of the components of the respiratory chain [111]. In addition to the availability of the components encoded in the nuclear and the mitochondrial compartments an appropriate assembly mechanism of these subunits is essential for the functionality of the oxidative phosphorylation system [110]. One possible candidate transcription factor able to orchestrate nuclear and mitochondrial gene expression is the glucocorticoid receptor which mediates gene expression of both nuclear and mitochondrial encoded genes [98, 99, 100, 102, 112, 113, 114, 115, 116].

In fact, dexamethasone has been shown to affect energy metabolism and the balance between OXPHOS and glycolysis [117, 118]. Also, evidence has been recently presented indicating that changes in metabolic patterns and cellular proliferation are key aspects of resistance to GC mediated apoptosis in ALL [39]. Elevated glycolytic rate due to increased expression of genes involved in glucose metabolism are associated with resistance to glucocorticoid induced apoptosis and this resistance can be reversed by inhibitors of glycolysis in ALL [119, 120]. Moreover, glucocorticoid induced apoptosis is regulated by genes involved in cellular energy metabolism [121, 122, 123, 124] suggesting that dexamethasone contributes to the apoptosis / survival decisions in ALL cells indirectly by modulating the balance between OXPHOS and glycolysis [15, 120]. Indeed coordination of oxidative phosphorylation and glycolysis by mechanisms involving glucocorticoid receptor mediated transcriptional regulation of genes encoding enzymes implicated in both pathways has been extensively reported in the literature [99, 125, 126]. Enzymes participating in the tricarboxylic acid cycle encoded by the nuclear genome such as malate dehydrogenase 1 (Mdh1) and succinyl coenzyme A synthetase (Suclg1) are GR transcriptional target genes [127]. In addition, several mitochondrial genes encoding subunits of the OXPHOS pathway possess one or more functional glucocorticoid responsive elements [99, 100, 102, 112, 113] implying that glucocorticoids exert direct effects on mitochondrial biogenesis and respiration. Key enzymes involved in glycolysis including 6-phosphofructo-2-kinase/fructose-2, 6-bisphosphatase [126] lactate dehydrogenase B (LdhB) and aldolase A (AldoA) [128] are under GR transcriptional control [120].

To shed light on the molecular mechanisms involved in GR mediated regulation of the OXPHOS pathway bioinformatic analysis using the TRED or CCTFSP software [129, 130, 131] was performed to identify potential glucocorticoid responsive elements (GREs) in the promoters of genes encoding Surf-1, and SCO2 enzymes which are essential for the assembly of the Cytochrome *c* Oxidase (COX) wholoenzyme [132, 133, 134]. Similar approaches were used to detect possible existence of potential GREs in the regulatory region of the promoter of the nuclear gene encoding COX-Va. Putative GREs were identified in the regulatory regions of the promoters of Surf-1, SCO2, and COX-Va using this approach. To test whether these GREs conferred glucocorticoid responsiveness to the expression of these genes, qRT-PCR experiments were performed to quantify their mRNA levels in untreated or dexamethasone treated CEM-C1-15 (resistant to glucocorticoid induced apoptosis) and CEM-C7-14 (sensitive to glucocorticoid induced apoptosis) ALL cells [135] (Figure 2).

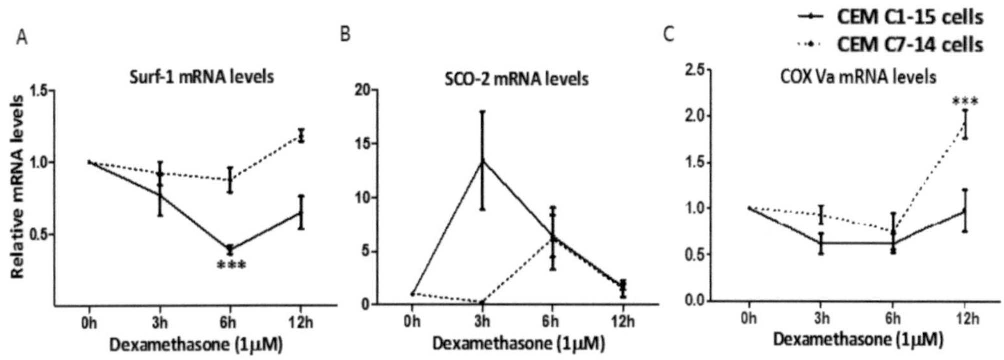

Figure 2. Relative mRNA levels of the COX assembly enzymes Surf-1 (A), SCO-2 (B), and the nuclear COX-Va (C) OXPHOS subunit were followed in the resistant CEM-C1-15 and the sensitive CEM-C7-14 to glucocorticoid induced apoptosis ALL cells treated with dexamethasone for the indicated time points by quantitative real-time PCR. Solid lines represent mRNA levels in CEM-C1-15 and dotted lines correspond to mRNA levels determined in CEM-C7-14 cells. Error bars represent standard error of the mean of five independent experiments and asterisks indicate statistical significance of $p<0.05$ compared to the untreated sample.

A marked reduction of Surf-1 mRNA levels in the resistant CEM-C1-15 cells was observed after 6 and 12 hours of dexamethasone treatment compared to the non-treated cells (Figure 2A, solid line). In contrast, in the sensitive to glucocorticoid-induced apoptosis CEM-C7-14 cells, Surf-1 mRNA levels remained constant during the first 6 hours of dexamethasone treatment and a moderate increase of Surf-1 mRNA levels was observed only 12h after the addition of the hormone (Figure 2A, dotted line). SCO-2 mRNA levels initially increased after 3h and 6h of dexamethasone treatment in CEM-C1-15 cells and later after 12h of dexamethasone treatment decreased to the level of that exhibited in the untreated cells (Figure 2B, solid line).

The fact that COX-Va expression is altered in various tumours and its association with Surf-1 in the formation of sub-complexes consisting of variable COX subunits such as

COX-I, COX-II, COX-III, and COX-IV [136] triggered our interest to investigate the regulation of the expression of the COX-Va gene. This investigation aimed to test whether differential COX-Va cellular levels in the resistant versus the sensitive CEM cells in response to glucocorticoid treatment was taking place in a similar way as that observed for Surf-1. COX-Va mRNA levels were higher in CEM-C7-14 compared to those detected in the CEM-C1-15 cells in all time points of dexamethasone treatment investigated in this study and the longer the incubation with the hormone the higher the COX-Va mRNA levels in the CEM-C7-14 cells (Figure 2C, compare dotted to solid line). Results shown in Figure 2A, 2B, and 2C support the notion that the Surf-1 and COX-Va genes encoded by the nuclear genome are under GR transcriptional control and their expression is higher in the sensitive to glucocorticoid induced apoptosis cells compared to the resistant CEM-C1-15 cells.

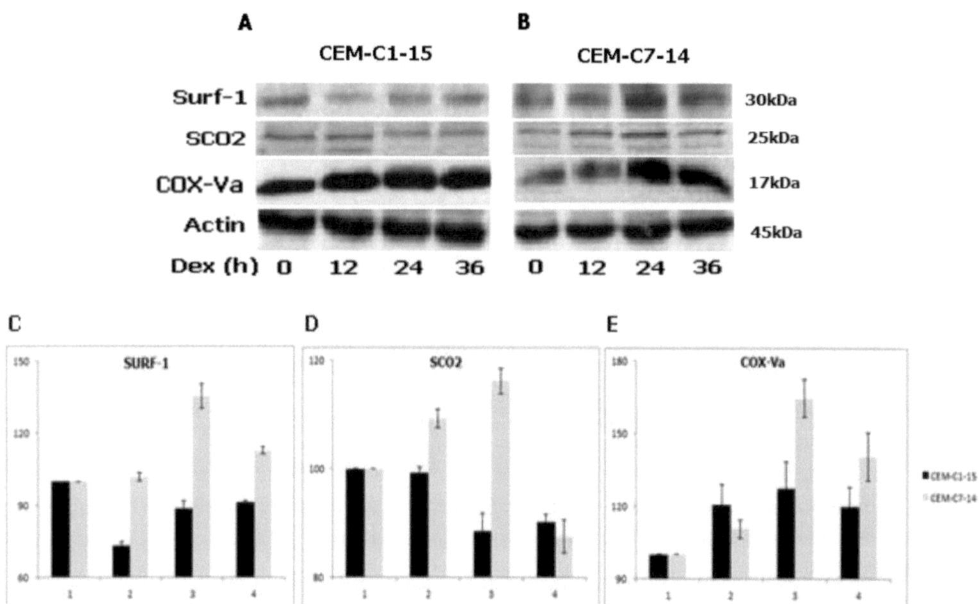

Figure 3. Western blot analysis of Surf-1, SCO-2, and COX-Va in CEM-C1-15 (A) and CEM-C7-14 (B) cells treated with dexamethasone for the indicated times. Actin was used as a loading control. Densitometric analysis of the western blots presented in A and B was carried out using Image J software. The intensity of the bands of Surf-1 (C), SCO2 (D) and COX-Va (E) at each time point was normalised to the intensity of the actin band at the respective time point and the obtained values were plotted. The intensity of the bands in the untreated cells normalised to the intensity of the actin band in the untreated cells was arbitrarily set to 100. The values representing the intensities of the bands in the treated cells were calculated as follows: Intensity of band in treated cells/intensity of actin band in treated cells x 100 / intensity of band in untreated cells/intensity of actin in untreated cells. Black bars represent the CEM-C1-15 cells and the grey bars the CEM-C7-14 cells.

The protein levels of Surf-1, SCO2 and COX-Va were also followed in CEM-C7-14 and CEM-C1-15 cells under the same conditions (Figure 3). Higher Surf-1 protein levels were observed in dexamethasone treated CEM-C7-14 cells compared to the non-treated cells for all time points tested (Figure 3A, B and C compare grey bars 2, 3 and 4 to grey bar 1). In contrast lower Surf-1 protein levels were observed in the dexamethasone treated CEM-C1-15 cells irrespectively of the length of the dexamethasone treatment compared to the untreated cells (Figure 3A, B and C compare black bars 2, 3 and 4 to black bar 1). In a similar manner to that observed for Surf-1, increasing SCO2 protein levels were observed in CEM-C7-14 cells treated with dexamethasone for 12h and 24h compared to the untreated cells (Figure 3A, B and D compare grey bars 2 and 3 to bar 1). On the contrary lower SCO2 protein levels were observed in CEM-C7-14 cells 36h after the addition of dexamethasone compared to the untreated cells (Figure 3A, B and D compare grey bar 4 to grey bar 1). On the other side the SCO2 protein levels in CEM-C1-15 cells were lower than those measured in the untreated cells for all the time points of dexamethasone treatment examined in this study (Figure 3A, B and D compare black bars 2, 3 and 4 to black bar 1). Finally the COX-Va protein levels were higher in both CEM-C1-15 and CEM-C7-14 cells treated with dexamethasone compared to the non-treated cells (Figure 3A, B and E compare black and grey bars 2, 3, and 4 to grey and black bars 1).

The expression of COX subunits and oxidative phosphorylation are affected by glucocorticoid treatment [137] possibly through the GR transcriptional activity. Given that some OXPHOS subunits are encoded by the nuclear genome, and others by the mitochondrial DNA, it was thought that glucocorticoids exert indirect effects on the regulation of transcription of mitochondrial encoded OXPHOS subunits by modulating the activity of nuclear factors involved in the gene expression of mitochondrial genes [101]. However, the identification of mitochondrial GR, and the existence of GRE-like domains in the mitochondrial genome [100, 101, 138] suggest that glucocorticoids exert direct effects on mitochondrial transcription. Taking into consideration the fact that glucocorticoid receptor potentially regulates the expression of several COX assembly factors and nuclear COX subunits (Figure 2A, 2B and 2C) it was interesting to investigate whether GR fine tunes the expression of OXPHOS genes in both nuclear and mitochondrial genomes. In order to assess this hypothesis, and in parallel, to strengthen the perception that energy metabolism is a possible pathway by which CEM cells determine resistance / sensitivity to glucocorticoid induced apoptosis we followed the mRNA levels of the mitochondrial OXPHOS subunits COX-I, COX-II and COX-III in CEM C1-15 and CEM C7-14 cells treated with dexamethasone (Figures 4A, 4B and 4C).

A similar picture to that observed for the nuclear OXPHOS components was observed for the mitochondrial OXPHOS subunits. Specifically higher cellular levels of the mitochondrial COX-I, COX-II and COX-III OXPHOS subunits were observed in CEM-C7-14 compared to CEM-C1-15 cells (Figure 4A-4C). Increased levels of COX-I mRNA in both cell lines after 12 hours of dexamethasone treatment were observed in both CEM-C1-15 and CEM-C7-14 cells (Figure 4A, compare solid with dotted line). COX-II mRNA expression initially decreased in both cell lines 3h after the addition of dexamethasone

(Figure 4B, compare solid and dotted lines 3h point) and then started to increase steadily at 6 and 12h after the treatment with the hormone but it reached higher levels in the CEM-C7-14 cells (Figure 4B, compare solid line with dotted line). COX-III gene expression remains unaffected by glucocorticoid treatment during the first 3 hours, in CEM-C1-15 cells, followed by two fold increase 6h and 12h after hormone addition (Figure 4C, solid line compare 0 time point with 6 and 12h time points). A similar pattern was evident in CEM-C7-14 cells where the induction of COX-III mRNA after 6h and 12h of dexamethasone treatment was four and five fold higher respectively compared to those detected in the untreated cells (Figure 4C, dotted line compare 0 time point with 6 and 12h time points).

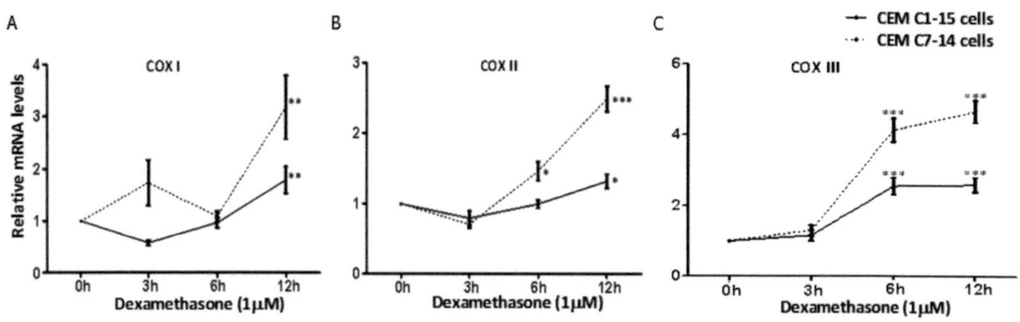

Figure 4. Relative mRNA levels of the mitochondrial OXPHOS subunits COX-I (A), COX-II (B), and COX-III (C) were followed in the resistant CEM-C1-15 and the sensitive CEM-C7-14 to glucocorticoid induced apoptosis ALL cells treated with dexamethasone for the indicated time points by quantitative real-time PCR. Solid lines represent mRNA levels in CEM-C1-15 and dotted lines correspond to mRNA levels determined in CEM-C7-14 cells. Error bars represent standard error of the mean of five independent experiments and asterisks indicate statistical significance of $p<0.05$ compared to the untreated sample.

Taken together, results presented in this manuscript endorse the hypothesis that the glucocorticoid resistance / sensitivity in CEM cells is determined by differences in the efficacy of the OXPHOS system to produce energy in the two cell lines. Support to this conclusion is lent by observations shown in Figure 2A, 2B and 2C indicating that the mRNA levels of nuclear encoded components of the OXPHOS system were higher in the sensitive CEM-C7-14 than in the resistant CEM-C1-15 cells. Higher levels of COX assembly factors in CEM-C7-14 cells imply a more efficient energy metabolism in these cells. This could be a result of distinct signalling pathways operating in the two cell lines giving rise to increased transactivation function of GR in CEM-C7-14 cells, where the receptor could be phosphorylated at S211 [58] and stimulate the expression of its potential transcription targets Surf-1 and COX-Va, whereas on the contrary, it is phosphorylated at S226 in CEM-C1-15 cells, thereby targeted to different subset of its transcriptional targets in these cells [58]. The link between altered metabolism in cancer cells and varying expression of COX subunits has been well established [139, 140, 141]. The presence of mitochondrial GR and of GRE-like domains in the mitochondrial genome [100, 102, 138, 142, 143, 144] and regulation of the mitochondrial COX subunits (COX-I, COX-II and COX-III) provide a probable mechanism explaining the dexamethasone dependent regulation of the mitochondrial COX subunits gene expression (Figure 4). In addition, differences in post translational modifications of the receptor, which in the case of CEM-C7-14 cells, allow activation [58] and possibly translocation of GR into mitochondria [96] while in CEM-C1-15 cells these events are not permissible could be an additional justification for these observations.

8. Conclusions and future perspectives

Resistance to glucocorticoid induced apoptosis in ALL has been attributed to several different processes and pathways including predominance of certain GR isoforms with reduced transcriptional activity [34, 145, 146], either due to altered binding capacity of the receptor to other transcription factors [147, 148, 149, 150] or co-regulators [81, 151], disparate expression and consequent dissimilar balance between pro- versus anti-apoptotic members of the Bcl-2 family [18], GR mitochondrial localisation [97], autophagy [72, 73, 74, 75], and post-translational modifications which affect GR transcription target selectivity and protein stability [22, 38, 89, 152, 153].

We have recently presented evidence to suggest that differential GR phosphorylation in resistant versus sensitive to glucocorticoid induced apoptosis ALL cells results in selective induction of anti-apoptotic and inhibition of pro-apoptotic Bcl-2 family members gene expression in the resistant cells [58]. Several reports have indicated the potential role of differential kinase activity in glucocorticoid resistant and sensitive cells in determining the GR subcellular localisation [96, 98, 154] and diverse effects on the induction of autophagy [72, 73, 74].

In this study we provide new evidence signifying the differential expression of OXPHOS components in glucocorticoid resistant versus sensitive ALL cells and we propose that resistant and sensitive CEM cells use different pathways to produce energy. These results are in accord with reports showing that resistance to GC in ALL is associated with increased glucose consumption [155] with concomitant induction of Mcl-1 expression and resistance to apoptosis [39]. In our anticipated model (Figure 5) in resistant lymphocytes the predominantly phosphorylated at S226 GR is possibly transcriptionally inactive and thus incapable to significantly induce OXPHOS assembly enzymes and COX subunits gene expression or translocate into mitochondria thereby exhibiting reduced oxidative phosphorylation consistent with a proliferative phenotype, and this is probably one of the mechanisms employed by the glucocorticoid-resistant CEM-C1-15 cells to survive GC treatment.

The results presented in this study endorse the hypothesis that differential GR phosphorylation affects components of cellular energy production pathways in distinct ways in resistant versus sensitive cells altering energy production and possibly ROS generation in unique ways in the two cell lines, suggesting that combination of kinase inhibitors, and glycolytic modulators together with dexamethasone could be a possible mean by which resistance to glucocorticoid induced apoptosis could be circumvented in ALL.

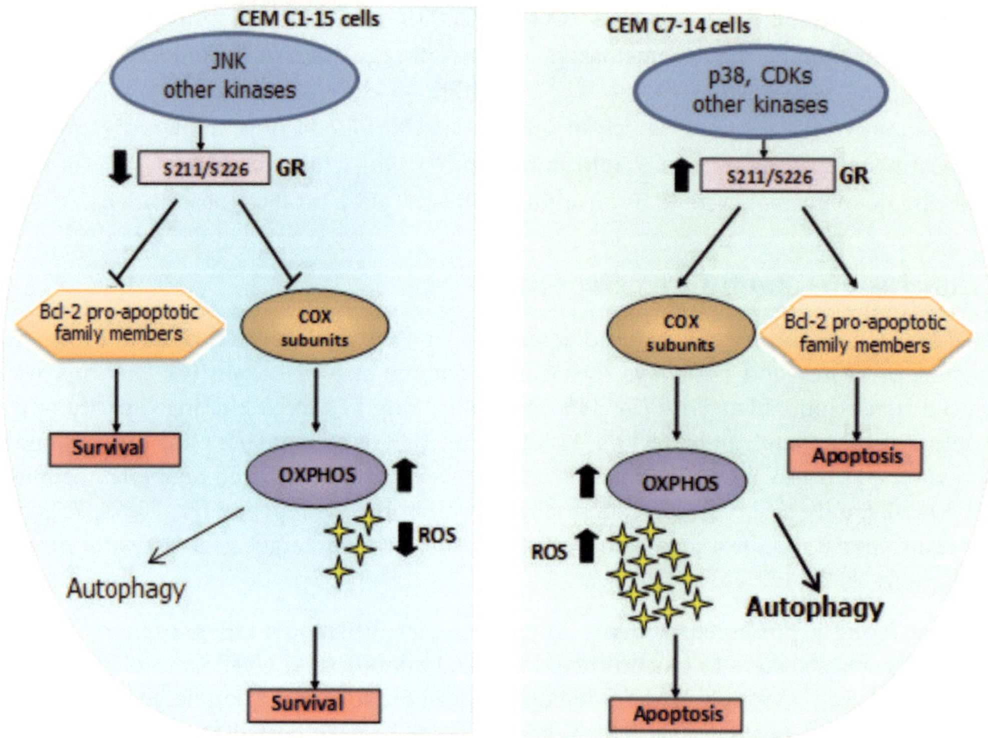

Figure 5. Model summarising the proposed mechanism determining resistance / sensitivity of CEM cells to glucocorticoid-induced apoptosis. Differential phosphorylation of GR in glucocorticoid resistant versus sensitive cells leads to the reduction of gene expression of OXPHOS subunits and pro-apoptotic Bcl-2 family members in the resistant cells (left panel) whereas the opposite is the case for the sensitive cells (right panel).

Author details

Ilhem Berrou, Marija Krstic-Demonacos, Constantinos Demonacos
University of Manchester, School of Pharmacy and Faculty of Life Sciences, Manchester, UK

9. References

[1] Buttgereit F, Saag KG, Cutolo M, da Silva JAP, Bijlsma JWJ (2005) The molecular basis for the effectiveness, toxicity, and resistance to glucocorticoids: focus on the treatment of rheumatoid arthritis. Scand J Rheumatol 34: 14-21.

[2] Sionov RV, Spokoini R, Kfir-Erenfeld S, Cohen O, Yefenof E (2008) Mechanisms regulating the susceptibility of hematopoietic malignancies to glucocorticoid-induced apoptosis. Adv Cancer Res 101: 127-248.

[3] Schmidt S, Rainer J, Ploner C, Presul E, Riml S, et al. (2004) Glucocorticoid-induced apoptosis and glucocorticoid resistance: molecular mechanisms and clinical relevance. Cell Death Differ 11 Suppl 1: S45-55.

[4] Losel R, Wehling M (2003) Nongenomic actions of steroid hormones. Nat Rev Mol Cell Biol 4: 46-56.

[5] Buttgereit F, Straub RH, Wehling M, Burmester GR (2004) Glucocorticoids in the treatment of rheumatic diseases: an update on the mechanisms of action. Arthritis Rheum 50: 3408-3417.

[6] Stellato C (2004) Post-transcriptional and nongenomic effects of glucocorticoids. Proc Am Thorac Soc 1: 255-263.

[7] Solito E, Mulla A, Morris JF, Christian HC, Flower RJ, et al. (2003) Dexamethasone induces rapid serine-phosphorylation and membrane translocation of annexin 1 in a human folliculostellate cell line via a novel nongenomic mechanism involving the glucocorticoid receptor, protein kinase C, phosphatidylinositol 3-kinase, and mitogen-activated protein kinase. Endocrinology 144: 1164-1174.

[8] Qiu J, Wang CG, Huang XY, Chen YZ (2003) Nongenomic mechanism of glucocorticoid inhibition of bradykinin-induced calcium influx in PC12 cells: possible involvement of protein kinase C. Life Sci 72: 2533-2542.

[9] Long F, Wang YX, Liu L, Zhou J, Cui RY, et al. (2005) Rapid nongenomic inhibitory effects of glucocorticoids on phagocytosis and superoxide anion production by macrophages. Steroids 70: 55-61.

[10] Liu L, Wang YX, Zhou J, Long F, Sun HW, et al. (2005) Rapid non-genomic inhibitory effects of glucocorticoids on human neutrophil degranulation. Inflamm Res 54: 37-41.

[11] Koukouritaki SB, Gravanis A, Stournaras C (1999) Tyrosine phosphorylation of focal adhesion kinase and paxillin regulates the signaling mechanism of the rapid nongenomic action of dexamethasone on actin cytoskeleton. Mol Med 5: 731-742.

[12] Löwenberg M, Stahn C, Hommes DW, Buttgereit F (2008) Novel insights into mechanisms of glucocorticoid action and the development of new glucocorticoid receptor ligands. Steroids 73: 1025-1029.

[13] Smith LK, Cidlowski JA (2010) Glucocorticoid-induced apoptosis of healthy and malignant lymphocytes. Prog Brain Res 182: 1-30.

[14] Frankfurt O, Rosen ST (2004) Mechanisms of glucocorticoid-induced apoptosis in hematologic malignancies: updates. Curr Opin Oncol 16: 553-563.

[15] Distelhorst CW (2002) Recent insights into the mechanism of glucocorticosteroid-induced apoptosis. Cell Death Differ 9: 6-19.

[16] Lepine S, Sulpice JC, Giraud F (2005) Signaling pathways involved in glucocorticoid-induced apoptosis of thymocytes. Crit Rev Immunol 25: 263-288.

[17] Thorburn A (2004) Death receptor-induced cell killing. Cell Signal 16: 139-144.

[18] Ploner C, Schmidt S, Presul E, Renner K, Schrocksnadel K, et al. (2005) Glucocorticoid-induced apoptosis and glucocorticoid resistance in acute lymphoblastic leukemia. J Steroid Biochem Mol Biol 93: 153-160.

[19] D'Adamio F, Zollo O, Moraca R, Ayroldi E, Bruscoli S, et al. (1997) A new dexamethasone-induced gene of the leucine zipper family protects T lymphocytes from TCR/CD3-activated cell death. Immunity 7: 803-812.

[20] Ashwell JD, Lu FW, Vacchio MS (2000) Glucocorticoids in T cell development and function. Annu Rev Immunol 18: 309-345.

[21] Planey SL, Abrams MT, Robertson NM, Litwack G (2003) Role of apical caspases and glucocorticoid-regulated genes in glucocorticoid-induced apoptosis of pre-B leukemic cells. Cancer Res 63: 172-178.

[22] Garza AS, Miller AL, Johnson BH, Thompson EB (2009) Converting cell lines representing hematological malignancies from glucocorticoid-resistant to glucocorticoid-sensitive: signaling pathway interactions. Leuk Res 33: 717-727.

[23] Almawi WY, Melemedjian OK, Jaoude MM (2004) On the link between Bcl-2 family proteins and glucocorticoid-induced apoptosis. J Leukoc Biol 76: 7-14.

[24] Bouillet P, Metcalf D, Huang DC, Tarlinton DM, Kay TW, et al. (1999) Proapoptotic Bcl-2 relative Bim required for certain apoptotic responses, leukocyte homeostasis, and to preclude autoimmunity. Science 286: 1735-1738.

[25] Shi Y (2004) Caspase activation, inhibition, and reactivation: a mechanistic view. Protein Sci 13: 1979-1987.

[26] Abrams MT, Robertson NM, Yoon K, Wickstrom E (2004) Inhibition of glucocorticoid-induced apoptosis by targeting the major splice variants of BIM mRNA with small interfering RNA and short hairpin RNA. J Biol Chem 279: 55809-55817.

[27] Iglesias-Serret D, de Frias M, Santidrian AF, Coll-Mulet L, Cosialls AM, et al. (2007) Regulation of the proapoptotic BH3-only protein BIM by glucocorticoids, survival signals and proteasome in chronic lymphocytic leukemia cells. Leukemia 21: 281-287.

[28] Wang Z, Malone MH, He H, McColl KS, Distelhorst CW (2003) Microarray analysis uncovers the induction of the proapoptotic BH3-only protein Bim in multiple models of glucocorticoid-induced apoptosis. J Biol Chem 278: 23861-23867.

[29] Elmore S (2007) Apoptosis: a review of programmed cell death. Toxicol Pathol 35: 495-516.

[30] Lauber K, Appel HA, Schlosser SF, Gregor M, Schulze-Osthoff K, et al. (2001) The adapter protein apoptotic protease-activating factor-1 (Apaf-1) is proteolytically processed during apoptosis. J Biol Chem 276: 29772-29781.

[31] Arai Y, Nakamura Y, Inoue F, Yamamoto K, Saito K, et al. (2000) Glucocorticoid-induced apoptotic pathways in eosinophils: comparison with glucocorticoid-sensitive leukemia cells. Int J Hematol 71: 340-349.

[32] Segal M, Niazi S, Simons MP, Galati SA, Zangrilli JG (2007) Bid activation during induction of extrinsic and intrinsic apoptosis in eosinophils. Immunol Cell Biol 85: 518-524.

[33] Kaufmann T, Tai L, Ekert PG, Huang DC, Norris F, et al. (2007) The BH3-only protein bid is dispensable for DNA damage- and replicative stress-induced apoptosis or cell-cycle arrest. Cell 129: 423-433.

[34] Oakley RH, Cidlowski JA (2011) Cellular processing of the glucocorticoid receptor gene and protein: new mechanisms for generating tissue-specific actions of glucocorticoids. J Biol Chem 286: 3177-3184.

[35] Evans RM (1988) The steroid and thyroid hormone receptor superfamily. Science 240: 889-895.

[36] Yamamoto KR (1985) Steroid receptor regulated transcription of specific genes and gene networks. Annu Rev Genet 19: 209-252.

[37] Ploner C, Rainer J, Niederegger H, Eduardoff M, Villunger A, et al. (2008) The BCL2 rheostat in glucocorticoid-induced apoptosis of acute lymphoblastic leukemia. Leukemia 22: 370-377.

[38] Kfir-Erenfeld S, Sionov RV, Spokoini R, Cohen O, Yefenof E (2010) Protein kinase networks regulating glucocorticoid-induced apoptosis of hematopoietic cancer cells: fundamental aspects and practical considerations. Leuk Lymphoma 51: 1968-2005.

[39] Beesley AH, Weller RE, Senanayake S, Welch M, Kees UR (2009) Receptor mutation is not a common mechanism of naturally occurring glucocorticoid resistance in leukaemia cell lines. Leuk Res 33: 321-325.

[40] Medh RD, Webb MS, Miller AL, Johnson BH, Fofanov Y, et al. (2003) Gene expression profile of human lymphoid CEM cells sensitive and resistant to glucocorticoid-evoked apoptosis. Genomics 81: 543-555.

[41] Herold MJ, McPherson KG, Reichardt HM (2006) Glucocorticoids in T cell apoptosis and function. Cell Mol Life Sci 63: 60-72.

[42] Helmberg A, Auphan N, Caelles C, Karin M (1995) Glucocorticoid-induced apoptosis of human leukemic cells is caused by the repressive function of the glucocorticoid receptor. EMBO J 14: 452-460.

[43] Zhou J, Cidlowski JA (2005) The human glucocorticoid receptor: one gene, multiple proteins and diverse responses. Steroids 70: 407-417.

[44] Oakley RH, Jewell CM, Yudt MR, Bofetiado DM, Cidlowski JA (1999) The dominant negative activity of the human glucocorticoid receptor beta isoform. Specificity and mechanisms of action. J Biol Chem 274: 27857-27866.

[45] Kino T, Liou SH, Charmandari E, Chrousos GP (2004) Glucocorticoid receptor mutants demonstrate increased motility inside the nucleus of living cells: time of fluorescence recovery after photobleaching (FRAP) is an integrated measure of receptor function. Mol Med 10: 80-88.

[46] Hillmann AG, Ramdas J, Multanen K, Norman MR, Harmon JM (2000) Glucocorticoid receptor gene mutations in leukemic cells acquired in vitro and in vivo. Cancer Res 60: 2056-2062.

[47] Zilberman Y, Zafrir E, Ovadia H, Yefenof E, Guy R, et al. (2004) The glucocorticoid receptor mediates the thymic epithelial cell-induced apoptosis of CD4+8+ thymic lymphoma cells. Cell Immunol 227: 12-23.

[48] Webster JC, Oakley RH, Jewell CM, Cidlowski JA (2001) Proinflammatory cytokines regulate human glucocorticoid receptor gene expression and lead to the accumulation of the dominant negative beta isoform: a mechanism for the generation of glucocorticoid resistance. Proc Natl Acad Sci U S A 98: 6865-6870.

[49] Youle RJ, Strasser A (2008) The BCL-2 protein family: opposing activities that mediate cell death. Nat Rev Mol Cell Biol 9: 47-59.

[50] Hartmann BL, Geley S, Loffler M, Hattmannstorfer R, Strasser-Wozak EM, et al. (1999) Bcl-2 interferes with the execution phase, but not upstream events, in glucocorticoid-induced leukemia apoptosis. Oncogene 18: 713-719.

[51] Broome HE, Yu AL, Diccianni M, Camitta BM, Monia BP, et al. (2002) Inhibition of Bcl-xL expression sensitizes T-cell acute lymphoblastic leukemia cells to chemotherapeutic drugs. Leuk Res 26: 311-316.

[52] Bailly-Maitre B, de Sousa G, Boulukos K, Gugenheim J, Rahmani R (2001) Dexamethasone inhibits spontaneous apoptosis in primary cultures of human and rat hepatocytes via Bcl-2 and Bcl-xL induction. Cell Death Differ 8: 279-288.

[53] Huang ST, Cidlowski JA (2002) Phosphorylation status modulates Bcl-2 function during glucocorticoid-induced apoptosis in T lymphocytes. FASEB J 16: 825-832.

[54] Lu J, Quearry B, Harada H (2006) p38-MAP kinase activation followed by BIM induction is essential for glucocorticoid-induced apoptosis in lymphoblastic leukemia cells. FEBS Lett 580: 3539-3544.

[55] Salomons GS, Brady HJM, Verwijs-Janssen M, Van Den Berg JD, Hart AAM, et al. (1997) The Baxα:Bcl-2 ratio modulates the response to dexamethasone in leukaemic cells and is highly variable in childhood acute leukaemia. Int J Cancer 71: 959-965.

[56] Wei G, Twomey D, Lamb J, Schlis K, Agarwal J, et al. (2006) Gene expression-based chemical genomics identifies rapamycin as a modulator of MCL1 and glucocorticoid resistance. Cancer Cell 10: 331-342.

[57] Alves NL, Derks IA, Berk E, Spijker R, van Lier RA, et al. (2006) The Noxa/Mcl-1 axis regulates susceptibility to apoptosis under glucose limitation in dividing T cells. Immunity 24: 703-716.

[58] Lynch JT, Rajendran R, Xenaki G, Berrou I, Demonacos C, et al. (2010) The role of glucocorticoid receptor phosphorylation in Mcl-1 and NOXA gene expression. Mol Cancer 9: 38.

[59] Jiang N, Koh GS, Lim JY, Kham SK, Ariffin H, et al. (2011) BIM is a prognostic biomarker for early prednisolone response in pediatric acute lymphoblastic leukemia. Exp Hematol 39: 321-329.

[60] Schmidt S, Rainer J, Riml S, Ploner C, Jesacher S, et al. (2006) Identification of glucocorticoid-response genes in children with acute lymphoblastic leukemia. Blood 107: 2061-2069.

[61] Bouillet P, Metcalf D, Huang DCS, Tarlinton DM, Kay TWH, et al. (1999) Proapoptotic Bcl-2 Relative Bim Required for Certain Apoptotic Responses, Leukocyte Homeostasis, and to Preclude Autoimmunity. Science 286: 1735-1738.

[62] Villunger A, Michalak EM, Coultas L, Mullauer F, Bock G, et al. (2003) p53- and drug-induced apoptotic responses mediated by BH3-only proteins puma and noxa. Science 302: 1036-1038.

[63] Herr I, Gassler N, Friess H, Büchler M (2007) Regulation of differential pro- and anti-apoptotic signaling by glucocorticoids. Apoptosis 12: 271-291.

[64] Memon SA, Moreno MB, Petrak D, Zacharchuk CM (1995) Bcl-2 blocks glucocorticoid- but not Fas- or activation-induced apoptosis in a T cell hybridoma. J Immunol 155: 4644-4652.

[65] Erlacher M, Michalak EM, Kelly PN, Labi V, Niederegger H, et al. (2005) BH3-only proteins Puma and Bim are rate-limiting for gamma-radiation- and glucocorticoid-induced apoptosis of lymphoid cells in vivo. Blood 106: 4131-4138.

[66] Real PJ, Tosello V, Palomero T, Castillo M, Hernando E, et al. (2009) Gamma-secretase inhibitors reverse glucocorticoid resistance in T cell acute lymphoblastic leukemia. Nat Med 15: 50-58.

[67] Hoijman E, Rocha Viegas L, Keller Sarmiento MI, Rosenstein RE, Pecci A (2004) Involvement of Bax protein in the prevention of glucocorticoid-induced thymocytes apoptosis by melatonin. Endocrinology 145: 418-425.

[68] Rathmell JC, Lindsten T, Zong WX, Cinalli RM, Thompson CB (2002) Deficiency in Bak and Bax perturbs thymic selection and lymphoid homeostasis. Nat Immunol 3: 932-939.

[69] Fésüs L, Demény MÁ, Petrovski G (2011) Autophagy shapes inflammation Antioxid Redox Signal 14: 2233-2243.

[70] Mizushima N (2007) Autophagy: process and function. Genes Dev 21: 2861-2873.

[71] Chen S, Rehman SK, Zhang W, Wen A, Yao L, et al. (2010) Autophagy is a therapeutic target in anticancer drug resistance. Biochim Biophys Acta 1806: 220-229.

[72] Grander D, Kharaziha P, Laane E, Pokrovskaja K, Panaretakis T (2009) Autophagy as the main means of cytotoxicity by glucocorticoids in hematological malignancies. Autophagy 5: 1198-1200.

[73] Laane E, Tamm KP, Buentke E, Ito K, Khahariza P, et al. (2009) Cell death induced by dexamethasone in lymphoid leukemia is mediated through initiation of autophagy. Cell Death Differ 16: 1018-1029.

[74] Bonapace L, Bornhauser BC, Schmitz M, Cario G, Ziegler U, et al. (2010) Induction of autophagy-dependent necroptosis is required for childhood acute lymphoblastic leukemia cells to overcome glucocorticoid resistance. J Clin Invest 120: 1310-1323.

[75] Heidari N, Hicks MA, Harada H (2010) GX15-070 (obatoclax) overcomes glucocorticoid resistance in acute lymphoblastic leukemia through induction of apoptosis and autophagy. Cell Death Dis 1: e76.

[76] Yu L, Wan F, Dutta S, Welsh S, Liu Z, et al. (2006) Autophagic programmed cell death by selective catalase degradation. Proc Natl Acad Sci U S A 103: 4952-4957.

[77] Luecke HF, Yamamoto KR (2005) The glucocorticoid receptor blocks P-TEFb recruitment by NFkappaB to effect promoter-specific transcriptional repression. Genes Dev 19: 1116-1127.

[78] De Bosscher K, Vanden Berghe W, Haegeman G (2000) Mechanisms of anti-inflammatory action and of immunosuppression by glucocorticoids: negative interference of activated glucocorticoid receptor with transcription factors. J Neuroimmunol 109: 16-22.

[79] Nawata H, Okabe T, Yanase T, Nomura M (2008) Mechanism of action and resistance to glucocorticoid and selective glucocorticoid receptor modulator to overcome glucocorticoid-related adverse effects. Clinical & Experimental Allergy Reviews 8: 53-56.

[80] Perissi V, Rosenfeld MG (2005) Controlling nuclear receptors: the circular logic of cofactor cycles. Nat Rev Mol Cell Biol 6: 542-554.

[81] Davies L, Paraskevopoulou E, Sadeq M, Symeou C, Pantelidou C, et al. (2011) Regulation of glucocorticoid receptor activity by a stress responsive transcriptional cofactor. Mol Endocrinol 25: 58-71.

[82] Nader N, Chrousos GP, Kino T (2009) Circadian rhythm transcription factor CLOCK regulates the transcriptional activity of the glucocorticoid receptor by acetylating its hinge region lysine cluster: potential physiological implications. FASEB J 23: 1572-1583.

[83] Matthews JG, Ito K, Barnes PJ, Adcock IM (2004) Defective glucocorticoid receptor nuclear translocation and altered histone acetylation patterns in glucocorticoid-resistant patients. J Allergy Clin Immunol 113: 1100-1108.

[84] Wallace AD, Cidlowski JA (2001) Proteasome-mediated glucocorticoid receptor degradation restricts transcriptional signaling by glucocorticoids. J Biol Chem 276: 42714-42721.

[85] Deroo BJ, Rentsch C, Sampath S, Young J, DeFranco DB, et al. (2002) Proteasomal inhibition enhances glucocorticoid receptor transactivation and alters its subnuclear trafficking. Mol Cell Biol 22: 4113-4123.

[86] Holmstrom S, Van Antwerp ME, Iniguez-Lluhi JA (2003) Direct and distinguishable inhibitory roles for SUMO isoforms in the control of transcriptional synergy. Proc Natl Acad Sci U S A 100: 15758-15763.

[87] Tian S, Poukka H, Palvimo JJ, Janne OA (2002) Small ubiquitin-related modifier-1 (SUMO-1) modification of the glucocorticoid receptor. Biochem J 367: 907-911.

[88] Le Drean Y, Mincheneau N, Le Goff P, Michel D (2002) Potentiation of glucocorticoid receptor transcriptional activity by sumoylation. Endocrinology 143: 3482-3489.

[89] Davies L, Karthikeyan N, Lynch JT, Sial EA, Gkourtsa A, et al. (2008) Cross talk of signaling pathways in the regulation of the glucocorticoid receptor function. Mol Endocrinol 22: 1331-1344.

[90] Krstic MD, Rogatsky I, Yamamoto KR, Garabedian MJ (1997) Mitogen-activated and cyclin-dependent protein kinases selectively and differentially modulate transcriptional enhancement by the glucocorticoid receptor. Mol Cell Biol 17: 3947-3954.

[91] Hoeck W, Groner B (1990) Hormone-dependent phosphorylation of the glucocorticoid receptor occurs mainly in the amino-terminal transactivation domain. J Biol Chem 265: 5403-5408.

[92] Ismaili N, Garabedian MJ (2004) Modulation of glucocorticoid receptor function via phosphorylation. Ann N Y Acad Sci 1024: 86-101.

[93] Beck IM, Vanden Berghe W, Vermeulen L, Yamamoto KR, Haegeman G, et al. (2009) Crosstalk in inflammation: the interplay of glucocorticoid receptor-based mechanisms and kinases and phosphatases. Endocr Rev 30: 830-882.

[94] Galliher-Beckley AJ, Cidlowski JA (2009) Emerging roles of glucocorticoid receptor phosphorylation in modulating glucocorticoid hormone action in health and disease. IUBMB Life 61: 979-986.

[95] Galliher-Beckley AJ, Williams JG, Cidlowski JA (2011) Ligand-independent phosphorylation of the glucocorticoid receptor integrates cellular stress pathways with nuclear receptor signaling. Mol Cell Biol 31: 4663-4675.

[96] Adzic M, Djordjevic A, Demonacos C, Krstic-Demonacos M, Radojcic MB (2009) The role of phosphorylated glucocorticoid receptor in mitochondrial functions and apoptotic signalling in brain tissue of stressed Wistar rats. Int J Biochem Cell Biol 41: 2181-2188.

[97] Sionov RV, Cohen O, Kfir S, Zilberman Y, Yefenof E (2006) Role of mitochondrial glucocorticoid receptor in glucocorticoid-induced apoptosis. J Exp Med 203: 189-201.

[98] Hock MB, Kralli A (2009) Transcriptional Control of Mitochondrial Biogenesis and Function. Ann Rev Physiol. Palo Alto: Annual Reviews. pp. 177-203.

[99] Scheller K, Sekeris CE (2003) The effects of steroid hormones on the transcription of genes encoding enzymes of oxidative phosphorylation. Exp Physiol 88: 129-140.

[100] Demonacos CV, Karayanni N, Hatzoglou E, Tsiriyiotis C, Spandidos DA, et al. (1996) Mitochondrial genes as sites of primary action of steroid hormones. Steroids 61: 226-232.

[101] Demonacos C, Tsawdaroglou NC, Djordjevic-Markovic R, Papalopoulou M, Galanopoulos V, et al. (1993) Import of the glucocorticoid receptor into rat liver mitochondria in vivo and in vitro. J Steroid Biochem Mol Biol 46: 401-413.

[102] Demonacos C, Djordjevic-Markovic R, Tsawdaroglou N, Sekeris CE (1995) The mitochondrion as a primary site of action of glucocorticoids: the interaction of the glucocorticoid receptor with mitochondrial DNA sequences showing partial similarity to the nuclear glucocorticoid responsive elements. J Steroid Biochem Mol Biol 55: 43-55.

[103] Sionov RV, Kfir S, Zafrir E, Cohen O, Zilberman Y, et al. (2006) Glucocorticoid-induced apoptosis revisited: a novel role for glucocorticoid receptor translocation to the mitochondria. Cell Cycle 5: 1017-1026.

[104] Kondoh H, Lleonart ME, Gil J, Wang J, Degan P, et al. (2005) Glycolytic enzymes can modulate cellular life span. Cancer Res 65: 177-185.

[105] Kwong JQ, Henning MS, Starkov AA, Manfredi G (2007) The mitochondrial respiratory chain is a modulator of apoptosis. J Cell Biol 179: 1163-1177.

[106] Cuezva JM, Krajewska M, de Heredia ML, Krajewski S, Santamaria G, et al. (2002) The bioenergetic signature of cancer: a marker of tumor progression. Cancer Res 62: 6674-6681.

[107] Lemarie A, Grimm S (2011) Mitochondrial respiratory chain complexes: apoptosis sensors mutated in cancer? Oncogene 30: 3985-4003.

[108] Tomiyama A, Serizawa S, Tachibana K, Sakurada K, Samejima H, et al. (2006) Critical role for mitochondrial oxidative phosphorylation in the activation of tumor suppressors Bax and Bak. J Natl Cancer Inst 98: 1462-1473.

[109] Huang G, Chen Y, Lu H, Cao X (2007) Coupling mitochondrial respiratory chain to cell death: an essential role of mitochondrial complex I in the interferon-[beta] and retinoic acid-induced cancer cell death. Cell Death Differ 14: 327-337.

[110] Coenen MJ, van den Heuvel LP, Smeitink JA (2001) Mitochondrial oxidative phosphorylation system assembly in man: recent achievements. Curr Opin Neurol 14: 777-781.

[111] Fontanesi F, Soto IC, Horn D, Barrientos A (2006) Assembly of mitochondrial cytochrome c-oxidase, a complicated and highly regulated cellular process. Am J Physiol Cell Physiol 291: C1129-C1147.

[112] Weber K, Brück P, Mikes Z, Küpper J-H, Klingenspor M, et al. (2002) Glucocorticoid hormone stimulates mitochondrial biogenesis specifically in skeletal muscle. Endocrinology 143: 177-184.

[113] Van Itallie CM (1992) Dexamethasone treatment increases mitochondrial RNA synthesis in a rat hepatoma cell line. Endocrinology 130: 567-576.

[114] Kulinsky V, Kolesnichenko L (2007) Regulation of metabolic and energetic functions of mitochondria by hormones and signal transduction systems. Biochemistry (Moscow) Supplemental Series B: Biomedical Chemistry 1: 95-113.

[115] Ritz P, Dumas JF, Ducluzeau PH, Simard G (2005) Hormonal regulation of mitochondrial energy production. Curr Opin Clin Nutr Metab Care 8: 415-418.

[116] Vijayasarathy C, Biunno I, Lenka N, Yang M, Basu A, et al. (1998) Variations in the subunit content and catalytic activity of the cytochrome c oxidase complex from different tissues and different cardiac compartments. Biochim Biophys Acta 1371: 71-82.

[117] Martens ME, Peterson PL, Lee CP (1991) In vitro effects of glucocorticoid on mitochondrial energy metabolism. Biochim Biophys Acta 1058: 152-160.

[118] Pandya JD, Agarwal NA, Katyare SS (2007) Dexamethasone treatment differentially affects the oxidative energy metabolism of rat brain mitochondria in developing and adult animals. Int J Dev Neurosci 25: 309-316.

[119] Holleman A, den Boer ML, Kazemier KM, Janka-Schaub GE, Pieters R (2003) Resistance to different classes of drugs is associated with impaired apoptosis in childhood acute lymphoblastic leukemia. Blood 102: 4541-4546.

[120] Hulleman E, Kazemier KM, Holleman A, VanderWeele DJ, Rudin CM, et al. (2009) Inhibition of glycolysis modulates prednisolone resistance in acute lymphoblastic leukemia cells. Blood 113: 2014-2021.

[121] Adebodun F (1999) Phospholipid metabolism and resistance to glucocorticoid-induced apoptosis in a human leukemic cell line: a 31P-NMR study using a phosphonium analog of choline. Cancer Lett 140: 189-194.

[122] Brown GC, Borutaite V (2008) Regulation of apoptosis by the redox state of cytochrome c. Biochim Biophys Acta 1777: 877-881.

[123] Carlet M, Janjetovic K, Rainer J, Schmidt S, Panzer-Grumayer R, et al. (2010) Expression, regulation and function of phosphofructo-kinase/fructose-biphosphatases (PFKFBs) in glucocorticoid-induced apoptosis of acute lymphoblastic leukemia cells. BMC Cancer 10: 638.

[124] Dong H, Zitt C, Auriga C, Hatzelmann A, Epstein PM (2010) Inhibition of PDE3, PDE4 and PDE7 potentiates glucocorticoid-induced apoptosis and overcomes glucocorticoid resistance in CEM T leukemic cells. Biochem Pharmacol 79: 321-329.

[125] Vander Kooi BT, Onuma H, Oeser JK, Svitek CA, Allen SR, et al. (2005) The glucose-6-phosphatase catalytic subunit gene promoter contains both positive and negative glucocorticoid response elements. Mol Endocrinol 19: 3001-3022.

[126] Lange AJ, Espinet C, Hall R, El-Maghrabi MR, Vargas AM, et al. (1992) Regulation of gene expression of rat skeletal muscle/liver 6- phosphofructo-2-kinase/fructose-2, 6-bisphosphatase: Isolation and characterization of a glucocorticoid response element in the first intron of the gene. J Biol Chem 267: 15673-15680.

[127] Datson NA, Van Der Perk J, De Kloet ER, Vreugdenhil E (2001) Identification of corticosteroid-responsive genes in rat hippocampus using serial analysis of gene expression. Eur J Neurosci 14: 675-689.

[128] Datson NA, Morsink MC, Meijer OC, de Kloet ER (2008) Central corticosteroid actions: Search for gene targets. Eur J Pharmacol 583: 272-289.

[129] Zhao F, Xuan Z, Liu L, Zhang MQ (2005) TRED: a Transcriptional Regulatory Element Database and a platform for in silico gene regulation studies. Nucleic Acids Res 33: D103-107.

[130] Marinescu VD, Kohane IS, Riva A (2005) MAPPER: a search engine for the computational identification of putative transcription factor binding sites in multiple genomes. BMC Bioinformatics 6: 79.

[131] Kolchanov NA, Merkulova TI, Ignatieva EV, Ananko EA, Oshchepkov DY, et al. (2007) Combined experimental and computational approaches to study the regulatory elements in eukaryotic genes. Brief Bioinform 8: 266-274.

[132] Yang H, Brosel S, Acin-Perez R, Slavkovich V, Nishino I, et al. (2010) Analysis of mouse models of cytochrome c oxidase deficiency owing to mutations in Sco2. Hum Mol Genet 19: 170-180.

[133] Fontanesi F, Soto IC, Horn D, Barrientos A (2006) Assembly of mitochondrial cytochrome c-oxidase, a complicated and highly regulated cellular process. Am J Physiol Cell Physiol 291: C1129-1147.

[134] Fernandez-Vizarra E, Tiranti V, Zeviani M (2009) Assembly of the oxidative phosphorylation system in humans: what we have learned by studying its defects. Biochim Biophys Acta 1793: 200-211.

[135] Harmon JM, Thompson EB (1981) Isolation and characterization of dexamethasone-resistant mutants from human lymphoid cell line CEM-C7. Mol Cell Biol 1: 512-521.

[136] Williams SL, Valnot I, Rustin P, Taanman JW (2004) Cytochrome c oxidase subassemblies in fibroblast cultures from patients carrying mutations in COX10, SCO1, or SURF1. J Biol Chem 279: 7462-7469.

[137] Rachamim N, Latter H, Malinin N, Asher C, Wald H, et al. (1995) Dexamethasone enhances expression of mitochondrial oxidative phosphorylation genes in rat distal colon. Am J Physiol 269: C1305-C1310.

[138] Sekeris CE (1990) The mitochondrial genome: a possible primary site of action of steroid hormones. In Vivo 4: 317-320.

[139] Herrmann JM, Funes S (2005) Biogenesis of cytochrome oxidase-sophisticated assembly lines in the mitochondrial inner membrane. Gene 354: 43-52.

[140] Krieg RC, Knuechel R, Schiffmann E, Liotta LA, Petricoin EF, 3rd, et al. (2004) Mitochondrial proteome: cancer-altered metabolism associated with cytochrome c oxidase subunit level variation. Proteomics 4: 2789-2795.

[141] Grandjean F, Bremaud L, Robert J, Ratinaud MH (2002) Alterations in the expression of cytochrome c oxidase subunits in doxorubicin-resistant leukemia K562 cells. Biochem Pharmacol 63: 823-831.

[142] Scheller K, Sekeris CE (2003) The effects of steroid hormones on the transcription of genes encoding enzymes of oxidative phosphorylation. Exp Physiol 88: 129-140.

[143] Chen JQ, Eshete M, Alworth WL, Yager JD (2004) Binding of MCF-7 cell mitochondrial proteins and recombinant human estrogen receptors α and β to human mitochondrial dna estrogen response elements. J Cell Biochem 93: 358-373.

[144] Chen JQ, Eshete M, Alworth WL, Yager JD (2004) Binding of MCF-7 cell mitochondrial proteins and recombinant human estrogen receptors alpha and beta to human mitochondrial DNA estrogen response elements. J Cell Biochem 93: 358-373.

[145] Pujols L, Xaubet A, Ramirez J, Mullol J, Roca-Ferrer J, et al. (2004) Expression of glucocorticoid receptors alpha and beta in steroid sensitive and steroid insensitive interstitial lung diseases. Thorax 59: 687-693.

[146] Rainer J, Lelong J, Bindreither D, Mantinger C, Ploner C, et al. (2012) Research resource: transcriptional response to glucocorticoids in childhood acute lymphoblastic leukemia. Mol Endocrinol 26: 178-193.

[147] De Bosscher K, Vanden Berghe W, Haegeman G (2003) The interplay between the glucocorticoid receptor and nuclear factor-kappaB or activator protein-1: molecular mechanisms for gene repression. Endocr Rev 24: 488-522.

[148] Ma J, Xie Y, Shi Y, Qin W, Zhao B, et al. (2008) Glucocorticoid-induced apoptosis requires FOXO3A activity. Biochem Biophys Res Commun 377: 894-898.

[149] Nicholson L, Hall AG, Redfern CP, Irving J (2010) NFkappaB modulators in a model of glucocorticoid resistant, childhood acute lymphoblastic leukemia. Leuk Res 34: 1366-1373.

[150] Tissing WJ, Meijerink JP, den Boer ML, Pieters R (2003) Molecular determinants of glucocorticoid sensitivity and resistance in acute lymphoblastic leukemia. Leukemia 17: 17-25.

[151] Sivils JC, Storer CL, Galigniana MD, Cox MB (2011) Regulation of steroid hormone receptor function by the 52-kDa FK506-binding protein (FKBP52). Curr Opin Pharmacol 11: 314-319.

[152] Chen W, Dang T, Blind RD, Wang Z, Cavasotto CN, et al. (2008) Glucocorticoid receptor phosphorylation differentially affects target gene expression. Mol Endocrinol 22: 1754-1766.

[153] Miller AL, Webb MS, Copik AJ, Wang Y, Johnson BH, et al. (2005) p38 Mitogen-activated protein kinase (MAPK) is a key mediator in glucocorticoid-induced apoptosis of lymphoid cells: correlation between p38 MAPK activation and site-specific phosphorylation of the human glucocorticoid receptor at serine 211. Mol Endocrinol 19: 1569-1583.

[154] Itoh M, Adachi M, Yasui H, Takekawa M, Tanaka H, et al. (2002) Nuclear export of glucocorticoid receptor is enhanced by c-Jun N-terminal kinase-mediated phosphorylation. Mol Endocrinol 16: 2382-2392.

[155] Bhadri VA, Trahair TN, Lock RB (2011) Glucocorticoid resistance in paediatric acute lymphoblastic leukaemia. J Paediatr Child Health.

Chapter 8

The Role of GILZ in Anti-Inflammatory and Immunosuppressive Actions of Glucocorticoids

Huapeng Fan and Eric F. Morand

Additional information is available at the end of the chapter

http://dx.doi.org/10.5772/52027

1. Introduction

Chronic inflammatory diseases place a social and financial burden on society. Glucocorticoids, a class of steroid hormones existing in almost every vertebrate, have been exploited for more than 60 years as a therapeutic option for the inflammatory diseases. For example, the therapeutic effects of synthetic glucocorticoids, first observed in rheumatoid arthritis (RA), led to the awarding of a Nobel prize in 1950 (Slocumb *et al.*, 1950). Based on their rapid, profound and wide-ranging effects, glucocorticoids are a mainstay of treatment for virtually all inflammatory diseases besides RA, and now are among the most frequently prescribed of all medications (Hillier, 2007). Indeed, a community practice survey in 2000 indicated that up to 1% of the entire adult population is taking systemic glucocorticoids at any given time (van Staa *et al.*, 2000). Glucocorticoids have widespread systemic effects, particularly on the inflammation and immune response (Barnes, 2006; Chrousos, 1995). However, glucocorticoids are associated with dose dependent side effects, including diabetes mellitus, osteoporosis, weight gain, and hypertension (Huscher *et al.*, 2009), as well as increased risk of cardiovascular events (Davis *et al.*, 2007). Much effort has been expended identifying glucocorticoid anti-inflammatory mechanisms of action (Barnes, 2006; Scha¨cke *et al.*, 2002). Understanding of the mechanism of action of glucocorticoids is essential in order to devise better ways to treat inflammatory disease, ideally retaining the beneficial effects of glucocorticoids but not their adverse effects.

The discovery of a glucocorticoid-induced protein that could emulate the beneficial, but not harmful, effects of glucocorticoids, would represent a landmark in inflammation translational research on a glucocorticoid alternative therapy. Glucocorticoid induced leucine zipper (GILZ) may be such a candidate molecule. GILZ was first identified in 1997 in a gene extraction library, where it was found to be dramatically induced by dexamethasone (D'Adamio *et al.*, 1997). Subsequent studies, mostly utilizing forced over expression of GILZ have ascertained that GILZ has anti-inflammatory functions that include interactions with the NF-κB and AP-1 pathways (Di Marco *et al.*, 2007; Mittelstadt & Ashwell, 2001), which closely mimics the anti-inflammatory effects of glucocorticoids. Moreover, it has recently been shown that GILZ is also expressed in rheumatoid arthritis (RA) synovial tissues, where it exerts inhibitory effects on cytokine expression, and inhibiting the expression of GILZ results in exacerbation of disease in a mouse model of RA. As we will summarise in this Chapter, GILZ is a pivotal endogenous regulator of inflammation and immune responses, which could represent a potential new therapeutic alternate to glucocorticoids.

2. GILZ structure and expression

2.1. Molecular structure of GILZ

As shown in **Fig 1**, GILZ, also named TSC22 domain family protein 3 (TSC22D3), is a 137-amino acid protein, consisting of three major domains: the N-terminal (1-75 aa), leucine zipper (76-97 aa), and C-terminal domains (98-137 aa) (Beaulieu & Morand, 2011). To date, four isoforms of GILZ have been characterized as splice variants from the *Tsc22d* gene and named GILZ1-4 (Soundararajan *et al.*, 2007). The leucine zipper motif of GILZ is located in the central part of the protein and mainly mediates the homodimerization of GILZ required for many of its functions (Di Marco *et al.*, 2007), while the other two domains are responsible for protein-protein interactions between GILZ and transcription factors and signaling molecules. For example, the C-terminal of GILZ is a proline-rich region necessary for direct binding of GILZ to the p65 subunit of NF-κB (Di Marco *et al.*, 2007; Riccardi *et al.*, 2001). In 2001, Aryoldi and colleagues showed that the over expression of GILZ in T cells inhibits the activation of NF-κB by binding the p65 subunit of NF-κB and preventing its nuclear translocation (Ayroldi *et al.*, 2001). GILZ was co-precipitated with the p65 subunit of NF-κB in macrophages stimulated with glucocorticoids, and expression of GILZ with an NF-κB reporter inhibits reporter activity (Berrebi *et al.*, 2003). The N-terminal domain of GILZ directly binds with the upstream MAP kinase pathway activating molecule Raf-1, to inhibit its function. The interaction between GILZ and c-Fos and c-Jun (two constituents of AP-1) also occurs via the N-terminal domain of GILZ. Moreover, GILZ also binds to Ras via its tuberous sclerosis complex (TSC) box (61-75 aa), or even interacts with Ras and Raf together to form a trimer.

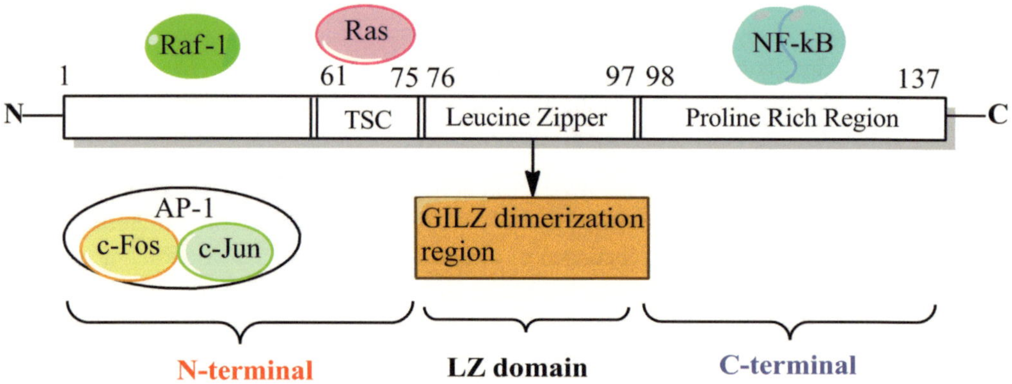

Figure 1. Functional domains of GILZ

2.2. Expression of GILZ

GILZ gene expression is exquisitely sensitive to induction by glucocorticoids. For example, in human RA synovial fibroblasts, dexamethasone (Dex), a synthetic drug derived from glucocorticoid class of steroid, induced a more than 10-fold increase in GILZ transcripts at a concentration of only 1 nM, while 100 nM dexamethasone increased GILZ mRNA by over 100-fold (Beaulieu *et al.*, 2010a). *In vivo*, exogenous glucocorticoids induce GILZ expression, while blockade of endogenous glucocorticoids inhibits GILZ expression in mouse, and GILZ expression is reduced in response to reductions in circulating cortisol in humans (Beaulieu *et al.*, 2010a; Lekva *et al.*, 2009). The dramatic effect of glucocorticoids on GILZ is mediated via the direct binding of the glucocorticoid/glucocorticoid receptor (GR) complex to six glucocorticoid-responsive elements (GREs) located in the promoter region of the *GILZ* gene. The *GILZ* promoter also contains two functional forkhead-responsive elements (FHREs), which when bound to the transcription factor forkhead box O 3 (FoxO3) facilitate maximal GILZ expression induced by glucocorticoid receptor binding (Asselin-Labat *et al.*, 2005b).

Although GILZ expression is mainly controlled by glucocorticoids (Beaulieu *et al.*, 2010b; Berrebi *et al.*, 2003; Eddleston *et al.*, 2007a), it is also modulated by a variety of cytokines (Eddleston *et al.*, 2007a). For example, GILZ is up-regulated by IL-10 (Berrebi *et al.*, 2003), IL-15 and TGF-β (Ayroldi & Riccardi, 2009; Cohen *et al.*, 2006a), whereas GILZ is down-regulated by IL-2 in some cell types. IL-2 can inhibit FoxO3 transcriptional activity, thus inhibiting glucocorticoid induced GILZ expression (Asselin-Labat *et al.*, 2005a). Some inflammatory stimuli, such as tumor necrosis factor (TNF) and lipopolysaccharide (LPS), were also found to reduce GILZ mRNA expression in fibroblast like synoviocytes (Beaulieu *et al.*, 2010b). GILZ expression can also be regulated by other anti-inflammatory molecule such as Annexin A1. Yang et al have reported that in Annexin A1 deficient cells, dexamethasone failed to significantly induce GILZ, in contrast to wild type cells (Yang *et al.*, 2009), which indicates a regulatory role of Annexin A1 on GILZ expression.

Interestingly, GILZ expression is also modulated by the oxygen environment. Wang and colleagues recently found that hypoxia not only remarkably upregulated the expression of GILZ, but also significantly enhanced Dex-induced expression of GILZ in macrophages and the spleen of rats (Wang *et al.*, 2011). They also reported ERK MAP kinase activity is involved in the upregulation of GILZ induced by hypoxia.

To date, GILZ has been discovered to be expressed in a variety of tissues (**Table 1**). This information indicates a widespread distribution of GILZ in the human body and suggests it is well placed for a role as a pivotal regulator of inflammation. Moreover, growing evidence showed that GILZ is present in a wide range of cell types that are sensitive to glucocorticoids *in vitro*. In 1997, GILZ was first identified in T cells, in which GILZ inhibited T cell receptor (TCR)-mediated T cell activation (D'Adamio *et al.*, 1997). Since then, GILZ has been shown to be expressed in other immune cells, including monocytes/macrophages, mast cells, and dendritic cells (Berrebi *et al.*, 2003; Cohen *et al.*, 2006b; Godot *et al.*, 2006; Hamdi *et al.*, 2007a), and to have numerous anti-inflammatory functions in these cells. These functions are outlined in the following sections. Besides immune cells, GILZ has also been shown to express in other cell types such as epithelial cells and bone-marrow-derived mesenchymal stem cells (MSCs). For example, GILZ was reported to inhibit NF-κB activation in epithelial cells and MSCs (Eddleston *et al.*, 2007b; Yang *et al.*, 2008). The studies also reported the expression of GILZ is necessary for dexamethasone-mediated inhibition of IL-8 production in respiratory epithelial cells and similarly for the dexamethasone-dependent inhibition of cyclo-oxygenase 2 expression in MSCs.

Tissue types	Expression of GILZ	Reference(s)
Lymphoid tissue	Lymphocytes mainly from thymus, spleen, and lymph nodes	(Asselin-Labat *et al.*, 2004; D'Adamio *et al.*, 1997; Riccardi *et al.*, 2001)
Brain	Ubiquitously expressed in rat brain	(van der Laan, 2008)
Renal epithelium	mammalian kidney epithelial cells	(Soundararajan *et al.*, 2009)
Collecting duct	the cortical collecting duct of the mouse kidney	(Robert-Nicoud *et al.*, 2001)
Ovaries	normal ovary and epithelial ovary cancer	(Redjimi *et al.*, 2009)
Bone tissue	fetal osteoblasts, mesenchymal stem cells, and osteoclasts	(Lekva *et al.*, 2010)
Skeletal muscle and cardiac tissue	skeletal muscle tissue and myoblasts	(Bruscoli *et al.*, 2010)

Table 1. Expression of GILZ in different tissues

3. Effects of GILZ on the immune response

3.1. Innate immunity

A variety of studies suggest that GILZ has critical inhibitory effects on the activity of the innate immune system. In a monocytic cell line (THP-1), RANTES (also known as CCL5) and MIP-1α (also known as CCL3), antigen presenting MHC class II molecules, B7 co-stimulatory molecules CD80 and CD86, and the the pathogen-associated molecular pattern (PAMP) receptor TLR2, are all modulated by GILZ, with an expected effect on reducing recruitment and activation of inflammatory cells (Berrebi *et al.*, 2003; Cohen *et al.*, 2006b). Furthermore, in liver disease, GILZ expression in Kupffer macrophages due to glucocorticoids treatment reduces the production of pro-inflammatory mediators in response to LPS (Hamdi *et al.*, 2007a). Besides macrophages and monocytes, GILZ is also expressed in human airway epithelial cells and inhibited by IL-1β, TNF and interferon (IFN)-γ, and overexpression of GILZ inhibited the activation of NF-κB by IL-1β and TLR ligands (Eddleston *et al.*, 2007b). Currently, it is known that GILZ expression is inhibited by different pro-inflammatory mediators. For example, GILZ was not produced in granulomas in Crohn disease and tuberculosis since the macrophages in the granulomas were activated with the strong expression of the RANTES gene (Berrebi *et al.*, 2003). By contrast, GILZ expression is retained in macrophages in Burkitt lymphomas, potentially contributing to the failure of the immune system to reject the tumor (Berrebi *et al.*, 2003). Taken together, these results above indicate a wide range of inhibitory effects of GILZ in a variety of innate immune responses. Clearly, immune responses, such as the expression of cytokines, chemokines and TLRs, are highly pertinent to the known pathology of inflammatory diseases such as RA. Of note, no *in vivo* studies of the role of GILZ in regulating classic innate immune responses, such as responses to endotoxin or other TLR ligands, have been reported.

3.2. Adaptive immunity

Parallel to innate immune responses, multiple critical functions of GILZ have been found which regulate the activity of antigen-presenting and effector cells of the adaptive immune response. For example, GILZ can mediate the effects of glucocorticoids on dendritic cells (DCs), whose maturation and antigen presentation are impaired in the presence of increased GILZ. Cohen *et al* demonstrated that GILZ over expression altered MHC and co-stimulatory molecule expression, resulting in reduced antigen presentation (Cohen *et al.*, 2006a), and subsequent decreased T lymphocyte activation. Moreover, the expression of GILZ is induced by glucocorticoids and transforming growth factor β (TGF-β) in immature DCs, and oral administration of glucocorticoids to patients increased the expression of GILZ in antigen-presenting cells (Cohen *et al.*, 2006b). The overexpression of GILZ is also able to drive the development of regulatory DCs, which secrete IL-10, and prevent the production of pro-inflammatory cytokines induced by CD40L. Furthermore, these GILZ-expressing regulatory DCs were found to induced $CD25^{hi}FoxP3^{+}CTLA\text{-}4^{+}$, IL-10 secreting T-regulatory cells from $CD4^{+}$ T-lymphocytes (Hamdi *et al.*, 2007b), resulting in inhibition of subsequent immune responses to specific antigens (Suffia *et al.*, 2006). Regulatory T cells (Tregs) that inhibit activation of other T lymphocytes are generated in response to GILZ over expressing dendritic cells (Hamdi *et al.*, 2007b), providing a further immunomodulatory effect of GILZ. This immunosuppressive effect of GILZ on DCs is extremely relevant in the context of inflammatory pathology since DCs determine whether antigen presentation will lead to an immune response or a tolerogenic response.

Additional knowledge of the effects of GILZ in adaptive immunity arises from studies of modified GILZ expression in T lymphocyte cells. For example, Cannarile and colleagues have demonstrated increased secretion of cytokines associated with a TH2 response, such as IL-4, IL-10, IL-5, and IL-13, and reduced expression of cytokines associated with a TH1 response such as IFN-γ in GILZ overexpressing cells compared with wild type T cells (Cannarile *et al.*, 2006a). In their study on GILZ transgenic T lymphocytes, they found there was decreased expression of T-box protein 21 (T-bet) (Cannarile *et al.*, 2006a), a transcription factor specifically associated with a TH1 response, and increased expression of the transcription factors GATA-3 and STAT6. As STAT6 modulates GATA3 which is important for polarization towards a TH2 phenotype (Wurster *et al.*, 2000; Zheng & Flavell, 1997), these studies indicate that the expression of GILZ promotes T lymphocyte development towards a

TH2 instead of TH1 phenotype. Moreover, mice transgenic for GILZ under the control of the CD2 promoter, that overexpresse GILZ in T cells, display a TH2-skewed phenotype, and are protected from the TH1-dependent model of dinitrobenzene sulfonic acid (DNBS)-induced colitis but exhibit an increase in the 'allergenic' TH2 Oxazolone-induced colitis (Cannarile *et al.*, 2009). Another study investigated the levels of inflammatory mediators in wild type and GILZ transgenic mice induced with DNBS, and were able to demonstrate a decrease in pro-inflammatory cytokines and NF-κB activation in GILZ transgenic mice compared to wild type. Furthermore, in T-cell specific GILZ transgenic mice, young animals do not exhibit a significant difference in thymic weight. However, there was a significant decrease in $CD4^+CD8^+$ double positive thymocytes. There was also a parallel increase in $CD4^-CD8^-$ double negative and $CD8^+$ T-cells, but no change in the $CD4^+$ population (Delfino *et al.*, 2004). In the aged mice, the $CD4^+$ population also increased in a significant manner, although not as dramatically as the $CD8^+$ or the $CD4^-CD8^-$ populations, signifying a disturbance in thymic maturation. The observation above is interesting since GILZ might mediate some of the glucocorticoid-triggered apoptotic effects during thymic development. Microarray studies also show that GILZ is expressed in resting B cells, and it is presumed that GILZ down-regulation facilitates B-cell activation (Glynne *et al.*, 2000).

4. Effect of GILZ on signalling pathways

4.1. NF-κB pathway

To date, much research has focused on the function of the NF-κB pathway in the anti-inflammatory effects of glucocorticoids (Auphan *et al.*, 1995; DeBosscher & Haegeman, 2009; Gossye *et al.*, 2009). Glucocorticoids are known as effective inhibitors of the NF-κB pathway, and considerable research directed at understanding the antagonistic effects of glucocorticoids on this pathway has been undertaken (De Bosscher *et al.*, 2003). As shown in **Fig 2**, GILZ, significantly up regulated in the presence of glucocorticoids, participates in the inhibition of NF-κB by glucocorticoids through a physical interaction with the NF-κB p65 subunit (Ayroldi *et al.*, 2001), preventing its nuclear translocation. The inhibition of GILZ is independent from other IκB- or Rel-related proteins, since GILZ was found to co-immunoprecipitate with NF-κB p65 subunit in the presence or absence of IκB (Ayroldi *et al.*, 2001). Subsequently, Yang *et a*l demonstrated the role of GILZ in the inhibition of the inflammatory mediator COX-2 in MCSs in response to IL-1α and TNF-α, by preventing NF-κB p65 subunit nuclear transport (Yang *et al.*, 2008). Similarly, the mechanism of GILZ-NF-κB mediated inhibition of COX-2 transcription has been shown in epithelial cells (Eddleston *et al.*, 2007b). The inhibition of NF-κB by GILZ has also been demonstrated *in vivo*, in a transgenic mouse model in which GILZ expression is driven by the CD2 promoter, resulting in the overexpression of GILZ in thymocytes (Delfino *et al.*, 2006). When subjected to T-cell receptor-triggered apoptosis, the nuclear translocation and DNA binding of NF-κB were impaired in T cells from GILZ transgenic mice, whereas the translocation of transcription factors belonging to the NFAT family was not affected. All the findings above arouse interest in GILZ and its function in the pathogenesis of NF-κB–related inflammatory diseases. For example, GILZ transgenic mice demonstrated reduced NF-κB activation in spinal cord injury in comparison to wild type mice, and overexpression of GILZ protects TH1 inflammatory responses in colitis associated with inhibition of nuclear and phosphorylated p65 (Cannarile *et al.*, 2009; Esposito *et al.* 2011). Moreover, Srinivasan and colleagues have described a novel NF-κB p65-binding GILZ-derived peptide which exhibited therapeutic potential as a small molecule NF-κB inhibitor in experimental autoimmune encephalomyelitis (EAE), a model of human multiple sclerosis (Srinivasan & Janardhanam, 2011a).

4.2. AP-1 pathway

The transcription factor AP-1 is another major participant in inflammatory and immune responses (Adcock & Caramori, 2001). AP-1, as a heterodimer of the c-Fos and c-Jun proteins, can be phosphorylated to significantly increase its transcriptional activity. The direct inhibitory effects of the glucocorticoid-glucocorticoid receptor complex on AP-1 signaling are well documented (De Bosscher *et al.*, 2003). It is also known that glucocorticoids lead to the repression of mitogen-activated protein kinase (MAPK) activity and hence AP-1 activation through the expression of phosphatases that exert inhibitory interactions with various MAPK members (Aeberli *et al.*, 2006). Of interest, Mittelstadt and colleagues showed direct binding of GILZ to the AP-1 components c-Jun and c-Fos (**Fig 2**) in Jurkat cells (an immortalized line of T cells) (Mittelstadt & Ashwell, 2001). The paper also showed GILZ is critical for the regulation of FasL expression in response to glucocorticoids. FasL is a promoter containing NFAT binding elements and under regulation of the NFAT/AP-1 complex signalling. FasL promoter and its enhancer elements, early growth response factor (Erg) -2 and Erg-3 were inhibited by transient transfection of GILZ in Jurkat cells. The authors demonstrated that c-Fos and c-Jun do in fact interact with N-terminal, but not the LZ or PER domains, of GILZ. Furthermore, Ayroldi et al. confirmed the interaction of GILZ with c-Fos and c-Jun, and further showed that GILZ expression interferes with c-Fos transcription in response to anti-CD3 stimulation of IL-2, but not c-Jun, and also by negatively interfering with upstream signalling of Raf-1-ERK pathway (Ayroldi *et al.*, 2002).

4.3. MAP kinase pathways

The MAP kinase family consists of extracellular signal-regulated kinase (ERK), p38 kinase, and JNK, all of which can be activated by upstream molecules such as Ras and Raf-1 (Rincon, 2001) and all of which phosphorylate downstream proteins in the respective cascades to regulate expression of a variety of genes related to inflammation, cell proliferation, differentiation and apoptosis. GILZ has also been shown to bind to both Raf-1 (Ayroldi *et al.*, 2002) and Ras (Ayroldi *et al.*, 2007) and thereby to modulate downstream signalling (**Fig 2**). Ayroldi and colleagues reported that GILZ overexpression in anti-CD3-stimulated T cells can bind to Raf-1, which inhibits phosphorylation of Raf-1 and results in suppression of MEK and ERK1/2 phosphorylation (Ayroldi *et al.*, 2002). They also found that GILZ can bind to Raf-1 via the NH_2-terminal region of GILZ and Ras via the TSC box of GILZ. The interaction of GILZ with Ras or Raf-1 has been shown to be dependent on the activation of Ras, where GILZ will bind predominately to Raf-1 in the absence of active Ras. However, as Ras is activated, Raf-1 will bind to Ras to a stronger degree than it will bind to GILZ. Furthermore, the affinity of GILZ to Ras will also increase, leading to predominately GILZ-Ras complexes (Ayroldi, 2007). GILZ may also form a trimer with both Ras and Raf-1, and this is also dependent on Ras activation. All the results above suggest that GILZ inhibits cell activation and inflammation via regulation of MAPK signaling molecules.

4.4. PI3K/Akt and apoptotic signalling pathways

The inhibition by GILZ of Ras and Raf-1 also decreases the activation of another downstream signalling pathway, the PI3 kinase (PI3K)/Akt pathway, which is involved in cell survival as well as activation. Recent studies have uncovered a crucial role for FoxO3 in mediation of PI3K/Akt pathway. In the cell, non-phosphorylated FoxO3 migrates into the nucleus and up-regulates several mediators of cell cycle progression, such as G1/S-specific cyclin-D1, $p27^{KIP1}$ (also known as cyclin-dependent kinase inhibitor 1B), Fas ligand (also known as tumor necrosis factor ligand superfamily member 6) and Bim (also known as Bcl-2-like protein 11), to inhibit cell proliferation (Schmidt *et al.*, 2002). Activation of Akt leads to the phosphorylation of FoxO3, which results in the nuclear exclusion of FoxO3 and thus leads to the inhibition of their cognate transcriptional targets. Interestingly, the gene encoding GILZ has been identified as a transcriptional target of FoxO3 (Asselin-Labat *et al.*, 2005b). Other studies have demonstrated that GILZ can inhibit its own expression through a negative feedback effect to promote nuclear exclusion of FoxO3 shown in **Fig 2** (Latre de Late et al., 2010). However, until now, the net effect of the PI3K/Akt-FoxO3–GILZ regulatory loop on cell proliferation has not yet been clearly defined.

GILZ has also been shown to modulate the expression of a variety of apoptosis pathway proteins in accordance with the observations that GILZ can prevent anti-CD3 mediated apoptosis (D'Adamio *et al.*, 1997). Asselin-Labat and colleagues showed that an increase in GILZ expression down-regulates the expression of Bim, a pro-apoptotic member of the Bcl-2 family, but has no effect on $Bcl\text{-}x_L$ protein, an anti-apoptotic Bcl-2 family protein, to prevent apoptosis. In the same study, they demonstrated that knockdown of GILZ accelerates IL-2-deprivation-mediated apoptosis in the IL-2-dependent, CTLL-2 cell line, through increased levels of Bim (Asselin-Labat *et al.*, 2004). Furthermore, they showed that GILZ acts on Bim through the transcriptional factor FoxO3. Using a Bim-promoter-luciferase construct, GILZ expression was shown to repress Bim transcription, and these effects were abrogated with the co-expression of FoxO3 (Asselin-Labat *et al.*, 2004). However, it had been previously shown in $CD4^+CD8^+$ double positive T cells that overexpression of GILZ leads to an increase in the spontaneous apoptosis, and an interaction with, and reduction of, $Bcl\text{-}x_L$. Furthermore, GILZ expression was associated with an increase in the activation of extrinsic apoptotic caspases -3 and -8, but not caspase-9, involved in the mitochondrial/cytochrome C pathway (Delfino *et al.*, 2004). The authors suggested that NF-κB inhibition is the mechanism by which TCR mediated apoptosis is inhibited by GILZ in over expression models, and that NF-κB may be involved in control of Bcl-xL (Delfino *et al.*, 2006). Whilst the mechanism of GILZ in regulation of cell apoptosis has yet to be well understood, it follows the general trend of GILZ to display a dual activity in regards to apoptosis and cell survival.

4.5. Other non-inflammatory signalling pathways

In addition to mediating glucocorticoid effects in inflammation and immunity, GILZ may also play a critical role in non-immune function such as adipogenesis and osteogenesis. For example, Shi *et al* reported that GILZ directly binds to CCAAT/enhancer-binding protein (C/EBP) DNA binding sites in the *PPAR-γ2* promoter, with consequent inhibition of mesenchymal cell adipogenesis (Shi *et al.*, 2003). Previously, glucocorticoids had been shown to activate C/EBP directly, and therefore promote PPAR-γ2 expression and adipocyte differentiation (Shi *et al.*, 2003). This observation thus suggests a potential role of GILZ as a direct transcriptional repressor of gene expression in a direction opposite to the effects of Glucocorticoids. Of note, this is in contrast to the effects of GILZ binding to pro-inflammatory transcription factors where it mimics the effects of glucocorticoids. Moreover, as PPAR-γ2 is a key regulator of adipogenesis, GILZ's prevention of C/EBP action inhibits adipogenesis, and thereby promotes osteogenesis (Zhang *et al.*, 2008b), again an effect opposite to those of glucocorticoids which promote osteoporosis. The findings offer the suggestion of a possible GILZ-based therapy wherein GILZ exhibits beneficial glucocorticoid anti-inflammatory actions without the negative side effects of adiposity and osteoporosis.

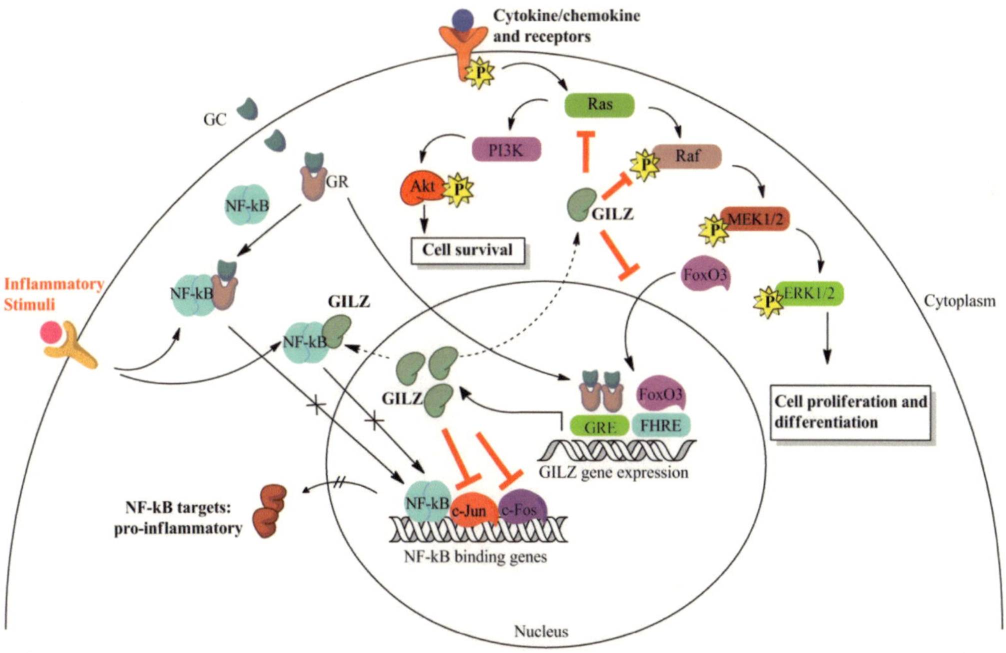

Figure 2. Roles of GILZ as a mediator in immune signaling pathways

NF-κB, activated by a variety of inflammatory stimulation, translocates into the nucleus and binds to target genes encoding pro-inflammatory factors. Glucocorticoid bound to the receptor GR can directly interact with NF-κB to prevent its nuclear translocation. In addition, the GC/GR complex can translocate into the nucleus and bind to glucocorticoid response elements on the *GILZ* gene to induce GILZ expression. GILZ in turn binds to NF-κB and prevents its nuclear translocation. GILZ can also directly bind to c-Jun and c-Fos, two constituents of AP-1, to inhibit their transcriptional activity and gene expression of pro-inflammatory molecules. The location, in the cytoplasm or nucleus, where GILZ binds to AP-1 subunits is still unknown. In the cytoplasm, GILZ also modulates cell survival by blocking Ras activation and the downstream PI3K/Akt signaling pathway. GILZ binds and inhibits Ras and Raf phosphorylation and thus inhibits downstream MEK-1/2 and ERK-1/2 activation. As part of a negative feedback loop, GILZ prevents nuclear translocation of FoxO3, which is in turn a key transcriptional factor to upregulate *GILZ* gene expression.

5. Effect of GILZ on inflammatory and autoimmune diseases

The reported actions of GILZ suggest GILZ may exert anti-inflammatory effects in immune and inflammatory diseases. Studies in animal disease models, or in human pathology, remain limited, but favour a role for GILZ as a modulator of immune-inflammatory responses. For example, Cannarile and colleagues reported GILZ effects on delayed-type hypersensitivity (DTH) responses in the GILZ transgenic mouse (Cannarile *et al.*, 2006b). In response to ovalbumin (OVA) immunization, GILZ overexpression mice exhibited significantly less swelling than wild type control, which indicates the essential role of GILZ in T cells in inhibiting TH1 dependent DTH responses. The authors also investigated a murine model of colitis, in which it was shown that significant inhibition was observed in mice overexpressing GILZ in T cells (Cannarile *et al.*, 2009). In addition, studies of these T cells showed reduction of the TH1 cytokine IFN-γ. Moreover, colon lysates from GILZ overexpressing mice have lower total and phosphorylated Ser536 NF-κB p65, which indicates that GILZ overexpression in T cells protects mice from TH1-mediated colitis disease by inhibition of NF-κB activity.

Recently, Beaulieu and colleagues investigated the role of endogenous GILZ in RA (Beaulieu *et al.*, 2010a). GILZ was potently induced by glucocorticoids in cultured human RA synovial cells *in vitro*, and in murine arthritis *in vivo*. GILZ silencing by *in vivo* siRNA administration resulted in increased severity of the collagen-induced model of RA in mice, and in parallel GILZ overexpression inhibited chemokine and cytokine expression in human synovial cells. These results suggest GILZ as a key endogenous regulatory molecule in RA. Another study showed that GILZ was noticeably absent in granulomas in Crohn disease and tuberculosis (Berrebi *et al.*, 2003), which suggests inhibitor regulation of GILZ in the presence of chronic inflammatory disease, while human asthma patients demonstrated increased GILZ expression in response to glucocorticoid therapy (Kelly *et al.*, 2011).

GILZ is also reported to attenuate experimental autoimmune encephalomyelitis (EAE), a disease model of human multiple sclerosis. Srinivasan and colleagues demonstrated that delivery of a GILZ-derived peptide is protective against EAE in mice (Srinivasan & Janardhanam, 2011b). The GILZ fragment they isolated, containing a proline rich domain, can directly interact with p65 NF-κB, thereby inhibiting p65 translocation from activated human $CD4^+$ T cells isolated from peripheral blood mononuclear cells (PBMCs) (Srinivasan & Janardhanam, 2011a). As T cells are a major target of glucocorticoids in EAE (Wust *et al.*, 2008), these data provide further evidence that exogenous GILZ could exert therapeutically useful anti-inflammatory properties.

6. Perspective and expectations: GILZ as a glucocorticoid sparing target

GILZ, a molecule mainly modulated by glucocorticoids, play a pivotal role in the regulation of inflammation and immune responses. Expressed in multiple cells and tissues, GILZ inhibits the expression of a variety of inflammatory mediators and modulates the immune response. In this chapter, we have summarised GILZ structure and function, the effects of GILZ in immune responses, and its interaction with a number of key transduction pathways pivotal to the pathogenesis of inflammatory diseases. The more recent observations that GILZ exerts immunomodulatory and anti-inflammatory effects *in vivo* that mimic the inhibitory actions of glucocorticoids strongly suggests GILZ is a potential substitute for glucocorticoids in the therapy of inflammatory diseases.

As we have noted, currently a number of important anti-inflammatory molecules, such as Annexin A1 and MKP-1, are induced by glucocorticoids, and evidence that synthetic glucocorticoids lose their effectiveness in the absence of these molecules has been adduced (Furst *et al.*, 2007; Ralph & Morand, 2008; Yang *et al.*, 2009; Yang *et al.*, 2004; Yang *et al.*, 2006). Attention to the molecules that glucocorticoids amplify the expression of will permit discovery of the means to develop a surrogate for glucocorticoids' beneficial impact on immune activation without their toxicity. Importantly, the presence of GILZ exerts immune and inflammation modulatory effects in the absence of glucocorticoids. A GILZ-based therapeutic approach, therefore, could potentially offer profound glucocorticoid-like regulatory effects in autoimmune disease. Investigation of the metabolic effects of any GILZ-based therapy is required in order to ensure that the undesirable effects of glucocorticoids are not recapitulated. Early results are encouraging in this regard. In mesenchymal stem cells, differentiation towards osteogenic precursors is enhanced by GILZ, whereas silencing of GILZ reduced osteogenic differentiation (Zhang *et al.*, 2008a), suggesting that a GILZ therapy might have protective rather than harmful effects on bone. GILZ expression was also associated with osteoblast development, and GILZ silencing increased osteoblast expression of OPG and RANKL in favour of osteoclastogenesis (Lekva *et al.*, 2010), further suggesting that GILZ-based therapy might have a bone-protective effect. Studies of the role of GILZ in glucocorticoid-induced osteoporosis *in vivo* are eagerly awaited.

GILZ-based therapies could be based around the administration of recombinant protein or NF-κB binding peptides. As we have introduced above, Srinivasan and colleagues have described a novel NF-κB p65 binding GILZ peptide which exhibited therapeutic potential as a NF-κB inhibitor in EAE (Srinivasan & Janardhanam, 2011b). Alternatively, a gene therapy approach, which has already been successfully used *in vivo* to suppress arthritis via delivery of the anti-inflammatory cytokine IL-10 (Apparailly *et al.*, 2002), could be applied to GILZ. Inducing GILZ expression other than through the use of glucocorticoids, for example by modifying activity of the transcription factor FoxO3, could represent a further means to increase available GILZ protein, as could inhibition of the as-yet unidentified mechanisms of GILZ protein turnover. Finally, structure-function analysis of the molecules with which GILZ interacts in order to achieve its immune modifying effects could reveal targets for synthetic GILZ mimetics. Although considerable work remains, the first proof of concept studies of an *in vivo* GILZ-based therapeutic approach is under development in the authors' laboratory (unpublished observations).

In conclusion, glucocorticoids remain among the most widely used drugs in human diseases, and in particular in autoimmune disease. Their effectiveness is increasingly well understood, based on their effects on inflammatory signal transduction, but their use is constrained by toxicity, which also relates to their specific physiological actions. GILZ is a key molecule in glucocorticoid biology, which now represents a candidate mediator of glucocorticoid regulation of immune and inflammatory responses, and deserves further investigation.

Author details

Huapeng Fan and Eric F. Morand
Centre for Inflammatory Diseases, Monash University, Australia

Acknowledgement

The authors are supported by a Project Grant from the National Health and Medical Research Council of Australia.

7. References

Adcock IM, Caramori G. Cross-talk between pro-inflammatory transcription factors and glucocorticoids. *Immunol Cell Biol* 79(4):376-384, 2001.

Aeberli D, Yang Y, Mansell A, Santos L, Leech M, Morand EF. Endogenous macrophage migration inhibitory factor modulates glucocorticoid sensitivity in macrophages via effects on MAP kinase phosphatase-1 and p38 MAP kinase. *FEBS Lett* 580(3):974-981, 2006.

Apparailly F, Millet V, Noel D, Jacquet C, Sany J, Jorgensen C. Tetracycline-inducible interleukin-10 gene transfer mediated by an adeno-associated virus: application to experimental arthritis. *Hum Gene Ther* 13(10):1179-1188, 2002.

Asselin-Labat M, Biola-Vidamment A, Kerbrat S, Lombes M, Bertoglio J, Pallardy M. Fox03 Mediates Antagonistic Effects of Glucocorticoids and Interleukin-2 on Glucocorticoid-Induced Leucine Zipper Expression. *Molecular Endocrinology* 19(7):1752-1764, 2005a.

Asselin-Labat ML, Biola-Vidamment A, Kerbrat S, Lombes M, Bertoglio J, Pallardy M. FoxO3 mediates antagonistic effects of glucocorticoids and interleukin-2 on glucocorticoid-induced leucine zipper expression. *Molecular endocrinology (Baltimore, Md* 19(7):1752-1764, 2005b.

Asselin-Labat ML, David M, Biola-Vidamment A, Lecoeuche D, Zennaro MC, Bertoglio J, Pallardy M. GILZ, a new target for the transcription factor FoxO3, protects T lymphocytes from interleukin-2 withdrawal-induced apoptosis. *Blood* 104(1):215-223, 2004.

Auphan N, Didonato JA, Rosette C, Helmberg A, Karin M. Immunosuppression by Glucocorticoids: Inhibition of NF-κB Activity Through Induction of IκB Synthesis. *Science* 270(5234):286-290, 1995.

Ayroldi E. GILZ mediates the antiproliferative activity of glucocorticoids by negative regulation of Ras signaling. *J. Clin. Invest.* 117:1605-1615, 2007.

Ayroldi E, Migliorati G, Bruscoli S, Marchetti C, Zollo O, Cannarile L, D'adamio F, Riccardi C. Modulation of T-cell activation by the glucocorticoid-induced leucine zipper factor via inhibition of nuclear factor kappaB. *Blood* 98(3):743-753, 2001.

Ayroldi E, Riccardi C. Glucocorticoid-induced leucine zipper (GILZ): a new important mediator of glucocorticoid action. *FASEB Journal* 23:1-10, 2009.

Ayroldi E, Zollo O, Bastianelli A, Marchetti C, Agostini M, Di Virgilio R, Riccardi C. GILZ mediates the antiproliferative activity of glucocorticoids by negative regulation of Ras signaling. *J Clin Invest* 117(6):1605-1615, 2007.

Ayroldi E, Zollo O, Macchiarulo A, Di Marco B, Marchetti C, Riccardi C. Glucocorticoid-induced leucine zipper inhibits the Raf-extracellular signal-regulated kinase pathway by binding to Raf-1. *Molecular and cellular biology* 22(22):7929-7941, 2002.

Barnes PJ. How corticosteroids control inflammation: Quintiles Prize Lecture 2005. *British Journal of Pharmacology* 148(3):245-254, 2006.

Beaulieu E, Morand EF. Role of GILZ in immune regulation, glucocorticoid actions and rheumatoid arthritis. *Nat Rev Rheumatol* advance online publication, 2011.

Beaulieu E, Ngo D, Santos L, Smith M, Jorgensen C, Escriou V, Scherman D, Courties G, Apparailly F, Morand EF. Glucocorticoid-induced leucine zipper is an endogenous anti-inflammatory mediator in arthritis. *Arthritis Rheum*, 2010a.

Beaulieu E, Ngo D, Santos L, Yang YH, Smith M, Jorgensen C, Escriou V, Scherman D, Courties G, Apparailly F, Morand E. Glucocorticoid- Induced Leucine Zipper is an Endogenous Antiinflammatory Mediator in Arthritis. *Arthritis and Rheumatism* 62(9), 2010b.

Berrebi D, Bruscoli S, Cohen N, Foussat A, Migliorati G, Bouchet-Delbos L, Maillot MC, Portier A, Couderc J, Galanaud P, Peuchmaur M, Riccardi C, Emilie D. Synthesis of glucocorticoid-induced leucine zipper (GILZ) by macrophages: an anti-inflammatory and immunosuppressive mechanism shared by glucocorticoids and IL-10. *Blood* 101(2):729-738, 2003.

Bruscoli S, Donato V, Velardi E, Di Sante M, Migliorati G, Donato R, Riccardi C. Glucocorticoid-induced leucine zipper (GILZ) and long GILZ inhibit myogenic differentiation and mediate anti-myogenic effects of glucocorticoids. *J Biol Chem* 285(14):10385-10396, 2010.

Cannarile L, Cuzzocrea S, Santucci L, Agostini M, Mazzon E, Esposito E, Muia C, Coppo M, Di Paola R, Riccardi C. Glucocorticoid-induced leucine zipper is protective in Th1-mediated models of colitis. *Gastroenterology* 136(2):530-541, 2009.

Cannarile L, Fallarino F, Agostini M, Cuzzocrea S, Mazzon E, Vacca C, Genovese T, Migliorati G, Ayroldi E, Riccardi C. Increased GILZ expression in transgenic mice up-regulates Th-2 lymphokines. *Blood* 107(3):1039-1047, 2006a.

Cannarile L, Fallarino F, Agostini M, Cuzzocrea S, Mazzon E, Vacca C, Genovese T, Migliorati G, Ayroldi E, Riccardi C. Increased GILZ expression in transgenic mice up-regulates Th-2 lymphokines. *Blood* 107(3):1039-1047, 2006b.

Chrousos G. The Hypothalamic-Pitutitary-Adrenal Axis and Immune Mediated Infalmmation. *The New England Journal of Medicine* 332(30):1351-1363, 1995.

Cohen N, Mouley E, Hamdi H, Maillot M, Pallardy M, Godot V, Capel F, Balian A, Naveau S, Galanaud P, Lemoine FM, Emilie D. GILZ expression in human dendritic cells redirects their maturation and prevents antigen-specific T lymphoctye response. *Blood* 107(5):2037-2044, 2006a.

Cohen N, Mouly E, Hamdi H, Maillot MC, Pallardy M, Godot V, Capel F, Balian A, Naveau S, Galanaud P, Lemoine FM, Emilie D. GILZ expression in human dendritic cells redirects their maturation and prevents antigen-specific T lymphocyte response. *Blood* 107(5):2037-2044, 2006b.

D'adamio F, Zollo O, Moraca R, Ayroldi E, Bruscoli S, Bartoli A, Cannarile L, Migliorati G, Riccardi C. A new dexamethasone-induced gene of the leucine zipper family protects T lymphocytes from TCR/CD3-activated cell death. *Immunity* 7(6):803-812, 1997.

Davis JM, 3rd, Maradit Kremers H, Crowson CS, Nicola PJ, Ballman KV, Therneau TM, Roger VL, Gabriel SE. Glucocorticoids and cardiovascular events in rheumatoid arthritis: a population-based cohort study. *Arthritis and rheumatism* 56(3):820-830, 2007.

De Bosscher K, Vanden Berghe W, Haegeman G. The interplay between the glucocorticoid receptor and nuclear factor-kappaB or activator protein-1: molecular mechanisms for gene repression. *Endocrine reviews* 24(4):488-522, 2003.

Debosscher K, Haegeman G. MInireview: Latest Perspectives on Antiinflammaotry Actions of GLucocorticoids. *Molecuar Endocrinology* 23(3):281-291, 2009.

Delfino DV, Agostini M, Spinicelli S, Vacca C, Riccardi C. Inhibited cell death, NF-kappaB activity and increased IL-10 in TCR-triggered thymocytes of transgenic mice overexpressing the glucocorticoid-induced protein GILZ. *International immunopharmacology* 6(7):1126-1134, 2006.

Delfino DV, Agostini M, Spinicelli S, Vito P, Riccardi C. Decrease of Bcl-xL and augmentation of thymocyte apoptosis in GILZ overexpressing transgenic mice. *Blood* 104(13):4134-4141, 2004.

Di Marco B, Massetti M, Bruscoli S, Macchiarulo A, Di Virgilio R, Velardi E, Donato V, Migliorati G, Riccardi C. Glucocorticoid-induced leucine zipper (GILZ)/NF-kappaB interaction: role of GILZ homo-dimerization and C-terminal domain. *Nucleic Acids Res* 35(2):517-528, 2007.

Eddleston J, Herschbach J, Wagelie-Steffen AL, Christiansen S, Zuraw BL. The anti-inflammatory effect of glucocorticoids is mediated by glucocorticoid-induced leucine zipper in epithelial cells. *Journal of Allergy and Clinical Immunology* 119(1):115-122, 2007a.

Eddleston J, Herschbach J, Wagelie-Steffen AL, Christiansen SC, Zuraw BL. The anti-inflammatory effect of glucocorticoids is mediated by glucocorticoid-induced leucine zipper in epithelial cells. *J Allergy Clin Immunol* 119(1):115-122, 2007b.

Esposito E, Bruscoli S, Mazzon E, Paterniti I, Coppo M, Velardi E, Cuzzocrea S, Riccardi C. Glucocorticoid-Induced Leucine Zipper (GILZ) Over-Expression in T Lymphocytes Inhibits Inflammation and Tissue Damage in Spinal Cord Injury. *Neurotherapeutics,* 2011.

Furst R, Schroeder T, Eilken HM, Bubik MF, Kiemer AK, Zahler S, Vollmar AM. MAPK phosphatase-1 represents a novel anti-inflammatory target of glucocorticoids in the human endothelium. *FASEB J* 21(1):74-80, 2007.

Glynne R, Ghandour G, Rayner J, Mack DH, Goodnow CC. B-lymphocyte quiescence, tolerance and activation as viewed by global gene expression profiling on microarrays. *Immunol Rev* 176:216-246, 2000.

Godot V, Garcia G, Capel F, Arock M, Durand-Gasselin I, Asselin-Labat ML, Emilie D, Humbert M. Dexamethasone and IL-10 stimulate glucocorticoid-induced leucine zipper synthesis by human mast cells. *Allergy* 61(7):886-890, 2006.

Gossye V, Elewaut D, Bougarne N, Bracke D, Calenbergh SV, Haegeman G, Debosscher K. Differential Mechanism of NF- B Inhibition by Two Glucocorticoid Receptor Modulators in Rheumatoid Arthritis Synovial Fibroblasts. *Arhtritis and Rheumatism* 60(11):3241-3250, 2009.

Hamdi H, Bigorgne A, Naveau S, Balian A, Bouchet-Delbos L, Cassard-Doulcier AM, Maillot MC, Durand-Gasselin I, Prevot S, Delaveaucoupet J, Emilie D, Perlemuter G. Glucocorticoid-induced leucine zipper: A key protein in the sensitization of monocytes to lipopolysaccharide in alcoholic hepatitis. *Hepatology (Baltimore, Md* 46(6):1986-1992, 2007a.

Hamdi H, Godot V, Maillot MC, Prejean MV, Cohen N, Krzysiek R, Lemoine FM, Zou W, Emilie D. Induction of antigen-specific regulatory T lymphocytes by human dendritic cells expressing the glucocorticoid-induced leucine zipper. *Blood* 110(1):211-219, 2007b.

Hillier SG. Diamonds are forever: the cortisone legacy. *The Journal of endocrinology* 195(1):1-6, 2007.

Huscher D, Thiele K, Gromnica-Ihle E, Hein G, Demary W, Dreher R, Zink A, Buttgereit F. Dose-related patterns of glucocorticoid-induced side effects. *Annals of the Rheumatic Diseases* 68(7):1119-1124, 2009.

Kelly M, King E, Rider C, Gwozd C, Holden N, Eddleston J, Zuraw B, Leigh R, O'byrne P, Newton R. Corticosteroid-induced gene expression in allergen-challenged asthmatic subjects taking inhaled budesonide. *Br J Pharmacol*, 2011.

Latre De Late P, Pepin A, Assaf-Vandecasteele H, Espinasse C, Nicolas V, Asselin-Labat ML, Bertoglio J, Pallardy M, Biola-Vidamment A. Glucocorticoid-induced leucine zipper (GILZ) promotes the nuclear exclusion of FOXO3 in a Crm1-dependent manner. *J Biol Chem* 285(8):5594-5605.

Lekva T, Bollerslev J, Kristo C, Olstad OK, Ueland T, Jemtland R. The Glucocorticoid-Induced Leucine Zipper Gene (GILZ) Expression Decreases after Successful Treatment of Patients with Endogenous Cushing's Syndrome and May Play a Role in Glucocorticoid-Induced Osteoporosis. *J Clin Endocrinol Metab*, 2009.

Lekva T, Bollerslev J, Kristo C, Olstad OK, Ueland T, Jemtland R. The glucocorticoid-induced leucine zipper gene (GILZ) expression decreases after successful treatment of patients with endogenous Cushing's syndrome and may play a role in glucocorticoid-induced osteoporosis. *J Clin Endocrinol Metab* 95(1):246-255, 2010.

Mittelstadt PR, Ashwell JD. Inhibition of AP-1 by the glucocorticoid-inducible protein GILZ. *J Biol Chem* 276(31):29603-29610, 2001.

Ralph JA, Morand EF. MAPK phosphatases as novel targets for rheumatoid arthritis. *Expert opinion on therapeutic targets* 12(7):795-808, 2008.

Redjimi N, Gaudin F, Touboul C, Emilie D, Pallardy M, Biola-Vidamment A, Fernandez H, Prevot S, Balabanian K, Machelon V. Identification of glucocorticoid-induced leucine zipper as a key regulator of tumor cell proliferation in epithelial ovarian cancer. *Mol Cancer* 8:83, 2009.

Riccardi C, Bruscoli S, Ayroldi E, Agostini M, Migliorati G. GILZ, a glucocorticoid hormone induced gene, modulates T lymphocytes activation and death through interaction with NF-[kappa]B. *Adv. Exp. Med. Biol.* 495:31-39, 2001.

Rincon M. MAP-kinase signaling pathways in T cells. *Curr Opin Immunol* 13(3):339-345, 2001.

Robert-Nicoud M, Flahaut M, Elalouf JM, Nicod M, Salinas M, Bens M, Doucet A, Wincker P, Artiguenave F, Horisberger JD, Vandewalle A, Rossier BC, Firsov D. Transcriptome of a mouse kidney cortical collecting duct cell line: effects of aldosterone and vasopressin. *Proc Natl Acad Sci U S A* 98(5):2712-2716, 2001.

Scha¨Cke H, Do¨Cke W, Asadullah* K. Mechanisms involved in the side effects of glucocorticoids. *Pharmacology and Therapeutics* 96:23-43, 2002.

Schmidt M, Fernandez De Mattos S, Van Der Horst A, Klompmaker R, Kops GJ, Lam EW, Burgering BM, Medema RH. Cell cycle inhibition by FoxO forkhead transcription factors involves downregulation of cyclin D. *Molecular and cellular biology* 22(22):7842-7852, 2002.

Shi X, Shi W, Li Q, Song B, Wan M, Bai S, Cao X. A glucocorticoid-induced leucine-zipper protein, GILZ, inhibits adipogenesis of mesenchymal cells. *EMBO Rep* 4(4):374-380, 2003.

Slocumb CH, Polley HF, Hench PS, Kendall EC. Effects of cortisone and ACTH on patients with rheumatoid arthritis. *Proc Staff Meet Mayo Clin* 25(17):476-478, 1950.

Soundararajan R, Melters D, Shih I-C, Wang J, Pearce D. Epithelial sodium channel regulated by differential composition of a signaling complex. *Proceedings of the National Academy of Sciences* 106(19):7804-7809, 2009.

Soundararajan R, Wang J, Melters D, Pearce D. Differential Activities of Glucocorticoid-induced Leucine Zipper Protein Isoforms. *The Journal of Biological Chemistry* 282(50):36303-36313, 2007.

Srinivasan M, Janardhanam S. Novel p65 binding GILZ peptide suppresses experimental autoimmune encephalomyelitis. *J Biol Chem*, 2011a.

Srinivasan M, Janardhanam S. Novel p65 binding GILZ peptide suppresses experimental autoimmune encephalomyelitis. *Journal of Biological Chemistry*, 2011b.

Suffia IJ, Reckling SK, Piccirillo CA, Goldszmid RS, Belkaid Y. Infected site-restricted Foxp3+ natural regulatory T cells are specific for microbial antigens. *The Journal of experimental medicine* 203(3):777-788, 2006.

Van Der Laan S. Chromatin immunoprecipitation scanning identifies glucocorticoid receptor binding regions in the proximal promoter of a ubiquitously expressed glucocorticoid target gene in brain. *J. Neurochem.* 106:2515-2523, 2008.

Van Staa TP, Leufkens HGM, Abenhaim L, Begaud B, Zhang B, Cooper C. Use of oral corticosteroids in the United Kingdom. *QJM* 93(2):105-111, 2000.

Wang Y, Ma Y-Y, Song X-L, Cai H-Y, Chen J-C, Song L-N, Yang R, Lu J. Upregulations of Glucocorticoid-Induced Leucine Zipper by Hypoxia and Glucocorticoid Inhibit Proinflammatory Cytokines under Hypoxic Conditions in Macrophages. *The Journal of Immunology*, 2011.

Wurster A, Tanaka T, Grusby MJ. The biology of Stat4 and Stat6. *Oncogene* 19:2577-2584, 2000.

Wust S, Van Den Brandt J, Tischner D, Kleiman A, Tuckermann JP, Gold R, Luhder F, Reichardt HM. Peripheral T cells are the therapeutic targets of glucocorticoids in experimental autoimmune encephalomyelitis. *J Immunol* 180(12):8434-8443, 2008.

Yang N, Zhang W, Shi XM. Glucocorticoid-induced leucine zipper (GILZ) mediates glucocorticoid action and inhibits inflammatory cytokine-induced COX-2 expression. *J Cell Biochem* 103(6):1760-1771, 2008.

Yang YH, Aeberli D, Dacumos A, Xue JR, Morand EF. Annexin-1 regulates macrophage IL-6 and TNF via glucocorticoid-induced leucine zipper. *J Immunol* 183(2):1435-1445, 2009.

Yang YH, Morand EF, Getting SJ, Paul-Clark M, Liu DL, Yona S, Hannon R, Buckingham JC, Perretti M, Flower RJ. Modulation of inflammation and response to dexamethasone by Annexin 1 in antigen-induced arthritis. *Arthritis and rheumatism* 50(3):976-984, 2004.

Yang YH, Toh ML, Clyne CD, Leech M, Aeberli D, Xue J, Dacumos A, Sharma L, Morand EF. Annexin 1 negatively regulates IL-6 expression via effects on p38 MAPK and MAPK phosphatase-1. *J Immunol* 177(11):8148-8153, 2006.

Zhang W, Yang N, Shi XM. Regulation of mesenchymal stem cell osteogenic differentiation by glucocorticoid-induced leucine zipper (GILZ). *J Biol Chem* 283(8):4723-4729, 2008a.

Zhang W, Yang N, Shi XM. Regulation of MSC osteogenic differentiation by glucocorticoid-induced leucine zipper (GILZ). *J. Biol. Chem.* 283:4723-4729, 2008b.

Zheng W, Flavell R. The Transcription Factor GATA-3 Is Necessary and Sufficient for Th2 Cytokine Gene Expression in CD4 T Cells. *Cell* 9:587-596, 1997.

Section 2

Glucocorticoids in Behaviour Models

Chapter 9

Glucocorticoids in Mate Choice

Fhionna R. Moore

Additional information is available at the end of the chapter

http://dx.doi.org/10.5772/51433

1. Introduction

Choosing the right mate is fundamental to reproductive success. Selecting the right genes with which to combine one's own increases the chances of offspring survival and reproduction. Choosing wisely, then, can increase the number of copies of genetic material being passed on to future generations. This means that it serves an individual well to signal their own strengths and qualities in order to attract mates, and it serves the opposite sex well to express preferences for honest signals of mate quality. As opposed to natural selection (the process by which traits which confer a survival advantage are selected for [1]), sexual selection is selection for those traits that confer benefits in terms of attracting, and mating with, members of the opposite sex [2]. Such sexually selected traits often serve to reduce the chances of survival and their adaptive function is solely to increase an individual's mating success. Classic examples are the peacock's extravagant tail plumage that dramatically increases chances of predation [3], and the display of the bowerbird, which bears a heavy energetic cost to construct [4]. These traits have evolved as the benefits of attracting members of the opposite sex outweigh the associated costs to survival. In order for these social signalling systems to work, however, the signal must provide an honest indication of quality [5, 6]. If it is possible to cheat, the system could not function: elaborate displays would no longer signal a genetic benefit for offspring.

Honest signals of mate-choice relevant qualities fall into two broad categories, both of which are impossible to fake. These are qualities that infer "indirect" benefits, which include heritable traits such as a strong immune system [7, 8], and those that infer "direct" benefits, such as the ability and willingness to provide resources and parental care. Over the last decade evidence has accumulated to suggest that the physiological stress response may be linked to both sets of characteristics. For one, the glucocorticoid hormones modulate the immune system, meaning that stress may influence health and condition which, in turn, influence the ability of an individual to mate successfully or to provision and care for offspring [9, 10]. Alternatively, between-individual variation in dimensions of the stress response such as the peak levels of glucocorticoids secreted in response to a stressor and the time taken for levels to return to baseline are heritable, meaning that individuals are likely to differ in their ability to cope effectively and efficiently with stress [11, 12]. There is a growing body of evidence that demonstrates that females assess the glucocorticoid status of potential opposite sex partners, and express preferences for cues to low stress.

Given the role of hormones in directing the allocation of energy to different physiological and behavioural functions, it is not surprising that they have received attention in the context of mate choice and sexual signalling. Testosterone has received by far the most attention in this domain due to evidence for its role in the development of those male traits used to attract females. Among many other traits testosterone is, for example, consistently found to relate to the vitality of sexually selected plumage colouration in birds (see for example [13, 14]), the size and strength of antlers in red deer stags (*Cervus elaphus*; see for example [15, 16]) and the intensity and complexity of bird song (see for example [17, 18]). In essence, high testosterone results in a strong signal that, in turn, translates into mating success. In the Immunocompetence Handicap Hypothesis of sexual selection [7], testosterone-dependent traits are proposed to provide an honest signal of the strength of a male's immune system due to the hormone's immunosuppressive actions. In other words, only those males who have inherited a robust immune system can afford the costs of the elevated testosterone required for development of extravagant sexual signals. A large antlered red deer stag, then, is signalling his superior immune system. This, in turn, should attract female mates who seek to acquire such "good genes" for their offspring. In the years since its inception, this model has generated a huge body of research, with a Google Scholar search for "Immunocompetence Handicap" returning ~2, 500 publications.

Despite providing an elegant explanation for the maintenance of variation in the expression of sexual signals as honest indicators of quality, and good evidence that such traits are linked to parasite resistance, however, one of the Immunocompetence Handicap model's fundamental assumptions fails to receive adequate support. Reviews show inconsistency in evidence for immunosuppression by testosterone [19]. As a consequence, biologists have attempted to address this weakness by identifying additional or alternative endocrinological factors that may contribute to the system. And this is where the glucocorticoids have attracted attention. These stress hormones are correlated with testosterone across species (albeit the direction of the relationship is variable; see for example [11, 20 – 23]) and modulate immune function [24] and body condition [9, 10]. In [11], for example, the authors demonstrated that an immunosuppressive effect of testosterone in the house sparrow (*Passer domesticus*) disappeared when the effects of the primary avian glucocorticoid corticosterone were controlled for statistically. They concluded that the effects of testosterone on the immune system may be mediated or moderated by co-occurring levels of glucocorticoids. More recently, it has been suggested that low levels of glucocorticoids may be preferable due to detrimental effects of high levels on body condition and health [10]. The following discussion addresses the evidence to date to suggest functions of glucocorticoids in mate choice and sexual selection.

2. How do glucocorticoids influence mate choice?

Human research offers excellent opportunities to test roles of stress in mate choice. There is evidence that cortisol (the primary human glucocorticoid) and testosterone are positively correlated [25], although this finding is not consistent (see for example [26, 27]) and may depend upon, for example, the intensity of recent exercise [28]. Sexually dimorphic facial characteristics derive from sex differences in the ratio of the male and female sex hormones that emerge at puberty (see for example [29]). A surge of testosterone in males during adolescence promotes cranio-facial bone growth resulting in heavier jaws and eyebrow ridges. These changes are inhibited in females by the action of oestrogen. In adulthood there are positive relationships between both circulating testosterone [30] and testosterone response to a challenge [31] and masculinity of the male face, as well as between oestrogen and femininity in female faces [32]. This means that there are cues to testosterone in the male face that we can parametrically manipulate using sophisticated digital face morphing techniques. Circulating levels of cortisol and testosterone can be measured using non-invasive methods that reduce activation of the stress response to provide an accurate estimate of baseline levels of the hormones. Furthermore, it is possible to obtain ratings by women of perceptions of facial stimuli that differ in cues to the hormones. These are luxuries not so easily afforded by work with other species and mean that we are able to identify any mediating or moderating role of cortisol on relationships between testosterone and attractiveness in a uniquely controlled way.

The relationship between sexual dimorphism and attractiveness is fairly consistent for female faces, with both men and women agreeing that the more feminine a face, the more attractive it is (see for example [33, 34]). For male faces, however, the story is more complicated, with variation in women's preferences suggestive of a trade-off in the relative importance of a committed, reliable partner versus a partner who signals "good genes". Given the relationship between testosterone and masculinity of the male face, masculine faced males may signal a robust immune system. While this is likely to be attractive to women seeking to secure a strong immune system for offspring, it must be balanced up against the negative personality characteristics that are attributed to the owners of masculine male faces, including dishonesty, low likelihood to commit to a relationship and aggression (see for example [35, 36]). This perhaps explains why women tend to prefer feminine-faced men who are attributed with honesty, commitment and good parenting in general, but to switch to preferences for more masculine faces at times when the chances of conception are high including the fertile phase of the menstrual cycle (see for example [37]), when commitment is less important to mate choice decisions, such as when faces are judged for a short term rather than a long term relationship (see for example [38]) and in societies in which there is greater competition for resources [39] or in which the costs of ill health are high [40].

In a sample of 69 Scottish male students, my colleagues and I measured testosterone and cortisol from saliva samples collected by passive drool at two time-points (one in the morning and one in the afternoon), to control for circadian fluctuations in both hormones, using enzyme-linked immunosorbant assays. Mean testosterone leves ranged from 0.07 – 0.63 ng/mL, and mean cortisol from 3.7 – 24.04 nmol/L. We also took facial photographs of participants under standardized conditions (e.g. with diffuse flash lighting, at the same distance from the camera and with glasses removed and neutral expression). We assessed the effects of testosterone and cortisol on facial attractiveness in two ways. First, we asked a sample of female participants to rate the faces for attractiveness, masculinity and health on 1 – 7 scales (1 = not at all attractive/masculine/healthy, 7 = extremely attractive/masculine/healthy). The faces of males with low cortisol were rated as significantly more attractive than those with high cortisol ($r^2 = -0.36$, $p = 0.027$). There were no relationships between cortisol, health and masculinity and, unlike previous studies ([37] for example), testosterone was not related to women's perceptions of the faces (all $p > 0.3$). Next, we used the face morphing software *Psychomorph* to create "composite" facial images which contained cues to combinations of high and low levels of testosterone and cortisol [41]. For this, we identified groups of 5 – 6 males with the following combinations of hormones, based on median splits: high testosterone and high cortisol, high testosterone and low cortisol, low testosterone and high cortisol, low testosterone and low cortisol. We then "averaged" together the faces of the participants in each of these groups to give composite stimuli containing cues to the 4 combinations of hormones (see Figure 1).

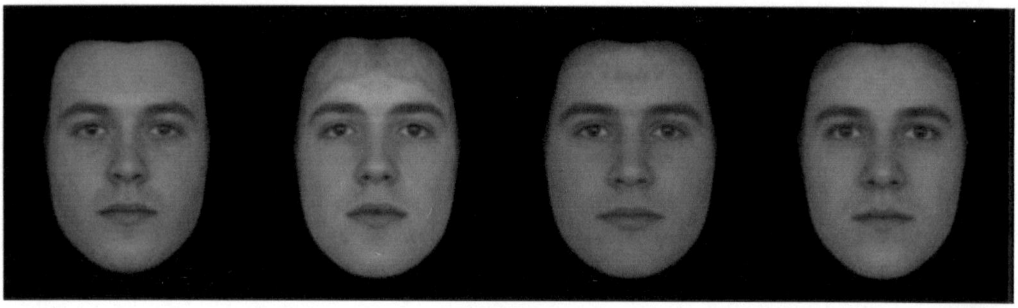

Figure 1. Composite male faces constructed to differ in combinations of testosterone and cortisol. From left to right: high testosterone with high cortisol, high testosterone with low cortisol, low testosterone with high cortisol, low testosterone with low cortisol. Taken from Moore et al. 2011. Proceedings of the Royal Society of London Series B, doi:10.1098/rspb.2010.1678.

The stimuli were then rated by a novel sample of female participants during the fertile and non-fertile phases of their menstrual cycles. Using mixed model Anova, we found that women consistently preferred the low cortisol composites ($F_{(1, 42)} = 5.11$, $p = 0.029$). Post hoc analyses revealed that this effect was significant in the fertile ($F_{(1, 42)} = 6.44$, $p = 0.015$), but not the non-fertile ($p > 0.1$) cycle phase (see Figure 2). We concluded that women can detect cues to cortisol in the male face, and that low cortisol is desirable in a male partner. We also suggested that low cortisol may be associated with beneficial heritable characteristics as women expressed the strongest preferences for facial cues to low cortisol at times when they were most likely to conceive [26].

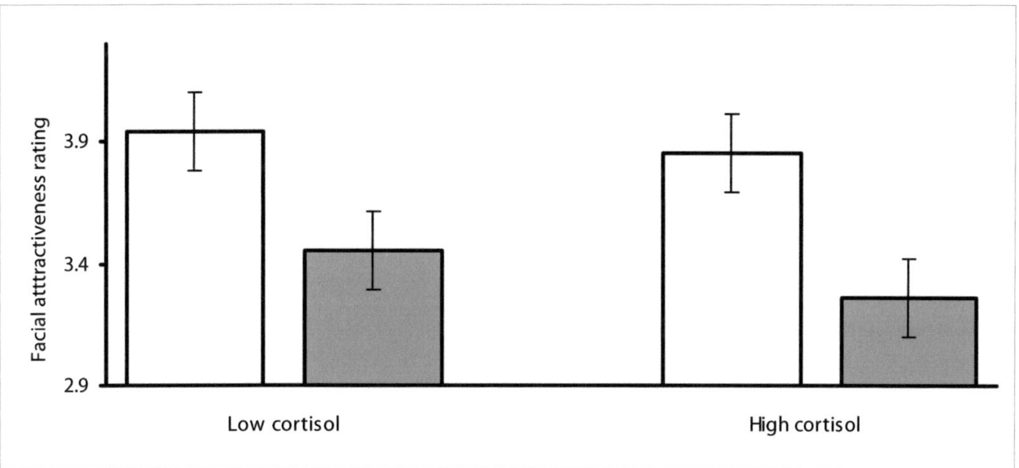

Figure 2. Mean attractiveness ratings of composite male faces constructed to differ in cues to cortisol by women during the non-fertile (empty bars) and fertile (filled bars) phases of their menstrual cycles with error bars showing +- 1 SE. In a mixed model anova there was a significant effect of cortisol on attractiveness ($F_{(1, 42)} = 5.11$, $p = 0.029$). Post hoc tests revealed that this effect was significant only during the fertile phase of the cycle ($F_{(1, 42)} = 6.44$, $p = 0.015$) [26].

We replicated this pattern of results in a different sample of faces with a novel sample of female raters, again recruited from UK student populations. Once again, women preferred the faces of males with low cortisol, and didn't express preferences for testosterone. In this second study, we also tested the effects of the hormones on perceived dominance and health, finding that low cortisol faces were also rated as more dominant and healthy than high cortisol faces [26, 27]. The findings of both studies are consistent with work in other species that shows that females prefer males with low levels of glucocorticoids. In [12], for example, the authors found that female zebra finch (*Tynopygea guttatta*) preferred males with low corticosterone, and expressed no preference for cues to testosterone. Spectrophotometric measures of plumage suggested that dimensions of plumage colour and brightness provided cues to the stress status of the male. Similarly, in [42] Leary and colleagues found that female great plains toads (*Bufo cognatus*) preferred the calls of males with low glucocorticoids. There is growing evidence, then, that glucocorticoids play a role in mate choice. Why this may be, however, is unclear.

Glucocorticoids and testosterone

One possibility is that the hormonal underpinnings in expression of sexual traits that have previously been attributed to testosterone are, in fact, due to the effects of the glucocorticoids (see for example [11]). If this were the case, however, we would expect to find effects of testosterone that disappear once glucocorticoids are controlled for statistically. Although this pattern of results was reported for a study of effects of the hormones on the immune function of the house sparrow, this has not been replicated in other species. It seems unlikely, then, that the role of stress is so straightforward. Rather than simple mediation of effects of testosterone by those of cortisol, in both of our studies described above we found an interaction between testosterone and cortisol, such that the detrimental effects of cortisol were stronger in those males with low testosterone compared to those with high testosterone (See Figure 3). We proposed that high testosterone males (i.e. those signalling the strength of their immune system) are better able to cope with the detrimental effects of stress [26, 27]. In order to test this explanation, however, it is necessary to experimentally manipulate stress in males who differ in their level of testosterone and test for any divergent effects on immune system and/or sexual signals.

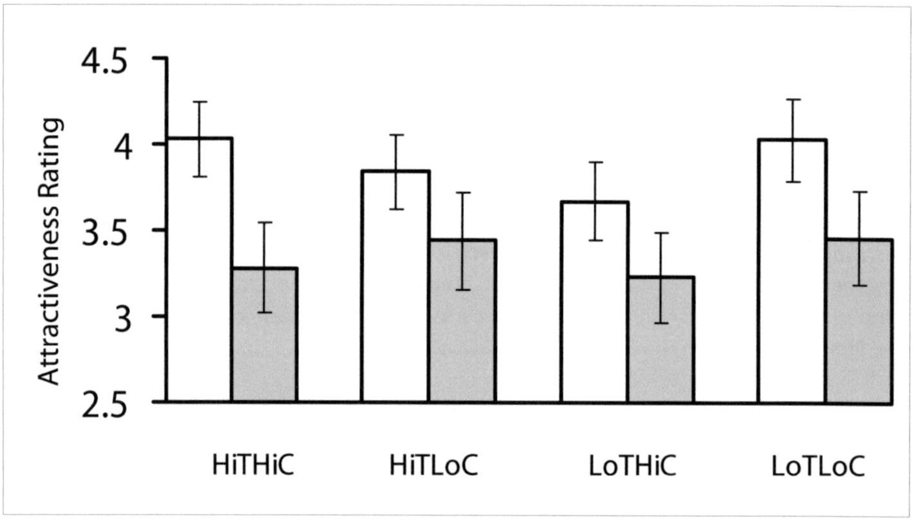

Figure 3. Mean attractiveness ratings of composite faces that differ in combinations of testosterone and cortisol (+1 s.e.) by women during the non-fertile (empty) and fertile (filled) phases of their menstrual cycles. The figure shows an interaction between the hormones, such that cortisol reduces attractiveness in males with low testosterone, but enhances it in males with high testosterone. Taken from Moore et al. 2011. Proceedings of the Royal Society of London Series B, doi:10.1098/rspb.2010.1678.

While we have replicated the interaction between testosterone and cortisol in two UK samples, in a recent attempt to determine whether our results extend across human populations, we found evidence to suggest that the effects of combinations of sex and stress hormones on facial appearance are population-dependent. In a third study, we tested relationships between testosterone, cortisol and facial attractiveness in a sample of 74 male students. This time we tested relationships across the faces of individual males, rather than in digitally manipulated composite faces and measured testosterone and cortisol from intravenous blood samples rather than from saliva as this allowed us to take simultaneous measurements of immune function. Contrary to previous studies, we found a positive relationship between testosterone and men's facial attractiveness, but no relationship between cortisol and attractiveness. While we found an interaction between testosterone and cortisol in effects on facial attractiveness, it's nature differed to that reported in our previous studies such that this time the positive relationship between testosterone and attractiveness was strongest in those males with low cortisol [43]. See Figure 4.

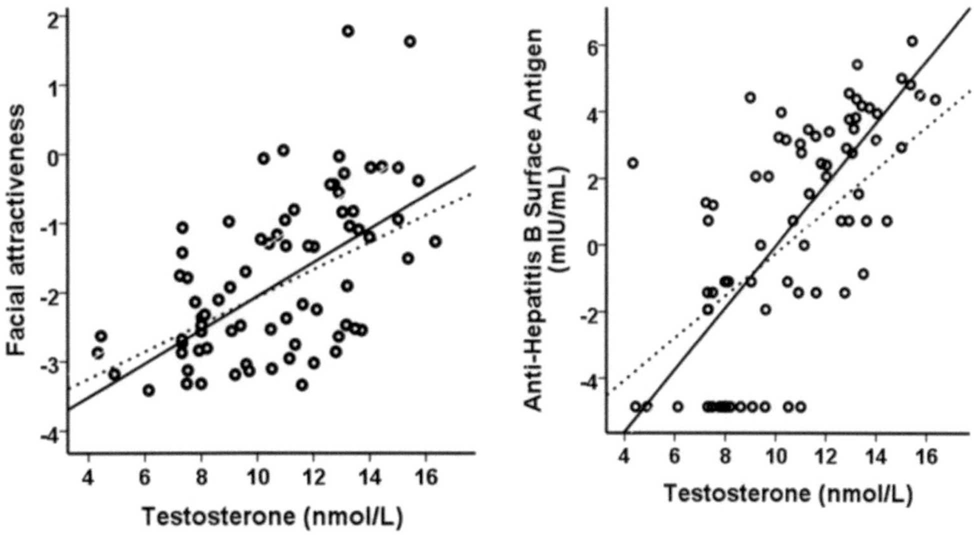

(a) (b)

Figure 4. Relationships between testosterone and (a) facial attractiveness in a sample of Latvian male students rated by female participants drawn from the same population, showing an interaction with cortisol such that the relationship was strongest in those males with low cortisol (solid line) and weakest in those with high cortisol (broken line) and (b) antibody response to a hepatitis B vaccine, showing an interaction with cortisol such that the relationship was strongest in those males with low cortisol (solid line) and weakest in those with high cortisol (broken line). From [43].

Why should we find differences in the nature of the interaction between testosterone and cortisol on facial attractiveness between our samples? It seems unlikely that we can attribute this to differences in our methods. In all 3 studies we tested for relationships between the hormones and face perceptions across individual faces and failed to find interactions between testosterone and cortisol in either of the first two studies. Does the construction of composites result in spurious results? Only further testing will adequately test this, but an alternative possibility is that societal-level factors cause systematic variation in the effects of sex- and stress- hormones (and combinations of the two) on attractiveness. While the samples in our first two studies were taken from populations of UK students, the sample for our third study – the one in which we found a different interaction between the hormones – was drawn from a sample of male students and female raters from the University of Daugavpils in Latvia. Could societal-level differences in the strategies employed by women to assess the attractiveness of male faces underpin the differences we report in the effects of sex- and stress-hormones on facial attractiveness? There is evidence to suggest that this could be the case. In [40], for example, Debruine and colleagues reported that societal level health measures were related to women's preferences for cues to testosterone in the male face. That is, women in societies in which the costs of ill health are high express stronger preferences for cues to high testosterone. Perhaps, then, cultural differences in the provision of healthcare, or in other social and economic factors, cause the female raters in our samples to express divergent preferences for cues to testosterone and/or cortisol, which in turn will influence the nature of the interaction between the two. This is insightful as identification of the socioecological factors that underpin variation in preferences for cues to the hormones can contribute to our understanding of the traits and characteristics that they signal. My collaborators and I are currently conducting further cross-cultural research to achieve this.

That population-level differences in socioecology could influence the nature of the role of stress in mate choice is further supported by cross-species differences in interactions between testosterone and glucocorticoids on sexual traits. Such interactions have been reported in several avian species. In the red grouse, for example, a positive relationship between testosterone and comb area was stronger in males with low levels of co-occurring glucocorticoids than in those with physiological markers of high stress [44]. Conversely, in the red bishop (*Euplectes orix*), the relationship between testosterone and plumage colour was inverse under high stress, but positive or non-significant under low stress [45]. Despite evidence, then, that testosterone-dependent signalling is contingent upon concurrent stress, the nature of interactions between sex and stress hormones is inconsistent.

In order to begin to interpret the meaning of this inconsistency, it is necessary to understand a little more about how the two hormones interact at a physiological level. One way is through competition for binding sites on the two types of glucocorticoid receptor. The first of these has a high affinity for the stress hormones, so glucocorticoids tend to bind to these first, meaning that the receptors are typically saturated at peak points in the circadian cycle and therefore serve primarily to regulate circadian rhythms. The second type, although more abundant, have a lower binding affinity, so tend to bind once all the first type are engaged. These, then, are the receptors that are bound during response to a stressor and regulate the stress response [46]. This means that baseline and peak response glucocorticoids can be conceptualized as different hormonal systems as their binding to different types of receptors results in divergent effects on physiology and behaviour [46]. As the proteins which bind glucocorticoids (corticosteroid binding globulins) can also bind testosterone, there may be competition between the hormones for binding sites – particularly in avian species who lack independent sex steroid binding globulins [47, 48]. It is possible, for example, that elevated glucocorticoids reduce the numbers of receptors available for testosterone, reducing bound levels and increasing free levels which may influence effects of testosterone on behaviour and signalling. Perhaps, then, relationships between testosterone and glucocorticoids, and their combined effects on sexual signals, depend upon the species and the dimension of the stress response that is measured (e.g. peak versus baseline).

Immunocompetence

The "stress-linked" model of hormonally-mediated sexual selection as originally proposed over a decade ago [11, 49], in acknowledgement of increasing awareness that extant endocrinological models did not sufficiently explain variation in the cross-species data, proposed that effects of glucocorticoids on sexual traits were likely to occur through their effects on the immune system. Despite evidence for an immunomodulatory role of stress, meaning that this seems to be a viable possibility, it poses a difficult problem to address, and an even more difficult system to model, as it is not simply the case that stress suppresses the immune system. Depending upon the nature, duration and predictability of a stressor, for example, stress can enhance, suppress or redistribute immune activity [24]. How, then, can we model and test roles of stress in sexual selection that are mediated by effects on the immune system? To date, a handful of studies of avian species have tested inter-relationships between stress, immune function and sexual signalling demonstrating complex relationships between immune function, stress and sexual signals. A study of red grouse, for example, reported a positive relationship between glucocorticoids and parasite load and an inverse relationship between parasite load, and testosterone-dependent ornament (i.e. supraorbital comb) area [44]. Similarly, a study of blue tits (*Cyanistes caeruleus*) demonstrated parasite load to be positively related to a physiological marker of stress (heat shock proteins) and inversely to sexually selected colouration [50]. Conversely, a study of song sparrows (*Melospiza melodia*) reported no relationship between stress and immune function [51], meaning that detrimental effects of stress on song repertoire were not mediated by immunocompetence. In our work with human faces, my colleagues and I found that the pattern of the interaction between testosterone and cortisol on attractiveness was mirrored by the same pattern in effects on antibody response to a vaccine [43]. See Figure 4b. While there is some evidence, then, to suggest that the combined effects of testosterone and cortisol on sexual signalling are concurrent with those on immune function, it seems likely that such results are dependent upon the arm of the immune system that is assessed as well as the measurement of stress.

Stress and body condition

Husak and Moore [10] suggested that glucocorticoids could influence the intensity of sexual signals via their detrimental effects on body condition. If stress reduces body condition (e.g. body mass and/or fat stores), an individual who is experiencing stress is less likely to be able to afford to allocate energy and metabolic resources to sexual signalling. Effects of stress on body condition, however, are inconsistent, with studies from some species showing that stress reduces body condition (song sparrow (*Melospiza melodia*) [51]; upland geese (*Chloephaga picta*) [52]; zebra finches [53]), others showing stress to increase body condition (Beldings ground squirrels (*Spermophilus beldingi*) [54]) and still others showing no effect (e.g. mallard ducks (*Anas platyrhynchos*) [55]). Furthermore, few studies have shown effects of stress on sexual signals that were consistent with those on condition. An exception is the red grouse, in which parasite load was shown to reduce body condition, increase physiological markers of stress and reduce the expression of plumage colouration [56]. The evidence, then, suggests that any effects of stress on sexual signals do not occur via its action on body condition. In fact, in some cases, stress may cause a reallocation of resources away from body condition and into sexual signalling. Positive relationships between stress and the expression of carotenoid – based colouration at the cost of condition have been reported in the zebra finch [53] and the common lizard [57]. This suggests that, in some cases, stress causes a redistribution of energy and resources away from long term goals and instead to short term priorities (e.g. mating). This would seem to be a sensible strategy when, for example, survival was threatened, which may be signalled by elevated stress hormones.

Stress &behaviour

In addition to sexual signals such as ornaments, colouration or song, stress also impacts upon behaviours relevant to reproduction. There may, then, be behavioural cues to glucocorticoid status which females make use of in their mate choice decisions, or stress-dependent sexual signals may provide insight into an individual's likely behaviour. Activation of the hypothalamic-pituitary-adrenal axis in response to stress suppresses the hypothalamic-pituitary-gonadal axis which is responsible for mediating sexual behaviour [58], resulting in reduced expression of sexual behaviours. One mechanism, for example, by which stress suppresses reproductive behaviour is via inhibition of the gonadotropin protein hormones which regulate reproductive function by glucocorticoids [59, 60]. It is well known that chronically elevated stress suppresses reproduction by, for example, reducing sex drive, courtship behaviour and fertility(see for example [61 - 63]). There is also evidence that acutely elevated glucocorticoids have a similar outcome with, for example, glucocorticoids elevated by fasting reducing courtship behaviour such as singing in the male zebra finch [64] and the locomotor activity that contributes to foraging and reproduction in male Allegheny dusky salamanders (*Desmognathus ochrophaeus*;[65]). Elevated glucocorticoids are also associated with reduced provisioning of offspring (see for example [66]).It is possible, then, that females attend to behavioural indications of high stress, or that stress-dependent sexual signals provide an indication of reproductive function and/or ability to provision offspring. Avoiding individuals who are currently experiencing stress will reduce the chances of attempting to mate with a member of the opposite sex with reduced reproductive function and/or ability to provision offspring, thereby allowing the female to maximise her reproductive success.

There are also relationships between stress and dominance, although these are typically complex and dependent upon, among many others, both the status of an individual in a hierarchy and the stability of the social structure. Attention to cues to stress, then, may enable an individual to select an opposite sex partner who occupies a high status position in a dominance hierarchy, with associated high status and access to premium resources, ensuring high status, well-provisioned offspring. It is not simply the case, however, that high stress is a cue to low rank in a hierarchy. Creel [67], for example, demonstrates that, although agonistic social interactions can provoke a large glucocorticoid response, in established social groups, where individuals know the hierarchy, such responses are not necessarily the case and in some cooperative breeding species (i.e. a social system in which individuals contribute to the care of others' offspring) such as the meerkat (*Suricata suricatta*), for example, dominant individuals may have higher glucocorticoids that subordinates. It seems likely that divergent levels of stress hormones in accordance with strata of the social structure are dependent upon both the nature of the hierarchy which is, in turn, dependent upon species socioecology but also upon stability of the hierarchy. In unstable structures, if dominant individuals are involved in the most agonistic encounters, then it is the dominant individuals who experience the highest levels of stress. In mallards and pintails (*Anas acuta;* [55]), bison (*Bison bison;* [68]) and ring necked pheasants (*Phasianus colchicus;* [56]), for example, dominant males have higher levels of glucocorticoids than subordinate males. It seems likely, then, that if cues to stress are used to infer information about a potential partner's dominance status or, vice versa, if dominance status influences stress levels, the direction of such relationships will be species dependent.

Future research

Despite evidence to suggest that glucocorticoids play a role in sexual selection and mate choice, the nature and function of that role remains unclear. The effects of stress, while typically serving to reduce male attractiveness and the expression of sexual signals, are not consistent with some studies showing positive effects. Furthermore, despite proposals that the effects of stress occur through its action on immune function and/or body condition, there is little evidence to support this. Therefore, while we know that females prefer males with cues to low levels of stress hormones, we do not yet know what cues they attend to or what is signalled by "low stress". Despite a growing body of research, then, we are still confronted by a number of unknowns. Is it the case, for example, that males signal their current stress status? Or do they rather signal their ability to respond optimally to a stressor (i.e. an adaptive response which promotes survival but reduces the detrimental costs to health)? Are all sexual traits and signals similarly influenced by stress? That is, does stress affect those traits which show great plasticity during adulthood (e.g. plumage colouration in birds, or skin health in humans) differently to those which emerge at set developmental stages (e.g. bird song or human facial sexual dimorphism). Is the link with immune function so complex that we have to look at redistribution of resources across the arms of the immune system in response to chronic versus acute, and predictable versus unpredictable stressors? To begin to answer these questions, and to model roles of stress in mate choice, it is now necessary to test the effects of baseline stress, and of dimensions of the stress response (e.g. total amount of glucocorticoids produced in response to a standardised stressor and time to return to baseline) on different types of sexual signals (e.g. those that are typically dependent upon current condition versus those that develop at set life history stages) and to interpret findings in the context of species and population ecology [69]. Cross-cultural and cross-species comparisons can likewise contribute to our understanding of the traits signalled by low glucocorticoids.

3. Conclusion

To summarise, then, there is a growing body of evidence to show that the glucocorticoid hormones are implicated in mate choice and sexual selection. Women prefer the faces of males with low levels of cortisol, for example, and female zebra finch prefer males with low levels of corticosterone. We do not know, however, why females express these preferences as it is not yet clear what characteristics are signalled by cues to low glucocorticoids. Suggestions in the literature are that stress reduces body condition or suppresses the immune system which, in turn, reduce the extent to which individuals seek to attract members of the opposite sex. The extant evidence, however, does not consistently support these theories. It has also been proposed that stress mediates the effect of testosterone on sexual signals. Again, there is little support for this with results instead suggesting an interaction between testosterone and glucocorticoids – the nature of which is dependent upon the species, population and, in all likelihood, current socioecological conditions. What is clear is that there is increasing evidence for stress in sexual selection. It is now necessary to seek to better understand and model its precise roles and functions by conducting research which clearly operationalises the dimension of the stress response and the type of trait under investigation.

Author details

Fhionna R. Moore
School of Psychology, College of Art and Social Science, University of Dundee, UK

Acknowledgement

I am grateful to Kate Buchanan for insightful comments on a related draft and to Indrikis Krams, Markus Rantala and Vinet Coetzee for interesting discussions on the roles of stress in sexual selection.

4. References

[1] Darwin C (1859) On the Origin of Species by Means of Natural Selection, or the Preservation of Favoured Races in the Struggle for Life. John Murray, London; modern reprint Charles Darwin, Julian Huxley.

[2] Darwin C (1871) The Descent of Man and Selection in Relation to Sex. John Murray, London

[3] Petrie M, Halliday T, Sanders C (1991) Peahens prefer peacocks with elaborate trains. Anim. Behav. 41: 323-331.

[4] Borgia G (1985) Bowers as markers of male quality. Tests of a hypothesis. Anim. Behav. 33: 266-271.

[5] Grafen A (1990) Biological signals as handicaps. J. Theor. Biol 144:517-546.

[6] Zahavi A (1975) Mate selection - a selection for a handicap. J. Theor. Biol. 53: 205-214.

[7] Folstad I, Karter A J (1992) Parasites, bright males and the immunocompetence handicap. Am. Nat. 139: 603-622.

[8] Hamilton W D, Zuk M (1982) Heritable true fitness and bright birds: a role for parasites? Science 218: 384-387.

[9] Buchanan K L (2000) Stress and the evolution of condition dependent signals. Trends Ecol. Evol. 15: 156-160.

[10] Husak J F, Moore I T (2008) Stress hormones and mate choice. Trends Ecol. Evol. 23: 532-534.

[11] Evans M R, Goldsmith A R, Norris, S R A (2000) The effects of testosterone on antibody production and plumage colouration in male house sparrows (*Passer domesticus*). Behav. Ecol. Sociobiol. 47: 156-163.

[12] Roberts M L, Buchanan K L, Bennett A T D, Evans M R (2007) Mate choice in zebra finches: does corticosterone play a role? Anim. Behav. 74: 921-929.

[13] Hill G E, McGraw K J (2006). Bird Coloration. Vol. 2: Function and Evolution. Cambridge, Massachusetts: Harvard University Press

[14] Lindsay W R, Webster M S, Schwabl H (2011) Sexually selected male plumage colouration is testosterone dependent in a tropical passerine, the red-backed fairy wren (*Malanus melanocephalus*). PLoS One 6: e26067.

[15] Malo A F, Roldan E R S, Garde J J, Soler A J, Vicente J, Gortazar C, Gomendio A (2009) What does testosterone do for red deer males? Proc. Roy. Soc. B 276: 971-980.

[16] Price J, Allen S (2004) Exploring the mechanism regulating regeneration of deer antlers. Phil. Trans. R. Soc. B 359: 809–822.

[17] Ritschard M, Laucht S, Dale J, Brumm H (2011) Enhanced testosterone levels affect singing motivation but not song structure in Bengalese finches. Physiol. Behav. 102: 31-35.

[18] Saldanha C, Clayton N, Schlinger B (1999) Androgen metabolism in the juvenile oscine forebrain: a cross-species analysis at neural sites implicated in memory function J. Neurobiol. 33: 619–631.

[19] Roberts M L, Buchanan K L, Evans M R (2004) Testing the immunocompetence handicap hypothesis: a review of the evidence. Anim. Behav. 68: 227-239.

[20]. Deviche P J, Hurley L L, Fokidis H B, Lerbour B, Silverin B, Silverin B, Sabo J, Sharp (2010). Acute stress rapidly decreases plasma testosterone in a free-ranging male songbird: Potential site of action and mechanism. Gen. Compar. Endocrin. 169: 82-90.

[21] Gratto-Trevor C L, Oring L W, Fivizzani A J (1991) Effects of blood sampling stress on hormone levels in the semipalmated sandpiper. J. Field Ornithol. 62: 19–27.

[22] Owen-Ashley N T, Hasselquist D, Wingfield J C (2004) Androgens and the immunocompetence handicap hypothesis: unravelling direct and indirect pathways in song sparrows. Am. Nat. 164: 490-505.

[23] Moore I T, Lerner J P, Lerner, D T, Maso R T (2000) Relationships between Annual Cycles of Testosterone, Corticosterone, and Body Condition in Male Red-Spotted Garter Snakes, *Thamnophis sirtalis concinnus*. Physiolog. Biochem. Zool. 73:307–312.

[24] Martin L B (2009) Stress and immunity in wild vertebrates: timing is everything. Gen. Compar. Endocrinol. 163: 70-76.

[25] Mehta P H , Josephs R A (2010) Testosterone and cortisol jointly regulate dominance: Evidence for a dual-hormone hypothesis. Horm. Behav.58: 898–906.

[26] Moore F R, Cornwell R E, Law Smith M J, Al Dujaili E A S, Sharp M, Perrett D I (2011) Tests of the stress-linked immunocompetence handicap hypothesis in human male faces. Proc. Roy. Soc. B278: 774-780.

[27] Moore F R, Al Dujaili E A S, Cornwell R E, Law Smith M J, Lawson J F, Sharp M, Perrett D I (2011) Cues to sex and stress hormones in the human male face: functions of glucocorticoids in the immunocompetence handicap hypothesis. Horm. Behav. 60: 269-274.

[28] Brownlee K K, Moore A W, Hackney A C (2005) Relationship between circulating cortisol and testosterone: influence of physical exercise. J. Sports Sci. Medicine 4: 76-83.

[29] Enlow D H (1990) Facial growth, 3rd edn. Philadelphia, PA: Harcourt Brace Jovanovich

[30] Penton-Voak I S& Chen J Y (2004) High salivary testosterone is linked to masculine male facial appearance in humans.Evol. Hum. Behav. *25:* 229-241.

[31] Pound N, Penton Voak I S, Surridge A K (2009) Testosterone responses to competition in men are related to facial masculinity. Proc. Roy. Soc. B. 276: 153-159.

[32] Law Smith M J, Perrett D I, Jones B C, Cornwell R E, Moore F R, Feinberg D R, Boothroyd L G, Stirrat M R, Whiten S, Pitman R M, Hillier S G (2006) Facial appearance is a cue to oestrogen levels in women. Proc. Roy. Soc. B 273: 135-140.

[33] Perrett D I, Lee K J, Penton-Voak I, Rowland D R, Yoshikawa S, Burt D M, Henzi S P, Castles D L, Akamatsu S (1998) Effects of sexual dimorphism on facial attractiveness. Nature 394: 884-887.

[34]Moore F R, Taylor V, Law Smith M J, Perrett D I (2011) Sexual dimorphism in the female face is a cue to health and social status but not age. Pers. Ind. Diff. 50: 1068-1073.

[35] Boothroyd L G, Jones B C, Burt D M, Perrett D I (2007) Partner characteristics associated with masculinity, health and maturity in male faces. Pers. Ind. Diffs. 43: 1161-1173.

[36] Swaddle J, Reierson G (2002) Testosterone increases perceived dominance but not attractiveness. Proc. Roy. Soc. B 269: 2285–2289.

[37] Penton Voak I S, Perrett D I, Castles D L, Kobayashi T, Burt D M, Murray L K, Minamisawa R (1999). Menstrual cycle alters face preferences. Nature *399:* 741-742.

[38] Waynforth D, Delwadia S, Camm. (2005). The influence of women's mating strategies on preference for masculine facial architecture. Evol. Human Behav. 26: 409–416.

[39] Brooks R, Scott I M, Maklakov A A, Kasumovic M M, Clark A P, Penton-Voak I S. 2011. National income inequality predicts women's preferences for masculinised faces better than health does. Proc. R. Soc. B 278: 810–812.

[40] DeBruine L M, Jones B C, Crawford J R, Welling L L M, Little A C (2010) The health of a nation predicts their mate preferences: cross-cultural variation in women's preferences for masculinized male faces. Proc. R. Soc. B 277: 2405–2410.

[41] Tiddeman B, Burt, M, Perrett, D I (2001) Prototyping and Transforming Facial Textures for Perception Research. IEEE Computer Graphics and Applications 21: 42-50.

[42] Leary C J, Jessop T S, Garcia A M, Knapp R (2004). Steroid hormone profiles and relative body condition of calling and satellite toads: implications for proximate regulation of behavior in anurans. Behav. Ecol. 15: 313-320.

[43] Rantala M J, Moore F R, Skrinda I, Krama T, Kivleniece I, Kecko S, Krams I (2012) Evidence for the stress-linked immunocompetence handicap hypothesis in humans. Nature Comms. DOI: 10.1038/ncomms1696.

[44] Bortolotti G R, Mougoet F, Martinez-Padilla J, Webster L M I, Piertney S B (2009) Physiological stress mediates the honesty of social signals. PloS One 4: e4983.

[45] Edler A V, Friedl T W P (2010) Individual quality and carotenoid-based plumage ornaments in male red bishops (*Euplectes orix*): plumage is not all that counts. Biol. J. Linn. Soc. 99: 384-397.

[46] Romero L M (2004) Physiological stress in ecology: lessons from biomedical research. Trends in Ecol Evol. 19: 249-255.

[47] Klukowski L A, Cawthorn J M, Ketterson E D, Nolan Jr. V (1997) Effects of experimentally elevated testosterone on plasma corticosterone and corticosteroid-binding globulin in dark-eyed juncos (*Junco hyemalis*). Gen. Comp. Endocrinol. 108: 141–151.

[48] Swett MB, Breuner CW (2008) Interaction of testosterone, corticosterone and corticosterone binding globulin in the white-throated sparrow (*Zonotrichia albicollis*). Comp Biochem Physiol A Mol Integr Physiol. 151: 226-31.

[49]Møller A P (1995) Hormones, handicaps and bright birds. Trends Ecol. Evol. 10: 121.

[50] del Cerro S, Merino S, Martinez-de la Puerte J, Lobato E, Ruiz-de-Castañeda Rivero-de Aguilar J Martinez J, Morales J, Tomás G, Moreno J (2010). Carotenoid-based plumage colouration is associated with blood parasite richness and stress protein levels in blue tits (*Cyanistes caeruleus*). Oecologia 162: 825-835.

[51] Pfaff J A, Zanette L, MacDougall-Shackleton S A, MacDougall-Shackleton E A (2007) Song repertoire size varies with HVC volume and is indicative of male quality in song sparrows (*Melospiza melodia*). Proc. R. Soc. B. 274: 2035-2040.

[52] Gladbach A, Gladbach D J, Quillfeldt P (2010) Variations in leukocyte profiles and plasma biochemistry are related to different aspects of parental investment in male and female upland geese *Chloephaga picta leucoptera*. Comp. Biochem. Physiol. A. 156: 269-277.

[53] McGraw K J, Lee K, Lewin A (2011) The effect of capture-and-handling stress on carotenoid-based beak coloration in zebra finches. J. Comp. Physiol. A. 197: 683-691.

[54] Nunes S, Pelz K M, Muecke E-M, Holekamp K E, Zucker I (2006). Plasma glucocorticoids concentrations and body mass in ground squirrels: seasonal variation and circannual organisation. Gen. Compar. Endocrin. 146: 136-143.

[55] Poisbleau M, Fritz H, Guillon N, Chastel O (2005) Linear social dominance hierarchies and corticosterone responses in male mallards and pintails. Horm. Behav. 47: 485-492.

[56] Mateos C (2005) The subordination stress paradigm and the relation between testosterone and corticosterone in male ring-necked pheasants. Anim. Behav. 69: 249-255.

[57] Cote J, Meylan S, Clobert J, Voituron Y (2010) Carotenoid-based colouration, oxidative stress and corticosterone in common lizards. J. Experiment. Biol. 213: 2116-2124.

[58] Breen K M, Stackpole C A, Clarke I J, Pytlak A V, Tilbrook, A J, Wagenmaker E R, Young E A, Karsch F J (2004) Does the type II glucocorticoid receptor mediate cortisol-induced suppression in pituitary responsiveness to gonadotropin-releasing hormone? Endocrinology 145: 2739–2746.

[59] Attardi B, Klatt B, Hoffman G E, Smith M S (1997) Facilitation or inhibition of the estradiol-induced gonadotropin surge in the immature rat by progesterone: regulation of GnRH and LH messenger RNAs andactivation of GnRH neurons. J. Neuroendocrinol. 9: 589–599.

[60] Attardi B, Pfaff D W, Fink G (1999) Actions of progesterone on the pituitary in relation to facilitation of the estradiol induced gonadotropin surge in the immature rat. Soc. Neurosci. Abstr. 582: 13.

[61] Greenburg N, Wingfield J C (1987) Stress and reproduction: reciprocal relationships. D.O. Norris, R.E. Jones (Eds.), Reproductive Endocrinology of Fishes, Amphibians and Reptiles, Wiley, New York, pp. 389–426

[62] Menendez-Patterson A, Florez-Lozano J A, Fernandez S, Marin B (1980) Stress and sexual behavior in male rats. Physiol. Behav. 24: 403–406.

[63] Moberg GP (1991) How behavioral stress disrupts the endocrine control of reproduction in domestic animals J. Dairy Sci. 74: 304–311.

[64] Lynn S E, Stamplis T B, Barrington W T, Weida N, Hudak C A (2010) Food, stress, and reproduction: Short-term fasting alters endocrine physiology and reproductive behavior in the zebra finch. Horm. Behav. 58: 214–222.

[65] Ricciardella L F, Bliely J M, Feth, C C, Woodley, S K (2010). Acute stressors increase plasma corticosterone and decrease locomotoractivity in a terrestrialsalamander (*Desmognathus ochrophaeus*). Physiol. Behav. 101: 81-86.

[66] Tilgar V, Moks K, Saag P (2011) Predator-induced stress changes parental feeding behavior in pied flycatchers.Behav. Ecol. 22:23-28.

[67] Creel S (2001) Social dominance and stress hormones. Trends in Ecol Evol. 18: 491-198.

[68] Mooring M S, Patton M L, Lance V A, Hall B M, Schaad E W, Fetter G A, Fortin S S, McPeak K M Glucocorticoids of bison bulls in relation to social status. Horm. Behav. 49: 369-375.

[69] Evans M R (2010) Why does testosterone influence morphology, behaviour and plasticity? Open Ornithol. J. 3: 21-26.

Chapter 10

Using Rodent Models to Simulate Stress of Physiologically Relevant Severity: When, Why and How

Carine Smith

Additional information is available at the end of the chapter

http://dx.doi.org/10.5772/52045

1. Introduction

Given the demands of modern life, it is no wonder that the concept of stress has become a household topic for discussion. Also in the academic realm the phenomenon which is stress, is topping the charts in terms of research interest. The short term costs as well as the long term maladaptive effects of stress have been a popular topic of research in especially physiology and psychology for the past few decades, ever since Hans Selye defined the term "stress" in 1956 (Selye, 1956). Stress-related chronic disease, such as cardiovascular disease, diabetes and depression, places an ever-increasing burden on society – medically, socially and financially. Therefore, if we are to limit the spread and impact of this "pandemic", it is imperative to properly manage the effects of stress on our bodies. This of course, is only possible if we have a complete understanding of the body's response to stress.

The response to stress is almost never localised and contained. Rather, a stress response is initiated in response to a local physical (e.g. contusion to skeletal muscle) or mental (e.g. the loss of a loved one) stressor, but always culminates in a wide-spread, systemic response process that affects many organs and systems. Consider for a moment a less complex research model in a different discipline. Metabolic pathways (e.g. the Krebs cycle or glycolysis) can easily be manipulated in cell culture assays using one single cell type at a time, since these pathways (including substrate supply and waste removal systems) are contained in its entirety within each cell. In contrast, with the stress response pathways this is clearly not the case.

The stress response is a complex network of events, which is directed via two interlinked pathways, one endocrine (the hypothalamic pituitary adrenal (HPA)-axis) and one neural (the locus coeruleus norepinephrine (LC-NE) or sympatho-adrenal medullary (SAM)-system). While the neural pathway is mainly activated neurally in response to stress perception, leading to the well-known "fight-or-flight" response, the endocrine pathway has many more triggers. Apart from neural activation, the HPA-axis is also activated by a large number of hormones and even chemical messengers, such as interleukin-6, a cytokine and mediator of inflammation, which is known to increase cortisol secretion. A contributing factor to the complexity of the HPA-axis is the fact that cortisol, the main end product of this stress response, has both endocrine and metabolic functions. Although cortisol is commonly known as the "stress hormone" in the context of psychological stress, its main function is actually metabolic – to maintain glucose supply to the brain. Therefore, the HPA-axis is structured not only for activation in response to perceived stress, but also to react to metabolic stimuli. Furthermore, while the stress response should be powerful and fast in an acute stress situation, the response should be controlled and relatively more limited in a situation of chronic stress, to prevent detrimental effects to the organism in the long term. One can appreciate therefore the need for relatively complex signalling networks in this regard, which serves to activate, limit or inhibit the stress response. To achieve this, numerous molecular mechanisms are in place, and react and interact in response to various stress signals. To give just one example, the glucocorticoid receptor, which is present on most cells to enable cortisol's effect on these cells, is up-regulated in response to acute stress, but down-regulated after a period of chronic stress.

Such complexities make the choice of a suitable stress research model both a difficult, and vital one. While some mechanisms, e.g. activation agents of specific adrenal or pituitary cell types, may be elucidated in cell culture, a whole-system model is required in order to assess the net effect of any stressor to these systems. This does not imply that there is no place for *ex vivo* or *in vitro* studies in the discipline of stress research, far from it! A large number of cell-based – and more recently organotypic culture-based – studies have contributed substantially to our understanding of specific mechanisms and/or partial pathways relevant to stress. The important point here is that ideally, *in vitro* work should at some point be followed up by *in vivo* investigations, in order to test the applicability of results obtained *in vitro*, to a whole system.

The importance of *in vivo* assessments, and the need for conducting them in a model specifically suitable to answer the question at hand, is clear when one considers the huge number of described animal models in the scientific literature. Apart from more conventional models using genetically "intact" rodents, recent advances in biotechnology have made possible research using non-physiological models such as gene-knock out animals. These animals may be genetically modified to erase the gene coding for a particular protein, so that the researcher may elect to produce animals completely lacking a particular protein of interest (e.g. IL-6 knockout mice), or in some cases lacking it in only one organ or system (e.g. STAT-3 knocked out or "switched off" in skeletal muscle only). These models may be used to shed light on various *in vivo* mechanisms which could previously not be properly elucidated using the conventional methods. However, these models have their limitations. For example, when doing research on inflammation, an animal in which a pro-inflammatory cytokine was knocked out, may display increased or decreased basal levels of other pro-inflammatory cytokines, or an altered anti-inflammatory cytokine profile, or even up- or down-regulated cytokine responses on activation, as a spontaneous compensatory mechanism. The resultant net effect of the genetic manipulation therefore may result in a model that is not physiologically accurate, and responses measured may not accurately reflect normal *in vivo* responses. Furthermore, these compensatory mechanisms and/or the mere absence of an important protein may also result in other – sometimes unanticipated – side-effects (such as severe constipation in IL-6 knockout mice). Apart from being a confounding factor in the intended study, in some cases these undesired outcomes may result in poor health or even shortened life expectancy of the experimental animal, so that it limits the application of such a model even further. Of course, chain-reaction compensatory responses will also limit the extent to which results obtained in such models, may be extrapolated to a (at least genetically) normal situation.

Relatively "old-fashioned", or more conventional methods, when applied optimally, therefore still have an important place in research, both in applied areas such as pharmacology and in areas of basic research. Only when a situation that is physiologically relevant is recreated or simulated, can one realistically assess either the response to a challenge, or the outcome of a remedial intervention.

Therefore, in this chapter, I would like to reflect on methods used to simulate a variety of stressors to the body, starting with a variety of models used to simulate psychological stress, ranging in severity from non-extreme (mild) psychological stress to extreme mental trauma. I will also discuss general considerations in picking the appropriate animal model to use, which may determine the difference between success and failure in your research. Details on the various models will be provided, including issues such as repeatability and standardisation. Models will also be discussed in terms of their suitability for different research approaches or objectives, as well as in terms of their limitations. Arguments for and against the use of any particular model will also be illustrated using actual research data.

2. General considerations when choosing a rodent stress model

Small rodents are an obvious choice for research models in need of a whole body system, since they are relatively small and prolifically reproducing mammals, making them relatively economical to breed and house. Although rats and mice are physiologically very similar to humans in terms of organs and systems implicated in their response to stress, there are some fundamental differences between rodents and humans that may greatly influence results obtained using such models. It is necessary to understand these differences and the impact that it may have on any particular study employing rodents, and to adapt protocols to accommodate these differences in order to maximise the validity of results obtained. Let us consider just a few general factors that have huge impact on study outcome, but which may often be ignored or overlooked.

2.1. When to stress: lights on or off?

The timing of stress exposure, interventions to relieve stress and sampling of blood or tissue for analysis is a vital consideration, with many confounders complicating the issue. Firstly, the rat is nocturnally active, while humans obviously are not naturally nocturnal. Therefore, the question arises of whether to stress the rats during their active time, at night, or during the day, when they are asleep – which would most accurately mimic the physiological responses of humans? One could argue that it would be more applicable to expose an animal to a psychological stressor while it is awake, i.e. in the darkness – after all, how can one stress a rat when it is half asleep during the day anyway? However, this seemingly logical argument is not correct, for a very simple reason. Whether the rodent is asleep or wide awake when exposed to an experimental stressor is not the determining factor – rather, the normal rhythmic changes of hormones over the course of a day hugely affects the ability to respond to stress.

A typical circadian rhythm graph for corticosterone is presented in Figure 1. The circadian rhythm illustrated is expected in experiments employing a normal light-dark cycle – convention would be a 12 hour light-dark cycle, with lights switched on at 7am, and off at 7pm. Reversal of the light cycle has significant effects on the circadian rhythms, the "pattern" of which follows the delay in timing from the conventional one. This effect of light and darkness may be partially explained by the fact that sympathetic input to the adrenal gland is photo-sensitive: in periods of darkness, a dramatic increase in basal norepinephrine secretions from sympathetic nerves occurs (Hashimoto et al., 1999), so that basal corticosterone secretion is up-regulated in periods of darkness. However, one can also see from the curve that corticosterone secretion starts to increase after the nadir at a time of day when there is still much light – this further illustrates the complexity of this regulation, pointing to the existence of additional important causative factors.

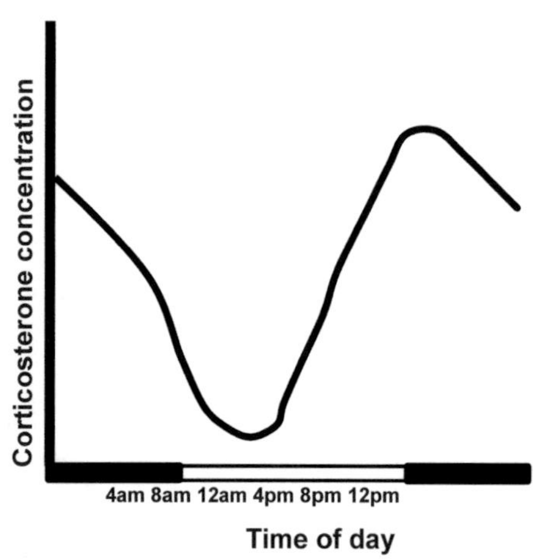

Figure 1. Expected circadian rhythm graph for corticosterone in rats. Dark bars at the bottom indicate "lights off" periods and open bar indicates the "lights on" period.

It is of importance to note that adaptation to changes in lighting conditions is not synchronised, and so does not occur within similar time frames, for all hormones. For example, while the corticosterone rhythm was shown to adapt to a 12-hour delay (phase reversal) and become constant after about 6 days, the rhythm for adrenaline only adapted after 10 days, indicating that the pituitary adrenocortical system adapts more readily to light-dark cycle shifts, while the sympatho-adrenal medullary system requires relatively more time (Miki and Sudo, 1996).

Researchers working on models using juvenile animals should also take note that the circadian rhythms for these hormone fluctuations are not fully developed at birth. The diurnal rhythm for corticosterone for example is only regular from about day 30-32 in rats (Allen and Kendall, 1967). Also, circadian rhythms are affected by many stress-related disorders – in this context, a chronic mild stress model of depression has been shown to cause fluctuations in corticosterone rhythm which only normalised after 8 weeks of chronic mild stress, and which was dependent on resilience of animals exposed to stress (Christiansen et al., 2012).

Therefore, in planning an experiment, it is most important to decide whether the stress exposure and sample collection should take place during the rising or falling phase of a hormone pulse. In the context of stress for example, one would time stress exposure and sample collection to coincide with the natural decrease of hormones expected to increase in response to stress, such as corticosterone and the catecholamines. Otherwise, if done at a time when hormone levels were increasing naturally, the circadian rhythm may effectively mask the acute response to stress. Even though these experiments should always include control samples taken from unstressed animals at the same time of day, unsynchronised sampling may still increase the variability of data, and thus decrease statistical power. This consideration is especially important in models employing physiologically relevant levels of stress, since the response seen is usually not enormous, and any potential confounders should be excluded as far as possible. Therefore, a suggestion is that all stress exposure interventions should be performed in the early morning hours, so that subsequent sample collection may to completed before noon, when the nadir for corticosterone occurs.

2.2. Metabolic rate

Another very important way in which rodents differ from humans is their much faster basal metabolic rate. Rats have a metabolic rate roughly 10 times and mice 30 times that of humans. This would obviously have huge implications for any study design with a pharmacological component. For example, when testing the potential of a stress relief medication, one would have to either increase the dose recommended by the manufacturer for human consumption, or decrease the dosage interval in rodents to ensure the maintenance of a therapeutic concentration of the drug at the level of the target tissue. Both these approaches have their drawbacks though. On the one hand, administration of a mega dose may result in intolerance reactions to the drug, most often including side effects such as gastroenteritis, with obvious confounding results given the interaction between inflammation and the glucocorticoid response. When choosing this method, parameters to monitor gut integrity, such as prostaglandin E2 levels or serum lipopolysaccharide levels, should ideally be included in the testing profile. On the other hand, decreasing the dosage interval requires more frequent handling of the experimental animals, which increases the possibility of an undesired stress response to the constant handling. This last obstacle can be partially overcome with the use of osmotic mini-pumps – these tiny pumps are implanted subcutaneously behind the neck of the rodent where it cannot reach, and releases the drug constantly at a pre-selected rate and over a pre-selected number of days. It is debatable however whether or not this method accurately reflects *in vivo* conditions for and effects of a drug that is, for example, intended to be administered orally once or twice a day, rather than continuously. A further limitation of this method is that labile substances can't be tested in this way, since the drug can only be maintained at body temperature (i.e. not cooled) for the duration of the infusion.

2.3. Social issues

A factor that should be of particular interest to researchers investigating effects of psychological stress, is the social hierarchy that exists within experimental rodent colonies. Rats in particular are a very social species, and individual housing of rats actually causes a degree of psychological stress. Therefore, standard practise is to house rats in groups of four to five, when using standard sized cages. This in itself is a limiting factor, since it is logistically not really possible to monitor appetite or food and water consumption of individual rats (which are usually done using metabolic cages in which rats are individually housed) without causing a stress response to housing conditions. Logistic factors aside, it is interesting to see that within these small groups, a social hierarchy quickly emerges, with some rats being submissive, while others are clearly dominant. Dominant rats have been shown to grow faster and to be relatively more resistant to stress interventions that submissive rats. This is both good and bad for the researcher. On the one hand, having this social hierarchy in a way simulates human situations, making the model more representative of the human population as a whole. On the other hand, the variation in the response to stress resulting from social hierarchy results in great variations in data obtained within the same experimental group, which could hide differences between experimental groups. This lowers the statistical power of any experiment, necessitating the use of larger experimental groups, which of course is more time and resource consuming. In our experience, experimental groups for the purpose of research into the psychological stress response should consist of at least 10-15 rats, on condition that all rats have been properly accustomed to the environment, handlers and protocols.

2.4. Practical tips

Apart from the factors discussed above, there are a few more general considerations to keep in mind when setting up an animal model of stress. I will touch on these just briefly. Research has shown that the mood (emotional state) of the animal handler(s) also affect the basal anxiety level of animals. Therefore some personality types may be more suited to work using animal models than others. For example, in our group we had two students conducting stress studies on sibling rats from the same litters. One student was completely at ease with the rats and handled them with natural ease, while the other student was very nervous around the rats and anxious about handling them. When assessing corticosterone levels in the control rats from the first student's study, serum concentrations were all lower than 10ng/ml. However, those from the more nervous student all had values in excess of 40ng/ml. (All samples were collected at the same time of day, so that diurnal variation did not play a role.) Of course, the fact that even unstressed animals had clearly elevated corticosterone levels, severely limits the conclusions that may be drawn from this specific experiment.

Different strains of animals have also been shown to vary substantially in their natural sensitivity to stress. This has been comprehensively reviewed elsewhere, in the context of neurobiology (Ellenbroek et al., 2005). Perhaps of specific interest for the stress researcher is the fact that these differences in stress sensitivity seems to be the effect of differences at adrenocortical level, rather than a central effect, since restraint were reported to elicit similar hippocampal and hypothalamic responses across five rat strains, although differences were quite clearly present at adrenal level (Gomez et al., 1996). An interesting fact is that some of these supposedly strain-dependent differences are more the result of nurture than nature: for example, if a spontaneously hypertensive rat (SHR) is reared by a Wistar-Kyoto rat (WKY), its hypertension is significantly less pronounced. One should therefore exercise caution in the selection of a strain to breed for the purpose of stress research. Furthermore, even within an established strain, differences occur. For example, first-time rat mothers have been shown to yield pups with relatively less resistance to stress, so that litters from first-time mothers should be avoided by the stress researcher. Also, a vital point to remember is that the experimental animal does not speak human! When conducting research in humans, it is possible – and ethically required – to explain to any volunteer the intervention that he or she will be subjected to, including expected risks. Therefore, when a human is stressed experimentally (e.g. by participating in a maths test or public speaking), although they will mount a psychological stress response, they also know that the test, or stressor, won't be permanently detrimental. A rodent on the other hand, has no way of knowing whether an acutely applied stressor will be lethal or not, so that even mild stressors are perceived as quite severe the first time. Therefore, if the requirement for research purposes is to simulate stress of a physiologically relevant severity in rodents, the stress intervention may actually seem relatively mild in comparison to what one might expect to be necessary.

From just these few considerations it is clear that the ideal *in vivo* model for psychological stress may simply not exist. However, if one is aware of potential confounders, the protocol may be optimised, and interpretation of results approached with the necessary caution, making in vivo models very valuable and realistic tools. So, how does one go about setting up the optimum model?

3. Design and setup of an animal model

Moving on to the actual setting up of a model, there are several precautions to include in the protocol, that are unique to studies on stress, especially psychological stress. For this section, I will limit myself to a discussion of rat models for stress, since this is the species of choice for this discipline, and also the species that I have most experience working with.

Putting first things first, one has to decide what situation of stress should be simulated. This is directly dependent on the research question. For example, if the question is related to the effect of a calming tablet administered to someone who has been exposed to a sudden trauma (e.g. car hi-jacking), a model where rats are subjected to a severe acute stressor is obviously the best choice. When a daily supplement is tested for stress relieving properties, or the effect of long-term occupational/stress on a specific organ is investigated, a model with multiple exposures to a relatively milder stressor would be more ideal. Sometimes, it may even be useful to combine protocols to achieve a mix of acute and chronic stress, in order to most accurately simulate actual human situations. Rats have been reported to be able to adjust to any mild stressor within a period of about 3 days (Garcia et al., 2000). Therefore, a study requiring mild stress to continue for a relatively long time, may require combination of a number of stressors in order to maintain a stressful environment.

3.1. What does a rat find stressful?

The decision of the type of stressor again depends on the situation being simulated. Stressors in real life vary from "mild irritation" to traumatic. Similar variety is therefore required in models for stress. Arguably the most popular simulation of prolonged trauma is a model known as maternal separation. Normally, pups remain with their mother throughout the first few weeks of their life until they are weaned at the age of 21-30 days, dependent on laboratory standard operating procedure. In the maternal separation model, rat pups are removed from their mother during a critical time in their development, usually during the first two or three weeks after birth, for a period of three hours per day. This traumatic separation is characterised by changes in both behavioural responses (such as anxious-like behaviour and hyperactivity in the open field test) and HPA-axis responses (such as decreased expression of glucocorticoid receptor in the hippocampus and ≈15% higher basal blood corticosterone concentrations) to stress, that persists into adulthood. These changes suggest an increased natural anxiety in response to chronic severe stress during early development. This technique is uniquely suited for and commonly used for investigating the development of psychiatric disorders such as anxiety and depression. Note that the endocrine responses seen in this model is relatively small in comparison to for example restraint stress models, even though it represents trauma, i.e. the most severe type of stress. One has to keep in mind though that these changes are assessed in the "rested" state, and reflects chronic changes, which are always smaller in magnitude than acute responses assessed directly after application of an acute stressor.

A somewhat milder form of stress may be simulated using restraint (sometimes called immobilisation). This technique is highly variable due to research group-specific differences in the execution of this technique. On the extreme end, animals are literally taped down on a flat board, immobilising them completely, for a period between one and two hours. Rats are fairly vocal in response to this particular protocol, so that it is advisable to conduct this particular protocol in soundproof facilities, to prevent negative effects on the rest of the animals housed in the same unit. A much milder form of restraint is to place rats in small cages that limit their movement. An example of a Perspex restraint cage (restraining up to 6 rats simultaneously) as used by our group is presented in Figure 2.

This particular cage has compartments 6cm wide x 7cm high x 18 cm long, and works best for restraint of mature Wistar rats, weighing around 300-350 g (this type of restraint is only successful when rats fit tightly into restraint compartments). Note the use of Perspex as material for the cages: this prevents the rats from having a stress response to being isolated from their group because they can still see their "neighbours". Also, body heat from peers warms the sides of the cages, creating a similar effect to when rats sleep clumped together, as they habitually do. When rats are put into these compartments, they typically turn around once or twice (invariably getting stuck halfway through the turn), and then stop trying to move. Grooming behaviour – a known self-pacifying behaviour in rats – indicates that rats are feeling claustrophobic, i.e. a psychological stress response can be expected. Rats are usually restrained for a period of 30 minutes to 2 hours once per day. During this time, they do not have access to food or water, but sufficient ventilation holes at both ends allow for normal ventilation. Keep in mind that when restraining nocturnal animals during light hours, they won't have a huge requirement to feed or drink, so that the absence of food and water is not perceived as stressful and does not impact significantly on their normal metabolism.

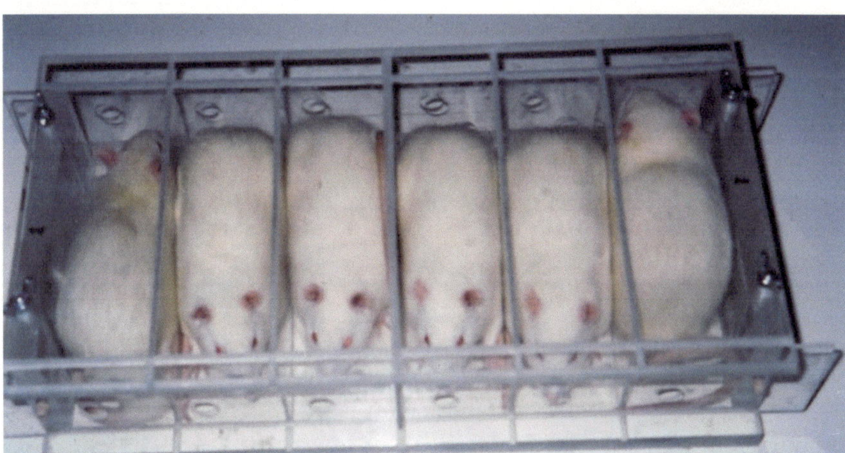

Figure 2. Restraint stress by confinement in purpose-designed Perspex cages elicits a mild form of psychological stress in rats. Adult male Wistar rats weighing more than 300g were used in this particular instance. Note the two rats on each side that were able to turn around in the cage once, but prefer not to attempt it again.

The response obtained using this model is of mild severity, and is ideal for studying normal adaptation to both acute and chronic stress. Given the wide relevance of this severity of stress to the human population, it is also a valuable model to use in the pharmacological, psychological and physiological testing of therapies, drugs and daily supplements intended to decrease stress levels or counter the side-effects of stress. This particular model is relatively easy to standardise in terms of diet, stress duration, light-dark cycle, etc. and is highly repeatable within a research group, as long as particular care is taken in selection of animal handlers and other factors already discussed. However, inter-research group differences do exist, so that care should be taken to consider changes in stress intervention protocols when comparing results reported by different laboratories. Commonly expected values with the restraint model used as an acute stress intervention lasting one hour, in our hands, are presented below (Figure 3) for changes in body mass, corticosterone, testosterone and the pro-inflammatory cytokine interleukin (IL)-1β.

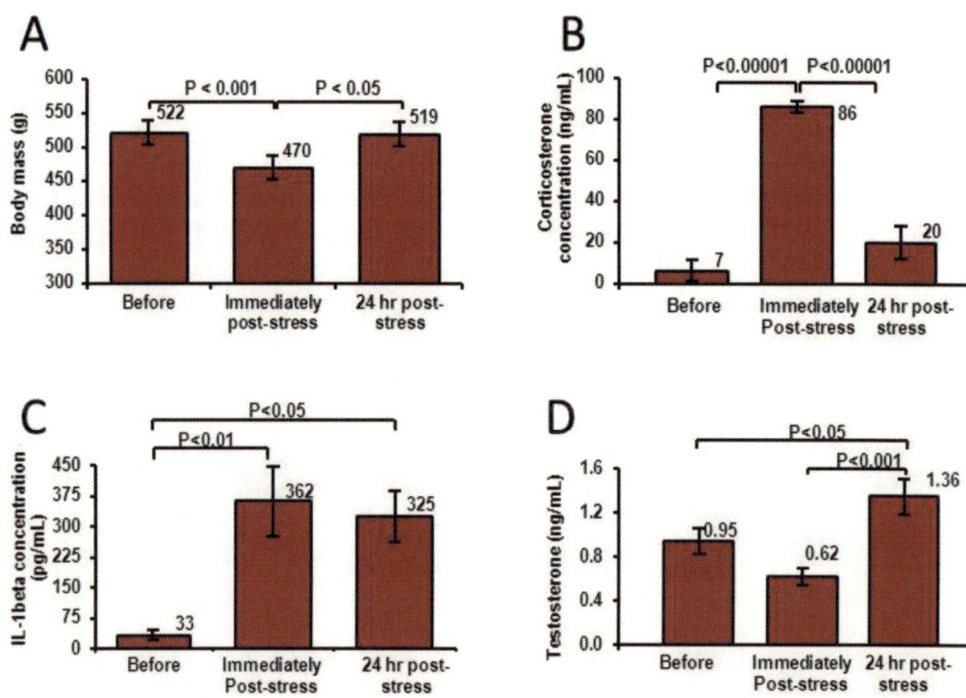

Figure 3. Effects of acute short-term restraint stress (1 hour) and recovery from stress on mean a) body mass, b) serum corticosterone, c) serum interleukin-1β and d) serum testosterone concentrations. Bars on graphs illustrate mean values, while error bars indicate standard deviations.

Body mass decreases significantly, but only transiently, in response to acute stress as applied by our group. This is mainly the result of increased defecation and urination. In terms of corticosterone, an acute increase of between 8-12-fold is seen. This response plateaus after one hour, and rats are able to recover from one exposure to restraint within one day. Testosterone concentrations are not acutely affected by acute stress, but it may increase during the recovery period. This effect is similar to that seen in athletes after a stressful bout of exercise, and may suggest an ability to cope and resist the stressful effects of the particular stressor.

In the chronic model, since the rat is not able to fully recover between stress exposure sessions when done daily for an extended time, testosterone levels do decrease with this model, resulting in a more catabolic state, and even up-regulation of the proteolytic pathways. In other words, although only mild in severity, this model is severe enough to result in undesirable side-effects in the longer term, making it an excellent simulation for chronic stress such as occupation-related stress in humans. From the cytokine data, restraint stress clearly has a pro-inflammatory effect as well, which makes this a particularly suitable model for investigations into the efficacy of e.g. anti-inflammatory interventions. Note that the IL-1β levels are still significantly elevated even after the recovery period – this is most likely due to the relatively long half-life of the cytokine. Again, in the long term, a shift toward a pro-inflammatory status is achieved.

Some groups have used involuntary swimming (forced swimming in a $1m^3$ swimming pool warmed to 24°C) as stressor. Although acute forced swimming is a recognised test to assess depressive-like behaviour (although this is being disputed), rats are natural swimmers, so it is doubtful whether this method – when applied chronically - is really a significant stressor. In fact, in the discipline of exercise science, researchers train rats to swim in order to study hypertrophy and metabolic adaptation to exercise training. These anabolic responses are the direct opposite of the catabolic response that is the stress response, further placing doubt on the use of this technique to realistically simulate chronic stress. Furthermore, in our experience, females are more willing swimmers than males. Males were found to simply climb onto the most submissive animal, which would then literally be drowned without investigator intervention. Alternatively, they might hold their breath and sit at the bottom of the pool for as long as they can before jumping/swimming up for a breath of air, rather than exercising the whole time. Although females tend to actually swim a lot better without the constant prodding required with males, their voluntary exercise capacity/willingness to exercise also varies dramatically. Therefore, as with voluntary running models (using purpose-designed running wheels), the "natural athletes" have to be selected from a larger cohort prior to the study. This then has the disadvantage of possible genetic pre-selection, which may yield data that is not widely applicable across the whole population. It is clear therefore, that this model has many limitations and should not be a first choice for simulation of psychological stress.

A number of other stressors may be employed, and some of these are not very labour-intensive, so that they are commonly used in combination with the stressors discussed above, to prevent adaptation, as mentioned earlier. These include soiled bedding, tail flick, and inversion or cage tilt. Bedding is soiled with water by simply pouring 300ml of water onto cage bedding and leaving rats to endure this discomfort for an hour before changing the bedding again. For the tail flick protocol, a rat is manually restrained and its tail placed in a water bath kept at 49 °C until the rat voluntarily flicks it out. For the cage tilt, the restraint cage is turned upside down for the duration of a restraint session which usually lasts from 30 minutes to an hour when used in combination with cage tilt. These are all examples of mild severity stressors. Extreme heat or cold are also referred to as stress models, but these stressors are more metabolic than psychological in nature.

3.2. Keeping experimental animal stress free

Although left for last in this section, the following point is perhaps the most important. When conducting any experiment investigating the response to stress, it is of major importance to keep all animals "otherwise" stress free. In other words, one has to ensure that rats are only exposed to the standardised stressors used as interventions in the study. Several precautions may be needed to prevent other stressors from confounding data. For example, vibration has recently been identified as a stressor in terms of the immune system. Animals exposed to constant low grade vibration may deplete their lymphocytes in as little as two to three weeks. Considering that lymphocytes make up the bulk of rat white blood cells (about 75%), it is clear that the end result is an immune-compromised animal with very abnormal cytokine profile. Therefore, while it may seem like a good idea to have a generator handy, the constant vibration it causes, may in fact be detrimental to your study.

Furthermore, new male rats should never be introduced to existing housing groups (e.g. if one rat dies, it should not be replaced with another adult rat), and adult male rats should not redistributed between cages after they have established their hierarchy. They have a social hierarchy and such changes will result in social stress, the result of which is difficult to determine before it is too late. Lastly, rodents in particular have to be handled to accustom them to their handlers. During this time, they also become used to the sounds and smells associated with their housing environment. Introduction of a new sound or smell may result in an uncontrolled, unstandardized stress response. In our laboratory, the simple guideline during acclimation of rats after arrival from the breeding unit, is to expose them to all sounds, smells (e.g. disinfectants used both during every day maintenance and during sample collection procedures), actions (e.g. weighing, sham injections, oral gavage with tap water only) and people required for the intervention study, with the exception of the intervention itself. During sacrifice, a meticulous procedure has to be followed: Firstly, all surfaces should be disinfected with a disinfectant the animal has been habituated to, in order to disguise any body odour from the previously sacrificed animal. Then, the rat is taken from its cage and euthanasia applied as soon as possible. Rats still in line for sacrifice have to be protected from any sound or smell that could alert them to what is happening; otherwise they will have a severe acute stress response. Sprague-Dawley rats for example has been shown to have increased heart rate and mean arterial blood pressure when present in the same room where other rats were being exposed to a variety of interventions, which included routine actions such as cage changes, but also experimental interventions such as decapitation (Sharp et al., 2002).

Interestingly in this study, witness rats that were individually housed, showed a greater stress response than rats group housed, further illustrating the additive effect of different stressors. The magnitude of this acute stress response can indeed be enormous. In a study by our group, corticosterone responses were determined in rats that could smell and hear experimental procedures for sacrifice. When sorted according to the order of sacrifice, it is clear that the rats waiting their turn were experiencing acute stress that accumulated with time (Figure 4).

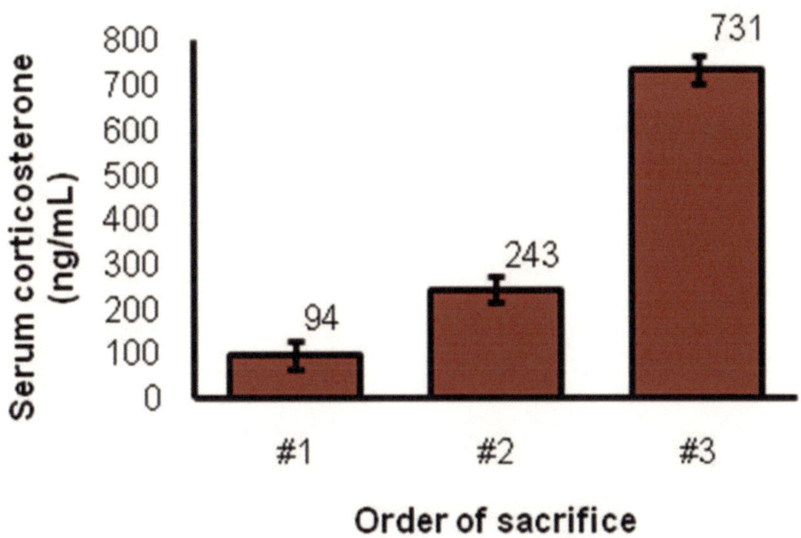

Figure 4. Cumulative corticosterone levels in an acute stress response that was elicited by witnessing the experimental killing of littermates in male Wistar rats killed approximately 15-20 minutes apart.

4. Quantifying stress responses

In terms of psychological stress, an obvious and very popular assessment technique in humans are the use of validated, standardised questionnaires designed to assess levels of perceived stress, anxiety, depression, hardiness, job satisfaction, etc. Quite clearly this method is not of use in animal models. Instead, tests to analyse and quantify stressed behaviour have been developed. The most common techniques in this context are the open field and elevated plus maze tests, as well as the forced swimming test mentioned earlier. To increase the accuracy of interpretations made from behavioural tests, it is advised to combine at least two behavioural tests, rather than to rely on the results from only one technique.

For the open field test, the researcher relies on the fact that rats naturally fear large open spaces, since this would expose them to predators. For this test, an "open field" of $1m^2$ with gridlines, with high walls around all sides, are used (Figure 5). The rat to be assessed is simply placed in the centre of the open field, and its exploratory behaviour assessed by quantification of movement frequency and distance. A variation of this test is to have a second open field test on a separate day, which involves placing a novel object in the centre of the open field – the number of approaches made to this object is recorded. The interpretation of the results is not without complexity though. While a greater degree of locomotor activity and more time spent in the inner zone is usually seen as indicative of a relaxed emotional state, this same result is obtained in young rats after the traumatic experience of maternal separation. The latter condition is seen as an anxious, hyperreactivity or hyperarousal state. The "novel object" open field test can distinguish between these two explanations for the same behavioural test result: while an emotionally relaxed rat would approach the novel object often to investigate, the hyperaroused rat would be much less keen to explore the novelty.

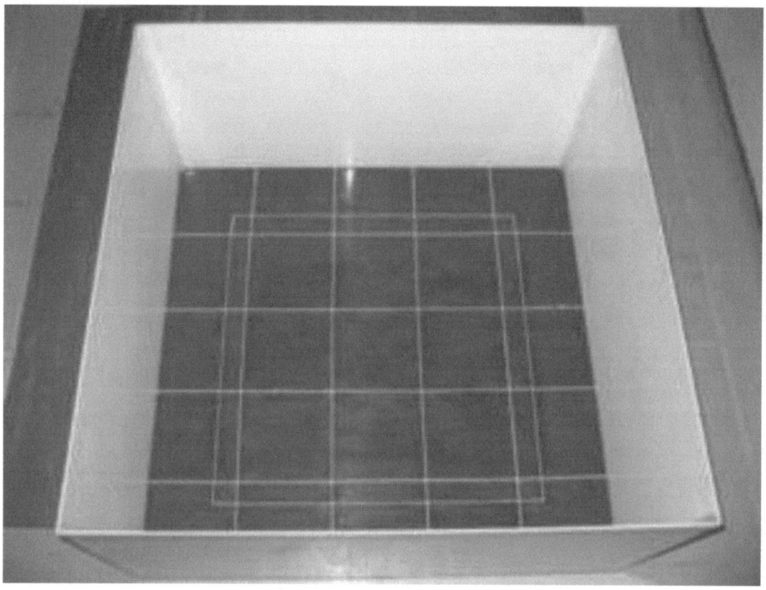

Figure 5. The open field test platform

The elevated plus maze test uses this same basic principle. The maze consist of a platform in the shape of a plus sign (+), with two opposite arms open (i.e. looking a bit like a diving platform) and the other arms closed along the sides. This platform is placed at a height of 0.5 m off the floor (Figure 6). Similar to the open field test, the rat is placed in the centre of the plus, and its courage to enter the open arms, *versus* the relatively safer closed arms (at least as perceived by a rodent), is assessed in terms of not only the number of times an open or closed arm is entered, but also the time spent in the respective arms, either moving about or sitting in one position, as well as the rat's aggressive (rearing) or self-soothing (grooming) behaviour while in the arms. In this way, a lot of data on behavioural changes may be generated, to use on its own, or to correlate with physiological data such as hormone levels. However, as with the open field test, the data is not easy to interpret. Therefore, again, no one measure should be considered as a stand-alone result.

It is of importance to note that the intervention protocol, or stress model used, may also dictate or limit the assessment techniques that are possible. Firstly, the behavioural tests are performed over the space of a few minutes. Therefore, if the investigation was related to the upstream stress responses to acute stress on the level of the brain, the physiological aspects of these responses need to be assessed immediately after exposure to the stressor. Doing a behavioural test first will result in central effects being missed, because the tissue sample will be collected too late. A suggestion to get around this is to perform the behavioural tests one day prior to the collection of tissue and blood samples for physiological and/or biochemical analyses. The use of appropriate control animals will prevent the behavioural tests from confounding results in such cases.

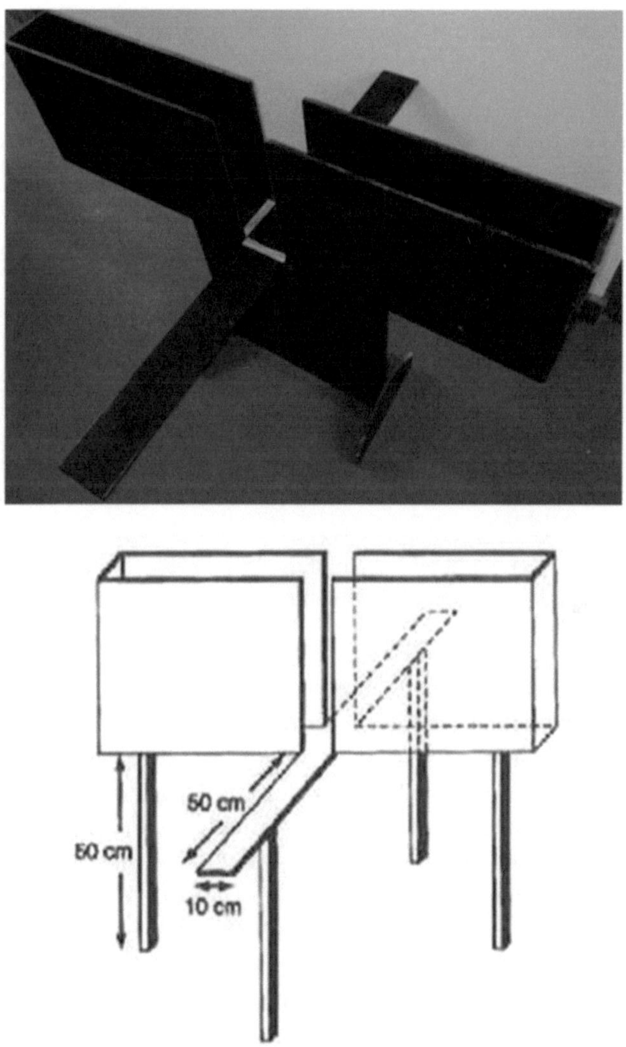

Figure 6. The elevated plus maze, with a technical drawing below to indicate dimensions.

Secondly, the type of stress intervention chosen may influence behaviour quite dramatically. For example, when considering the elevated plus maze, an anxious or stressed rat does not move about freely and would prefer the closed arms of the elevated plus maze, while an emotionally relaxed animal will exhibit more exploratory behaviour, and be more willing to enter and explore the open arms. However, when testing stressed or anxious behaviour in a rat that has just been restrained for an hour, the opposite effect is seen: an example of behavioural data illustrating this phenomenon in an elevated plus maze test is provided in Table 1. Data show that stressed rats chose to enter open arms more frequently than controls, which in this case may be interpreted as a counter reaction to having been confined to a small space during restraint. The latter explanation is very feasible, since the restraint stressed rats entered the closed arms less frequently than the controls. Although this decision would normally indicate a relaxed state, one has to keep in mind that the normally comforting closed arms would now resemble the restraint cage unit the rat had just "escaped" from, so that the rat, even though stressed, decided that the open arms are the safer option. The third parameter illustrated in Table 1, grooming, which is a self-soothing behaviour as stated earlier, clearly shows that despite the atypical result just described, the restrained rats were indeed stressed, since they spent more than four times as long trying to calm themselves than the control animals.

	Number of entries into open arms	Number of entries into closed arms	Time spent grooming (in seconds)
Control	4.3 ± 0.5	8.3 ± 0.7	11.3 ± 2.3
Stressed	5.9 ± 0.6*	6.1± 0.5*	49.8 ± 8.5**

Table 1. Selected parameters indicating behavioural responses to repeated restraint stress in male Wistar rats. Asterisks indicate values significantly different from controls (ANOVA with Bonferroni *post hoc* tests: *P<0.05; **P<0.001).

In terms of physiological assessment, stress can be assessed in terms of neuronal and endocrine pathways, as well as signalling proteins such as cytokines. Factors which may impact significantly on the quality of data is the method and timing of sacrifice and of sample collection. Recent studies on rodents commonly use intraperitoneal injection of a sodium pentabarbitone overdose. This is relatively painless and the animal loses consciousness fairly quickly. This method is also useful in the context of stress, with the exception of studies with the aim of investigating central changes. The reason for this is that the rodent will perceive the "loss of control" when losing consciousness, resulting in a central stress effect. While this effect may not reach downstream tissues in time to affect the outcome of analyses significantly, definite changes will be seen in the brain itself. Therefore, when conducting *in vivo* studies in the field of neurophysiology, it may be advisable to rather use cervical dislocation or decapitation techniques. The timing of sample a sample is of course vital. Sample collection for hormones should take into account diurnal variation in glucocorticoid levels, as discussed earlier. (For rodents, corticosterone is the glucocorticoid produced in highest quantities, whereas in humans it is cortisol.) For example, samples for determination of corticosterone levels should all be taken at the same time of day AND at the same period of recovery after the last stress exposure, so that the experiment may require quite a bit of logistical synchronisation. Also, the biological half-life of parameters of interest should be considered. For example, while corticosterone is a down-stream output of the stress pathways and has a relatively long half-life, ACTH is secreted fairly early in the stress response and has a half-life of less than 15 minutes, so that samples obtained at the end of a two-hour restraint protocol will probably not have detectable levels of ACTH, but sufficient corticosterone to be able to quantify the stress response. The design of stress protocols will therefore have different endpoints, depending on the aim of the investigation, for example a short restrain period may be more ideal for detection of upstream events in the stress pathways, while a longer one may be required for down-stream parameters to become available in circulation. Therefore, in order to time the sacrifice of an animal and collection of samples optimally, it is necessary to understand the basic biochemistry and/or pharmacology of parameters of interest.

In some instances it may be even more useful to determine down-stream effects related to earlier events, rather than trying to "catch" upstream parameters in circulation at an optimal time. This is also true when the parameter of interest can have its origin from more than one source. For example, when considering the inflammatory component of the response to stress – which has been linked to many chronic diseases recently – it is difficult to pinpoint the origin of cytokines when only assessed in blood, since most of them are released from a wide variety of cells. Also, since some cytokines, such as IL-6, have an autocrine-type action, its level in circulation is often not indicative of events at cellular level. In these instances, immunostaining of tissue levels of these parameters are very useful. Indirect measurements of e.g. inflammatory responses can also inform on the response to stress. For example, instead of measuring TNF-α levels in blood, activity of the proteolytic pathways in tissue may be employed as indirect indicator of TNF-α activity, which known to play an important role in muscle wasting, or cachexia. In this way, the timing of sampling become less critical, and the effect at the level of the target tissue, may be directly elucidated.

5. Characterisation and standardisation of stress models

The severity of the stressor will determine the extent of acute activation of the HPA-axis and/or SAM pathway, as well as the adaptability of the animal to the stressor, i.e. the chronic response to any particular stressor. This necessitates the standardisation and characterisation of any particular model by researchers prior to its application for research purposes. Our group have characterised our model of restraint stress in terms of a variety of parameters. One of these is the corticosterone response, which is presented for protocols of different durations in Figure 7.

This figure illustrates the significant difference in the response to a specific stressor acutely, and after chronic intermittent exposure, after which one may expect habituation to the stressor. One can see from these data that the stressor employed was indeed mild; although there was a substantial increase in corticosterone concentration in serum immediately after the restraint (at the "acute" time point), the rat was able to completely recover its corticosterone levels to control levels one day after the single restraint session. The data further indicates the effectiveness of this model to induce chronic stress: the value labelled "4 days" indicates that 3 restraint stress sessions over 3 days resulted in a corticosterone response that the rats could not completely recover from overnight, resulting in a significantly elevated corticosterone level even after a period of recovery, albeit not as highly elevated as in the acute version of the model.

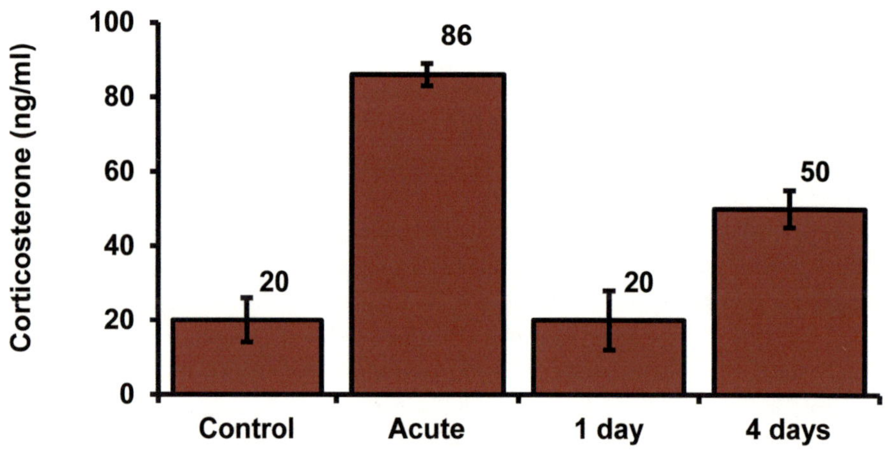

Figure 7. Corticosterone responses to one hour of restraint stress daily, for protocols of different durations. Values are means for at least n=10 rats per experimental group.

However, as discussed earlier, these results in its entirety will probably only be valid for the model as executed in our hands. Although the same trend should be seen – e.g. the increased corticosterone levels in stressed rats – the magnitude of this response as well as the animal's ability to habituate to it, is largely dependent on the execution of the model by various research groups, who each adapts the protocol to be best suited for their own particular research interests. Therefore, it is vital to include sufficient control groups for all interventions, in order to facilitate cross-group comparisons of results.

6. Conclusion

Conducting research using experimental animal models is a complex endeavour, with many considerations, adaptations to make and precautions to take. However, when applied by researchers with the ability to adapt a protocol to make the most of it, results achieved are very satisfactory in terms of quality, repeatability and direct applicability to actual physiological situations. Therefore, in conclusion, cell-based scientists and systems biologists should combine efforts to successfully counter the effects of stress.

Author details

Carine Smith
Stellenbosch University, South Africa

Acknowledgement

I would like to acknowledge all the postgraduate students and collaborators of the Interdisciplinary Stress Biology Group at the Department Physiological Sciences at Stellenbosch University, South Africa, who contributed to the experience gained and lessons learnt through working in rodent models of stress.

7. References

Allen C and Kendall JW (2005) Maturation of the circadian rhythm of plasma corticosterone in the rat. *Endocrinology* 80 (5): 926-930.

Christiansen S, Bouzinova EV, Palme R, Wiborg O (2012) Circadian activity of the hypothalamic-pituitary-adrenal axis is differentially affected in the rat chronic mild stress model of depression. *Stress* (epub Feb 23) PMID 22217141.

Ellenbroek BA, Geven EJ, Cools AR (2005) Rat Strain Differences in Stress Sensitivity, In: *Handbook of Stress and the Brain,* volume 15, chapter 14, Steckler T, Kalin NH, Reul JMHM, Elsevier B.V.

Garcia A, Marti O, Valles A, Dal-Zotto S, Armario A (2000) Recovery of the Hypothalamic-pituitary-adrenal Response to Stress. Effect of Stress Intensity, Stress Duration and Previous Stress Exposure. *Neuroendocrinology* 72(2): 114-125.

Gomez F, Lahmane A, de Kloet ER, Armario A (1996) Hypothalamic-pituitary-adrenal Response to Chronic Stress in Five Inbred Rat Strains: Differential Responses are Mainly Located at the Adrenocortical Level. *Neuroendocrinology* 63(4):327-337.

Hashimoto M, Kuwahara M, Tsubone H, Sugano S (1999) Diurnal Variation of Autonomic Nervous Activity in the Rat. *Journal of Electrocardiology* 32(2):167-171.

Miki S and Sudo A (1996) Adaptation of circadian corticosterone and catecholamine rhythms to light-dark cycle reversal in the rat. *Industrial Health* 34: 134-138.

Selye H. (1956). *The Stress of Life*, McGrawHill, New York. (Revised edition: 1976)

Sharp J, Zammit T, Azar T, L. Dawson D (2002) Does Witnessing Experimental Procedures Produce Stress in Male Rats? *Contemp Top Lab Anim Sci* 41: 8 -12.

Section 3

Glucocorticoids in Metabolism and Energy Cycling

Chapter 11

Novel Aspects of Glucocorticoids Actions on Energy Homeostasis and Hydromineral Balance

Silvia Graciela Ruginsk, Rodrigo Cesar Rorato,
Beatriz de Carvalho Borges, Ernane Torres Uchoa,
Lucila Leico Kagohara Elias and Jose Antunes-Rodrigues

Additional information is available at the end of the chapter

http://dx.doi.org/10.5772/53266

1. Introduction

Glucocorticoids can readily diffuse into the cells due to their lipophilic nature and bind to glucocorticoid (GR) and mineralocorticoid (MR) receptors, which, in the inactive form, are associated with other proteins in the cytosol. MR was shown to bind most of the glucocorticoids under basal conditions. However, after an increase in the circulating levels of glucocorticoids (i.e. caused by exposure to stress or during the circadian and ultradian peaks of glucocorticoid secretion) GRs are predominantly activated (de Kloet et al., 2005). The activated receptor undergoes conformational changes followed by the translocation of the ligand-bound complex to the nucleus. Within this subcellular compartment, this complex can form homo or heterodimers and bind to responsive elements (GREs) in the promoter region of target genes, a mechanism known as transactivation, or interact with transcription factors as monomers to modulate the transcription of responsive genes, a mechanism known as transrepression. The main transcriptional factors involved in these responses are the nuclear factor kappa B (NFκB) and the AP-1 protein family.

More recently, it has been suggested that nontranscriptional actions may account for the very rapid effects observed with acute glucocorticoid treatment (Limbourg & Liao, 2003). These actions differ from the classic genomic responses by the targets, type of interaction and period of action, being detected within few minutes after hormone secretion (Mikics et al., 2004; Sandi et al., 1996). The administration of high doses of dexamethasone was shown to protect the myocardial tissue from infarction and stroke through the prompt activation of endothelial nitric oxide (NO) system (Hafezi-Moghadam et al., 2002). During the 1990's, NO has been identified as a potent vasodilatatory gas. Its properties in decreasing blood pressure are still clinically explored by the use of NO donors as anti-hypertensive drugs.

More recently, NO has also been implicated in neuromodulation, exerting its actions in an autocrine or paracrine manner in the central nervous system (CNS).

In general, these rapid effects mediated by glucocorticoids seem to modulate signaling (through actions on ion channels, neuromodulators, neurotransmitters and other receptors systems), being very distinctive depending on the brain areas involved. It is generally accepted that glucocorticoids increase the excitability in some areas, like hippocampus and amygdala, and potentially decrease neuronal activity in others, such as the hypothalamus. Since the expression of glucocorticoid receptors vary considerably in the CNS, glucocorticoids are likely to modulate not only the activity of the hypothalamic-pituitary-adrenal (HPA) axis, but also indirectly modify the inputs to hypothalamic neurons, projecting from the limbic system and cerebral cortex.

The classic glucocorticoid receptors GR and MR have already been identified in neuronal and non-neuronal cellular membranes, although their involvement in these nongenomic responses is still controversial (Gametchu et al., 1993; Lipositis & Bohn, 1993). In pituitary-derived cells, the use of a GR antagonist prevented the dexamethasone-induced translocation of annexin-1, which was implicated in the rapid inhibition of adrenocorticotrophic hormone (ACTH) release (Buckingham et al., 2003; Solito et al., 2003; Tierney et al., 2003). Nevertheless, a GR-independent pathway has been also reported in the fast feedback mechanism at the pituitary level *in vivo* (Hinz & Hirschelmann, 2000).

Another line of evidence suggests that most of nongenomic responses are mediated by the glucocorticoid binding to G-coupled protein receptors (Liu & Chen, 1995; Orchinik et al., 1991). In tumor-derived cells, a receptor coupled to an inhibitory G-protein (Gi) has been implicated in the glucocorticoid-induced inhibition of ACTH release (Iwasaki et al., 1997). In the hypothalamus, however, the production and release of neuromodulators (endocannabinoids and NO) seem to be driven by the activation of a membrane receptor associated with a stimulatory G-protein (Gs) (Di et al., 2009). Endocannabinoids were shown to mediate most of the nongenomic actions of the glucocorticoids, including the rapid negative feedback on the HPA axis (Evanson et al., 2010). Accordingly, several signaling pathways have been implicated in the responses induced by glucocorticoids downstream from the putative membrane receptors, mainly including protein kinase A (PKA)- and protein kinase C (PKC)-derived mechanisms (Han et al., 2002, 2005; Lou & Chen, 1998; Qiu et al, 1998, 2003).

2. Glucocorticoids and energy balance

2.1. The control of food intake by glucocorticoids: novel aspects

The motivated behaviour of eating comprises one of the most primordial responses in all species. It is regulated by several factors, including adiposity (leptin and insulin) and satiety signals (such as mechanical and chemical stimulation of stomach and small intestine), as well as hormones [such as cholecystokinin (CCK)] (Schwartz et al., 2000). The adiposity factors are involved in the long-term control of energy balance and act primarily in hypothalamic neurons expressing orexigenic or anorexigenic neuropeptides (Schwartz et al., 2000). Neuropeptide Y (NPY) and agouti related protein (AgRP) in the arcuate nucleus of the hypothalamus (ARC), and orexins and melanin-concentrating hormone (MCH) in the lateral hypothalamic area (LHA), represent the main hypothalamic orexigenic neuropeptides (Gehlert, 1999; Smith & Ferguson, 2008; Valassi et al., 2008). In contrast, proopiomelanocortin (POMC) and cocaine and amphetamine-regulated transcript (CART) in the ARC, and corticotrophin-releasing factor (CRF) and oxytocin (OT) in the paraventricular nucleus of the hypothalamus (PVN) are the main mediators involved in the inhibition of food intake (Schwartz et al., 2000; Valassi et al., 2008). The localization of the above mentioned neuropeptides in hypothalamic nuclei is summarized in Table 1. The satiety signals, in turn, are implicated in the short-term control of food intake and have their actions mediated by brainstem areas, primarily by the nucleus of the solitary tract (NTS), which is implicated in the control of meal size (Havel, 2001). It is well established that the hypothalamic nuclei involved in the control of food intake have reciprocal connections with the brainstem (Sawchenko & Swanson, 1982; Swanson & Kuypers, 1980). This evidence provides the neuroanatomical basis for the hypothesis that adiposity signals may modulate satiety (Matson & Ritter, 1999; Wang et al., 2000).

Neuropeptides	Localization in the hypothalamus
NPY	ARC
AgRP	ARC
Orexins	LHA and PFA
MCH	LHA
POMC	ARC
CART	ARC, PVN and SON
CRF	PVN
OT	PVN and SON

Table 1. Hypothalamic localization of the neuropeptides involved in the control of food intake. NPY, neuropeptide Y; ARC, arcuate nucleus of the hypothalamus; AgRP, agouti related protein; LHA, lateral hypothalamic area; PFA, perifornical area; MCH, melanin-concentrating hormone; POMC, proopiomelanocortin; CART, cocaine and amphetamine-regulated transcript; PVN, paraventricular nucleus of the hypothalamus; SON, supraoptic nucleus of the hypothalamus; CRF, corticotrophin-releasing factor; OT, oxytocin.

Glucocorticoids play an important role in the control of energy balance (La Fleur, 2006). It is well established that a peak in the concentration of glucocorticoids occurs immediately before or at the onset of the activity period, with a progressive decrease in the HPA axis activity being detected over the remaining period within 24 hours, resulting in the classic circadian rhythm (Moreira & Leal, 1997). In addition, this rhythm occurs due to glucocorticoids release from the adrenal gland in discrete pulses, which results in an ultradian rhythm. Changes in the amplitude of these pulses, and to a lesser extent in their frequency, determine the pattern of the circadian rhythm (Lightman et al., 2008). In fact, it has been also demonstrated that feeding is a major synchronizer of the HPA axis rhythmicity (Leal & Moreira, 1997), being the size of the meal directly related to glucocorticoid secretion (Honma et al., 1983). At the same time, increased food intake and body weight gain have been observed in humans following glucocorticoid treatment (Tataranni et al., 1996). Stress conditions, characterized by elevated circulating glucocorticoids levels, are also associated with increased food intake, body weight gain and obesity (Dallman et al., 2003; La Fleur, 2006; Spencer & Tilbrook, 2011).

Consistent with the importance of glucocorticoids on energy homeostasis are two very prevalent clinical conditions: 1) Cushing's syndrome, which is characterized by clinical findings that include abnormalities in the HPA axis rhythmicity, insulin resistance and hyperglycaemia secondary to hypercortisolism. The most common cause of Cushing's syndrome is the administration of pharmacological doses of oral, parenteral and, rarely, by topical glucocorticoids. Endogenous glucocorticoid excess may arise from ACTH–secreting pituitary tumors, ectopic (nonpituitary) ACTH production, or adrenal tumors. Hypercortisolaemia is associated with increased glucose production, decreased glucose transport and utilization, decreased protein synthesis, increased protein degradation in muscle and body weight gain (Nieuwenhuizen & Rutters, 2008; Shibli-Rahhal et al., 2006); (2) Addison's disease or primary adrenal insufficiency, first described by Addison in 1855, is characterized by an inability of the adrenal cortex to synthesize and secrete glucocorticoids and mineralocorticoids. Chronically, the main clinical findings observed in patients with Addison's disease include malaise, fatigue, anorexia, weight loss, darkening of the skin, hyponatraemia, hypoglycaemia and hyperkalaemia (Nieman and Chanco Turner, 2006).

It has been shown that the effects of glucocorticoids on food intake can vary according to their concentration in the circulation (Devenport et al., 1989). Low doses of corticosterone administered to adrenalectomized (ADX) rats activate MR and induce a stimulatory effect on fat intake, body weight gain and fat depot, being these effects prevalent at the late phase of the feeding period, the same period in which HPA axis activity is reduced during the circadian variation (Tempel & Leibowitz, 1994, 1989; Tempel et al., 1991). In contrast, GRs are activated by higher doses of circulating corticosterone, being this effect observed just before or at the first hours after the beginning of the feeding period, mimicking the peak of glucocorticoids secretion within the 24 hours of circadian rhythm. Such high levels of circulating glucocorticoids produce an increase in carbohydrate ingestion and metabolism (Goldstein et al., 1993; Kumar & Leibowitz, 1988; Kumar et al., 1988; Tempel & Leibowitz, 1994, 1989; Tempel et al., 1993). In addition, extremely high corticosterone plasma concentrations, such as those observed in response to stress or food restriction, stimulate fat and protein catabolism (mainly from muscular source) and, consequently, body weight loss, which increases the availability of gluconeogenesis substrates and enhances glucose plasma concentrations (Tempel & Leibowitz, 1994; Tomas et al., 1979).

Historically, the brain has been considered the main regulator of hunger and satiety. However, the existence of a unique hypothalamic satiety or hunger center, as proposed a few decades ago, is no longer acceptable. It has been demonstrated that dexamethasone injection into the lateral ventricle not only stimulates food intake but also enhances body weight gain in rats, being these effects accompanied by hyperleptinaemia and hyperinsulinaemia (Cusin et al., 2001; Zakrzewska et al., 1999). These central effects of glucocorticoids seem to be mediated by their interaction with neurons co-expressing glucocorticoid receptors and neuropeptides involved in the control of energy homeostasis (Aronsson et al., 1988; Hisano et al., 1988). This hypothesis has been evaluated by Zakrzewska and co-workers (1999), who demonstrated that the hypothalamic levels of NPY and CRF were, respectively, increased and decreased in response to the intracerebroventricular administration of dexamethasone. In addition, circulating glucocorticoids were shown to be required for the feeding-induced decrease in the expression of orexigenic neuropeptides in the ARC, as well as for the increased expression of the anorexigenic neuropeptide POMC in the same nucleus (Uchoa et al., 2012). It has been hypothesized by these authors that these effects would occur either by a direct effect of glucocorticoids on ARC neurons or indirectly by the feeding-induced secretion of leptin and insulin.

The removal of endogenous glucocorticoids induced by bilateral ADX surgery is one of the most used experimental models for replicating the human Addison's disease. The food intake and body weight gain are reduced in ADX animals, being these effects reversed by glucocorticoid replacement (Freedman et al., 1985; Uchoa et al., 2009a, 2009b, 2010). Furthermore, ADX is effective in diminishing hyperphagia and obesity under diverse experimental conditions (Bruce et al., 1982; Dubuc and Wilden, 1986; Yukimura et al., 1978). The ADX-induced hypophagia has been associated with a decrease of hypothalamic NPY and AgRP mRNA expression (Strack et al., 1995; Uchoa et al., 2012). Conversely, ADX induces an increase in the expression of CRF and OT in PVN (Uchoa et al., 2009b and 2010). The actions on these two peptides in the control of food intake were confirmed by the central administration of OT and CRF-2 receptor antagonists, which were able to reverse the ADX-induced hypophagic effect (Uchoa et al., 2009b and 2010).

It has been hypothesized that the stimulatory action of glucocorticoids on food intake may involve an increased drive for eating. Accordingly, it is believed that the ADX-induced hypophagia is caused, at least in part, by a reduction of this motivated behaviour. However, there are few evidences concerning the role of glucocorticoids on the satiety-related responses. Recent studies have demonstrated that the hypophagic response induced by ADX is associated with increased activation of satiety-related responses mediated by brainstem and hypothalamic circuits (Uchoa et al., 2009a, 2009b). Accordingly, the activation of NTS neurons, assessed by the increased number of cells expressing the nuclear c-Fos protein, is increased in ADX animals after feeding, indicating that this nucleus may be involved in the increased satiety responses following glucocorticoid deficiency (Uchoa et al., 2009a). Interestingly, the activation of CRF and OT neurons was also enhanced in the PVN of fed ADX rats, indicating that, besides the brainstem, the hypothalamus may be also involved in these satiety-related responses. Furthermore, this increased activation of satiety-related responses in the NTS following ADX is reversed by CRF_2 receptor antagonist, indicating that CRF also plays an important functional neuromodulatory role in the brainstem (Uchoa et al., 2010).

In addition to the reduced drive to eat and the increased satiety observed in ADX animals, a change in both the concentration as well as in the sensitivity to peripheral factors seems to underlie the hypophagic effect of glucocorticoid deficiency. Accordingly, ADX reduces plasma leptin levels in *ad libitum* rats (Germano et al., 2007; Savontaus et al., 2002), as well as the meal-induced insulin secretion (Germano et al., 2008; Uchoa et al., 2012), whereas glucocorticoid treatment increases leptin secretion and leptin expression in adipocytes (Jahng et al., 2008; Slieker et al., 1996; Zakrzewska et al., 1999). Furthermore, the sensitivity to insulin and leptin seems to be enhanced after ADX (Chavez et al., 1997; Zakrzewska et al., 1997), although CCK administration did not significantly alter food intake in ADX rats (Uchoa et al, 2009a). Another hormone that arises as a candidate for the modulation by glucocorticoids is ghrelin, although the effects of this hormone on food intake may also be produced independently of glucocorticoid action.

The physiological instinct of obtaining energy through food intake is parallel to the equally important development of satiation signals, which may terminate the ingestive behaviour as soon as the organism is replenished. Glucocorticoids have a well established role in both processes, contributing to the enhanced drive to eat as well as to the reduction of satiety-related responses. However, it is believed that, particularly in humans, the initiation of a meal often starts in the absence of any depletion signal, which means that it is possible for other brain areas such as the cortex and the limbic system to overcome the inputs coming from the hypothalamus and the brainstem, turning the organism into an ingestive mode, which actually exceeds its needs. Accordingly, both real and potential challenges that activate the HPA axis and, consequently, alter the secretion of glucocorticoids, may also disrupt this balance.

2.2. Glucocorticoids in the interface of immune challenges and food intake

Under acute immune challenges, the body produces a strong inflammatory response to the pathogens. This generalized reaction, triggered by the organism in order to safeguard the host homeostasis, comprises physiological and behavioural changes (Langhans, 2000). However, in a severe condition in which the overwhelming infection leads to life-threatening low blood pressure and decreased tissue perfusion, a medical emergency known as septic shock may contribute to organ damage and death. Microbial products such as lipopolisaccharides (LPS) from the outer lipid bilayer of gram-negative bacteria cell walls are commonly used to model acute illness, leading to the development of sepsis or endotoxaemia, depending on the dose of the endotoxin (Borges et al., 2007; 2011; Giusti-Paiva et al., 2002).

Hypophagia is part of the acute-phase response to illness. During endotoxaemia, food intake is limited and there is an impairment of energy expenditure. Experimental models have demonstrated that LPS dramatically reduces food consumption (Gautron et al., 2005; Sachot et al., 2004), being this hypophagic effect mainly elicited by the production of proinflammatory cytokines (Johnson, 1998; Wise et al., 2006). Consistent with the contribution of proinflammatory cytokines to this illness-induced hypophagia are the studies showing that their peripheral or central administration restrains eating, and that the acute antagonism of their actions attenuates this anorexic response (Asarian & Langhans, 2010).

The systemic administration of LPS triggers the synthesis and release of interleukin (IL)-1β, IL-6 and tumor necrosis factor (TNF)-α by monocytes and macrophages. In turn, these cytokines can exert local actions as signaling molecules to activate the immune system and the HPA axis (Turnbull and Rivier, 1999; Turnbull et al., 1998). Accordingly, it has been demonstrated that cytokines induce intense nuclear c-Fos immunoreactivity in CRF parvocellular neurons of the PVN (Matsunaga et al., 2000). Endotoxin also increases CRF synthesis and secretion, stimulating ACTH release from the pituitary corticotrophs and, consequently, the secretion of glucocorticoids from the adrenal cortex (Borges et al., 2007; Turnbull & Rivier, 1999). In turn, glucocorticoids inhibit the induction of proinflammatory cytokines, mostly by interacting with the intracellular GR, which culminates with the activation of NFκB and AP-1 (Jonat et al., 1990; Munoz et al., 1996). After glucocorticoid binding to the cytosolic GR, the activated complex is translocated to the cell nucleus, where it interacts with the specific transcription factors AP-1 and NF-κB and prevents the transcription of targeted genes, in a process called transrepression. Glucocorticoids are able to prevent the transcription of many inflammation-associated genes, such as those ones encoding cytokines, including interleukins IL-1B, IL-4, IL-5 and IL-8, chemokines, arachidonic acid metabolites and adhesion molecules. The immunosuppressant action exerted by glucocorticoids may be also evidenced by the increased hypothalamic messenger RNA (mRNA) expression of cytokines and IL-1β plasma levels observed in response to LPS administration to ADX rats (Goujon et al., 1996).

Within this context, glucocorticoids appear as crucial hormones involved in the mobilization of stored peripheral energy, directing the metabolism to the production of key substrates utilized by the liver to sustain gluconeogenesis. Studies performed in rats show that the search and consumption of palatable foods are stimulated by corticosterone in a dose-related fashion (Dallman et al., 2007). Accordingly, these authors have also demonstrated that ADX rats exhibit poor weight gain, low fat content and increased sympathetic and HPA axis outflow, effects that are, in general, reversed by replacement with corticosterone. The removal of the negative feedback exerted by glucocorticoids in ADX animals has been also implicated in the increased expression of CRF mRNA in the PVN (Herman & Morrison, 1996; Rorato et al., 2008). In addition to its essential function in the control of HPA axis activity, CRF also has a physiological role in the control of food intake, as evidenced by the anorexigenic response induced by central administration of CRF and CRF-related peptides to experimental animals (Kalra et al., 1999; Richard et al., 2002), as previously discussed in this chapter. Furthermore, the use of a CRF receptor antagonist partially reverses the reduction in food intake induced by different stress paradigms (Hotta et al., 1999; Krahn et al., 1986). Accordingly, Borges and coworkers (2007) observed that increased CRF mRNA expression in the PVN precedes LPS-induced anorexia. Hence, an interchange between feeding control and HPA axis activity is conceivable to operate in basal conditions as well as following an immune challenge.

Recently, Saito and Watanabe (2008) have described that dexamethasone treatment attenuates the production of multiple proinflammatory cytokines by the brain and liver, suggesting a potential preventive effect of glucocorticoids on the LPS-induced hypophagia.

Furthermore, Rorato and coworkers (2008) reported that the anorexigenic effect induced by LPS is amplified in ADX rats and that the ADX-induced glucocorticoid deficiency promotes an increased activation of hypothalamic CRF and POMC neurons. It has been already demonstrated that the activation of POMC neurons promotes the release of α-melanocyte stimulating hormone (α-MSH), which, in turn, activates melanocortin 4 receptor (MC4R) (Cone, 2005). Melanocortin has been also implicated in the LPS-induced hypophagia, since the administration of exogenous α-MSH intensified, whereas the antagonism of MC4R attenuated the inhibitory effect of LPS on food intake (Fan et al., 1997; Huang et al., 1999). Within this context, glucocorticoids appear as negative regulators of melanocortin signaling, since ADX was shown not only to reduce AgRP expression in the hypothalamus of wild type mice, but also to reverse obese phenotype and restore hypothalamic melanocortin tone to control levels in leptin-deficient *ob/ob* mice (Makimura et al., 2000).

A growing body of evidence has recently linked obesity to a chronic low-grade inflammatory state (Paternain et al., 2011; Trayhurn & Wood, 2005). In fact, inflammation may contribute to a range of metabolic disturbances related to obesity, such as diabetes mellitus and cardiovascular diseases (Oren et al., 2007). Rats fed with high-fat diet express high levels of TNF-α, IL-6 and IL-1β in the hypothalamus, which is consistent with the development of an inflammatory process (Milanski et al., 2009). Cani and coworkers (2007) have demonstrated that endotoxaemia dysregulates the inflammatory tone and induces body weight gain and diabetes in mice, showing that a 4-week high-fat diet induced a two to three-fold increase in plasma LPS concentrations. The bacterial endotoxin is normally present in the human intestinal tract (Kelly et al., 2012). Accordingly, LPS is detectable in the circulation of both healthy and obese individuals, but it may transiently raises following energy-rich meals. It has also been shown that the intake of fat-rich diet acts as an inducer of chronic stress, elevating basal glucocorticoid levels and enhancing HPA axis responses to stress (Tannenbaum et al., 1997), suggesting that glucocorticoids are likely to participate in the pathogenesis of metabolic syndrome and obesity (Milagro et al., 2007; Paternain et al., 2011), even though obese individuals and patients with metabolic syndrome do not necessarily show elevated systemic glucocorticoid concentrations (Pereira et al., 2012).

In face of these findings, efforts are now being turned to clarify the significance of glucocorticoids in counteracting the pathophysiology of illness-induced hypophagia. The better understanding of these processes may place glucocorticoids as important pharmacological targets to deal with obesity and metabolic syndrome, in which inflammatory modulators seem to play a key role.

3. Endocannabinoids as potential intermediates of glucocorticoids actions

3.1. Endocannabinoids: general aspects

The pharmacological properties of the plant *Cannabis sativa* are knwon since ancient times. The first cannabinoid receptor (CB1R) was characterized in 1988 and its predominant distribution through the CNS initially suggested a relationship with the control of cognitive function. However, over the past few years, the number of studies investigating the participation of CB1R in several areas has increased dramatically. Pioneer studies revealed that the exogenous administration of "cannabis-like" compounds inhibits the activity of diverse neuroendocrine functions (Lomax, 1970; Rettori et al., 1990; Tyrey, 1978). Accordingly, it has been demonstrated that the mRNA for the CB1R is expressed in the hypothalamus and in the external layer of the median eminence of rodents (Herkenham et al., 1991; Wittmann et al., 2007), as well as in both the anterior and intermediate lobes of the human pituitary gland (Pagotto et al., 2001). The evidence of the local production of endocannabinoids provided by this later group further suggested a role for these substances on the direct control of pituitary function.

In this context, the CB1R has been implicated in most, if not all, the actions of endogenously produced cannabinoids in neurotransmission. It has been also demonstrated that hippocampal astrocytes functionally express the CB1R and respond with elevations in intracellular calcium concentrations to the stimulation by neurotransmitters released locally from neuronal sources (Navarrete & Araque, 2008). This evidence suggests that non-neuronal populations can also contribute to the complexity of the responses elicited by endocannabinoids within the CNS. Differently from CB1R, the second cannabinoid receptor (CB2R) was identified in immune cells, being predominantly distributed in the peripheral organs, but not restricted to them. Most of the actions of the endocannabinoid system are mediated by the interaction of endogenous ligands with CB1R or CB2R, although the precise actions of orphan receptors, such as GPR55, still remain to be elucidated.

The identification of this receptor system, as well as the description of well-known effects induced by the consumption or administration of "cannabis-like" substances in humans, suggested the existence of endogenous ligands to be discovered. Anandamide (AEA) was the first one, followed by 2-araquidonoilglicerol (2-AG), the main endocannabinoids studied so far. AEA binds to CB1R with high affinity and regulates the signaling cascade as a partial agonist (Bouaboula et al., 1995). On the other hand, 2-AG, besides being the most abundant endocannabinoid produced by the CNS, has a lower affinity for CB1R when compared to AEA but stimulates the intracellular signaling pathway as a full agonist (Mechoulam et al., 1995). Both AEA and 2-AG are synthesized on demand from membrane phospholipids after the activation of membrane-associated glucocorticoid receptors. AEA and 2-AG are also metabolized by independent enzymatic pathways (Freund et al., 2003). Indeed, AEA acts as a very promiscuous ligand, since it can also bind to type 1 vanilloid (TRPV1) receptors with high affinity (Tóth et al., 2005). Accordingly, some of the effects induced by AEA cannot be mimicked by the administration of the synthetic cannabinoid agonist WIN55,212-2 (Al-Hayani et al., 2001) and the well-known AEA-induced antinociception is still preserved in experimental animals lacking the CB1R gene (Di Marzo et al., 2000).

3.2. Endocannabinoids and the ingestive behaviour

3.2.1. Food intake

It has been demonstrated that glucocorticoids increase endocannabinoid levels in hypothalamic PVN slices, supporting the hypothesis that at least part of the effects induced by glucocorticoids on food intake are mediated by these lipid-derived mediators (Malcher-Lopes et al., 2006). In this study, Malcher-Lopes and colleagues also demonstrated that the glucocorticoid-mediated activation of a membrane receptor coupled to a $G\alpha_s$–cAMP–PKA signaling cascade leads to an increase in endocannabinoid synthesis. Accordingly, increased hypothalamic levels of endocannabinoids have been also observed *in vivo* following glucocorticoid treatment (Hill et al., 2010).

Both endocannabinoids and glucocorticoids injected into hypothalamic areas induce similar effects on eating behaviour, increasing food consumption (Jamshidi & Taylor, 2001; Tempel et al., 1992). The synthesis of endocannabinoids in the hypothalamus and the expression of both endocannabinoids and glucocorticoid receptors in synapses and in hypothalamic neurons that synthesize peptides with a key role in food consumption reinforce this assumption (Castelli et al., 2007; Cota et al., 2003; Deli et al. 2009; Di Marzo et al., 2001; Malcher-Lopes et al., 2006). In fact, the neuropeptides CRF, OT and TRH, which have well described anorexigenic properties (Arletti et al., 1989, 1990; Morley et al., 1983; Steward et al., 2003), appear as potential targets for endocannabinoid-mediated actions induced by glucocorticoids. Therefore, the glucocorticoid-mediated blockade of excitatory glutamatergic synapses induced by endocannabinoids via CB1R has been already described in CRF, OT and TRH hypothalamic neurons (Di et al., 2003).

Although feeding is one of the main synchronizers of the HPA axis activity and both the endocannabinoid system and glucocorticoids seem to drive the organism into an increased ingestive behaviour under physiological conditions, several studies reported both stimulatory and inhibitory roles for endocannabinoids in the control of stress responses. In the experiments conducted by Patel and co-workers (2004), mice pretreated with a CB1R antagonist exhibited a robust increase in the restraint-induced glucocorticoid release and c-Fos immunolabeling in the PVN. In addition, the administration of a CB1R agonist, an inhibitor of endocannabinoid transport or a FAAH inhibitor attenuated the restraint-induced increase in glucocorticoid secretion. Although these authors hypothesized that the activation of endogenous CB1R may negatively modulate the HPA axis activity, they also demonstrated that the hypothalamic contents of 2-AG were, respectively, decreased and enhanced after acute and sustained stress. This finding is not consistent with an endocannabinoid-mediated inhibition of the HPA axis activity, but rather indicates that glucocorticoids may centrally inhibit the production of endocannabinoids. Similar results were obtained by Borges and colleagues (2011), who reported decreased hypothalamic 2-AG contents after acute LPS administration. Additionally, increased CRF mRNA expression, glucocorticoid plasma concentrations and hypophagia were found by this group in experimental animals submitted to a single LPS injection, being all these responses completely restored to basal levels following repeated LPS administration.

Conversely, an increase in hypothalamic 2-AG levels after acute restraint stress has also been recently reported (Evanson et al., 2010). According to these findings, these authors proposed that the CB1R-mediated signaling is required for glucocorticoid negative feedback, but not for the initial HPA axis response to restraint. In addition, a down-regulation of CB1R and an impaired glucocorticoid-mediated inhibition of excitatory inputs to parvocellular PVN neurons were observed in hypothalamic slices from rats submitted to repeated immobilization stress (Wamsteeker et al., 2010). Interestingly, application of a CB1R agonist to the bath did not suppress the excitatory inputs onto PVN neurons, suggesting that the CB1R-mediated signaling may be disrupted after prolonged exposure to stress. It has been recently reported by our group that the pharmacological blockade of the CB1R-mediated signaling during LPS-induced endotoxaemia produces a remarkable increase in the activation of CRF neurons in the parvocellular subdivision of the PVN, which is associated with a pronounced hypophagia (Rorato et al., 2011). Although further studies are needed to clarify the precise actions of endocannabinoids on stress responses, the majority of studies suggest that the endocannabinoid system may mediate the fast negative feedback exerted by glucocorticoids at both hypothalamic and pituitary levels, avoiding the overloading of this system and making it continuously responsive to other potential challenges.

It has been also observed that the peripheral nutrition-related hormone leptin reverses the increases in PVN endocannabinoid levels induced by glucocorticoids, indicating a central crosstalk between glucocorticoids and this satiety signal (Malcher-Lopes et al., 2006). In fact, Obese Zucker rats, which do not express leptin receptors, are hyperphagic and exhibit elevated glucocorticoid plasma levels (Ahima, 2000; Freedman et al., 1985) and increased hypothalamic levels of endocannabinoids (Di Marzo et al., 2001; Kirkham et al., 2002). Within this context, the study of the CB1R-mediated signaling has a great clinical relevance and expectation, since obesity is emerging as a very concerning heath problem worldwide, either considered alone or in association with other chronic degenerative diseases. Accordingly, an increasing number of recent studies have focused on the glucocorticoid-related effects mediated by CB1R, such as the central control of food consumption (Di Marzo et al., 2001) and satiety (Matias & Di Marzo, 2007), as well as the peripheral control of adiposity, a predictor of several chronic metabolic disorders (Westerink & Visseren, 2011).

Although the endocannabinoid system has been implicated in several physiological and pathological functions related to the control of food intake and body weight by glucocorticoids (Ameri, 1999; Bisogno et al., 2005; Di Marzo & Matias, 2005; Marco et al., 2011), it has been also demonstrated that these lipid-derived mediators can act independently of the glucocorticoid-mediated signalling (Jamshidi & Taylor, 2001; Kirkham & Williams, 2001; Williams & Kirkham, 1999; Williams et al. 1998). Most of these effects are also mediated by the activation of the CB1R, since the administration of the CB1R antagonist rimonabant reverses the cannabinoid-induced increase in food intake (Jamshidi & Taylor, 2001; Williams & Kirkham, 2002). Consistent with the CB1R-mediated orexigenic effects of endocannabinoids, transgenic mice that lack this receptor subtype or experimental animals treated with the CB1R antagonist exhibit decreased food consumption (Colombo et al. 1998; Di Marzo et al. 2001; Pertwee, 2005).

This rimonabant-induced decrease in food intake is, at least in part, mediated by changes in endocannabinoid signalling within the hypothalamus (Cota et al., 2003; Mailleux & Vanderhaeghen, 1992; Marsicano & Lutz, 1999). It has been already reported that the CB1R is co-expressed with several anorexigenic peptides such as CART and CRF (Asakawa et al.,

2001; Cota et al., 2003; Füzesi et al., 2008; Morley et al., 1983; Vrang et al., 2000). Accordingly, CB1R knockout mice exhibit increased CRF mRNA expression in the PVN (Cota et al., 2003). It has been also demonstrated that acute rimonabant treatment induces an increase in the co-localization of c-Fos with CART in the PVN and ARC and with POMC in the ARC, as well as promotes a decrease in both the protein and the mRNA for NPY in the ARC (Verty et al., 2009a). Conversely, no changes in NPY or POMC mRNA expression were found in the ARC of lean rats treated with rimonabant (Doyon et al., 2006), although the administration of AM251, a selective CB1R antagonist, blocked NPY release from hypothalamic explants (Gamber et al., 2005) and the POMC-expressing neurons were shown to release endocannabinoids under basal conditions (Hentges et al. 2005).

In the brainstem, the CB1R and the enzyme that metabolizes AEA, fatty acid amide hydrolase (FAAH), are expressed in the dorsal vagal complex, which includes the NTS (Van Sickle et al., 2001). In addition, peripheral vagal afferents expressing CB1R and the local production of AEA by the gastrointestinal tract are important food-stimulated signals involved with the control of food intake and meal size (Burdyga et al., 2004, 2010; Gómez et al., 2002; Jelsing et al., 2009a,b). Accordingly, our group has recently demonstrated that the previous CB1R blockade potentiates LPS-induced increase in the number of TH-expressing neurons of the NTS co-localizing c-Fos, suggesting that endocannabinoids may modulate satiety during an immune challenge.

Endocannabinoids can also modulate the hedonistic component of food intake. It has been demonstrated that the cannabinoid agonist THC increases the motivation to eat palatable food (Gallate et al., 1999), whereas the CB1R antagonism reduces this response (Simiand et al., 1998). Changes in content of endocannabinoids in the limbic forebrain regions were shown to be correlated with the nutritional status in experimental animals (Kirkham et al., 2002). Furthermore, the expression of the CB1R in the accumbens shell nucleus (NAcS), a key structure involved with motivation and reward, reinforce this hypothesis (Di Marzo et al., 2009). It is already known that dopamine release within NAcS is associated with rewarding associated with the addictive properties of abuse drugs (Volkow et al., 2007). Interestingly, it was observed that the administration of a CB1R antagonist attenuates the increases in dopamine release within this nucleus induced by a novel high palatable food (Melis et al., 2007), indicating that endocannabinoids may account for the integrated control of feeding-associated motivated behaviour.

In addition to their central effects on the control of hunger and satiety, the endocannabinoid signalling has been also implicated in the peripheral control of body weight through changes in energy storage and expenditure (Silvestri et al., 2011). Interestingly, SV40 immortalised murine white and brown adipocytes treated with rimonabant show increased uncoupling protein 1 (UCP1) expression (Perwitz et al., 2010), which is associated with the preferential production of heat. Furthermore, Quarta and colleagues (2010) have demonstrated that mice lacking CB1R exhibit a lean phenotype due to an increased lipid oxidation and thermogenesis. Accordingly, prolonged rimonabant administration was shown to increase lipolysis and decrease fat storage in white adipose tissue of mice with diet-induced obesity (Jbilo et al., 2005). A recent report from Verty and co-workers (2009b) has proposed that this response may be mediated by the autonomic nervous system, since the denervation of the sympathetic afferents blocked the effect of rimonabant on body weight.

3.2.2. *Fluid intake*

Although the endocannabinoid system has a great impact on the regulation of energy homeostasis, its participation in the control of fluid intake remains elusive. A pioneer study has demonstrated that the exogenous administration of compounds derived from the plant *Cannabis sativa* inhibits water intake (Sofia & Knobloch, 1976). On the other hand, the CB1R blockade significantly reduced water intake in the experiments conducted by Gardner & Mallet (2006). Recent studies have also reported that endocannabinoids increase the preference for palatable solutions such as sucrose (Higgs et al., 2003; Jarrett et al., 2005), without altering the drinking of salty solutions or distilled water induced by fluid deprivation (Yoshida et al., 2010). However, these conflicting results could be explained, at least in part, by the parallel effects of the endocannabinoid system in the control of locomotor activity, which could directly interfere with the search for eating and drinking.

The specific appetite for sodium and water is a very important adaptative response recruited to restore body fluid homeostasis. However, the excessive intake of sodium in industrialized food has a great impact in modern society, since it may be directly associated with the impairment of cardiovascular and renal functions. The neuropeptide OT appears as an important negative modulator of salt appetite in rats, being particularly relevant in osmolality- but not in the sodium-dependent inhibition of this ingestive behaviour (Blackburn et al., 1993). Furthermore, OT has been implicated in the central inhibition of water intake induced by water deprivation, hypertonic saline administration and angiotensin II injection (Arletti et al., 1990). More recently, studies developed by Verty and co-workers (2004) revealed that these effects of OT on water intake may be partially mediated by CB1R.

An empirical and very interesting observation is that animals that undergo periods of restricted or no access to water also reduce their food consumption, being this anorexic state as long as the water restriction persists. It is believed that this reduction in food intake is a compensatory mechanism, since a slight change in the osmolality of the gastrointestinal tract circulation may be detected after the beginning of the digestive process. This would contribute to a further increase in the already enhanced plasma osmolality, constituting a very life-threatening situation. Although some studies suggest the participation of central increases in CRF in this anorexic response induced by chronic exposure to osmotic stress (Koob et al., 1993; Krahn et al., 1986; Morley, 1987), it is clear that this decreased food intake occurs earlier than the activation of the HPA axis. Accordingly, no changes in c-Fos/CRF immunoreactivity or CRF mRNA expression were found in the hypothalamus of animals submitted to 24 hours (h) water restriction, despite the fact that the anorexigenic response, as well as the decrease in body weight, had already been observed after this short period (Ruginsk et al., 2011).

Furthermore, it has been also demonstrated by Ruginsk and coworkers (2011) that the number of CART neurons activated to produce c-Fos is increased in the hypothalamus of 24h water-deprived rats. Since CART is a well-known anorexigenic peptide, these results suggest a possible intersection between pathways controlling food and fluid intake. These results further propose the existence of an osmolality-related mechanism in this interface, since the immunoreactivity for c-Fos/CART and the CART mRNA expression in the PVN and supraoptic (SON) nuclei of the hypothalamus were increased after hypertonic but not isotonic extracellular volume expansion (Ruginsk et al., 2011).

4. Endocannabinoids and the control of hydromineral homeostasis

The magnocellular neurosecretory system consists of a group of neurons whose cell bodies are located at the PVN and SON in the hypothalamus and whose terminals, located at the neurohypophysis, release vasopressin (AVP) and OT in response to depolarization. Both neuropeptides act in the kidneys to control the excretion of water and electrolytes. AVP is mostly known for its antidiuretic and vasoconstrictor effects, while OT, together with atrial natriuretic peptide (ANP) produced by the heart, are the two major circulating hormones stimulating natriuresis and diuresis.

Immunohistochemical studies have revealed that GR and MR are co-localized in the parvocellular subdivision of the PVN, but not in magnocellular neurons, which predominantly express MR (Han et al., 2005). Accordingly, it has been demonstrated that high doses of dexamethasone can inhibit OT but not AVP secretion in response to hypertonic extracellular volume expansion (Durlo et al., 2004; Ruginsk et al., 2007) and central cholinergic, angiotensinergic and osmotic stimulation (Lauand et al., 2007). These effects were also correlated with immunohistochemical data, showing that the magnocellular neurons of the PVN and SON are inhibited by dexamethasone administration (Ruginsk et al., 2007).

More recently, the activation of membrane-associated glucocorticoid receptors has been proposed using hypothalamic slice preparations. It has been demonstrated that glucocorticoids could activate at least two divergent intracellular pathways mediated by $G_{\alpha}s$ and $G_{\beta\gamma}$ subunits. The local production of endocannabinoids and NO would then result in two synapse-specific mechanisms, respectively: 1) suppression of excitatory (glutamatergic) synaptic inputs and 2) facilitation of inhibitory (GABAergic) synaptic inputs to the hypothalamic magnocellular neurosecretory system (Di et al., 2003, 2005, 2009), consequently decreasing AVP and OT release from neurohypophyseal terminals. These actions on glutamatergic neurotransmission would be dependent on the activation of the CB1R, located mainly at presynaptic terminals. Accordingly, it has been recently demonstrated that the administration of rimonabant potentiates AVP and OT release as well as the number of c-Fos/AVP and c-Fos/OT double immunoreactive neurons in the PVN and SON of experimental animals submitted to hypertonic extracellular volume expansion (Ruginsk et al., 2010). Furthermore, the participation of the CB1R in the glucocorticoid-induced inhibition of the magnocellular neurosecretory system was clearly demonstrated by the same group, since the previous administration of rimonabant reversed the inhibitory effects of dexamethasone on hormone release (Ruginsk et al., 2012).

Although many brain regions seem to share similar cellular mechanisms triggered by endocannabinoids, their central actions can vary widely within the CNS. Several studies suggest that the endocannabinoid system can mediate not only the central effects of glucocorticoids but also independently modulate the excitability of postsynaptic terminals after the dendritic-mediated release of neuropeptides like OT (Hirasawa et al., 2004; McDonald et al., 2008; Oliet et al., 2007). This mechanism is likely to be implicated in the intra-hypothalamic feedback on hormone release and neuroplasticity (de Kock et al., 2003). The CB1R is also expressed in the NTS (Tsou et al., 1998), a key structure involved in the control of cardiovascular function that projects to the hypothalamus. Accordingly, the central administration of CB1R agonists was shown to reduce blood pressure and heart rate (Lake et al., 1997), while the microinjection of a CB1R antagonist into the NTS resulted in prolonged hypotension after activation of the baroreflex in experimental animals (Rademacher et al., 2003).

Besides participating in the central control of cardiovascular function, recent reports also suggest a role for peripherally-synthesized cannabinoids in the control of blood pressure. This hypothesis is supported by the evidence that the CB1R is expressed by human, rat and guinea-pig atria (Bonz et al., 2003; Kurz et al., 2008; Sterin-Borda et al., 2005). Within the heart, the activation of the CB1R induces a negative inotropic response on muscular fibers, thus reducing blood pressure. This is of particular interest for the study of the integrated cardiovascular and neuroendocrine responses to an increase in the circulating volume, since the distension of cardiac chambers (especially the right atria) in response to such experimental condition is the main stimulus for ANP secretion. Indeed, a role for the CB1R in ANP release has been recently proposed (Ruginsk et al., 2012), although further studies are needed to support this hypothesis.

5. Conclusions and perspectives

Besides the well-known effects on energy homeostasis and metabolism, the ability of glucocorticoids to suppress inflammatory responses has been extensively explored in therapeutics during the last fifty years. However, the clinical potential of glucocorticoids has not been fully achieved because of the severe dose-limiting side effects as well as the development of glucocorticoid resistance. More recently, a lot of expectation was put on characterization of non-steroidal dissociated GR agonists and modulators, which try to uncouple the desired and adverse effects of glucocorticoid administration based on the type of GR interaction with the DNA (transactivation and trasnrepression). However, the difficulty to transpose the effects to *in vivo* set-ups and their still unproved long-term safety have limited the use of these drugs in clinical practice so far.

In this context, different approaches to improve the benefit/risk ratio of glucocorticoids also include the development of drugs that selectively target the activation of membrane-associated GRs and its downstream nongenomic events, without evoking adverse effects, primarily attributed to the activation of genomic pathways. Therefore, the study of the nongenomic actions of glucocorticoids has introduced a novel player in the complexity of the circuitries regulated by the HPA axis and the integrated control of homeostasis. The endocannabinoid system appears as an important mediator of both central and peripheral effects of glucocorticoids, constituting a possible target by which several aspects of stress-mediated responses and energy acquisition/expenditure could be manipulated under diverse physiological and pathological conditions.

Author details

Silvia Graciela Ruginsk, Rodrigo Cesar Rorato, Beatriz de Carvalho Borges,
Ernane Torres Uchoa, Lucila Leico Kagohara Elias and Jose Antunes-Rodrigues
Department of Physiology, School of Medicine of Ribeirao Preto, University of Sao Paulo, Brazil

6. References

Al-Hayani, A., Wease, K.N., Ross, R.A., Pertwee, R.G., Davies, S.N. (2001). The endogenous cannabinoid anandamide activates vanilloid receptors in the rat hippocampal slice. *Neuropharmacology* Vol.41, No.8, pp. 1000-1005, ISSN 0028-3908

Ahima, R.S. (2000). Leptin and the neuroendocrinology of fasting. *Frontiers of Hormone Research* Vol.26, pp. 42-56, ISSN 0301-3073

Ameri, A. (1999). The effects of cannabinoids on the brain. *Progress in Neurobiology* Vol.58, No.4, pp.315-348, ISSN 0301-0082

Arletti, R., Benelli, A. & Bertolini, A. (1989). Influence of oxytocin on feeding behavior in the rat. *Peptides* Vol.10, No.1, pp. 89-93, ISSN 0196-9781

Arletti, R., Benelli, A.& Bertolini, A. (1990). Oxytocin inhibits food and fluid intake in rats. *Physiology and Behavior* Vol.48, No.6, pp. 825-830, ISSN 0031-9384

Aronsson, M., Fuxe, K., Dong, Y., Agnati, L.F., Okret, S., Gustafsson, J.A. (1988). Localization of glucocorticoid receptor mRNA in the male rat brain by in situ hybridization. *Proceedings of the National Academy of Sciences of the United States of America* Vol. 85, No. 23, pp. 9331-9335, ISSN 1091-6490

Asakawa, A., Inui, A., Yuzuriha, H., Nagata, T., Kaga, T., Ueno, N., Fujino, M.A., Kasuga, M. (2001). Cocaine-amphetamine-regulated transcript influences energy metabolism, anxiety and gastric emptying in mice. *Hormone and Metabolic Research* Vol.33, No.9, pp. 554–558, ISSN 1439-4286

Asarian, L., Langhans, W. (2010). A new look on brain mechanisms of acute illness anorexia. *Physiology and Behavior* Vol.100, No.5, pp. 464-471, ISSN: 0031-9384

Bisogno, T., Ligresti, A. & Di Marzo, V. (2005). The endocannabinoid signalling system: biochemical aspects. *Pharmacology, Biochemistry and Behavior* Vol.81, No.2, pp. 224-238, ISSN 0091-3057

Blackburn, R.E., Samson, W.K., Fulton, R.J., Stricker, E.M., Verbalis, J.G. (1993). Central oxytocin inhibition of salt appetite in rats: evidence for differential sensing of plasma sodium and osmolality. *Proceedings of the National Academy of Sciences of the United States of America* Vol.90, No.21, pp. 10380-10384, ISSN 0027-8424

Bonz, A., Laser, M., Küllmer, S., Kniesch, S., Babin-Ebell, J., Popp, V., Ertl, G., Wagner, J.A. (2003). Cannabinoids acting on CB1 receptors decrease contractile performance in human atrial muscle. *Journal of Cardiovascular Pharmacology* Vol.41, No.4, pp. 657-664, ISSN 1533-4023

Borges, B.C., Antunes-Rodrigues, J., Castro, M., Bittencourt, J.C., Elias, C.F., Elias, L.L. (2007). Expression of hypothalamic neuropeptides and the desensitization of pituitary-adrenal axis and hypophagia in the endotoxin tolerance. *Hormones and Behavior* Vol.52, No.4, pp. 508-519, ISSN: 0018-506X

Borges, B.C., Rorato, R., Avraham, Y., da Silva, L.E., Castro, M., Vorobiav, L., Berry, E., Antunes-Rodrigues, J., Elias, L.L. (2011). Leptin resistance and desensitization of hypophagia during prolonged inflammatory challenge. *American Journal of Physiology. Endocrinology and Metabolism* Vol.300, No.5, pp. E858-869, ISSN 1522-1555

Bouaboula, M., Poinot-Chazel, C., Bourrié, B., Canat, X., Calandra, B., Rinaldi-Carmona, M., Le Fur, G., Casellas, P. (1995). Activation of mitogen-activated protein kinases by stimulation of the central cannabinoid receptor CB1. *Biochemical Journal* Vol.312, No. 2, pp. 637-641, ISSN 0264-6021

Bruce, B.K., King, B.M., Phelps, G.R., Veitia, M.C. (1982). Effects of adrenalectomy and corticosterone administration on hypothalamic obesity in rats. *American Journal of Physiology* Vol. 243, No. 2, pp. E152-157, ISSN 0002-9513

Buckingham, J.C., Solito, E., John, C., Tierney, T., Taylor, A., Flower, R., Christian, H., Morris, J. (2003). Annexin 1: a paracrine/juxtacrine mediator of glucorticoid action in the neuroendocrine system. *Cell Biochemistry and Function* Vol.21, pp. 217–221, ISSN 1099-0844

Burdyga, G., Lal, S., Varro, A., Dimaline, R., Thompson, D.G., Dockray, G.J. (2004). Expression of cannabinoid CB1 receptors by vagal afferent neurons is inhibited by cholecystokinin. *The Journal of Neuroscience* 2004 Vol.24, No.11, pp. 2708-2715, ISSN 0270-6474

Burdyga, G., Varro, A., Dimaline, R., Thompson, D.G., Dockray, G.J. (2010). Expression of cannabinoid CB1 receptors by vagal afferent neurons: kinetics, and role in influencing neurochemical phenotype. *American Journal of Physiology. Gastrointestinal and Liver Physiology* Vol.299, No.1, pp. G63-G69, ISSN 1522-1547

Cani, P.D., Amar, J., Iglesias, M.A., Poggi, M., Knauf, C., Bastelica, D., Neyrinck, A.M., Fava, F., Tuohy, K.M., Chabo, C., Waget, A., Delmée, E., Cousin, B., Sulpice, T., Chamontin, B., Ferrières, J., Tanti, J.F., Gibson, G.R., Casteilla, L., Delzenne, N.M., Alessi, M.C., Burcelin, R. (2007). Metabolic endotoxemia initiates obesity and insulin resistance. *Diabetes* Vol.56, No.7, pp. 1761-1772, ISSN: 1939-327X

Castelli, M.P., Piras, A.P., Melis, T., Succu, S., Sanna, F., Melis, M.R., Collu, S., Ennas, M.G., Diaz, G., Mackie, K., Argiolas, A. (2007). Cannabinoid CB1 receptors in the paraventricular nucleus and central control of penile erection: immunocytochemistry, autoradiography and behavioral studies. *Neuroscience* Vol.147, No.1, pp. 197-206, ISSN 0306-4522

Chavez, M., Seeley, R.J,, Green, P.K., Wilkinson, C.W., Schwartz, M.W., Woods, S.C. (1997). Adrenalectomy increases sensitivity to central insulin. *Physiology and Behavior* Vol. 62, No. 3, pp. 631-634, ISSN 1873-507X

Colombo, G., Agabio, R., Diaz, G., Lobina, C., Reali, R., Gessa, G.L. (1998). Appetite suppression and weight loss after the cannabinoid antagonist SR 141716. *Life Sciences* Vol.63, No.8, pp. PL113–PL117, ISSN 0024-3205

Cone, D.R. (2005). Anatomy and regulation of the central melanocortin system. *Nature Neuroscience* Vol.8, No.5, pp. 571-578, ISSN: 1546-1726

Cota, D., Marsicano, G., Tschöp, M., Grübler, Y., Flachskamm, C., Schubert, M., Auer, D., Yassouridis, A., Thöne-Reineke, C., Ortmann, S., Tomassoni, F., Cervino, C., Nisoli, E., Linthorst, A.C., Pasquali, R., Lutz, B., Stalla, G.K., Pagotto, U. (2003). The endogenous cannabinoid system affects energy balance via central orexigenic drive and peripheral lipogenesis. *The Journal of Clinical Investigation* Vol.112, No.3, pp. 423-431, ISSN 0021-9738

Cusin, I., Rouru, J., Rohner-Jeanrenaud, F. (2001). Intracerebroventricular glucocorticoid infusion in normal rats: induction of parasympathetic-mediated obesity and insulin resistance. *Obesity Research* Vol. 9, No. 7, pp. 401-406, ISSN 1550-8528

Dallman, M.F., Pecoraro, N., Akana, S.F., La Fleur, S.E., Gomez, F., Houshyar, H., Bell, M.E., Bhatnagar, S., Laugero, K.D., Manalo, S. (2003). Chronic stress and obesity: a new view of "comfort food". *Proceedings of the National Academy of Sciences of the United States of America* Vol. 100, No. 20, pp. 11696-11701, ISSN 1091-6490

Dallman, M.F., Akana, S.F., Pecoraro, N.C., Warne, J.P., La Fleur, S.E., Foster, M.T. (2007). Glucocorticoids, the etiology of obesity and the metabolic syndrome. *Current Alzheimer Research* Vol.4, No.2, pp. 199-204, ISSN: 1875-5828

De Kloet, E.R., Joëls & M., Holsboer, F. (2005). Stress and the brain: from adaptation to disease. *Nature Reviews Neuroscience* Vol.6, No.6, pp. 463-475, ISSN 1471-003X

De Kock, C.P., Wierda, K.D., Bosman, L.W., Min, R., Koksma, J.J., Mansvelder, H.D., Verhage, M., Brussaard, A.B. (2003). Somatodendritic secretion in oxytocin neurons is upregulated during the female reproductive cycle. *The Journal of Neuroscience* Vol.23, No.7, pp. 2726-2734, ISSN 0270-6474

Deli, L., Wittmann, G., Kalló, I., Lechan, R.M., Watanabe, M., Liposits, Z., Fekete, C. (2009). Type 1 cannabinoid receptor-containing axons innervate hypophysiotropic thyrotropin-releasing hormone-synthesizing neurons. *Endocrinology* Vol.150, No.1, pp. 98-103, ISSN 1945-7170

Devenport, L., Knehans, A., Sundstrom, A., Thomas, T. (1989). Corticosterone's dual metabolic actions. *Life Science* Vol. 45, No. 15, pp. 1389-1396, ISSN 1879-0631

Di, S., Malcher-Lopes, R., Halmos, K.C., Tasker, J. (2003). Nongenomic glucocorticoid inhibition via endocannabinoid release in the hypothalamus: a fast feedback mechanism. *The Journal of Neuroscience* Vol.23, No.12, pp. 4850-4857, ISSN 0270-6474

Di, S., Malcher-Lopes, R., Marcheselli, V.L., Bazan, N.G., Tasker, J.G. (2005). Rapid glucocorticoid-mediated endocannabinoid release and opposing regulation of glutamate and γ-aminobutiric acid inputs to hypothalamic magnocellular neurons. *Endocrinology* Vol.145, No.10, pp. 4292-4301, ISSN 1945-7170

Di, S., Maxson, M.M., Franco, A., Tasker, J.G. (2009). Glucocorticoids regulate glutamate and GABA synapse-specific retrograde transmission via divergent nongenomic signaling pathways. *The Journal of Neuroscience* Vol.29, No.2, pp. 393-401, ISSN 0270-6474

Di Marzo, V., Breivogel, C.S., Tao, Q., Bridgen, D.T., Razdan, R.K., Zimmer, A.M., Zimmer, A., Martin, B.R. (2000). Levels, metabolism, and pharmacological activity of anandamide in CB(1) cannabinoid receptor knockout mice: evidence for non-CB(1), non-CB(2)receptor-mediated actions of anandamide in mouse brain. *Journal of Neurochemistry* Vol.75, No.6, pp. 2434-2444, ISSN 1471-4159

Di Marzo, V., Goparaju, S.K., Wang, L., Liu, J., Batkai, S., Jarai, Z., Fezza, F., Miura, G.I., Palmiter, R.D., Sugiura, T., Kunos, G. (2001). Leptin-regulated endocannabinoids are involved in maintaining food intake. *Nature* Vol.410, pp. 822-825, ISSN 0028-0836

Di Marzo, V. & Matias, I. (2005). Endocannabinoid control of food intake and energy balance. *Nature Neuroscience* Vol.8, No.5, pp. 585-589, ISSN 1546-1726

Di Marzo, V., Ligresti, A. & Cristino, L. (2009). The endocannabinoid system as a link between homoeostatic and hedonic pathways involved in energy balance regulation. *International Journal of Obesity* Vol.33, No.2, pp. S18-S24, ISSN 1476-5497

Doyon, C., Denis, R.G., Baraboi, E.D., Samson, P., Lalonde, J., Deshaies, Y., Richard, D. (2006). Effects of rimonabant (SR141716) on fasting-induced hypothalamic-pituitary-adrenal axis and neuronal activation in lean and obese Zucker rats. *Diabetes* Vol.55, No.12, pp. 3403-3410, ISSN 1939-327X

Dubuc, P.U., Wilden, N.J. (1986). Adrenalectomy reduces but does not reverse obesity in ob/ob mice. *International Journal of Obesity* Vol. 10, No. 2, pp. 91-98, ISSN 0307-0565

Durlo, F.V., Castro, M., Elias, L.L.K., Antunes-Rodrigues, J. (2004). Interaction of prolactin, ANPergic, oxytocinergic and adrenal systems in response to extracellular volume expansion in rats. *Experimental Physiology* Vol.89, No.5, pp. 541-548, ISSN 1469-445X

Evanson, N.K., Tasker, J.G., Hill, M.N., Hillard, C.J., Herman, J.P. (2010). Fast feedback inhibition of the HPA axis by glucocorticoids is mediated by endocannabinoid signaling. *Endocrinology* Vol.151, No.10, pp. 4811-4819, ISSN 1945-7170

Fan,W., Boston, B.A., Kesterson, R.A., Hruby,W.J., Cone, R.D. (1997). Role of melanocortinergic neurons in feeding and the agout obesity syndrome. *Nature* Vol.385, No.6612, pp. 165–168, ISSN: 1476-4687

Freedman, M.R., Castonguay, T.W. & Stern, J.S. (1985). Effect of adrenalectomy and corticosterone replacement on meal patterns of Zucker rats. *The American Journal of Physiology* Vol.249, R584-R594, ISSN 0002-9513

Freund, T.F., Katona, I. & Piomelli, D. (2003). Role of endogenous cannabinoids in synaptic signaling (review). *Physiological Reviews* Vol.83, pp. 1017-1066, ISSN 1522-1210

Füzesi, T., Sánchez, E., Wittmann, G., Singru, P.S., Fekete, C., Lechan, R.M. (2008). Regulation of cocaine- and amphetamine-regulated transcript-synthesising neurons of the hypothalamic paraventricular nucleus by endotoxin; implications for lipopolysaccharide-induced regulation of energy homeostasis. *Journal of Neuroendocrinology* Vol.20, No.9, pp. 1058-1066, ISSN 1365-2826

Gallate, J.E., Saharov, T., Mallet, P.E., McGregor, I.S. (1999). Increased motivation for beer in rats following administration of a cannabinoid CB1 receptor agonist. *European Journal of Pharmacology* Vol.370, No.3, pp. 233-240, ISSN 0014-2999

Gamber, K.M., Macarthur, H. & Westfall, T.C. (2005). Cannabinoids augment the release of neuropeptide Y in the rat hypothalamus. *Neuropharmacology* Vol.49, No.5, pp. 646-652, ISSN 0028-3908

Gametchu, B., Watson, C.S. & Wu, S. (1993). Use of receptor antibodies to demonstrate membrane glucocorticoid receptor in cells from human leukemic patients. *The FASEB Journal* Vol.7, No.13, pp. 1283-1292, ISSN 1530-6860.

Gardner, A. & Mallet, P.E. (2006). Supression of feeding, drinking, and locomotion by a putative cannabinoid receptor 'silent antagonist'. *European Journal of Pharmacology* Vol.530, pp. 103-106, ISSN 0014-2999

Gautron, L., Mingam, R., Moranis, A., Combe, C., Laye, S. (2005). Influence of feeding status on neuronal activity in the hypothalamus during lipopolysaccharide-induced anorexia in rats. *Neuroscience* Vol.134, No.3, pp. 933-946, ISSN: 0306-4522

Gehlert, D.R. (1999). Role of hypothalamic neuropeptide Y in feeding and obesity. *Neuropeptides* Vol. 33, No. 5, pp. 329-338, ISSN 0143-4179

Germano, C.M., Castro, M., Rorato, R., Laguna, M.T., Antunes-Rodrigues, J., Elias, C.F., Elias, L.L. (2007). Time course effects of adrenalectomy and food intake on cocaine- and amphetamine-regulated transcript expression in the hypothalamus. *Brain Research* Vol. 1166, pp. 55-64, ISSN 1872-6240

Germano, C.M., Castro, M., Rorato, R., Costa, D.B., Antunes-Rodrigues, J., Elias, C.F., Elias, L.L. (2008). Downregulation of melanocortin-4 receptor during refeeding and its modulation by adrenalectomy in rats. *Hormone and Metabolic Research* Vol. 40, No. 12, pp. 842-847, ISSN 1439-4286

Giusti-Paiva, A., De Castro, M., Antunes-Rodrigues, J., Carnio, E.C. (2002). Inducible nitric oxide synthase pathway in the central nervous system and vasopressin release during experimental septic shock. *Critical Care Medicine* Vol.30, No.6, pp. 1306–1310, ISSN: 1530-0293

Goldstein, R.E., Wasserman, D.H., McGuinness, O.P., Lacy, D.B., Cherrington, A.D., Abumrad, N.N. (1993). Effects of chronic elevation in plasma cortisol on hepatic carbohydrate metabolism. *American Journal of Physiology* Vol. 264, No. 1 Pt 1, pp. E119-E127, ISSN 0002-9513

Gómez, R., Navarro, M., Ferrer, B., Trigo, J.M., Bilbao, A., Del Arco, I., Cippitelli, A., Nava, F., Piomelli, D., Rodríguez de Fonseca, F. (2002). A peripheral mechanism for CB1 cannabinoid receptor-dependent modulation of feeding. *The Journal of Neuroscience* Vol.22, No.21, pp. 9612-9617, ISSN 0270-6474

Goujon, E., Parnet, P., Laye, S., Combe, C., Dantzer, R. (1996). Adrenalectomy enhances pro-inflammatory cytokines gene expression, in the spleen, pituitary and brain of mice in response to lipopolysaccharide. *Brain Research* Vol.36, No.1, pp. 53–62, ISSN: 0006-8993

Hafezi-Moghadam, A., Simoncini, T., Yang, Z., Limbourg, F.P., Plumier, J.C., Rebsamen, M.C., Hsieh, C.M., Chui, D.S., Thomas, K.L., Prorock, A.J., Laubach, V.E., Moskowitz, M.A., French, B.A., Ley, K., Liao, J.K. (2002). Acute cardiovascular protective effects of corticosteroids are mediated by non-transcriptional activation of endothelial nitric oxide synthase. *Nature Medicine* Vol.8, No.5, pp. 473-479, ISSN 1078-8956

Han, J.Z., Lin, W., Lou, S.J., Qiu, J., Chen, Y.Z. (2002). A rapid, nongenomic action of glucocorticoids in rat B103 neuroblastoma cells. *Biochimica et Biophysica Acta* Vol.1591, pp. 21–27, ISSN 0006-3002

Han, J.Z., Lin,W. & Chen, Y.Z. (2005). Inhibition of ATP-induced calcium influx in HT4 cells by glucocorticoids: involvement of protein kinase A. *Acta Pharmacologica Sinica* Vol.26, pp. 199–204, ISSN 1745-7254

Han F, Ozawa H, Matsuda K, Nishi M, Kawata M. (2005). Colocalization of mineralocorticoid receptor and glucocorticoid receptor in the hippocampus and hypothalamus. *Neuroscience Research* Vol.51, No.4, pp. 371-381, ISSN 0168-0102

Havel, P.J (2001). Peripheral signals conveying metabolic information to the brain: short-term and long-term regulation of food intake and energy homeostasis. *Experimental Biology and Medicine* Vol. 226, No. 11, pp. 963-977, ISSN 1535-3699

Hentges, S.T., Low, M.J. & Williams, J.T. (2005). Differential regulation of synaptic inputs by constitutively released endocannabinoids and exogenous cannabinoids. *The Journal of Neuroscience* Vol.25, No.42, pp. 9746-9751, ISSN 0270-6474

Herkenham, M., Lynn, A.B., Johnson, M.R., Melvin, L.S., de Costa, B.R., Rice, K.C. (1991). Characterization and localization of cannabinoid receptors in rat brain: a quantitative in vitro autoradiographic study. *The Journal of Neuroscience* Vol.11, No.2, pp. 563-83, ISSN 0270-6474

Herman, J.P., Morrison, D.G. (1996). Immunoautoradiographic and in situ hybridization analysis of corticotropin-releasing hormone biosynthesis in the hypothalamic paraventricular nucleus. *Journal of Chemical Neuroanatomy* Vol.11, No.1, pp. 49–56, ISSN: 0891-0618

Higgs, S., Williams, C.M. & Kirkham, T.C. (2003). Cannabinoid influences on palatability: Microstructural analysis of sucrose drinking after delta(9)-tetrahydrocannabinol, anandamide, 2-arachidonoyl glycerol and SR141716. *Psychopharmacology (Berlin)* Vol.165, pp. 370–377, ISSN 0033-3158

Hill, M.N., Karatsoreos, I.N., Hillard, C.J., McEwen, B.S. (2010). Rapid elevations in limbic endocannabinoid content by glucocorticoid hormones in vivo. *Psychoneuroendocrinology* Vol.35, No.9, pp. 1333-1338, ISSN 0306-4530

Hinz, B., Hirschelmann, R. (2000). Rapid non-genomic feedback effects of glucocorticoids on CRF-induced ACTH secretion in rats. *Pharmaceutical Research* Vol.17, No.10, pp. 1273-1277, ISSN 1573-904X

Hirasawa, M., Schwab, Y., Natah, S., Hillard, C.J., Mackie, K., Sharkey, K.A., Pittman, Q.J. (2004). Dendritically released transmitters cooperate via autocrine and retrograde actions to inhibit afferent excitation in rat brain. *The Journal of Physiology* Vol.559, No.2, pp. 611-624, ISSN 1469-7793

Hisano, S., Kagotani, Y., Tsuruo, Y., Daikoku, S., Chihara, K., Whitnall, M.H. (1988). Localization of glucocorticoid receptor in neuropeptide Y-containing neurons in the arcuate nucleus of the rat hypothalamus. *Neuroscience Letters* Vol. 95, No. 1-3, pp.13-18, ISSN 1872-7972

Honma, K.I., Honma, S., Hiroshige, T. (1983). Critical role of food amount for prefeeding corticosterone peak in rats. *American Journal of Physiology* Vol. 245, No. 3, pp. R339-R344, ISSN 0002-9513

Hotta, M., Shibasaki, T., Arai, K., Demura, H. (1999). Corticotropin-releasing factor receptor type 1 mediates emotional stress-induced inhibition of food intake and behavioral changes in rats. *Brain Research* Vol.823, No. 1-2, pp. 221–225, ISSN: 0006-8993

Huang, Q.H., Hruby, V.J., Tatro, J.B. (1999). Role of central melanocortins in endotoxin-induced anorexia. *American Journal of Physiology – Regulatory, Integrative and Comparative Physiology* Vol.276, No.3, pp. 864–871, ISSN: 1522-1490

Iwasaki, Y., Aoki, Y., Katahira, M., Oiso, Y., Saito, H. (1997). Non-genomic mechanisms of glucocorticoid inhibition of adrenocorticotropin secretion: possible involvement of GTP-binding protein. *Biochemical and Biophysical Research Communications* Vol.235, pp. 295–299, ISSN 0006-291X

Jahng, J.W., Kim, N.Y., Ryu, V., Yoo, S.B., Kim, B.T., Kang, D.W., Lee, J.H. (2008). Dexamethasone reduces food intake, weight gain and the hypothalamic 5-HT concentration and increases plasma leptin in rats. *European Journal of Pharmacology* Vol. 581, No. 1-2, pp. 64-70, ISSN 1879-0712

Jamshidi, N. & Taylor, D.A. (2001). Anandamide administration into the ventromedial hypothalamus stimulates appetite in rats. *British Journal of Pharmacology* Vol.134, No.6, pp. 1151-1154, ISSN 1476-5381

Jbilo, O., Ravinet-Trillou, C., Arnone, M., Buisson, I., Bribes, E., Péleraux, A., Pénarier, G., Soubrié, P., Le Fur, G., Galiègue, S., Casellas, P. (2005). The CB1 receptor antagonist rimonabant reverses the diet-induced obesity phenotype through the regulation of lipolysis and energy balance. *FASEB Journal* Vol.19, No.11, pp. 1567-1569, ISSN 1530-6860

Jarrett, M.M., Limebeer, C.L. & Parker, L.A. (2005). Effect of Delta9-tetrahydrocannabinol on sucrose palatability as measured by the taste reactivity test. *Physiology and Behavior* Vol.86, pp. 475–479, ISSN 0031-9384

Jelsing, J., Galzin, A.M., Guillot, E., Pruniaux, M.P., Larsen, P.J., Vrang, N. (2009a). Localization and phenotypic characterization of brainstem neurons activated by rimonabant and WIN55,212-2. *Brain Research Bulletin* Vol.78, No.4-5, pp. 202-210, ISSN 0361-9230

Jelsing, J., Larsen, P.J., Vrang, N. (2009b). The effect of leptin receptor deficiency and fasting on cannabinoid receptor 1 mRNA expression in the rat hypothalamus, brainstem and nodose ganglion. *Neuroscience Letters* Vol.463, No.2, pp. 125-129, ISSN 0304-3940

Johnson, R.W. (1998). Immune and endocrine regulation of food intake in sick animals. *Domestic Animal Endocrinology* Vol.15, No.5, pp. 309-319, ISSN: 0739-7240

Jonat, C., Rahmsdorf, H.J., Park, K.K., Cato, A.C.B., Gebel, S.,Ponta, H., Herrlich, P. (1990). Antitumor promotion and antiinflammation: down-modulation of AP-1 (Fos/Jun) activity by glucocorticoid hormone. *Cell* Vol.62, No.6, pp. 1189–1204, ISSN: 0092-8674

Kalra, S.P., Dube, M.G., Pu, S., Xu, B., Horvath, T.L., Kalra, P.S. (1999). Interacting appetite-regulating pathways in the hypothalamic regulation of body weight. *Endocrine Reviews* Vol.20, No.1, pp. 68–100, ISSN: 1945-7189

Kelly, C.J., Colgan, S.P., Frank, D.N. (2012). Of Microbes and Meals: The Health Consequences of Dietary Endotoxemia. *Nutrition in Clinical Practice* [Epub ahead of print], ISSN: 1941-2452

Kirkham, T.C. & Williams, C.M. (2001). Endogenous cannabinoids and appetite. *Nutrition Research Reviews* Vol.14, No.1, pp. 65-86, ISSN 1475-2700

Kirkham, T.C., Williams, C.M., Fezza, F., Di Marzo, V. (2002). Endocannabinoid levels in rat limbic forebrain and hypothalamus in relation to fasting, feeding and satiation: stimulation of eating by 2-arachidonoyl glycerol. *British Journal of Pharmacology* Vol.136, No.4, pp. 550-557, ISSN 1476-5381

Koob, G.F., Heinrichs, S.C., Merlo Pich, E., Menzaghi, F., Baldwin, H., Miczek, K., Britton, K.T. (1993). The role of corticotropin releasing factor in behavioural responses to stress. In: *Corticotropin Releasing Factor,* Ciba Foundation Symposium, Wiley, Chichester, UK, pp. 277-295.

Krahn, D.D., Gosnell, B.A., Grace, M., Levine, A.S. (1986). CRF antagonist partially reverses CRF- and stress-induced effects on feeding. *Brain Research Bulletin* Vol.17, pp. 285-289, ISSN 0361-9230

Kumar, B.A., Leibowitz, S.F. (1988). Impact of acute corticosterone administration on feeding and macronutrient self-selection patterns. *American Journal of Physiology* Vol. 254, No. 2 Pt 2, pp. R222-R228, ISSN 0002-9513

Kumar, B.A., Papamichael, M., Leibowitz, S.F. (1988). Feeding and macronutrient selection patterns in rats: adrenalectomy and chronic corticosterone replacement. *Physiology and Behavior* Vol. 42, No. 6, pp. 581-589, ISSN 1873-507X

Kurz, C.M., Gottschalk, C., Schlicker, E., Kathmann, M. (2008). Identification of a presynaptic cannabinoid CB1 receptor in the guinea-pig atrium and sequencing of the guinea-pig CB1 receptor. *Journal of Physiology and Pharmacology* Vol.59, No.1, pp. 3-15, ISSN 0867-5910

La Fleur, S.E., (2006). The effects of glucocorticoids on feeding behavior in rats. *Physiology and Behavior* Vol. 89, No. 1, pp.110-114, ISSN 1873-507X

Lake, K.D., Compton, D.R., Varga, K., Martin, B.R., Kunos, G. (1997). Cannabinoid-induced hypotension and bradycardia in rats mediated by CB1-like cannabinoid receptors.

Journal of Pharmacology and Experimental Therapeutics Vol.281, No.3, pp. 1030-1037, ISSN 1521-0103

Langhans, W. (2000). Anorexia of infection: current prospects. *Nutrition* Vol.16, No.10, pp. 996-1005, ISSN: 0899-9007

Lauand, F., Ruginsk, S.G., Rodrigues, H.L., Reis, W.L., De Castro, M., Elias, L.L., Antunes-Rodrigues, J., 2007. Glucocorticoid modulation of atrial natriuretic peptide, oxytocin, vasopressin and Fos expression in response to osmotic, angiotensinergic and cholinergic stimulation. *Neuroscience* Vol.147, No.1, pp. 247-257, ISSN 0306-4522

Leal, A.M., Moreira, A.C. (1997). Food and the circadian activity of the hypothalamic-pituitary-adrenal axis. *Braz. J. Med. Biol. Res.*, Vol. 30, No. 12, pp. 1391-1405, ISSN 1414-431X Limbourg, F.P. & Liao, J.K. (2003). Nontranscriptional actions of the glucocorticoid receptor. *Journal of Molecular Medicine (Berlin)* Vol.81, No.3, pp. 168-174, ISSN 1432-1440

Lightman, S.L., Wiles, C.C., Atkinson, H.C., Henley, D.E., Russell, G.M., Leendertz, J.A., McKenna, M.A., Spiga, F., Wood, S.A., Conway-Campbell, B.L. (2008). The significance of glucocorticoid pulsatility. *European Journal of Pharmacology* Vol.583, No.2-3, pp. 255-262, ISSN 1879-0712

Liposits, Z. & Bohn, M.C. (1993). Association of glucocorticoid receptor immunoreactivity with cell membrane and transport vesicles in hippocampal and hypothalamic neurons of the rat. *Journal of Neuroscience Research* Vol.35, No.1, pp. 14-19, ISSN 1097-4547

Liu, X. & Chen, Y.Z. (1995). Membrane mediated inhibition of corticosterone on the release of arginine vasopressin from rat hypothalamic slices. *Brain Research* Vol.704, No.1, pp. 19-22, ISSN 0006-8993

Lomax, P., 1970. The effect of marihuana on pituitary-thyroid activity in the rat. *Agents and Actions* Vol.1, No.5, pp. 252-257, ISSN 0065-4299

Lou, S.J. & Chen, Y.Z. (1998). The rapid inhibitory effect of glucocorticoid on cytosolic free Ca^{2+} increment induced by high extracellular K and its underlying mechanism in PC12 cells. *Biochemical and Biophysical Research Communications* Vol.244, pp. 403–407, ISSN 0006-291X

Mailleux, P. & Vanderhaeghen, J.J. (1992). Distribution of neuronal cannabinoid receptor in the adult rat brain: a comparative receptor binding radioautography and in situ hybridization histochemistry. *Neuroscience* Vol.48, No.3, pp. 655–668, ISSN 0306-4522

Makimura, H., Mizuno, T.M., Roberts, J., Silverstein, J., Beasley, J., Mobbs, C.V. (2000). Adrenalectomy reverses obese phenotype and restores hypothalamic melanocortin tone in leptin-deficient ob/ob mice. *Diabetes* Vol.49,No.11, pp. 1917–1923, ISSN: 1939-327X

Malcher-Lopes, R., Di, S., Marcheselli, V.S., Weng, F.J., Stuart, C.T., Bazan, N.G., Tasker, J.G. (2006). Opposing crosstalk between leptin and glucocorticoids rapidly modulates synaptic excitation via endocannabinoid release. *The Journal of Neuroscience* Vol.26, No.24, PP. 6643-6650, ISSN 0270-6474

Marco, E.M., García-Gutiérrez, M.S., Bermúdez-Silva, F.J., Moreira, F.A., Guimarães, F., Manzanares, J., Viveros, M.P. (2011). Endocannabinoid system and psychiatry: in search of a neurobiological basis for detrimental and potential therapeutic effects. *Frontiers in Behavioral Neuroscience* [Epub ahead of print], ISSN 1662-5153

Marsicano, G. & Lutz, B. (1999). Expression of the cannabinoid receptor CB1 in distinct neuronal subpopulations in the adult mouse forebrain. *The European Journal of Neuroscience* Vol.11, No.12, pp. 4213-4225, ISSN 1460-9568

Matias, I. & Di Marzo, V. (2007). Endocannabinoids and the control of energy balance. *Trends in Endocrinology and Metabolism* Vol.18, No.1, pp. 27-37, ISSN 1043-2760

Matias, I., Cristinol, L. & Di Marzo, V. (2008). Endocannabinoids: Some like it fat (and sweet too). *Journal of Neuroendocrinology* Vol.20, No.1, pp. 100-109, ISSN 1365-2826

Matson, C.A., Ritter, R.C., (1999). Long-term CCK-leptin synergy suggests a role for CCK in the regulation of body weight. *American Journal of Physiology* Vol. 276, No. 4 Pt 2, pp. R1038-R1045, ISSN 0002-9513

Mechoulam, R., Ben-Shabat, S., Hanus, L., Ligumsky, M., Kaminski, N.E., Schatz, A.R., Gopher, A., Almog, S., Martin, B.R., Compton, D.R., et al., 1995. Identification of an endogenous 2-monoglyceride, present in canine gut, that binds to cannabinoid receptors. *Biochemical Pharmacology* Vol.50, No.1, pp. 83-90, ISSN 0006-2952

Melis, T., Succu, S., Sanna, F., Boi, A., Argiolas, A., Melis, M.R. (2007). The cannabinoid antagonist SR 141716A (Rimonabant) reduces the increase of extra-cellular dopamine release in the rat nucleus accumbens induced by a novel high palatable food. *Neuroscience Letters* Vol.419, No.3, pp. 231–235, ISSN 0304-3940

Mikics, E., Kruk, M.R. & Haller, J. (2004). Genomic and non-genomic effects of glucocorticoids on aggressive behavior in male rats. *Psychoneuroendocrinology* Vol.29, No.5, pp. 618-635, ISSN 0306-4530

Milagro, F.I., Campion, J., Martinez, J.A. (2007). 11-Beta hydroxysteroid dehydrogenase type 2 expression in white adipose tissue is strongly correlated with adiposity. *The Journal of Steroid Biochemistry and Molecular Biology* Vol.104 , No.1–2, pp. 81–84, ISSN: 0960-0760

Milanski, M., Degasperi, G., Coope, A., Morari, J., Denis, R., Cintra, D.E., Tsukumo, D.M., Anhe, G., Amaral, M.E., Takahashi, H.K., Curi, R., Oliveira, H.C., Carvalheira, J.B., Bordin, S., Saad, M.J., Velloso, L.A. (2009). Saturated fatty acids produce an inflammatory response predominantly through the activation of TLR4 signaling in hypothalamus: implications for the pathogenesis of obesity. *The Journal of Neuroscience* Vol.29, No.2, pp. 359-370, ISSN: 1529-2401

Morley, J.E., Levine, A.S. & Rowland, N.E. (1983). Minireview: stress-induced eating. *Life Sciences* Vol.32, No.19, pp. 2169–2182, ISSN 0024-3205

Morley, J.E. (1987). Neuropeptide regulation of appetite and weight. *Endocrine Reviews* Vol.8, pp. 256-287, ISSN 1945-7189

Munoz, C., Pascual-Salcedo, D., Castellanos, M.C., Alfranca,A., Aragones, J., Vara, A., Redondo, J.M., de Landázuri, M.O. (1996). Pyrrolidine dithiocarbamate inhibits the production of interleukin-6, interleukin-8, and granulocyte-macrophage colony-stimulating factor by human endothelial cells in response to inflammatory mediators: modulation of NF-κB and AP-1 transcription factors activity. *Blood* Vol.88, No.9, pp. 3482–3490, ISSN: 1528-0020

Navarrete, M., Araque, A., 2008. Endocannabinoids mediate neuron-astrocyte communication. *Neuron* Vol.57, No.6, pp. 883-893, ISSN 0896-6273

Nieman, L.K., Chanco Turner, M.L. (2006). Addison's disease. *Clinics in Dermatology* Vol. 24, No. 4, pp. 276-280, ISSN 1879-1131

Nieuwenhuizen, A.G., Rutters, F. (2008). The hypothalamic-pituitary-adrenal-axis in the regulation of energy balance. *Physiol. Behav.*, Vol. 94, No.2, pp.169-177, ISSN 1873-507X Oliet, S.H., Baimoukhametova, D.V., Piet, R., Bains, J.S., 2007. Retrograde regulation of GABA transmission by the tonic release of oxytocin and endocannabinoids governs postsynaptic firing. *The Journal of Neuroscience* Vol. 27, No.6, pp. 1325-1333, ISSN 0270-6474

Orchinik, M., Murray, T.F. & Moore, F.L. (1991). A corticosteroid receptor in neuronal membranes. *Science* Vol.252, No.5014, pp. 1848-1851, ISSN 1095-9203

Oren, H., Erbay,A.R., Balci, M., Cehreli, S.(2007). Role of novel biomarkers of inflammation in patients with stable coronary heart disease. *Angiology* Vol.58, No.2, pp. 148–155, ISSN: 0003-3197

Pagotto, U., Marsicano, G., Fezza, F., Theodoropoulou, M., Grübler, Y., Stalla, J., Arzberger, T., Milone, A., Losa, M., Di Marzo, V., Lutz, B., Stalla, G.K. (2001). Normal human pituitary gland and pituitary adenomas express cannabinoid receptor type 1 and synthesize endogenous cannabinoids: first evidence for a direct role of cannabinoids on hormone modulation at the human pituitary level. *The Journal of Clinical Endocrinology and Metabolism* Vol.86, No.6, pp. 2687-2696, ISSN 0021-972X

Patel, S., Roelke, C.T., Rademacher, D.J., Cullinan, W.E., Hillard, C.J. (2004). Endocannabinoid signaling negatively modulates stress-induced activation of the hypothalamic-pituitary-adrenal axis. *Endocrinology* Vol.145, No.12, pp. 5431-5438, ISSN 1945-7170

Paternain, L., García-Diaz, D.F., Milagro, F.I., González-Muniesa, P., Martinez, J.A., Campión, J. (2011). Regulation by chronic-mild stress of glucocorticoids, monocyte chemoattractant protein-1 and adiposity in rats fed on a high-fat diet. *Physiology and Behavior* Vol.103, No.2, pp. 173-180, ISSN: 0031-9384

Pereira, C.D., Azevedo, I., Monteiro, R., Martins, M.J. (2012). 11β-Hydroxysteroid dehydrogenase type 1: relevance of its modulation in the pathophysiology of obesity, the metabolic syndrome and type two diabetes mellitus. *Diabetes, Obesity and Metabolism* [Epub ahead of print], ISSN: 1463-1326

Pertwee, R.G. (2005). Inverse agonism and neutral antagonism at cannabinoid CB1 receptors. *Life Sciences* Vol.76, No.12, pp. 1307-1324, ISSN 0024-3205

Perwitz, N., Wenzel, J., Wagner, I., Büning, J., Drenckhan, M., Zarse, K., Ristow, M., Lilienthal, W., Lehnert, H., Klein, J. (2010). Cannabinoid type 1 receptor blockade induces transdifferentiation towards a brown fat phenotype in white adipocytes. *Diabetes, Obesity and Metabolism* Vol.12, No., pp. 158-166, ISSN 1463-1326

Qiu, J., Lou, L.G., Huang, X.Y., Lou, S.J., Pei, G., Chen, Y.Z. (1998). Nongenomic mechanisms of glucocorticoid inhibition of nicotine-induced calcium influx in PC12 cells: involvement of protein kinase C. *Endocrinology* Vol.139, pp. 5103–5108, ISSN 1945-7170

Qiu, J., Wang, C.G., Huang, X.Y., Chen, Y.Z. (2003). Nongenomic mechanism of glucocorticoid inhibition of bradykinin-induced calcium influx in PC12 cells: possible involvement of protein kinase C. *Life Science* Vol.72, pp. 2533–2542, ISSN 0024-3205

Quarta, C., Bellocchio, L., Mancini, G., Mazza, R., Cervino, C., Braulke, L.J., Fekete, C., Latorre, R., Nanni, C., Bucci, M., Clemens, L.E., Heldmaier, G., Watanabe, M., Leste-Lassere, T., Maitre, M., Tedesco, L., Fanelli, F., Reuss, S., Klaus, S., Srivastava, R.K., Monory, K., Valerio, A., Grandis, A., De Giorgio, R., Pasquali, R., Nisoli, E., Cota, D., Lutz, B., Marsicano, G., Pagotto, U. (2010). CB(1) signaling in forebrain and sympathetic neurons is a key determinant of endocannabinoid actions on energy balance. *Cell Metabolism* Vol.11, No.4, pp. 273-285, ISSN 1550-4131

Rademacher, D.J., Patel, S., Hopp, F.A., Dean, C., Hillard, C.J., Seagard, J.L. (2003). Microinjection of a cannabinoid receptor antagonist into the NTS increases baroreflex duration in dogs. *American Journal of Physiology - Heart and Circulatory Physiology* Vol.284, pp. H1570–H1576, ISSN 1522-1539

Rettori, V., Aguila, M.C., Gimeno, M.F., Franchi, A.M., McCann, S.M., 1990. In vitro effect of delta 9-tetrahydrocannabinol to stimulate somatostatin release and block that of luteinizing hormone-releasing hormone by suppression of the release of prostaglandin E2. *Proceedings of the National Academy of Sciences of the United States of America* Vol.87, No.24, pp. 10063-10066, ISSN 0027-8424

Richard, D., Lin, Q., Timofeeva, E. (2002). The corticotropin-releasing factor family of peptides and CRF receptors: their roles in the regulation of energy balance. *European Journal of Pharmacology* Vol.440, No.2-3, pp. 189–197, ISSN: 0014-2999

Rorato, R., Castro, M., Borges, B.C., Benedetti, M., Germano, C.M., Antunes-Rodrigues, J., Elias, L.L. (2008). Adrenalectomy enhances endotoxemia-induced hypophagia: higher activation of corticotrophin-releasing-factor and proopiomelanocortin hypothalamic neurons. *Hormomes and Behavior* Vol.54, No.1, pp. 134-142, ISSN: 0018-506X

Rorato, R., Reis, W.L., Carvalho Borges, B.D., Antunes-Rodrigues, J., Kagohara Elias, L.L. (2011). Cannabinoid CB(1) receptor restrains accentuated activity of hypothalamic corticotropin-releasing factor and brainstem tyrosine hydroxylase neurons in endotoxemia-induced hypophagia in rats. *Neuropharmacology* [Epub ahead of print], ISSN 0028-3908

Ruginsk, S.G., Oliveira, F.R.T., Margatho, L.O., Vivas, L., Elias, L.L.K., Antunes-Rodrigues, J., 2007. Glucocorticoid modulation of neuronal activation and hormone secretion induced by blood volume expansion. *Experimental Neurology* Vol.206, No.2, pp. 192-200, ISSN 0014-4886

Ruginsk, S.G., Uchoa, E.T., Elias, L.L., Antunes-Rodrigues, J. (2010). CB(1) modulation of hormone secretion, neuronal activation and mRNA expression following extracellular volume expansion. *Experimental Neurology* Vol.224, No.1, pp. 114-122, ISSN 0014-4886

Ruginsk, S.G., Uchoa, E.T., Elias, L.L., Antunes-Rodrigues, J., Llewellyn-Smith, I.J. (2011). Hypothalamic cocaine- and amphetamine-regulated transcript and corticotrophin releasing factor neurons are stimulated by extracellular volume and osmotic changes. *Neuroscience* Vol.186, pp. 57-64, ISSN 0306-4522

Ruginsk, S.G., Uchoa, E.T., Elias, L.L.K., Antunes-Rodrigues, J. (2012). Cannabinoid CB(1) receptor mediates glucocorticoid effects on hormone secretion induced by volume and osmotic changes. *Clinical and Experimental Pharmacology and Physiology* Vol.39, No.2, pp. 151-154, ISSN 1440-1681

Sachot, C., Poole, S., Luheshi, G.N. (2004). Circulating leptin mediates lipopolysaccharide-induced anorexia and fever in rats. *The Journal of Physiology* Vol.15, No.561 , pp. 263-272, ISSN: 1469-7793

Saito, M., Watanabe, S. (2008). Differential modulation of lipopolysaccharide- and zymosan-induced hypophagia by dexamethasone treatment. *Pharmacology, Biochemistry and Behavior* Vol.90, No.3, pp. 428-433, ISSN: 0091-3057

Sandi, C., Venero, C. & Guaza, C. (1996). Novelty-related rapid locomotor effects of corticosterone in rats. *European Journal of Neuroscience* Vol.8, No.4, pp. 794-800, ISSN 1460-9568

Savontaus, E., Conwell, I.M., Wardlaw, S.L. (2002). Effects of adrenalectomy on AGRP, POMC, NPY and CART gene expression in the basal hypothalamus of fed and fasted rats. *Brain Research* Vol. 958, No. 1, pp. 130-138, ISSN 1872-6240

Sawchenko, P.E., Swanson, L.W. (1982). The organization of noradrenergic pathways from the brainstem to the paraventricular and supraoptic nuclei in the rat. *Brain Research* Vol. 257, No. 3, pp. 275-325, ISSN 1872-6240

Schwartz, M.W., Woods, S.C., Porte Jr., D., Seeley, R.J., Baskin, D.G. (2000). Central nervous system control of food intake. *Nature* Vol.404, pp. 661–671, ISSN 1476-4687

Silvestri, C., Ligresti, A. & Di Marzo, V. (2011). Peripheral effects of the endocannabinoids system in energy homeostasis: Adipose tissue, liver and skeletal muscle. *Reviews in Endocrine and Metabolic Disorders* Vol.12, No.3, pp. 153-162, ISSN 1573-2606

Simiand, J., Keane, M., Keane, P.E., Soubrié, P. (1998). SR 141716, a CB1 cannabinoid receptor antagonist, selectively reduces sweet food intake in marmoset. *Behavioural Pharmacology* Vol.9, No.2, pp. 179-181, ISSN 1473-5849

Shibli-Rahhal, A., Van Beek, M., Schlechte, J.A. (2006). Cushing's syndrome. *Clinics in Dermatology* Vol. 24, No. 4, pp.260-265, ISSN 1879-1131

Slieker, L.J., Sloop, K.W., Surface, P.L., Kriauciunas, A., LaQuier, F., Manetta, J., Bue-Valleskey, J., Stephens, T.W. (1996). Regulation of expression of ob mRNA and protein by glucocorticoids and cAMP. *The Journal of Biological Chemistry* Vol. 271, No. 10, pp. 5301-5304, ISSN 1083-351X

Smith, P.M., Ferguson, A.V. (2008). Neurophysiology of hunger and satiety. *Developmental Disabilities Research Reviews* Vol.14, No. 2, pp. 96-104, ISSN 1940-5529

Sofia, R.D. & Knobloch, L.C. (1976). Comparative effects of various naturally occurring cannabinoids on food, sucrose and water consumption by rats. *Pharmacology Biochemistry and Behavior* Vol.4, pp. 591-599, ISSN 0091-3057

Solito, E., Mulla, A., Morris, J.F., Christian, H.C., Flower, R.J., Buckingham, J.C. (2003). Dexamethasone induces rapid serine-phosphorylation and membrane translocation of annexin 1 in a human folliculostellate cell line via a novel nongenomic mechanism involving the glucocorticoid receptor, protein kinase C, phosphatidylinositol 3-kinase, and mitogen-activated protein kinase. *Endocrinology* Vol.144, pp. 1164–1174, ISSN 1945-7170

Spencer, S.J., Tilbrook, A. (2011). The glucocorticoid contribution to obesity. *Stress* Vol. 14, No. 3, pp. 233-246, ISSN 1607-8888

Sterin-Borda, L., Del Zar, C.F. & Borda, E. (2005). Differential CB1 and CB2 cannabinoid receptor-inotropic response of rat isolated atria: endogenous signal transduction pathways. *Biochemical Pharmacology* Vol.69, No.12, pp. 1705-1713, ISSN 0006-2952

Steward, C.A., Horan, T.L., Schuhler, S., Bennett, G.W., Ebling, F.J. (2003). Central administration of thyrotropin releasing hormone (TRH) and related peptides inhibits feeding behavior in the Siberian hamster. *Neuroreport* Vol.14, No.5, pp. 687-691, ISSN 1473-558X

Strack, A.M., Sebastian, R.J., Schwartz, M.W., Dallman, M.F. (1995). Glucocorticoids and insulin: reciprocal signals for energy balance. *American Journal of Physiology* Vol. 268, No. 1 Pt 2, pp. R142-R149, ISSN 0002-9513

Swanson, L.W., Kuypers, H.G. (1980). The paraventricular nucleus of the hypothalamus: cytoarchitectonic subdivisions and organization of projections to the pituitary, dorsal vagal complex, and spinal cord as demonstrated by retrograde fluorescence double-labeling methods. *The Journal of Comparative Neurology* Vol. 194, No. 3, pp. 555-570, ISSN 1096-9861

Tannenbaum, B.M., Brindley, D.N., Tannenbaum, G.S., Dallman, M.F., McArthur, M.D., Meaney, M.J. (1997). High-fat feeding alters both basal and stress-induced hypothalamic–pituitary–adrenal activity in the rat. *American Journal of Physiology, Endocrinology and Metabolism* Vol.273, No.6, pp. 1168–1177, ISSN: 1522-1555

Tataranni, P.A., Larson, D.E., Snitker, S., Young, J.B., Flatt, J.P., Ravussin, E. (1996). Effects of glucocorticoids on energy metabolism and food intake in humans. *American Journal of Physiology* Vol. 271, No. 2 Pt 1, pp. E317-E325, ISSN 0002-9513

Tempel, D.L., Leibowitz, S.F. (1989). PVN steroid implants: effect on feeding patterns and macronutrient selection. *Brain Research Bulletin* Vol. 23, No. 6, pp. 553-560, ISSN 1873-2747

Tempel, D.L., McEwen, B.S. & Leibowitz, S.F. (1992). Effects of adrenal steroid agonists on food intake and macronutrient selection. *Physiology and Behavior* Vol.52, No.6, pp. 1161-1166, ISSN 0031-9384

Tempel, D.L., McEwen, B.S., Leibowitz, S.F. (1993). Adrenal steroid receptors in the PVN: studies with steroid antagonists in relation to macronutrient intake. *Neuroendocrinology* Vol. 57, No. 6, pp. 1106-1113, ISSN 1423-0194

Tempel, D.L, Leibowitz, S.F. (1994). Adrenal steroid receptors: interactions with brain neuropeptide systems in relation to nutrient intake and metabolism. *Journal of Neuroendocrinology* Vol. 6, No. 5, pp. 479-501, ISSN 1365-2826

Tierney, T., Christian, H.C., Morris, J.F., Solito, E., Buckingham, J.C. (2003). Evidence from studies on co-cultures of TtT/GF and AtT20 cells that Annexin 1 acts as a paracrine or juxtacrine mediator of the early inhibitory effects of glucocorticoids on ACTH release. *Journal of Neuroendocrinology* Vol.15, pp. 1134–1143, ISSN 1365-2826

Tomas, F.M., Munro, H.N., Young, V.R. (1979). Effect of glucocorticoid administration on the rate of muscle protein breakdown in vivo in rats, as measured by urinary excretion of N tau-methylhistidine. *Biochemistry Journal* Vol. 178, No. 1, pp. 139-146, ISSN 1470-8728

Tóth, A., Boczán, J., Kedei, N., Lizanecz, E., Bagi, Z., Papp, Z., Edes, I., Csiba, L., Blumberg, P.M., 2005. Expression and distribution of vanilloid receptor 1 (TRPV1) in the adult rat brain. *Brain research. Molecular brain research* Vol.135, No.1-2, pp. 162-168, ISSN 0169-328X

Trayhurn, P., Wood, I.S. (2005). Signalling role of adipose tissue: adipokines and inflammation in obesity. *Biochemical Society Transactions* Vol.33, No.5, pp. 1078–1081, ISSN: 0300-5127

Tsou, K., Brown, S., Sanudo-Pena, M., Mackie, K., Walker, J. (1998). Immunohistochemical distribution of cannabinoid CB1 receptors in the rat central nervous system. *Neuroscience* Vol.83, No.2, pp. 393-411, ISSN 0014-4886

Turnbull, A.V., Lee, S., Rivier, C. (1998). Mechanisms of hypothalamic-pituitary-adrenal axis stimulation by immune signals in the adult rat. *Annals of the New York Academy of Sciences* Vol.840, pp. 434-443, ISSN: 1749-6632

Turnbull, A.V., Rivier, C.L. (1999). Regulation of the hypothalamic-pituitary-adrenal axis by cytokines: actions and mechanisms of action. *Physiology Reviews* Vol.79, No.1, pp. 1–71. ISSN: 1522-1210

Tyrey, L., 1978. Delta-9-Tetrahydrocannabinol suppression of episodic luteinizing hormone secretion in the ovariectomized rat. *Endocrinology* Vol.102, No.6, pp. 1808-1814, ISSN 1945-7170

Uchoa, E.T., Sabino, H.A., Ruginsk, S.G., Antunes-Rodrigues, J., Elias, L.L. (2009a). Hypophagia induced by glucocorticoid deficiency is associated with an increased activation of satiety-related responses. *Journal of Applied Physiology* Vol. 106, No. 2, pp. 596-604, ISSN 1522-1601

Uchoa, E.T., Silva, L.E., de Castro, M., Antunes-Rodrigues, J., Elias, L.L. (2009b). Hypothalamic oxytocin neurons modulate hypophagic effect induced by adrenalectomy. *Hormones and Behavior* Vol. 56, No. 5, pp. 532-538, ISSN 1095-6867

Uchoa, E.T., Silva, L.E., de Castro, M., Antunes-Rodrigues, J., Elias, L.L. (2010). Corticotrophin-releasing factor mediates hypophagia after adrenalectomy, increasing meal-related satiety responses. *Hormones and Behavior* Vol. 58, No. 5, pp. 714-719, ISSN 1095-6867

Uchoa, E.T., Silva, L.E., de Castro, M., Antunes-Rodrigues, J., Elias, L.L. (2012). Glucocorticoids are required for meal-induced changes in the expression of hypothalamic neuropeptides. *Neuropeptides* Vol.46, No.3, pp. 119-124, ISSN 1532-2785

Valassi, E., Scacchi, M., Cavagnini, F. (2008). Neuroendocrine control of food intake. *Nutrition, Metabolism and Cardiovascular Diseases* Vol. 18, No. 2, pp. 158-168, ISSN 1590-3729

Van Sickle, M.D., Oland, L.D., Ho, W., Hillard, C.J., Mackie, K., Davison, J.S., Sharkey, K.A. (2001). Cannabinoids inhibit emesis through CB1 receptors in the brainstem of the ferret. *Gastroenterology* Vol.121, No.4, pp. 767-774, ISSN 0016-5085

Verty, A.N., McFarlane, J.R., McGregor, I.S., Mallet, P.E. (2004). Evidence for an interaction between CB1 cannabinoid and oxytocin receptors in food and water intake. *Neuropharmacology* Vol.47, No.4, pp. 593-603, ISSN 0028-3908

Verty, A.N., Boon, W.M., Mallet, P.E., McGregor, I.S., Oldfield, B.J. (2009a). Involvement of hypothalamic peptides in the anorectic action of the CB receptor antagonist rimonabant (SR 141716). *The European Journal of Neuroscience* Vol.29, No.11, pp. 2207-2016, ISSN 1460-9568

Verty, A.N., Allen, A.M. & Oldfield, B.J. (2009b). The effects of rimonabant on brown adipose tissue in rat: implications for energy expenditure. *Obesity* Vol.17, No.2, pp. 254-261, ISSN 1930-739X

Volkow, N.D., Fowler, J.S., Wang, G.J., Swanson, J.M. (2004). Dopamine in drug abuse and addiction: results from imaging studies and treatment implications. *Molecular Psychiatry* Vol.9, No.6, pp. 557-569, ISSN 1359-4184

Vrang, N., Larsen, P.J., Kristensen, P., Tang-Christensen, M. (2000). Central administration of cocaine-amphetamine-regulated transcript activates hypothalamic neuroendocrine neurons in the rat. *Endocrinology* Vol.141, No.2, pp. 794-801, ISSN 1945-7170

Wamsteeker, J.I., Kuzmiski, J.B. & Bains, J.S. (2010). Repeated stress impairs endocannabinoid signaling in the paraventricular nucleus of the hypothalamus. *The Journal of Neuroscience* Vol.30, No.33, pp. 11188-11196, ISSN 0270-6474

Wang, L., Barachina, M.D., Martínez, V., Wei, J.Y., Taché, Y. (2000). Synergistic interaction between CCK and leptin to regulate food intake. *Regulatory Peptides* Vol. 92, No. 1-3, pp. 79-85, ISSN 1873-1686

Westerink, J. & Visseren, F.L. (2011). Pharmacological and non-pharmacological interventions to influence adipose tissue function. *Cardiovascular Diabetology* Vol.10, No.1, pp. 13, ISSN 1475-2840

Williams, C.M., Rogers, P.J. & Kirkham, T.C. (1998). Hyperphagia in pre-fed rats following oral delta9-THC. *Physiology and Behavior* Vol.65, No.2, pp. 343-346, ISSN 0031-9384

Williams, C.M. & Kirkham, T.C. (1999). Anandamide induces overeating: mediation by central cannabinoid (CB1) receptors. *Psychopharmacology* Vol.143, No.3, pp. 315-317, ISSN 1432-2072

Williams, C.M. & Kirkham, T.C. (2002). Reversal of delta 9-THC hyperphagia by SR141716 and naloxone but not dexfenfluramine. *Pharmacology, Biochemistry and Behavior* Vol.71, No.1-2, pp. 333-340, ISSN 0091-3057

Wisse, B.E., Ogimoto, K., Schwartz, M.W. (2006). Role of hypothalamic interleukin-1beta (IL-1beta) in regulation of energy homeostasis by melanocortins. *Peptides* Vol.27, No.2, p. 265-273, ISSN: 0196-9781

Wittmann, G., Deli, L., Kalló, I., Hrabovszky, E., Watanabe, M., Liposits, Z., Fekete, C. (2007). Distribution of type 1 cannabinoid receptor (CB1)-immunoreactive axons in the mouse hypothalamus. *The Journal of Comparative Neurolology* Vol.503, No.2, pp. 270-9, ISSN 1096-9861

Yoshida, R., Ohkuri, T., Jyotaki, M., Yasuo, T., Horio, N., Yasumatsu, K., Sanematsu, K., Shigemura, N., Yamamoto, T., Margolskee, R.F., Ninomiya, Y. (2010). Endocannabinoids selectively enhance sweet taste. *Proceedings of the National Academy of Sciences of the United States of America* Vol.107, No.2, pp. 935-939, ISSN 0027-8424

Yukimura, Y., Bray, G.A., Wolfsen, A.R. (1978). Some effects of adrenalectomy in the fatty rat. *Endocrinology* Vol. 103, No.5, pp. 1924-1928, ISSN 1945-7170

Zakrzewska, K.E., Cusin, I., Sainsbury, A., Rohner-Jeanrenaud, F., Jeanrenaud, B. (1997). Glucocorticoids as counterregulatory hormones of leptin: toward an understanding of leptin resistance. *Diabetes* Vol. 46, No. 4, pp. 717-719, ISSN 1939-327X

Zakrzewska, K.E., Cusin, I., Stricker-Krongrad, A., Boss, O., Ricquier, D., Jeanrenaud, B., Rohner-Jeanrenaud, F. (1999). Induction of obesity and hyperleptinemia by central glucocorticoid infusion in the rat. *Diabetes* Vol. 48, No. 2, pp. 365-370, ISSN 1939-327X

Chapter 12

Role of Glucocorticoids in Regulation of Iodine Metabolism in Thyroid Gland: Effects of Hyper-And Hypocorticism

Liliya Nadolnik

Additional information is available at the end of the chapter

http://dx.doi.org/10.5772/52043

1. Introduction

A close relationship between the key bodily regulatory systems, hypophysis-adrenal and hypophysis-thyroid systems, is fairly well-known.

However, the mechanisms of their interaction at different levels have not been conclusively established. This is of considerable interest due to glucocorticoids and thyroid hormones playing a key role in regulation of the most important systems of vital activity and adaptation. The role of glucocorticoids in regulation of thyroid cell function is interesting due to marked growth of thyroid pathology in different world's regions, along with considerably improved iodine prevention [1], as well as an increased level of environmental stressogenicity. One should also note an increased tension in life of the individual and the society on the whole (psychological, social and other types of stress). The development of the society has actually created a new human environment with a raised level of stressogenic factors. The chronic stress –induced development of hypercorticism can play a significant pathogenetic role in the changed thyroid function which does not only depend on bodily iodine allowances.

Thyroid-stimulating hormone (TSH) [2, 3, 4], iodine [4, 5], thyroglobulin (ThG) [6], estrogens [7], cytokines [8] and other biologically active molecules play an important role in regulation of thyroid cell functions. It is interesting that deficiency of iodine, the key substrate for synthesis of thyroid hormones, decreases the activity of the HPA-axis. It was found [9] that rats with chronic iodine deficiency showed the absence of a normal circadian rhythm of corticosterone secretion and a weakened secretory rise of a corticosterone level under stress that remains to be diminished in amplitude during a month following restoration of the iodine status.

Thyroid cell function can be regulated by glucocorticoids via changes in the concentrations of the pivotal bioregulators: thyroid-stimulating hormone, TSH, iodine and thyroglobulin. The mechanisms and effects of these interactions call for further studies. Thyrocytes express glucocorticoid receptors, alpha (GR-alpha) and beta (GR-beta), which seem to play an important role in differentiation of thyroid cells since cells of thyroid adenoma demonstrated a decrease of mRA GR-alpha and an increase in GR-beta [10].

1.1. Relationships between regulatory effects of hypothalamic and hypophyseal hormones of hypothalamo-hypophyseal-adrenal and hypothalamo-hypophyseal-thyroid axes

Relationships between the hypothalamo-hypophyseal-adrenal (HHA) and hypothalamo-hypophyseal-thyroid (HHT) systems were established at different regulatory levels. Administration of a thyrotropin-releasing hormone (TRH) was accompanied by a decreased adrenocorticotropic hormone (ACTH) level in blood serum of stressed rats [11]. Corticotropin-releasing hormone (CRH) increased plasma TSH and T4 [12]. Banos C. et al. [13] demonstrated that administration of 2 mg ACTH to healthy volunteers decreased the TSH response to TRH. These results characterize certain antagonism between TSH and ACTH.

1.2. Effects of glucocorticoids on TRH and TSH levels

TSH synthesis is determined by balance of positive regulation and negative regulation by TRH and triiodothyronine (T3), respectively; in addition, somatostatin and dopamine also exert inhibitory control (Diagram 1). Glucocorticoids decreased serum TSH in animals and humans. Administration of a high dose of dexamethasone not only suppressed TSH but also decreased the TSH response to TRH administration [14]; the suppressive effect of dexamethasone on TSH decreased in elderly people [15].

Administration of a single dose of hydrocortisone (500 mg) increased both TSH production and stimulation by TRH [16]; only long-term hypocorticism (Cushing's disease) may be a cause for decreased TSH level. The earlier recovery (up to control values) of the diurnal rhythm of TSH than that of cortisol suggests that the TSH rhythm is not under the direct control of circulating cortisol [17]. In adrenalectomized rats the TSH level decreased in serum but not in the pituitary gland [18]. Glucocorticoids decrease blood serum TSH concentrations in humans and animals. Dexamethasone administration to hypothyroid rats decreased serum TSH; dexamethasone augmented a T3-induced decrease of TSH. However, changes in pituitary TSH α- and β-subunit mRNA concentrations were not found [19].

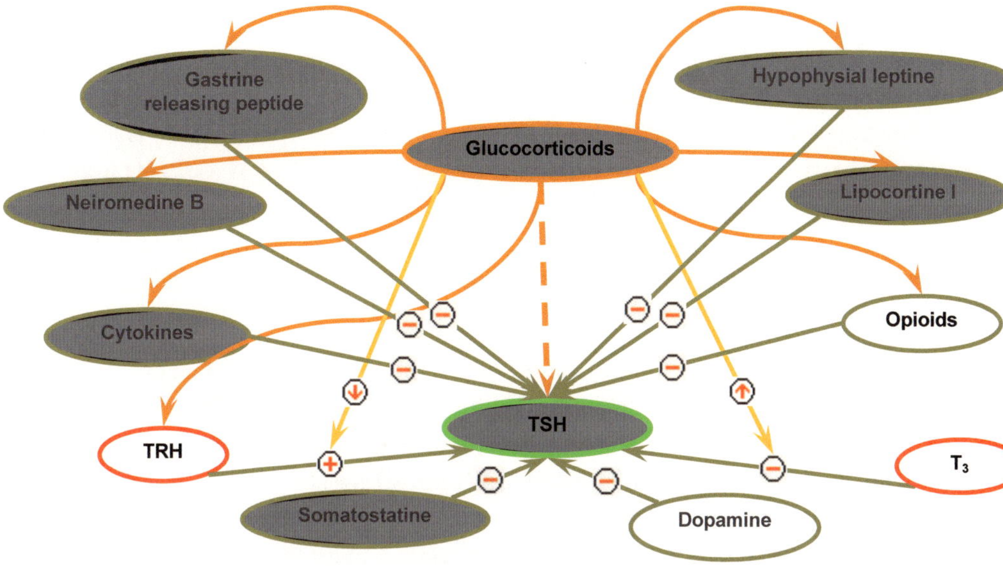

Scheme 1. Effect of glucocorticoids on TSH. +, stimulatory effect; -, inhibitory effect; ↓– weakening of stimulatory effect; ↑– enhancement of inhibitory effect

Kakucska I. et al. obtained clearer results on the effects of glucocorticoids on the hypothalamo-pituitary-thyroid axis [20]. In the paraventricular hypothalamic nuclei of adrenalectomized rats, an increase in corticotropin releasing hormone (CRH) mRNA occurred in parallel to the increase (68.3%) in pro-TRH mRNA. On the contrary, administration of corticosterone or dexamethasone caused a marked decrease in CRH mRNA and pro-TRH mRNA by 43.2 and 73.3%, respectively. Insignificant changes in pro-TRH mRNA were found in the lateral hypothalamus.

Mechanisms of the stress-induced decrease in TRH/TSH secretion possibly involve glucocorticoids, cytokines, and opioids. Recently, a new regulatory mechanism, involving pituitary neuromedin B, gastrin-releasing peptide, and pituitary leptin, acting as local inhibitors of TSH release, has been proposed [21]. In vitro studies have shown that the lipocortin-1 (LC1) protein is a mediator of the glucocorticoid-induced suppression of TSH secretion by the anterior pituitary [53]. Treatment of anterior pituitary cells with 0.1 μM dexamethasone significantly increased the amount of LC1, associated with the outer surface of the pituitary cells and decreased the intracellular content of LC1. Addition of an N-terminal LC1 fragment (residues 1-188) decreased TSH release mediated by vasoactive intestinal peptide and forskolin, but failed to influence those initiated by 10 μM BAYK 8644, the calcium channel stimulator. The inhibitory action of dexamethasone was substantially reversed by a specific monoclonal anti-LC1 antibody [22]. The inhibitory effect of dexamethasone was used for monitoring of subclinical hypothyroidism in obese patients. Administration of TRH after dexamethasone increased the TSH level only in hypothyroid patients but not in euthyroid obese patients [23].

1.3. Effect of glucocorticoids on iodine uptake by the thyroid gland

Iodine uptake is the most important function of thyroid cells; it is controlled by TSH, which stimulates ^{131}I uptake in vivo and in vitro and also expression of sodium-iodide symporter (NIS) in the culture of human thyrocytes [24]. Sodium-iodide symporter (NIS) is located on the apical membrane of thyrocytes; its activity is coupled to Na+,K+-ATPase. TSH influences transcription of NIS gene through Pax-8 and factors activated by intercellular interaction during folliculogenesis [25]. High iodine doses directly inhibit iodide uptake by influencing regulation of NIS protein and mRNA expression [26, 27].

Immobilization stress and also ACTH administration to rats with pituitary damages increased ^{131}I uptake by the thyroid gland in vitro [28]. Cultivation of FRTL-5 thyrocytes under hypoxic conditions was accompanied by increase iodide uptake [29]; heat stress (15 min at 45°C) eliminated this effect. Using culture of ewe thyroid gland follicles it was found that combination of TSH and 10 nM cortisol was optimal for stimulation of iodide uptake without additive and synergistic effects; this effect was also reproduced by combination of TSH with dexamethasone [30]. In addition, the stimulating effect of TSH was potentiated by physiological concentrations of insulin and insulin-like growth factors (IGF I and IGF II). Subsequent studies demonstrated a direct biphasic effect of hydrocortisone on metabolism of thyroid gland cells. Physiological concentrations of hydrocortisone (1—1000 nM) in a dose-dependent manner stimulated TSH- and 8-bromo-cAMP-induced iodide uptake, realized via increased production of cAMP and activation of cAMP-dependent metabolic pathways in the primary cultures of porcine thyrocytes [31]. The stimulating effect of hydrocortisone in combination with TSH was inhibited by the glucocorticoid antagonist RU486; the specific hydrocortisone effect appears to be mediated by a thyrocyte glucocorticoid receptor.

It is suggested that the stimulating effect of glucocorticoids on ^{131}I uptake may be used for treatment for breast cancer [32] and prostate cancer [33]. Incubation of NP-1 cells with dexamethasone (10^{-8}–10^{-6} M) caused a 1.5-fold increase in iodide uptake, and a 1.7-fold increase in expression of Na^{+}/I^{-}- simporter (NIS) mRNA and protein concentration; NP-1 cell death increased from 55 to 95%, thus suggesting increased cytotoxicity of ^{131}I. These studies (employing clonogenic assay and nonradioactive proliferation assay) also revealed that treatment of NP-1 cells decreased proliferation of prostate cancer cells. Thus, stress (at least acute stress) may be considered as a factor activating iodide content in the thyroid gland; however, univocal solution of this problem requires further investigations because of multilevel effects of glucocorticoids on thyroid homeostasis

1.4. Effects of glucocorticoids on iodine oxidation and organification in thyrocytes

Single reports on the effect of stress or glucocorticoids on iodide oxidation by thyroperoxidase (TPO), thyroglobulin iodination and subsequent thyroid hormone secretion are available in the literature. Corticosterone administration for 10 days in three different doses (25, 50, 100 mg per 100 g of body weight) inhibited thyroid gland TPO of juvenile female turtles [34], but the mechanism of the inhibitory effect was not studied. Studies in this direction are especially important due to the key role of TPO in thyroid hormone biosynthesis.

The electron microscopy study of thyrocytes revealed accumulation of colloidal droplets in follicle cytoplasm; this suggests that prednisone may decrease basal secretion of thyroid hormones by inhibiting lysosomal hydrolysis of colloid in the follicular cells [35].

1.5. Role of glucocorticoids in the regulation of thyroid hormone receptors

It is known that most of T3 effects are realized via nuclear receptors of thyroid hormones. T3 and glucocorticoid hormones synergistically interact in biosynthesis of growth hormone in the rat pituitary and in the T3-induced metamorphoses in amphibians. Glucocorticoid hormones potentiated metabolic effect of T3 [36]. Dexamethasone increased rat liver specific receptor binding of thyroid hormones. Dexamethasone administration to adrenalectomized rats increased the concentration of protein and mRNA of beta 1 receptor [36]. Molecular studies employing transfection of COS-7 cells revealed that dexamethasone increased transcription activity of thyroid hormone receptor beta 1 promoter [36].

1.6. Effect of stress on peripheral metabolism of thyroid hormones (deiodinase activity in target tissues)

Brain, liver, kidney, heart, muscles, and immune system are the most important targets for thyroid hormones. It is possible that glucocorticoids control tissue levels of T3. Acute stress (footshock) increased the brain T3 content in male and female rats by 12—19% [37]. Two days of total water and food deprivation as stress increased the thymus lymphocyte T3 content in weanling and adult female rats [38], which was normalized after 48 h [39]. It is known that thyroxine (T4) is the main hormone produced by the thyroid gland, however, since it does not exhibit biological activity and therefore thyroxin may be considered as a prohormone or a plasma storage form of thyroid hormones, which plays an important physiological role. A family of selenocysteine oxidoreductases known as iodothyronine deiodinases (D) plays the major role in T4 activation. Three types of these enzymes (mainly determining realization of the hormonal effect of thyroid hormones) have been identified. Their localization and activity are tissue-specific (Scheme 2, 3).

Glucocorticoids exhibit differentiated tissue- and age-specific effects on various tissue deiodinases [40, 41]; they also regulate deiodinases during embryogenesis. Dexamethasone administration to pregnant ewes increased activity of DI in the fetal liver and decreased DIII activity in fetal kidneys [42]. In 20-day-old fetuses, glucocorticoids had no effects on circulating thyroid hormone levels despite their clear decrease in the activity of hepatic and renal deiodinases and an increased activity in the brain, thereby indicating that in this age

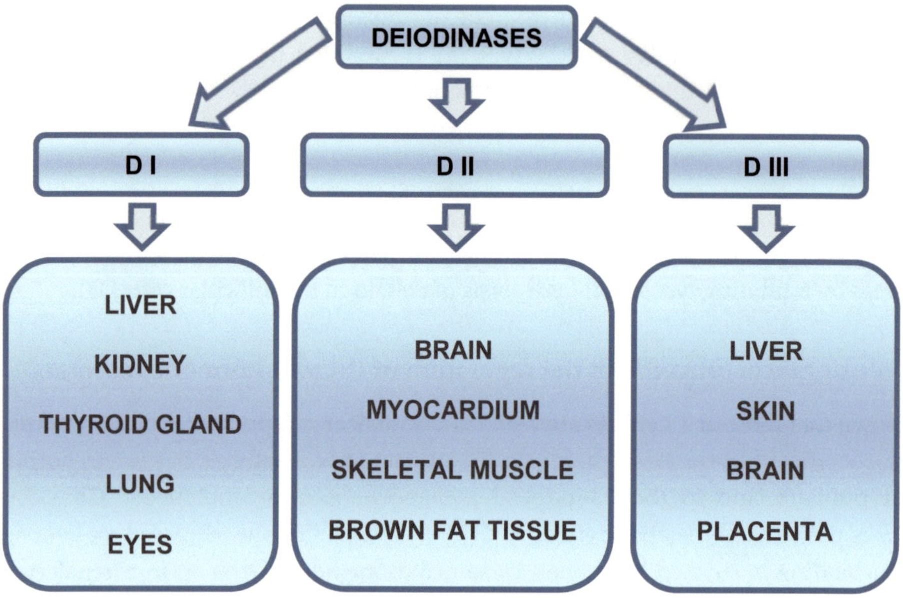

Scheme 2. Tissue distribution of deiodinases

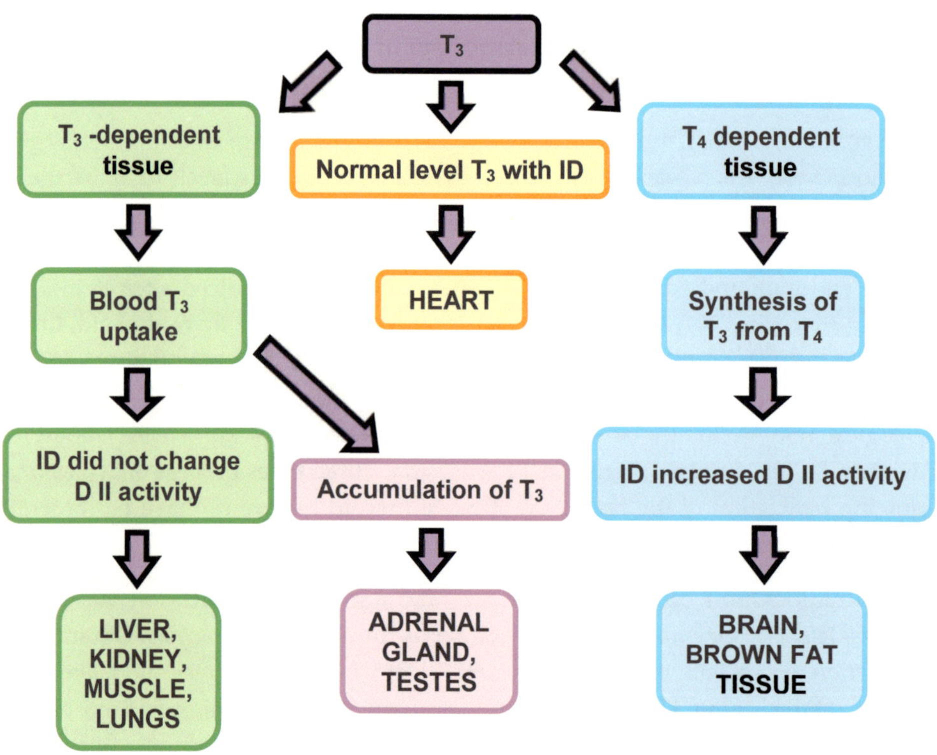

Scheme 3. Forms of thyroid hormone utilization by various

Types of deiodinases	Target tissues	Effect	Reference
DI	fetal liver, ewes	↑	[42]
DIII	fetal kidneys, ewes	↓	[42]
DIII	5-day-pups liver, rat	↑	[43]
DIII	5-day-pups kidneys, rat	↑	[43]
DIII	5-day-pups brain, rat	–	[43]
DIII	brown adipose tissue, rat	↓	[58]
DII	brain, rat	↑	[44]
DI	liver, rat	↓	[51]
DI	kidneys, rat	↓	[52]
DI	hepatocytes in vitro	↑	[54]

Table 1. Effect of GC and stress on activities of various types of deiodinases in rat tissues (↑– stimulatory effect; ↓ inhibitory effect; – no effect)

thyroid circulating thyroid hormone levels are more dependent on thyroidal secretion than on peripheral deiodination. In 5-day-pups, dexamethasone increased blood T3 and T4 and DII activity in the liver, kidney but not in the brain; however, in 12-day-old pups, the dexamethasone effects were maintained only on liver and kidney DIII activity [43].

Effects of stress on deiodinase activity in various tissues still require better elucidation. The most significant effect of glucocorticoids was found on brain DII activity. Even mild, short-term stress (intraperitoneal injection of saline, intragastric intubation, and two different forms of handling (being grasped as for intraperitoneal injection and being moved from one cage to another, and a 2-h period spent in a slowly rotating drum) caused a significant increase in brain DII activity [44], this was accompanied by a 300%-increase in T3 concentration. These effects were not found in the liver and no changes of DI activity were found in the brain and liver. Dexamethasone caused up-regulation of DII activity [45]. Administration of steroidogenesis inhibitors (aminoglutethimide and metyrapone) to rats decreased adrenal DII activity both in physiological rest and under stress [46]; this suggests normal corticosterone levels required for a deiodinase response to the stress treatment. It appears that the glucocorticoid regulation of DII is the most differentiated. Recent in vitro data obtained using mouse and rat pituitary cells demonstrated that addition of glucocorticoids increased the activity of this enzyme and its mRNA [47], whereas the opposite effect was obtained in mouse mammary gland epithelial cells [48]. In the AtT-20 mouse pituitary tumor cells, glucocorticoids and CRH stimulated expression of mRNA and activity of DII [49]. Effects of glucocorticoids, found in experiments on cultivated hypophyseal cells, confirm their important stimulatory role in the metabolism of thyroid hormones in the CNS.

A decrease in blood thyroid hormones and TRH mRNA seen in fasting and food deprivation was accompanied by the increase DII activity and DII mRNA. Studies of mechanisms of DII activation during fasting revealed that the decrease in leptin levels plays a permissive role during glucocorticoid-induced regulation of the DII enzyme [50].

There are contradictory data on the effects of glucocorticoids on DI activity in various tissues. Cold stress of rats either for 24 h or 28 days (as well as that combined with immobilization) significantly reduced DI activity in the liver [51]. Immobilization of rats for 6 - 8 h was accompanied by the decrease in DI activity in the liver and kidneys; this was attributed to the decrease in the enzyme activity rather than to decreased substrate availability because serum T4 concentration remained unchanged [52]. In adult rats, glucocorticoids decreased DI activity in the liver [53]. In vitro studies on the cultured rat hepatocytes revealed the opposite effects: glucocorticoids increased DI activity and expression of DI mRNA [54]. In kidney NRK 52E cells, dexamethasone increased DI activity and expression of DI mRNA, while in cultured pituitary tumor cells, glucocorticoids did not influence DI mRNA [55]. In the fish *Nile tilapia*, dexamethasone decreased activity of DI and DII in the liver; long-term administration of this hormone increased availability of circulating T3 [56].

The decrease in plasma T3 and the increase in rT3 concentrations observed in stress may be associated with glucocorticoid stimulation of DIII [57]. Regulatory mechanisms of effects of thyroid hormones in various tissue cells have not been conclusively established. Glucocorticoids decreased DIII expression in rat brown adipose tissue [58]. The study of deiodinase activities in human cell lines revealed that estradiol increased DIII activity in ECC-1 cells, dexamethasone inhibited DIII in WRL-68 cells only in the presence of fetal calf serum in the medium [59]. Dexamethasone in a dose-dependent manner decreased the stimulatory effect of T3 on ICAM-1 protein in human ECV 304 cells [74].

All these results indicate that glucocorticoids modulate effects of thyroid hormones by influencing deiodinase activity in various target tissues. They cause significant increase of DII activity in the brain (and thus increase brain T3 level); stress exhibited inhibitory effect on DI activity in the liver and kidneys. Nevertheless, mechanisms underlying glucocorticoid regulation of T4 deiodination in various tissues require further investigation.

1.7. Thyroid gland function under impaired adrenal functions

Taking into consideration the multilevel effects of glucocorticoids on the thyroid status and peripheral metabolism of thyroid hormones, a study of functional activity of the thyroid gland under conditions of adrenal impairments appears to quite reasonable.

Adrenalectomy in rats increased thyroid gland stimulation by TSH and its secretory activity [60]. In patients with adrenal insufficiency cessation of replacement glucocorticoid therapy resulted in an increase of T3 and a decrease of (reversive triiodothyronine) rT3 concentrations, whereas the level of T4 and TSH remained basically unchanged [61].

There are clinical case reports on impairments of thyroid function in patients with hypercorticism before and after adrenalectomy and with adrenal insufficiency. The state of the pituitary-adrenal axis mainly determines the thyroid status in humans. Under hypercorticism in patients with Cushing's syndrome there were decreased serum concentrations of thyroid hormones and TSH; in addition, in 56.2--66.6% there was a prevalence of thyroid nodular disease; this was significantly higher than in the control group [63]. Long-term hypercorticism in patients with Cushing's syndrome was accompanied by inhibition of basal and TRH-stimulated TSH secretion [62]. These patients had an attenuated pituitary response to TRH administration and there was a negative correlation between plasma levels of TSH and cortisol (but not T3); after convalescence the reaction to TRH normalized [64]. There was a single case report on the development of Graves's disease characterized by pronounced hyperthyroidism after a successful surgical operation in a patient with Cushing's syndrome [65]. Authors suggest that suppression of hypercorticism activated latent autoimmune processes in the thyroid gland. Graves's disease with hyperthyroidism manifestations was diagnosed 9 months after unitaleral adrenalectomy in a woman with Cushing's syndrome [66]. In some patients subjected to surgical adrenalectomy for hypercorticism transitory dysfunction of the thyroid gland with symptoms of hypo- or hyperthyroidism developed [67]. Silent thyroiditis developed in a female patient after unilateral adrenalectomy for treatment of Cushing's syndrome followed by a gradual tapering of replacement dose of prednisolone to 5 mg/day; thus thyroiditis was characterized by low TSH, increased thyroid hormone levels, extremely low iodine uptake and increased titers of antimicrosomal and antithyroglobulin antibodies [68]. Recent observations have demonstrated that secondary hypothyroidism and hypercalciemia are consequences of the glucocorticoid deficiency developed after adrenalectomy for Cushing's syndrome [69].

In 103 patients with ACTH deficiency Murakami T. et al. [70] found signs of hypothyroidism (a decrease in free T3 and T4 concentrations, high TSH) and characteristic symptoms of clinical manifestations of thyroid insufficiency (cold intolerance, muscle rigidity, loss of interest in life). After hydrocortisone therapy all signs of impairments of the pituitary-thyroid axis disappeared in more than 70% cases; this suggests that glucocorticoid insufficiency is one of reasons underlying thyroid dysfunction. A high TSH level was found in patients with Addison's disease; administration of glucocorticoids caused dose-dependent inhibition of TRH-induced stimulation of TSH secretion; it is possible that glucocorticoids regulate pituitary sensitivity to TRH [71].

Moderate hypothyroidism is a consequence of exogenous or endogenous hypercorticism. In prepubertal children with nonclassical congenital adrenal hyperplasia (NCCAH) TSH and cortisol were secreted in a pulsatile and circadian fashion with a clear nocturnal TSH surge; daytime TSH levels were lower in the NCCAH group than in control children. The cross-correlation analysis of the 24-h raw data demonstrated that TSH and cortisol were negatively correlated, with a 2.5-h lag time [72].

Adrenalectomy not only reduced plasma corticosterone levels to almost zero, but also decreased plasma T3 and T4 levels, but diurnal rhythms of the HPT axis did not depend on rhythms of the HPA axis [73]. In pregnant female rats adrenalectomized on gestation day 8 there was a decrease in TRH mRNA, increase in serum TSH, and a decrease of T3 only in females [74]; it appears that maternal glucocorticoids determine the development of the hypothalamic-pituitary-thyroid axis in progeny.

Conclusion. The analysis of the literature data shows that the role of glucocotricoids in regulation of iodine metabolism in thyroid cells as well as their effects on the HHT system have not been conclusively established. Very few data are available on early changes in thyrocyte iodine metabolism induced by psychoemotional stress which characterize triggering of adaptation in metabolic systems. The idea is very important of the mechanisms of iodine oxidation and organification and the function of the key enzyme in thyroid hormone biosynthesis, TPO, with the activity governing synthesis of thyroid hormones. This seems to be especially topical in relation to increased levels of stressogenic factors in human environment and functions of all the systems under the stress of hypocoticism.

The goal of the above research is to assess the effects of glucocorticoids on the activities of the main steps of thyroid iodine metabolism and to study the features of iodine metabolism under exposure to short-term and chronic psychoemotional stresses.

2. Materials and methods

Experimental animal models. All the experiments were carried out on Wistar female rats (160-180g body weight) which were fed on a standard laboratory diet. Control and experimental groups contained 10-12 animals.

Acute unavoidable psychoemotional stress. This model was aimed at simulation of negative emotions in rats (fear, alarm, anger and aggression). To this end, we used the modified techniques of Desiderato O. [75] and Tolmachev D.A. [76]. The rats were exposed to a combined stress (each animal was placed in an individual box) in a special chamber whose metallic floor was penetrated with 5-mA electric current. The mild painless irritation of the low extremities was accompanied by interrupted noise (electric bell) and light (100-Wt electric bulb) during 20 min or 5-60 min singly. Stress was always given at the same time from 9.00 to 10.00 o'clock in the morning. No manipulations were carried out before placing the animals to penal cells and taking them out. The number of animals in the groups was 8 to 10.

Short-term repeated psychoemotional stress was simulated using the modified techniques of Desiderato O. [75] and Tolmachev D.A. [76] but the exposure was repeated: 20 min daily during 28 days. Animals with normal thyroid status were subjected to multiple exposures to psychoemotional stress.

Simulation of hypocorticism in rats. To simulate glucocorticoid deficiency, the animals were subjected to bilateral adrenalectomy (AE) (n=10). The surgery was performed by a conventional method [30] under ester anaesthesia. After the surgery, the animals were fed on the standard laboratory diet and received a 0.9 sodium chloride solution as a drinking fluid. The animals were selected for experimental groups after a 3-day recovery period following the surgery.

Administration of high doses of potassium iodide to animals with normal and reduced glucocorticoid status.

Single administration. A KI solution was administered by a gastric tube at doses of 0.7; 7.0 and 70.0 mg/kg B.W. (which corresponds to 10, 100 and 1000 daily KI doses [77] or 0.54; 5.35; 53.51 mg iodide/kg B.W.) in the volume of 0.4-0.6 ml. The control rats received distilled water (0.5 ml). The animals were decapitated after 24 h following the administration.

Multiple administration. Potassium iodide was administered by a gastric tube at doses of 0.07, 0.21, 0.70 and 7.0 and 35 mg/kg body weight (which corresponds to 1, 3, 10, 100 and 500 daily doses of potassium iodide or 0.05, 0.16, 0.64, 5.35 and 27.76 mg iodine / kg body weight) in a volume of 0.4-0.6 ml at 9 o'clock daily over 14 days. The control rats received distilled water in a volume of 0.5 ml. After 24 h following the last (14th) administration of KI, the animals were decapitated.

Studies on thyroid iodine metabolism. Determination of total (It), protein-bound (Ib) and free iodine (If) in rat thyroid tissue. The method for determination of total iodine and its protein-bound and free fractions in thyroid tissue was developed directly for this research applying a commonly used catalytic cerium-arsenite method for measurement of iodine in the urine [78]. To determine the total iodine content, 0.125 ml of thyroid homogenate (1:2000) was placed to a test-tube and 0.3 ml of concentrated HClO3 and HClO4 (5:1) was added. The samples were incubated at 110°C for 60 min. They were cooled to a room temperature and 1 ml of a 0.5% sodium arsenite solution was added. The samples were shaken, and after 20 min, 0.5 ml of 1.2% cerium ammonium sulfate was added. Optical density was measured after 20 min at a wavelength of 400 nm. Iodine concentration was calculated by a calibration curve. To construct the calibration curve, we used KIO4 at concentrations of 0, 20, 50, 100, 150 and 200 μg/l.

To measure the contents of protein-bound and free iodine in the thyroid homogenate, the proteins were sedimented with 5.2% perchloric acid and 0.125 ml of the supernatant was used to determine free iodine concentration, the sediment was used to measure protein-bound iodine concentration. After the separation of the iodine fractions, the procedure of measurement corresponded to that described above (I total).

Determination of urinary total iodine concentration in rats. To determine urinary iodine concentration, 0.125 ml of urine from the morning portion (collected between 7 and 9 a.m.) was used. At high iodine concentrations, the samples were diluted 5-, 10-fold and over. Then the urine was burned in a mixture of concentrated HClO3 and HClO4 and the sample was assayed for iodine content as was described above.

Determination of TPO activity. To determine TPO activity, we used the method based on reactions of iodine enzymatic oxidation [79]. 2.8 ml of 0.05 M of sodium phosphate buffer,

0.05 ml of 0.6 M KI and 0.1 ml of thyroid homogenate (1:80) or its microsomal fraction were placed in a 1-cm thermostatically controlled cell. The reaction mixture was stirred and incubated for 15 min at temperature of 28°C. The reaction was started by addition of 0.05 ml of 12 μM H_2O_2. The reaction rate was recorded for 1 min at a wavelength of 353 nm using a Cary-100 spectrophotometer. The TPO activity was calculated using the molar extinction coefficient of ε =22900 M^{-1} x cm^{-1} for the product formed [77]. Enzyme activity was expressed as μmol/min x g protein.

Determination of thyroid hormone concentration in blood serum. The concentrations of total T_4 and total and free blood serum T_3 were measured radioimmunologically using RIA-T4 –CT and RIA-T3-CT kits (Institute of Bioorganic Chemistry, National Academy of Sciences of Belarus, Republic of Belarus).

Determination of total corticosterone concentration in rat blood serum. Blood serum total corticosterone concentration was measured by high performance liquid chromatography (HPLC). The assay was carried out using 0.2 ml of blood serum which was placed to a test-tube with a ground stopper, 1.0 ml of chloroform and 10 μM dexamethasone solution were added (as an internal standard) followed by addition of 40 μl of fresh 1.0 M solution of sodium hydroxide. Corticosteroids were extracted for 1 min. The test-tubes were centrifuged for 3 min at 600 g and then the lower (chloroform) fraction was carefully collected. The chloroform fraction was evaporated to dryness in a nitrogen flow. The samples were dissolved in 20 μl of the mobile phase and applied on a column. The steroids were separated on KAX-1-64-3 columns (2x64 mm) filled with a Silasorb -600 (LC) normal-phase sorbent with the particle diameter of 5 μm (Lachema, Czech Republic). The mixture of hexan-chloroform-methanol in the volume ratio of 7:1:1 was used as the mobile phase [80]. A Milikhrom liquid microcolumn chromatograph (Russia) was used for detection in a UV-detector at a wavelength of 246 nm. The rate of the eluent supply was 200 μl/min. Steroids were identified from the retention time. Corticosterone concentration was calculated from the calibration curve and expressed as nM. A corticosterone (Sigma) solution was used to construct the calibration curve and a dexamethasone (Sigma) solution was used as an internal standard.

Statistical analysis. The data were processed statistically using Mann-Whitney's U-test. The results are presented as means (M) ± standard deviation of the mean. * $P<0,05$; ** $P<0,01$; *** $P<0,001$. The critical value for the significance level was taken to be 5%.

3. Results

3.1. Studies on iodine metabolism under hypercorticism (stress and post-stress periods)

Under psychoemotional stress, the corticosterone content was most elevated (405.8-447.7%) for 15-60 min. It was decreased following 2 hours after stress cessation (2.9-fold) and increased after 6 hours (2.1-fold) at the post-stress period (Fig. 1). Analysing the wave-like dynamics of changes in corticosterone concentration at the post-stress period, we should note that the rats were stressed in the morning (9.00 to 10.00 a.m.) and the rise in corticosterone concentration at the post-stress period was not related to its circadian rhythm (since the circadian rhythm of corticosterone is characterized by maxima per 20.00 hour). The corticosterone concentration was observed to increase in the afternoon (16.00 p.m.) after 6 hours following the post-stress period, and this elevation of serum corticosterone is a characteristic manifestation of a regulatory feedback mechanism. As a response to a marked reduction of corticosterone concentration after 2 hours following stress, the ACTH concentration elevated, which induced a new wave in increasing blood and adrenal corticosterone concentration that is a manifestation of the adaptation syndrome.

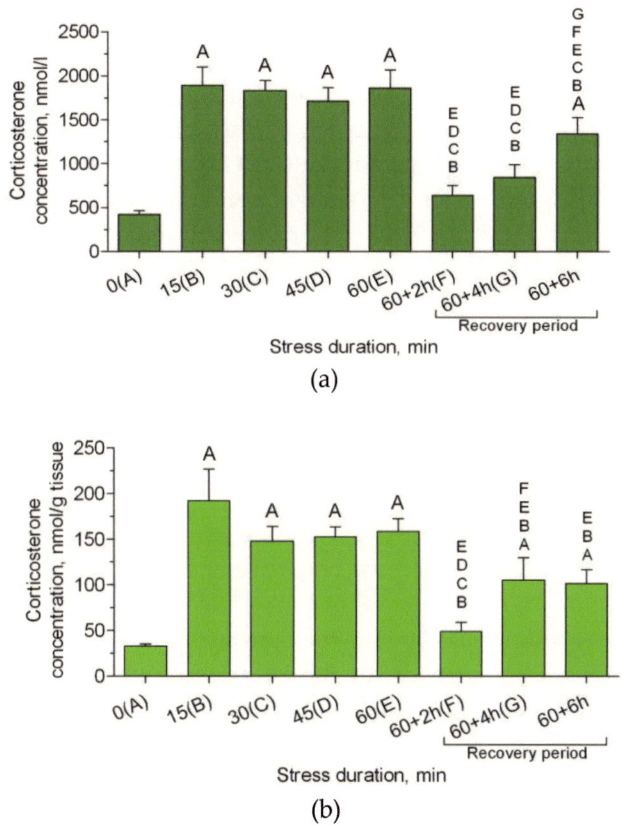

Figure 1. Blood serum (A) and adrenal (B) corticosterone concentrations in rats at acute stress and post-stress periods, after exposure to psychoemotional stress (n=8).
A, B, C, D, E, F, G are groups of animals, respectively. The letters under each column indicate statistically significant changes in the parameter (p<0.05) compared to the corresponding group (e.g., in Fig.1A, the parameter for Groups 15B, 30C, 45D, 60E is statistically significant compared to Group A). The same designations are in Figures 2-4.

The dynamics of changes in the parameters characterizing thyroid iodine metabolism was of a wave-like pattern, which indicates a pronounced response of the rat thyroid to stress. This was most pronounced for changes

in the index If, which is quite explicable. During 15-30 min of stress the thyroid total iodine concentrations remained unchanged (176.9-234.9 μg/g tissue). However, after 60 min, its content was 39.3% decreased in comparison with 15-and 30-min stress (Fig. 2A). During the acute stress phase (15-30 min), intensification of iodide organification was noticed: the concentration of its protein-bound fraction was 37.6% elevated, and the ratio of protein-bound I to total I was 1.2-fold increased (Fig. 2B). The 70.5% elevation of free iodide concentration in the thyroid gland (Fig. 2C) was probably due to activation of proteolytic processes in thyroglobulin and thyroid hormone formation. We cannot also exclude activation of iodine uptake with consideration for the absence of iodine supply to the body during stress, which can be due to increased activities of tissue deiodinases. Along with this, in spite of the evidence for Na^{+}/I^{-}- simporter expression in some cells (salivary and mammary glands) the literature lacks information about other iodine depots in addition to the TG. After 60-min stress, the thyroid showed diminished concentrations of free and protein-bound iodine, which seemed to be a consequence of highly active secretory processes and inhibition of iodine organification, TPO activity (Fig. 3) remained at a level of control values during 30-min exposure to stress, decreasing by 34.8% after 45 min, which was accompanied by a 16.8% reduction of protein-bound I concentration. The stress-induced drop in TPO activity can be due to changed kinetic parameters of the enzyme. TPO was found to be sensitive to elevation of ROS concentrations and aldehyde products of lipid peroxidation in thyroid cells [81]. Moreover, an important role in this case can be played by a decreased TSH level that regulates key processes in the TG. Taking into consideration the antagonistic relations between ACTH and TSH, one can suggest the metabolic changes in the TG to be caused by a stress-induced increase of the ACTH level which can induce a decrease of TSH production.

The correlation analysis of the results did not show a correlation between thyroid TPO activities and glucocorticoid levels in the blood serum and adrenal glands. After 60-min stress, a negative correlation was found between the total thyroid iodide and adrenal corticosterone ($r = -0.952$, $p = 0.003$). In the control group, the content of adrenal corticosterone positively correlated with the protein-bound I to total I ratio ($r = 0.955$, $p = 0.01$), which indicates involvement of glucocorticoids in regulation of iodine homeostasis in the TG.

The decrease in corticosterone concentration after 2 h following the stress exposure was followed by activation of TPO (3.6-fold) as opposed to 60-min stress and control (3.4-fold). The TPO activation at the post-stress period suggests the presence of regulatory mechanisms for its activity which are related to a corticosterone level since it is at that period that its blood and adrenal concentrations were diminished most appreciably. The subsequent elevation of corticosterone concentrations in 4 and 6 h within the recovery period was followed by a dramatic decrease of thyroid TPO activity.

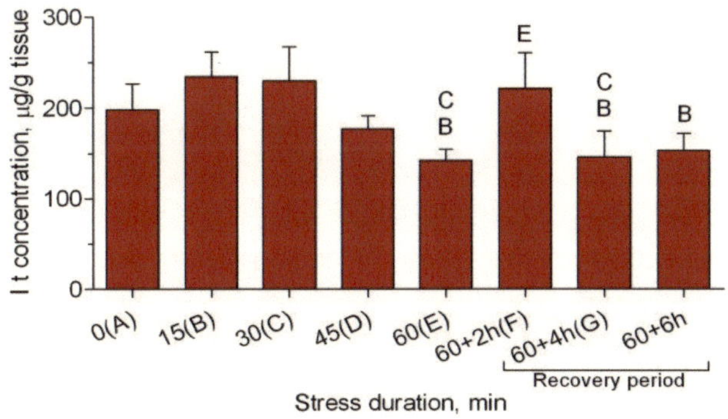

(a)

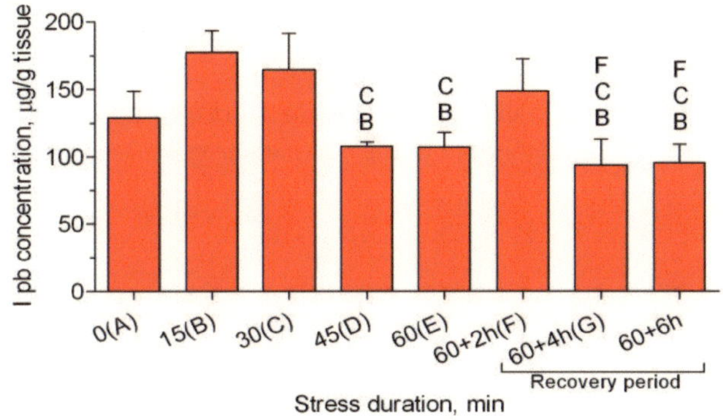

(b)

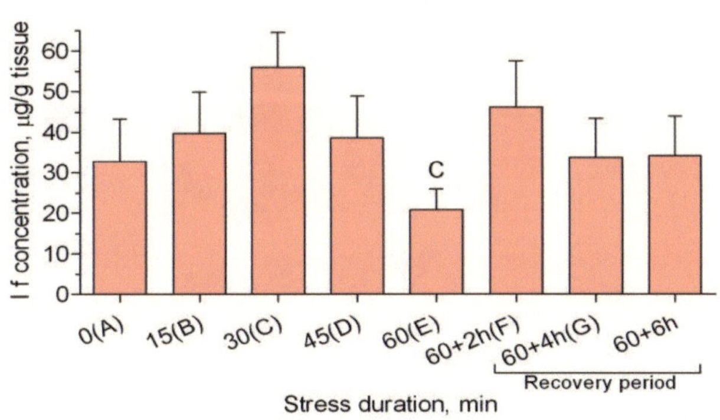

(c)

Figure 2. Rat thyroid total (A), protein-bound (B), and free (C) concentration of iodine during acute stress and post-stress periods.
A, B, C, D, E, F, G represent respective designations for groups of animals.
B, C, E. F represent statistically significant change in the parameter ($p < 0.05$) compared to the corresponding group

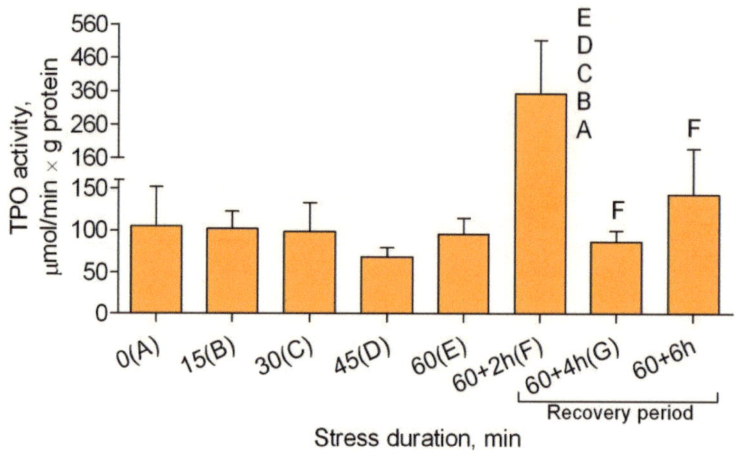

Figure 3. Rat thyroid TPO activity at acute stress and post-stress periods.
A, B, C, D, E, F, G represent corresponding designations for animal groups.
A, B, C, D, E represent statistically significant changes in parameter ($p<0.05$) compared to the corresponding group.

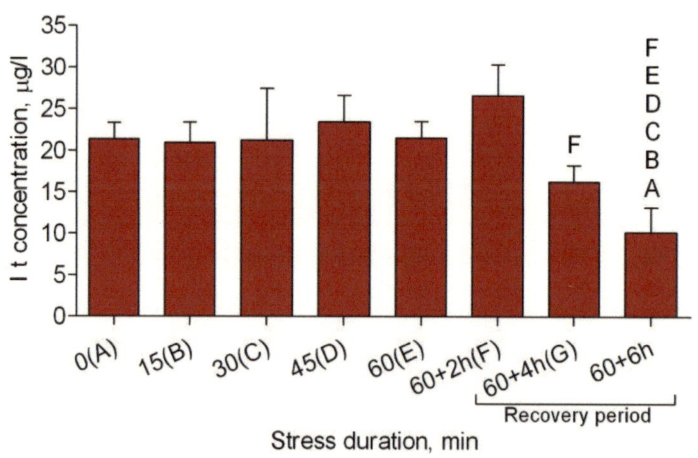

Figure 4. Rat blood iodine concentration at acute stress and post-stress periods.
A, B, C, D, E, F, G represent corresponding designations for animal groups.
A, B, C, D, E, F represent statistically significant changes in the parameter ($p<0.05$) compared to the corresponding group.

The iodine status restoration after the 2- h post-stress period is characterized by elevated concentrations of total I, protein-bound I and free I (55.5, 38.3 and 40.8%, respectively). A marked restoration to the control values of all the thyroid parameters studied was noticed after 4-6 h following the cessation of stress exposure. Under physiological conditions, the blood serum iodine content was not high (approx. 20 μg/l). However, acute stress diminished its level (52.3%) at the post-stress recovery period (after 6 h following stress), which can be a consequence of restoration of the iodine status in the thyroid (Fig. 4).

	Control	Stress, 15 min	Stress, 30 min	Stress, 45 min
Groups	A	B	C	D
T_4 total, nM	59.4±4.1	60.6±3.6	60.5±2.4	59.09±4.4
T_3 free, nM	2.9±0.22	2.9±0.21	2.3±0.12	2.3±0.20^{A,B}

	Stress, 60 min	Stress, 60 min + 2-hour post-stress periods	Stress, 60 min + 4-hour post-stress periods	Stress, 60 min + 6-hour post-stress periods
Groups	E	F	G	H
T_4 total, nM	58.7±3.5	59.1±2.2	64.8±6.0	51.6±4.5
T_3 free, nM	2.1±0.21^{A,B}	2.7±0.29	2.1±0.13^{A,B,F}	2.0±0.26^{A,B,F}

^{A,B,F} $P<0.05$ compared to control.

Table 2. Rat blood T_4 and T_3 concentrations at acute stress and post-stress periods

The stress exposure did not produce significant changes in the concentration of blood serum total T_4. However, the free T_3 content lowered at the 30th minute of stress and remained to be 18.6 to 28.5% lowered throughout the experiment. It was not until 2 hours later that it increased up to the control values (Table 1).

Our findings show involvement of the TG in adaptation of the body to acute stress. We should note the thyroid ability to a rapid recovery of the iodine status at the post-stress period. Throughout a short period of time (15-30 min), the acute stress induced activation and uptake of iodide and thyroid hormone secretion.

However, oxidation of iodide was inhibited and the contents of total I, protein-bound I and free I were decreased after 45 and, significantly, after 60 min.

The 60-min exposure to psychoemotional stress revealed a negative correlation between the concentration of total I in the thyroid and the corticosterone concentration in the adrenals ($r=-0.952$, $p=0.003$). This shows that overproduction of glucocorticoids under stress induces a decrease of thyroid iodine content, resulting in a negative iodine balance at the post-stress period. The 2-hour recovery period is characterized by a pronounced activation of thyroid iodine metabolism (TPO activity rose over 3-fold), and the partial restoration of the thyroid iodine status (after 4-6 hours) was accompanied by a decreased blood serum iodine content.

The following correlations were established at the post-stress recovery period:

- after 4 hours, the blood serum iodide concentration negatively correlated with the corticosterone concentration ($r=-0.831$, $p=0.040$);
- after 6 hours, there was a highly significant correlation ($r=0.937$, $p=0.006$) between the blood corticosterone level and the ratio of protein-bound I to total I;

The data for the recovery period demonstrate that the blood corticosterone level can be viewed as a factor inducing a decrease of blood iodine concentration in rats.

Thus, the short-term stress (5-30 min) induced activation of biosynthesis and secretion of thyroid hormones. The most important regularity of the post-stress period is restoration of the thyroid iodine status due to activation of iodine uptake and organification as well as the presence of a close negative correlation between the thyroid concentration of I total and the adrenal corticosterone concentration ($r= -0.956$, $p=0.003$). After 6 h of the recovery period, the concentration of blood corticosterone was positively correlated to the ratio of protein-bound I/total I in the TG ($r=0.937$, $p=0.006$). A close correlation found between the levels of corticosterone and iodine in the thyroid gland may primarily show possible regulatory effects of glucocorticoids on iodine uptake. But no effects of glucocorticoids on TPO were found, which definitely indicates the absence of direct interactions. However, elevation of thyroid iodine concentration, induced by glucocorticoids, can activate TPO.

The above findings show that the exposure to stress induced a marked imbalance in the thyroid iodine status which was rapidly recovered at the post-stress period due to the decreased blood serum iodine concentration and that the restoration of the thyroid iodine status is most closely related to the glucocorticoid status.

3.2. Studies on the effect of acute exposure to stress on the kinetics of iodine metabolism in rats after administration of physiological potassium iodide doses

We studied the effects of 30-min psychoemotional stress on the iodine metabolism after administration of three daily doses of potassium iodide (KI was administered directly before the exposure to stress). The administration of three daily doses of KI increased 4.3-fold the blood iodine level within 6 hours. This concentration was decreased to the control values after 24 h (Fig. 5). In the group of rats subjected to stress, the iodine content also increased (296.7%) after 30 min following the administration of 3 daily doses of KI. In contrast to the control rats, the stressed rats showed a pronounced maximum of blood iodine concentration after 6 h (839.4% elevation, 170.7μg/l). After 24 h, the level of blood iodine in the stressed rats did not differ from that in the controls. The stress-induced changes in the kinetics of blood iodine concentration are a consequence of a disturbed regulation of iodine homeostasis. The dramatic, over 800%, elevation of blood iodine concentration can be due to an imbalance in the activity of its uptake: lowering of uptake in the TG and activation of uptake in the gastrointestinal tract at the post-stress period. It should be noted that it is at that period that the rat blood showed an increase in the corticosterone concentration (Table 2). A comparative examination of the curves characterizing changes in thyroid iodine concentrations in two animal groups (Fig. 5 B) shows that after 24 h, the thyroid iodine concentration elevated 1.7-fold in the control rats and remained essentially unchanged in the stressed rats (1.2-fold increase).

The 30-min psychoemotional stress leveled off the increase in the thyroid iodine status after administration of 3 daily KI doses. The changed concentrations of thyroid protein-bound I and free I (Fig. 5, B and C) reflect changes in TPO activity in the thyroid gland (Fig. 5D). The administration of 3 daily KI doses was accompanied by activation of its organification in the group of control rats within 1 h (the level of protein-bound I was increased by 54.1%) and elevation of its concentration by 74.3% after 24 h.

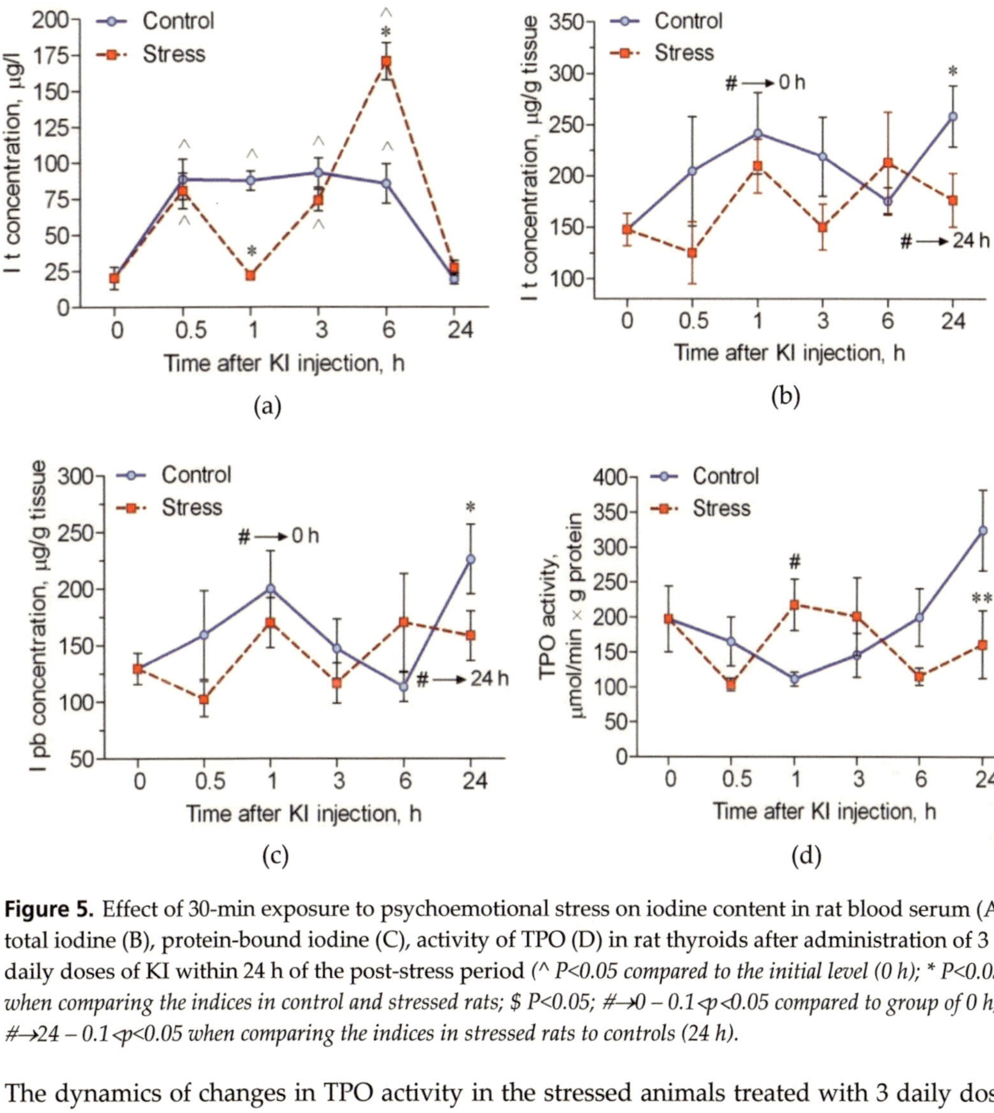

Figure 5. Effect of 30-min exposure to psychoemotional stress on iodine content in rat blood serum (A), total iodine (B), protein-bound iodine (C), activity of TPO (D) in rat thyroids after administration of 3 daily doses of KI within 24 h of the post-stress period (*^ P<0.05 compared to the initial level (0 h); * P<0.05 when comparing the indices in control and stressed rats; $ P<0.05; #→0 – 0.1<p<0.05 compared to group of 0 h; #→24 – 0.1<p<0.05 when comparing the indices in stressed rats to controls (24 h).*

The dynamics of changes in TPO activity in the stressed animals treated with 3 daily doses of KI had an essentially opposite character in comparison with the controls (Figure 5D). The post-stress increase in TPO activity after 1 h was accompanied by 41.5% decrease of its activity by 6 h as opposed to the initial level. As compared to the control animals, the activity of TPO in the thyroid of the stressed rats diminished over 2-fold , whereas the concentration of protein-bound I decreased 1.4-fold after 24 h following the administration of 3 daily KI doses.

The data obtained indicate that the 30-min exposure to stress after the administration of 3 daily KI doses changed the kinetics of iodine metabolism in rats within 24 h of the post-stress period. These data reflect complex relationships between the regulatory effects of the pituitary-thyroid and pituitary-adrenal systems as well as the whole complex of metabolic stress changes in the organism in respect to the key steps in thyroid iodine metabolism. Stress enhances the iodine inhibitory effect.

	Before KI administration	After KI administration				
		30 min	1 h	3 h	6 h	24 h
Blood corticosterone, nM	302.8±28.5	1279.1± 101.6*	1580.4± 118.9*	2135.8± 260.7*	1778± 194.9*	472.7± 47.4
	Before stress	After administration of KI and exposure to stress				
		30 min	1 h	3 h	6 h	24 h
Blood corticosterone, nM	302.8±28.5	2571.6± 282.7*	867.8± 104.5*	664.3± 100.5*	1661.8± 272.5*	697.7± 75.9*

Table 3. Effect of 30-min stress exposure on corticosterone concentration in rat blood after administration of 3 daily doses of KI within 24 h of post-stress period

The most pronounced stress-induced changes in iodine metabolism after administration of physiological KI doses (3 daily doses) are characterized by:

- abnormal kinetics of changes in blood iodine concentration within 24 h after administration of KI, which was manifested by accumulation of blood iodine (839.4% elevation) after 6 h at the post-stress period;
- changes in the kinetics of iodine uptake and oxidation in the TG, which results in a decreased content of total I and protein-bound I in thyroids of stressed rats after administration of 3 daily doses of KI as opposed to the control group which showed an increase of these parameters.

3.3. Effect of unavoidable repeated short-term psychoemotional stress on the functional activity of the rat thyroid

A research was carried out into a short-term stress effect (daily, over a long period of time) on the activities of the key steps in iodine metabolism in the rat thyroid. The data obtained indicate that daily 20-min exposure to stress (4 weeks) induced pronounced changes in thyroid iodine metabolism.

Figure 6 shows that the total thyroid iodine content in stressed animals was elevated 1.97-fold as opposed to controls and amounted to 491.8±15.5 μg/g tissue. The contents of its protein-bound and free fractions corresponded to 329.9±8.3 μg/g tissue and 161.8±18.4 μg/g tissue, which was 1.6-and 3.1-fold higher compared to the controls. The increased thyroid iodine concentration was accompanied by a changed ratio of its various fractions (Table 3). The 2-fold elevated free I/protein-bound I ratio and the lowered protein-bound I/total I ratio

(1.18-fold) are indicative of a lowered efficiency of thyroid iodine organification under stress.

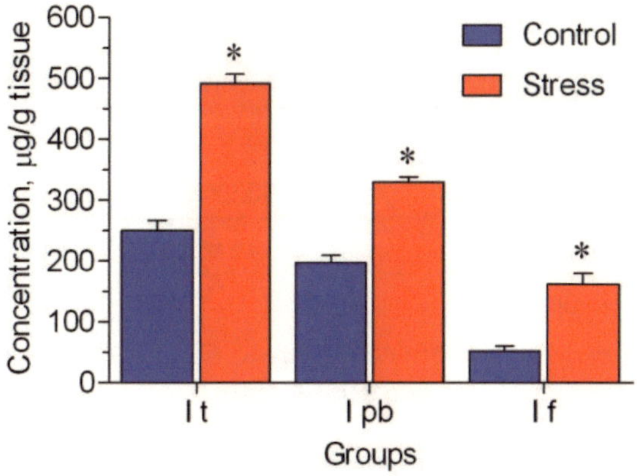

*statistically significant changes vs control group ($p<0.05$)

Figure 6. Effect of 4-week psychoemotional stress (20 min, daily) on contents of total I, protein-bound I and free I in the rat thyroid

Indices	Control	Stress
Free I/protein-bound I	0.26±0.034	0.50±0.066*
Protein-bound I/total I	0.79±0.021	0.67±0.028*
Urinary I, µg/l	17.9±2.29	22.2±1.94

* $P<0.05$ compared to control.

Table 4. Effect of short-term daily psychoemotional stress on the ratio of different rat thyroid iodine fractions and urinary iodine excretion

Indices	Control	Stress
T4 total, nM	49.2±2.82	51.7±3.34
T3 total, nM	1.2±0.06	1.3±0.07
TPO, µmol/min x g tissue	23.4±2.70	20.9±2.91
Thyroid weight, mg	15.7±0.63	13.3±0.47*
Thyroid cytosolic protein, mg/g tissue	158.5±3.6	137.9±5.3*

* $P<0.05$ compared to control.

Table 5. Effect of short-term daily psychoemotional stress on the concentration of blood thyroid hormones, TPO activity, thyroid weight and thyroid protein concentration

No changes were found in the activity of TPO, the key enzyme of thyroid hormone biosynthesis (Table 5). The thyroid weight in stressed rats was lowered by 18%, whereas the protein concentration in the thyroid cytosolic fraction – by 13%. The blood thyroid hormone content at the post-stress period was maintained at the level of control values (Table 5), the level of corticosterone was increased by 32.8% (Table 6) and the weight of the adrenal glands rose by 13%.

Indices	Control	Stress
Blood serum corticosterone, nM	383.2±65.9	509.2±90.0#
Adrenal corticosterone, nmol/g tissue	152.8±17.9	176.2±30.8
Adrenal weight, mg	46.6±1.9	52.7±2.5*

* P<0.05; # P<0.1 compared to control.

Table 6. Effects of short-term daily psychoemotional stress on adrenal weight, blood corticosterone concentration and corticosterone concentration in rat adrenals.

As our data show, stress caused multidirectional changes in the activities of the key steps of thyroid iodine metabolism. The elevated content of the total and free iodine is a consequence of stimulation of its absorption at the post-stress period [28]. The decreased efficiency of iodine organification may be due to TPO inhibition and lowering of thyroglobulin concentration. The stress-induced lowering of thyroid TPO activity was shown earlier. As Table 7 demonstrates, the repeated exposure to short-term stress during 7 days and over was accompanied by a decrease of thyroid TPO activity both directly after exposure to stress (46.9-56.6%) and after 24 h following its cessation (59.2-60.7%).

Index	Control	Stress, 7 days		Stress, 14 days	
		A	Б	A	Б
TPO, μmol/min g protein	153.5±15.2	81.4±21.43*	60.2±4.9*	66.6±9.4*	62.6±18.22*

Group A animals were decapitated directly after the last exposure to stress; Group B animals were decapitated 24 h after the last exposure to stress. * P<0.05 compared to control.

Table 7. Effect of short-term (20 min) psychoemotional stress (daily, 7, 14 days) on thyroid TPO activity

Effects of stress on iodine oxidation and organification in thyroid cells have not been virtually investigated. We found only one study on female tortoises. Thyroid TPO activity in young female tortoises was lowered after ten-fold administration of corticosterone (25, 50, 100 μg/100 g body weight) [34]. Nothing has been known of the effect of stress on thyroglobulin biosynthesis. However, the diminished level of thyroid protein-bound I can be stipulated by its impaired biosynthesis. Moreover, a consequence of stress was a 13%-decreased total protein concentration in the thyroid cytosolic fraction. This certainly applies to thyroglobulin, taking into consideration that it amounts to 75-80% and up of the total thyroid protein.

The main regulator of TPO and thyroglobulin synthesis is TSH whose secretion is inhibited by glucocorticoids [20], which can induce depression of thyroid hormone synthesis. Stress is suggested to cause a decrease of TSH production via pituitary neuromedin B, gastrin-releasing peptide and pituitary leptin acting as local inhibitors of TSH release under stress [21]. It was found that lipocortin -1 is a mediator of glucocorticoid-induced suppression of TSH secretion by the anterior lobe of the pituitary gland [21].

The inhibitory effect of stress seems to be followed by activation of thyroid metabolism at the post-stress period and the restoration of thyrocyte function is related to activation of thyroid hormone secretion, which is confirmed by resorption of colloid and depletion of thyroid follicules. These conditions disturb the thyroglobulin synthesis/secretion balance. As a result, the thyrocytes and follicular lumen accumulate a considerable amount of non-organified iodine, which is confirmed by our findings. Stress decreases thyroid weight, which can be both a consequence of its hypersecretion and destructive processes; the mechanism of this change is certainly interesting.

The experimental findings show that a consequence of the repeated exposures to psychoemotional stress are pronounced structural and metabolic changes in the TG that are characterized by an elevated iodine content, a decreased extent of its organification, development of oxidative stress and lymphocyte infiltration along with the impaired thyroid follicular structure. The mechanisms of the regularities found call for detailed research and are of great interest to disclose the pathogenesis of autoimmune thyroiditis, thyroid carcinoma as well as the contribution of the thyroid component to development of endemic and nodular goiters.

There are presently no unambiguous data on the role of stress in induction of thyroid pathology in humans. Individual cases have been described of autoimmune thyroiditis developed after surgical treatment of hypercorticism (Cushing's syndrome) [65]. A pronounced stress effect can be an onset of Graves' disease [82]. There were reports about relationships between stress and Hashimoto's thyroiditis [83]. According to Polish researchers [84] secondary adrenal deficiency can be a cause of autoimmune thyroid diseases in humans: stress affects the immune system, and immunologic modulations are considered to be a factor inducing autoimmune thyroiditis in genetically prone individuals [85]. Stress hormones, affecting antigen-presenting immune cells, can influence the differentiation of bipolar T-helpers from Th1 to Th2 phenotype, which causes suppression of cellular immunity and enhancement of humoral immunity. Stress is likely to contribute to the development of Graves' disease by shifting the Th1/Th2 ratio from Th1 to Th2. Recovery after stress or immunosuppressive effect of pregnancy can induce a "reverse shift" in Th2 → Th1, causing autoimmune (sporadic) thyroiditis [85].

Stress-induced impairment of thyroid function characterized by development of oxidative and iodine stress is likely to be viewed as a main mechanism of thyroid ageing in humans and, consequently, to be a cause of diseases of age related to thyroid deficiency [86, 87]. Further studies are needed to disclose the mechanisms of stress-induced impairment of thyroid functions.

3.4. Studies on rat thyroid iodine metabolism under hypocorticism (after adrenalectomy)

The above findings confirm that stress considerably changes thyroid iodine metabolism, affecting its uptake and organification. Since all the experimental studies were carried out using models characterizing hyperfunction of the adrenal glands (stress), a comparative investigation of iodine metabolism in rats with adrenal deficiency should be done in order to establish the biochemical mechanisms.

The glucocorticoid status in rats was assessed by the level of corticosterone which was lowered 4.4 to 6.4-fold in adrenalectomized (AE) rats compared to controls. Adrenal deficiency was a cause of 44.2 % - decreased thyroid TPO activity (Fig. 7B). The administration of 1000 daily doses of KI (a dose=70 mg/kg) decreased thyroid TPO activity in the TG of the control rats and elevated it in the glucocorticoid-deficient animals with to the control values. The administration of 1000 daily doses of KI was accompanied by increases in thyroid total I (42.2%), protein-bound I (19.1%) and free I (90.6%) in AE rats (Fig. 8). This indicates that under hypocorticism the regulatory mechanisms for thyrocyte functions can be disturbed by high iodine doses.

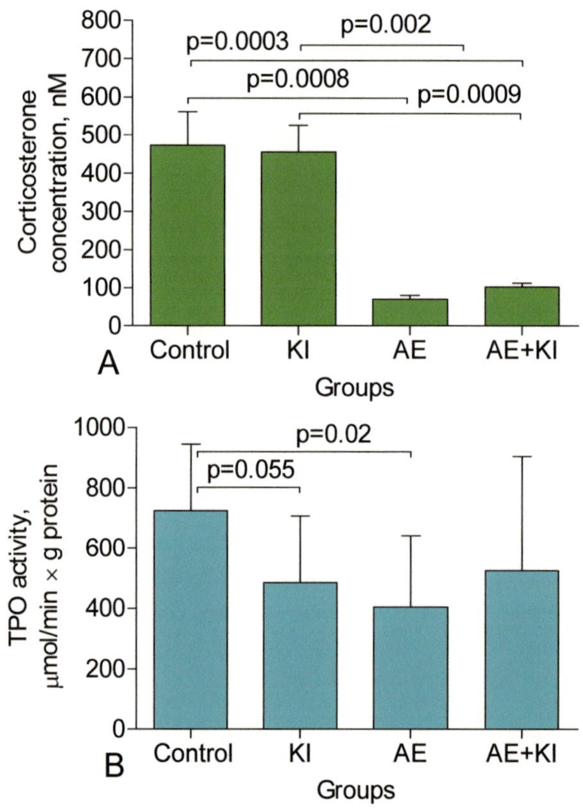

Figure 7. Effect of single administration of 1000 daily doses of KI on concentration of blood serum corticosterone (nM) (A) and TPO activity (µmol/min x g protein) in thyroids of intact and AE rats (B)

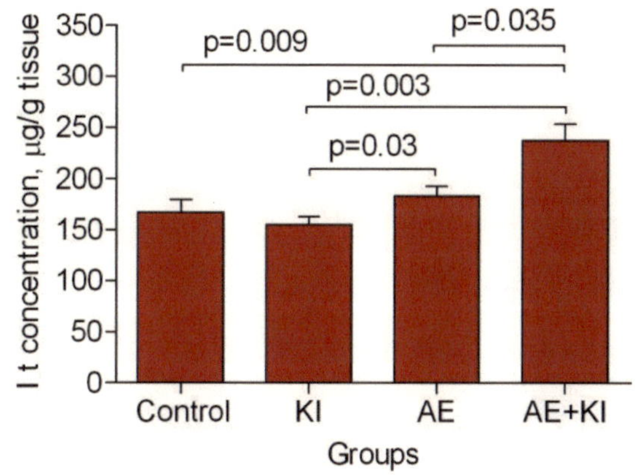

(a)

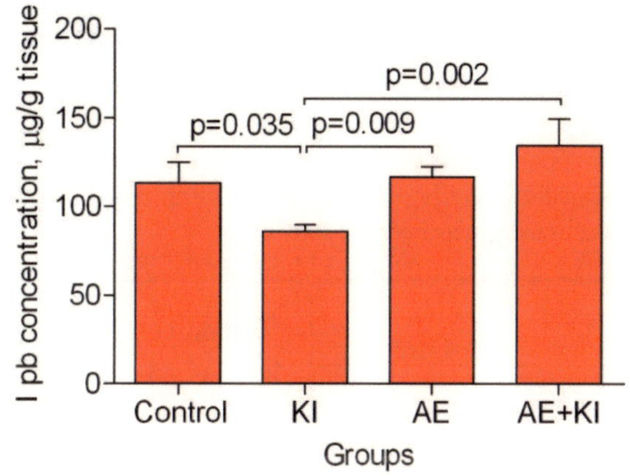

(b)

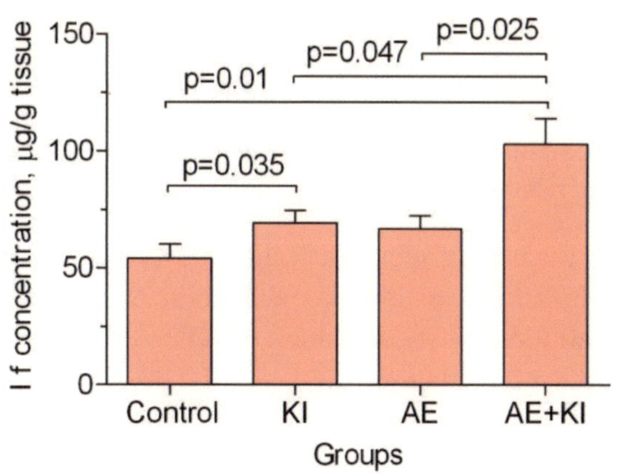

(c)

Figure 8. Effect of single administration of 1000 daily KI doses on contents of total I, protein-bound I and free I in thyroids of rats with normal and decreased glucocorticoid statuses

The blood thyroid hormone levels in AE rats were above the control values (27% for T_4 and 35% for T_3), but administration of KI lowered the concentrations of T_4 by 41.1% and T_3 by 34% compared to the AE animals. T_4 was 29% decreased even in comparison with the controls (Fig. 9).

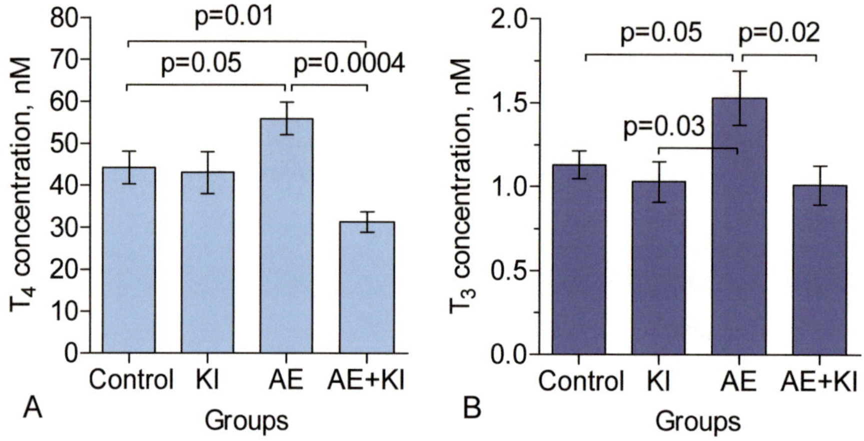

Figure 9. Effect of single administration of high KI dose on concentrations of total blood serum T4 and T3 in rats with normal and decreased glucocorticoid statuses

Index	Control	1000 daily doses of KI	AE	AE+1000 daily doses of KI
	A	B	C	D
TBARS, nmol/g tissue	131.2±8.9	212.5±22.9^{A}	150.4±15.0	115.5±9.6^{B,C}
Catalasa, μmol/min×g protein	36.8±1.3	40.0±1.6	32.2±0.8^{A,B}	33.7±1.7^{B}
SOD, activity u./min×g protein	43.2±4.2	56.8±1.4^{A}	51.1±2.0^{A,B}	48.9±2.9^{B}
GR, μmol/min×g protein	24.0±1.2	22.7±1.0	26.7±1.0^{B}	25.5±1.5

Table 8. Effect of single administration of 1000 daily doses of KI on TBARS levels and antioxidant enzyme activities in thyroids of rats with normal and decreased glucocorticoid statuses

In contrast to the rats with the normal glucocorticoid status, in which the administration of KI inhibited the thyroid function and induced activation of oxidative processes (62.0% elevation of TBARS concentration, 54.3% activation of SOD), the adrenalectomized rats did not show activation of lipid peroxidation (the level of TBARS was decreased by 23.2%, Table 8).

The AE animals demonstrated elevated concentrations of T_3 and T_4 in the blood serum (Fig. 9). These changes seemed to be caused by alterations in thyroid iodine metabolism since the contents of its different fractions did not change under decreased glucocorticoid status (Fig. 8). It was found earlier that AE caused enhancement of liver thyroxin-binding globulin synthesis and its binding capacity in the blood [88] as well as inhibition of the peripheral metabolism of thyroid hormones. Enhancement of deposition of blood thyroid hormones and, consequently, inhibition of their metabolism may cause elevation of thyroid hormone concentrations.

Most interesting changes were found after administration of high iodine doses to rats. In contrast to control animals with the characteristic acute Wolff – Chaikoff's effect, we did not observe inhibition of iodide organification in this group. Moreover, a pronounced lowering of T_4 and T_3 concentrations in the blood serum of AE rats after the administration of high iodine doses suggests that the cause of the absence of the Wolff-Chaikoff's effect under hypocorticism can be impaired maturing of the prohormone, thyroglobulin, and abnormal secretion of thyroid hormones to the blood, which provides for elevated concentration of protein-bound I in this group. Elevated TSH concentrations and enhanced NIS expression and, consequently, increased uptake of iodide absorption by the TG are also possible.

Our findings show that the effects of the single administration of the high KI dose on the activity of hormonogenesis in thyroids from normal and AE animals are multidirectional. Thyroids from the intact rats show inhibition of iodide organification accompanied by induction of oxidative stress, whereas the hypocorticoid rats demonstrate a reverse effect: activation of iodide uptake and organification as well as a decrease in the intensity of lipid peroxidation. These results are of a considerable interest in relation to some clinical studies which prove that impairments in the glucocorticoid status can be linked to development of autoimmune thyroid diseases. Lowering of the functional activity in the hypophyseal link (ACTH) and/or the adrenal (cortisol) link was noted in patients with autoimmune tyroiditis [89, 90]. It was shown that autoimmune tyroiditis and diabetes mellitus are developed on the average 7 years after autoimmune damage of the adrenal glands [91]. In patients suffering from hypercorticism of different genesis, AE contributes to development of autoaggression in their thyroids [68, 66, 92]. It is suggested that puerperal thyroiditis, as a consequence of a temporary decrease of the glucocorticoid status in females at the puerperal period [93], is due to ACTH-releasing hormone inhibition of the synthesis and secretion of maternal hypothalamic ACTH-releasing hormone and that this inhibition is of a placental origin. It should be mentioned that impaired functional activities of the pituitary-adrenal axis are also noted in other autoimmune diseases [94]. The mechanisms of the regularities found certainly require further studies since the literature lacks information on this problem.

3.5. Excess administration of iodine induces development of hyperthyroiditis in rats with glucocorticoid deficiency

Glucocorticoid deficiency is a cause for impairments of the adequate regulation of the thyroid status and thyroid iodine metabolism. It was interesting to study the properties of the iodine metabolism after its repeated administration to rats with adrenal deficiency.

After 2 weeks following AE, the blood serum thyroid hormone concentrations in operated animals were partially restored and amounted to 23.7-42.3% of the control values (Fig. 10)

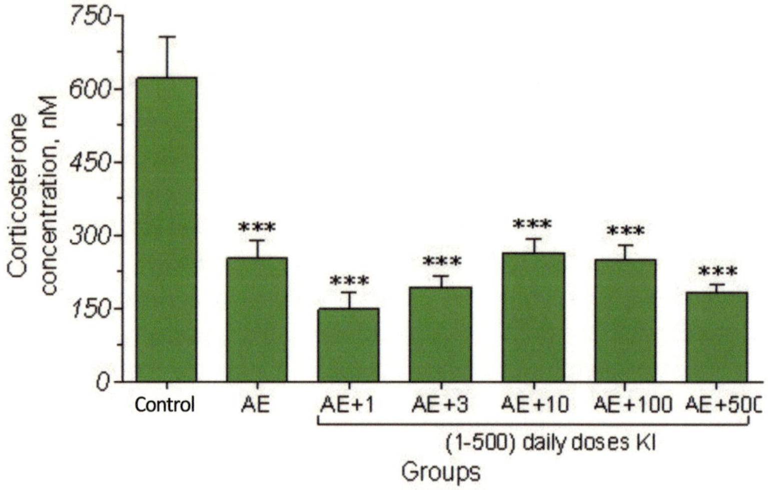

*** statistically significant changes vs control group (p<0.001)

Figure 10. Effect of 14-day administration of 1-500 daily doses of KI on blood serum corticosterone concentration in AE rats.

Studies on the thyroid iodine metabolism showed that repeated administration of high KI doses resulted in 46.9-115.7% increased concentrations of total I and caused 120.4 to 223.9% elevations of free I in all the experimental groups (Fig. 11). Glucocorticoid hormones are likely to inhibit iodide uptake by erythrocytes since the levels of nonorganified iodine were 1.2-fold increased after AE in rats which did not receive supplementary KI. One more confirmation is a more considerable growth of free I concentrations in thyroids of rats with hypocorticism (120.4-223.9%, Fig. 11) compared to controls (94.8-128.0%) after administration of KI at the same doses. Iodine organification in AE rats was enhanced by 32-86% in rats treated with 3 to 500 daily doses of KI (Fig. 11). TPO activity in AE rats was 29.4% elevated and 2.4, 3.9 and 3.7-fold increased (Table 9) after administration of 3, 100 and 500 KI daily doses.

	Control	Daily doses of KI administered to AE animals				
		No administration	1	3	100	500
TPO, μmol/min× g protein	173.9±22.5	193.8±10.3	275.4±77.4	387.9±78.4*	616.5±178.1*	579.7±120.6*

Table 9. Effect of 2-week administration of 1 to 500 daily doses of potassium iodide on TPO activity (μm/min×g tissue) in thyroids of AE rats

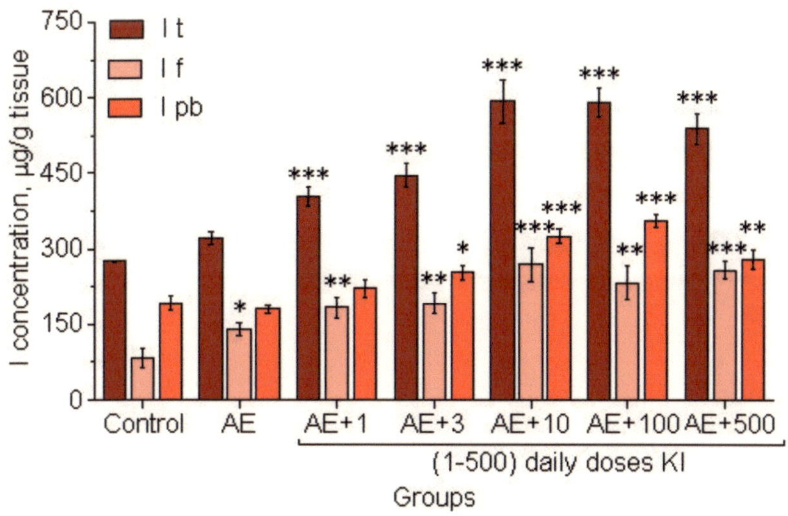

*statistically significant changes vs control group (p<0.05), **p<0.01; ***p<0.001

Figure 11. Effect of 14-day administration of 1-500 daily doses of KI on the concentrations of total I, protein-bound I and free I in thyroids of AE rats

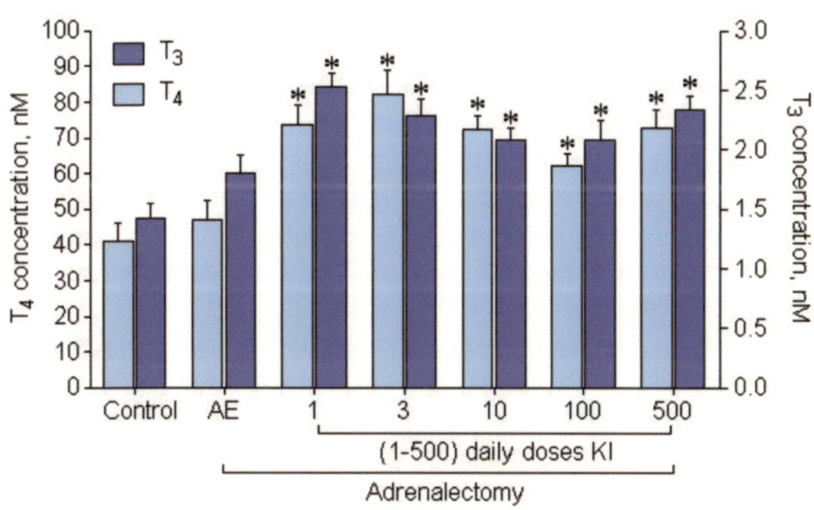

* statistically significant changes vs control group (p<0.05)

Figure 12. Effect of 14-day administration of 1 to 500 daily doses of potassium iodide on the concentrations of total T_4 and T_3 in the blood serum of rats with normal and lowered glucocorticoid statuses

The repeated and single administrations of excess potassium iodide to rats with hypocorticism were characterized by activation of iodide metabolism in the TG, which was followed by development of pronounced hyperthyroidism in AE animals. The blood serum total T_4 concentration (Fig. 12) was increased by 52-100% in rats with adrenal deficiency treated with KI for 14 days compared to control animals. The T_3 concentration (Fig. 12) reached 145.5-177.5% of the control level.

In this situation, a pronounced disturbance in the regulatory mechanisms of the pituitary-thyroid axis may be observed, which is accompanied by development of hypothyroidism and indicates a permissive (coordinating) role of glucocorticoids in regulation of thyroid homeostasis.

Our findings indicate that regulation of iodide uptake is very closely related to the state of the pituitary-adrenal system. Excess iodine intake under hypocorticism causes development of hyperthyroiditis.

4. Conclusion

1. Short-term stress (5-30 min) induced activation of biosynthesis and secretion of thyroid hormones. The most important established regularity of the post-stress period is restoration of the iodine thyroid status due to activation of uptake and organification of iodine as well as a negative correlation between the total thyroid concentration and adrenal corticosterone concentration ($r= -0.952$, $p=0.003$), which indicates participation of glucocorticoids in regulation of iodine thyroid homeostasis.
2. The most pronounced stress-induced changes in iodine metabolism after the treatment by physiological KI doses (3 daily doses) are characterized by:
   - disturbed kinetics of blood iodine content within 24 h following the KI treatment, which was characterized by accumulation of blood iodine (826%) after 6 hours following the post-stress period;
   - changed dynamics of thyroid uptake and oxidation of iodine, which caused a decrease in the concentrations of total I and protein-bound I in thyroids of stressed rats after the treatment with 3 daily doses of KI in contrast to the control group which showed elevation of these indices.
3. It was shown that repeated exposure to short-term psychoemotional stress (for 4 weeks) induced pronounced structural and metabolic changes in the thyroid gland that were characterized by elevated iodine content, as well as a decrease of the extent of its organification and development of oxidative stress.
4. The lowered glucocorticoid status in rats is characterized by increased blood thyroid hormone concentrations and decreased TPO activity (44.2%). In contrast to the animals with normal glucocorticoid status, the AE rats did not show any inhibitory effect of high iodine doses (Wolff-Chaikoff's effect) after the single administration of 1000 daily doses of KI, and activation of thyroid iodide uptake and organification was observed.
5. The 2-week administration of KI (1-500 daily doses) to rats with glucocorticoid deficiency increased the levels of free iodine (120-224%) and protein-bound iodine (32-86%) as well as thyroid TPO activity. In contrast to controls, this was followed by development of pronounced hyperthyroiditis (T_4 amounts to 152-200% and T_3 – 145 to

177% of the control values), which is a consequence of impairments in the key mechanisms of thyrocyte regulation and shows a permissive (coordinating) role of glucocorticoids in respect to the given effects.

The state of chronic stress may be a cause of impaired iodine metabolism in thyroid cells, which can induce development of hypothyroiditis and autoimmune thyroid pathology. Deficiency of the pituitary-adrenal system enhances the probability of development of hyperthyroiditis.

Author details

Liliya Nadolnik
Department of Bioregulators, Institute of Bioorganic Chemistry National Academy of Sciences of Belarus, Belarus

Acknowledgement

We are grateful to her colleagues and post –graduate students at the Institute of Pharmacology and Biochemistry of the National Academy of Sciences of Belarus, Dr. Sergey Chumachenko (Ph.D. in Biology), Dr. Sergey Lupachik (Ph.D. in Biology), Ms. Daria Goreva and Ludmila Kiryukhina for the assistance in the implementation of this project.

5. References

[1] Derwahl M, Seto P, Rapoport B (1989) Complete nucleotide sequence of the cDNA for thyroidperoxidase in FRTL-5 rat thyroid cells. Nucleic Acids Res. 17: 8380-8384.

[2] Kaminsky S, Levy O, Salvador C, Dai G, Carrasco N (1994) Na^+/I^- symporter activity is present in membrane vesicles from TSH-deprived non I^- transporting cultured thyroid cells. Proc. Natl. Acad. Sci. USA. 91: 3789-3793.

[3] Nikiforov Y (2006) Radiation-induced thyroid cancer: what we have learned from Chernobyl. Endocr. Pathol. 17: 307-317.

[4] Uyttersprot N, Pelgrims N, Carrasco N, Gervy C, Maenhaut C, Dumont J, Miot F (1997) Moderate doses of iodide in vivo inhibit cell proliferation and the expression of thyroperoxidase and Na+/I- symporter mRNAs in dog thyroid. Mol. Cell Endocrinol. 131: 195-203.

[5] Espinoza C, Schmitt L, Loos U (2001) Thyroid transcription factor 1 and Pax8 synergistically activate the promot er of the human thyroglobulin gene. J. Mol. Endocrinol. 27: 59–67.

[6] Lagorce J, Thomes J, Catanzano G, Buxeraud J, Raby M, Raby C (1991) Formation of molecular iodine during oxidation of iodide by the peroxidase/H2O2 system. Implications for antithyroid therapy. Biochem. Pharmacol. 42: S89-S92.

[7] Hahn F, McClellan R, Boecker B, Muggenburg B (1988) Future development of biological understanding of radiation protection: implications of nonstochastic effects. Health. Phys. 55: 303-313.

[8] Schumm-Draeger P (2001) Sodium/iodide symporter (NIS) and cytokines. Exp. Clin. Endocrinol. Diabetes. 109: P. 32-34.

[9] Bjorkman U, Ekholm R, Denef J (1981) Cytochemical localization of hydrogen peroxide in isolated thyroid follicles J. Ultrastruct. Res. 74: 105-115.

[10] Zang X, Li Y, Wang Z, Li P (2006) Glucocorticoids receptor subunit gene expression in thyroid gland and adenomas. Acta Oncol. 45: 1073-1078.

[11] Liu Z (1992) Effect of TRH on anti-restraint stress in rats. Zhongguo Yi Xue Ke Xue Yuan Xue Bao. 14: 118-121.

[12] Kuhn E, Geris K, Van der Geyten S, Mol K, Darras V (1998) Inhibition and activation of the thyroidal axis by the adrenal axis in vertebrates. Comp. Biochem. Physiol. A Mol. Integr. Physiol. 120: 169-174.

[13] Bános C, Takó J, Salamon F, Györgyi S, Czikkely R (1979) Effect of ACTH-stimulated glucocorticoid hypersecretion on the serum concentrations of thyroxine-binding globulin, thyroxine, triiodothyronine, reverse triiodothyronine and on the TSH-response to TRH. Acta Med. Acad. Sci. Hung. 36: 381-394.

[14] Re R, Kourides I, Ridgway E, Weintraub B, Maloof F (1976) The effect of glucocorticoid administration on human pituitary secretion of thyrotropin and prolactin. J. Clin. Endocrinol. Metab. 43: 338-346.

[15] Iovino M., Steardo L, Monteleone P (1991) Impaired sensitivity of the hypothalamo-pituitary-thyroid axis to the suppressant effect of dexamethasone in elderly subjects Psychopharmacology (Berl.). 1105: 481-484.

[16] Rubello D, Sonino N, Casara D, Girelli M, Busnardo B, Boscaro, M (1992) Acute and chronic effects of high glucocorticoid levels on hypothalamic-pituitary-thyroid axis in man. J. Endocrinol. Invest. 15: 437-441.

[17] Azukizawa M, Mori S, Ohta H, Matsumura S, Yoshimoto H, Uozumi T, Miyai K, Kumahara Y (1979) Effect of a single dose of glucocorticoid on the diurnal variations of TSH, thyroxine, 3,5,3'-triiodothyronine, 3,3',5'-triiodothyronine and cortisol in normal men. Endocrinol. Jpn. 26: P. 719-723.

[18] Fang V, Shian L (1981) Adrenal influence on pituitary secretion of thyrotropin and prolactin in rats. Endocrinology. 108: 1545-1551.

[19] Ahlquist J, Franklyn J, Ramsden D, Sheppard M (1989) The influence of dexamethasone on serum thyrotrophin and thyrotrophin synthesis in the rat. Mol. Cell Endocrinol. 64: 55-61.

[20] Kakucska I, Qi Y, Lechan R (1995) Changes in adrenal status affect hypothalamic thyrotropin-releasing hormone gene expression in parallel with corticotropin-releasing hormone. Endocrinology. 136: 2795-2802.

[21] Van der Geyten, S., Byamungu, N., Reyns, G.E., Kühn, E.R., and Darras, V.M (2005) Iodothyronine deiodinases and the control of plasma and tissue thyroid hormone levels in hyperthyroid tilapia (Oreochromis niloticus). J. Endocrinol. 184: 467-479.

[22] Taylor A, Flower R, Buckingham J (1995) Dexamethasone inhibits the release of TSH from the rat anterior pituitary gland in vitro by mechanisms dependent on de novo protein synthesis and lipocortin 1. J. Endocrinol. 147: 533-544.

[23] Coiro V, Volpi R, Capretti L, Speroni G, Pilla, S, Cataldo S, Bianconcini M, Bazzani E, Chiodera P (2001) Effect of dexamethasone on TSH-secretion induced by TRH in human obesity. Investig. Med. 49: P. 330-334.

[24] Saito T, Endo T, Kawaguchi A, Ikeda M, Nakazato M, Kogai T, Onaya T (1997) Increased expression of the Na/I symporter in cultured human thyroid cells exposed to thyrotropin and in Graves' thyroid tissue. J. Clin. Endocrinol. Metab. 82: 3331-3336.

[25] Bernier-Valentin F, Trouttet-Masson S, Rabilloud R, Selmi-Ruby S, Rousset B (2006) Three-dimensional organization of thyroid cells into follicle structures is a pivotal factor in the control of sodium/iodide symporter expression. Endocrinology. 147: 2035-2042.

[26] Ferreira A, Lima L, Araújo R, Müller G, Rocha R, Rosenthal D, Carvalho D. (2005) Rapid regulation of thyroid sodium–iodide symporter activity by thyrotrophin and iodine. J. Endocrinol. 184: P. 69-76.

[27] Tonacchera M, Pinchera A, Dimida A, Ferrarini E, Agretti P, Vitti P, Santini F, Crump K, Gibbs J (2004) Relative potencies and additivity of perchlorate, thiocyanate, nitrate, and iodide on the inhibition of radioactive iodide uptake by the human sodium iodide symporter. Thyroid. 14: 1012-1019.

[28] Knopp J, Kvetnansky R, Murgas M, Knopp J. (1978) The changes of in vitro ^{131}-iodine uptake in the thyroid gland of rats exposed to septal lesions and immobilization stress. Physiol. Bohemoslov. 27: 329-332.

[29] Kiang J, Wang X, Ding X, Gist I, Smallridge R (1996) Heat shock inhibits the hypoxia-induced effects on iodide uptake and signal transduction and enhances cell survival in rat thyroid FRTL-5 cells. Thyroid. 6: 475-483.

[30] Becks G, Buckingham D, Wang J, Phillips I, Hill D (1992) Regulation of thyroid hormone synthesis in cultured ovine thyroid follicles. Endocrinology. 130: 2789-2794.

[31] Takiyama Y, Tanaka H, Makino I (1994) The effects of hydrocortisone and RU486 (mifepristone) on iodide uptake in porcine thyroid cells in primary culture. Endocrinology. 135: 1972-1979.

[32] Unterholzner S, Willhauck M, Cengic N, Schütz M, Göke B, Morris J, Spitzweg C (2006) Dexamethasone stimulation of retinoic Acid-induced sodium iodide symporter expression and cytotoxicity of 131-I in breast cancer cells. J. Clin. Endocrinol. Metab. 91: 69-78.

[33] Scholz I, Cenqic N, Göke B, Morris J, Spitzweg C. (2004) Dexamethasone enhances the cytotoxic effect of radioiodine therapy in prostate cancer cells expressing the sodium iodide symporter. J. Clin. Endocrinol. Metab. 89: 1108-1116.

[34] Ray P, Sarkar S, Sengupta A, Chaudhuri-Sengupta S, Maiti B (2006) Roles of thyroid, adrenal and pancreatic hormones on thyroid activity of the soft-shelled turtles Lissemys punctata punctata Bonnoterre. Folia Biol. (Krakow). 54: 93-102.

[35] Woltz H, Thompson F, Kemppainen R, Munnell J, Lorenz M (1983) Effect of prednisone on thyroid gland morphology and plasma thyroxine and triiodothyronine concentrations in the dog. Am. J. Vet. Res. 44: 2000-2003.

[36] Montesinos M, Pellizas C, Velez M, Susperreguv S, Masini-Repiso A, Coleoni A (2006) Thyroid hormone receptor beta 1 gene expression is increased by Dexamethasone at transcriptional level in rat liver. Life Sci. 78: 2584-2594.

[37] Friedman Y, Bacchus R, Raymond R, Joffe R, Nobrega J (1999) Acute stress increases thyroid hormone levels in rat brain. Biol. Psychiatry. 45: 234-237.

[38] Csaba G, Kovacs P, Tothfalusi L, Pallinger E. (2005) Prolonged effect of stress (water and food deprivation) at weaning or in adult age on the triiodothyronine and histamine content of immune cells. Horm. Metab. Res. 37: 711–715.

[39] Pallinger E, Csaba G (2005) Influence of acute stress on the triiodothyronine (T_3) and serotonin content of rat's immune cells. Acta Physiol. Hung. 92: 47-52.

[40] Darras V, Kotanen S, Geris K, Berghman L, Kühn E (1996) Plasma thyroid hormone levels and iodothyronine deiodinase activity following an acute glucocorticoid challenge in embryonic compared with posthatch chickens Gen. Comp. Endocrinol. 104: 203-212.

[41] Van der Geyten S, Segers I, Gereben B, Bartha T, Rudas P, Larsen P, Kühn E, Darras V (2001) Transcriptional regulation of iodothyronine deiodinases during embryonic development. Molecular and Cellular Endocrinology. 183: 1-9.

[42] Forhead A, Jellyman J, Gardner D, Giussani D, Kaptein E, Visser T, Fowden A (2007) Differential effects of maternal dexamethasone treatment on circulating thyroid hormone concentrations and tissue deiodinase activity in the pregnant ewe and fetus. Endocrinology. 148: 800-805.

[43] Van der Geyten S, Darras V (2005) Developmentally defined regulation of thyroid hormone metabolism by glucocorticoids in the rat. J. Endocrinol. 185: 327-336.

[44] Baumgartner A, Hiedra L, Pinna G, Eravci M, Prengel H, Meinhold H (1998) Rat brain type II 5'-iodothyronine deiodinase activity is extremely sensitive to stress. J. Neurochem. 71: 817-826.

[45] Verhoelst C,Van der Geyten S, Roelens, S, Darras V, (2005) Regulation of thyroid hormone availability by iodothyronine deiodinases at the blood-brain barrier in birds. Ann. N.Y. Acad. Sci. 1040: 501-503.

[46] Anguiano B, Valverde C (2001) Cold-induced increment in rat adrenal gland type II deiodinase is corticosterone dependent. Endocrine. 15: 8-91.

[47] Kim S, Harney J, Larsen P (1993) Hormonal regulation of thyroglobulin export from the endoplasmic reticulum of cultured thyrocytes. J. Biol. Chem. 268: 4873-4879.

[48] Song S, Oka T (2003) Regulation of type II deiodinase expression by EGF and glucocorticoid in HC11 mouse mammary epithelium. American Journal of Physiology Endocrinology and Metabolism. 284: E1119-E1124.

[49] Araki O, Morimura T, Ogiwara T, Mizuma H, Mori M, Murakami M (2003) Expression of type 2 iodothyronine deiodinase in corticotropin-secreting mouse pituitary tumor cells is stimulated by glucocorticoid and corticotropin-releasing hormone. Endocrinology. 144: 4459-4465.

[50] Coppola A, Meli R, Diano S (2005) Inverse shift in circulating corticosterone and leptin levels elevates hypothalamic deiodinase type 2 in fasted rats. Endocrinology. 146: 2827-2833.

[51] Brtko J, Macejova D, Knopp J, Kvetnansky R (2004) Stress is associated with inhibition of type I iodothyronine 5'-deiodinase activity in rat liver. Ann. N.Y. Acad. Sci. 1018: P. 219-223.

[52] Bianco A, Nunes M, Hell N, Maciel R (1987) The role of glucocorticoids in the stress-induced reduction of extrathyroidal 3,5,3'-triiodothyronine generation in rats. Endocrinology. 120: 1033-1038.

[53] Balsam A, Ingbar S (1978) The influence of fasting, diabetes, and several pharmacological agents on the pathways of thyroxine metabolism in rat liver. Joural of Clinical Investigation. 62: 415-424.

[54] Menjo M, Murata Y, Fujii T, Nimura Y, Seo H (1993) Effects of thyroid and glucocorticoid hormones on the level of messenger ribonucleic acid for iodothyronine type I 5_-deiodinase in rat primary hepatocytes grown as spheroids Endocrinology. 133: 2984-2990.

[55] Maia A, Harney J, Larsen P, Maia A (1995) Pituitary cells respond to thyroid hormone by discrete, gene-specific pathways. Endocrinology. 136: 1488-1494.

[56] Walpita C, Grommen S, Darras V, Van der Geyten S (2007) The influence of stress on thyroid hormone production and peripheral deiodination in the Nile tilapia (Oreochromis niloticus). Gen. Comp. Endocrinol. 150: 18-25.

[57] Van der Geyten S, Darras V (2005) Developmentally defined regulation of thyroid hormone metabolism by glucocorticoids in the rat. J. Endocrinol. 185: 327-336.

[58] Hernandez A, St Germain D (2002) Dexamethasone inhibits growth factor-induced type 3 deiodinase activity and mRNA expression in a cultured cell line derived from rat neonatal brown fat vascular-stromal cells. Endocrinology. 143: 2652-2658.

[59] Kester M, Kuiper G, Versteeg R, Visser T (2006) Regulation of type III iodothyronine deiodinase expression in human cell lines. Endocrinology. 147: 5845-5854.

[60] Malendowicz L, Filipiak B (1975) The effects of adrenalectomy and hydrocortisone replacement on the thyroid of the adult male rat I. Morphometrical data and histochemistry of some oxidative enzymes. Endokrinologie. 64: 223-231.

[61] Grubeck-Loebenstein B, Vierhapper H, Vierhapper H, Waldhäusl, W., Nowotny P (1983) Thyroid function in adrenocortical insufficiency during withdrawal and re-administration of glucocorticoid substihetion. Acta. Endocrinol. (Copenh). 103: 254-258.

[62] Rubello D, Sonino N, Casara D, Girelli M, Busnardo B, Boscaro M, Acute and chronic effects of high glucocorticoid levels on hypothalamic-pituitary-thyroid axis in man. J. Endocrinol. Invest. 15: 437-441.

[63] Invitti C, Manfrini R, Romanini B, Cavagnini F (1995) High prevalence of nodular thyroid disease in patients with Cushing's disease. Clin. Endocrinol. (Oxf.). 43: 359-363.

[64] Benker G, Raida M, Olbricht T, Wagner R, Reinhardt W, Reinwein D (1990) TSH secretion in Cushing's syndrome: relation to glucocorticoid excess, diabetes, goitre, and the - sick euthyroid syndrome. Clin. Endocrinol. (Oxf.). 33: 777-786.

[65] Morita H, Isaji M, Mune T, Daido H, Isomura Y, Sarui H, Tanahashi T, Takeda N, Ishizuka T, Yasuda K (2002) Transient Graves disease developing after surgery for Cushing disease. Am. J. Med. Sci. 323: 162-165.

[66] Arikan E, Guldiken S, Altun B.U, Kara M, Tugrul A (2004) Exacerbations of Graves' disease after unilateral adrenalectomy for Cushing's syndrome. J. Endocrinol. Invest. 27: 574-576.

[67] Takasu N, Ohara N, Yamada T, Komiya I (1993) Development of autoummune thyroid dysfunction after bilateral adrenalectomy in a patient with Corney's complex and after removal of ACTH-producing pituitary adenoma in a patient with Cushing's desease. J. Endocrinol. Invest. 16: 697-702.

[68] Yamakita N, Sakata S, Hayashi H, Maekawa H, Miura K (1993) Case report: silent thyroiditis after adrenalectomy in a patient with Cushing's syndrome. Am. J. Med. Sci. 305: 304-306.

[69] Katahira M, Yamada T, and Kawai M (2004) A case of cushing syndrome with both secondary hypothyroidism and hypercalcemia due to postoperative adrenal insufficiency. Endocr. J. 51: P. 105-113.

[70] Murakami T, Wada S, Katayama Y, Nemoto Y, Kugai N, Nagata N (1993) Thyroid dysfunction in isolated adrenocorticotropic hormone (ACTH) deficiency: case report and literature review. Endocr. J. 40: 473-478.

[71] Hangaard J, Andersen M, Grodum E, Koldkjaer O, Hagen C (1996) Pulsatile thyrotropin secretion in patients with Addison's disease during variable glucocorticoid therapy. J. Clin. Endocrinol. Metab. 81: 2502-2507.

[72] Ghizzoni L, Mastorakos G, Street M.E, Vottero A, Mazzardo G, Vanelli M, Chrousos G, Bernasconi S (1997) Spontaneous thyrotropin and cortisol secretion interactions in patients with nonclassical 21-hydroxylase deficiency and control children. J. Clin. Endocrinol. Metab. 82: 3677-3683.

[73] Ooka-Souda S, Draves D, Timiras P (1979) Diurnal rhythm of pituitary-thyroid axis in male rats and the effect of adrenalectomy. Endocr. Res. Commun. 6: 43-56.

[74] Slone-Wilcoxon J, Redei E (2004) Maternal-fetal glucocorticoid milieu programs hypothalamic-pituitary-thyroid function of adult offspring. Endocrinology. 145: 4068-4072.

[75] Desiderato O,. MacKinnon J, Hissom H (1974) Devolopment of gastric ulcers in rats following stress termination. J. Compar. Physiol. Psychol. 87: 208-214.

[76] Tolmachev D (1991) A technique for modelling chronic psychoemotional stresses in experimental toxicological conditions. Gig. Tr. Prof. Zabol. 8: 26-28.

[77] Boltze C, Brabant G, Dralle H, Gerlach R, Roessner A, Hoang-Vu C (2002) Radiation–induced thyroid carcinogenesis as a function of time and dietary iodine supply: an in vivo model of tumorigenesis in the rat. Endocrinology. 143: 2584-2592.

[78] Dunn J, Crutchfield H, Gutekunst R, Dunn A (1993) Two simple methods for measuring iodine in urine. Thyroid. Summer. 3:119-123.

[79] Alexander N (1962) Spectrophotometric assay for iodide oxidation by thyroid peroxidase. Analytical Biochem. 4: 341-345.

[80] Yamada Y, Aizawa A (1984) Simple and convenient method for quantitation of corticosterone by high–performance liquid chromatography – ultraviolet detection. J. Pharmac. Methods. 11: P. 291-297.

[81] Sugawara M, Sugawara Y, Wen K, Giulivi C (2002) Generation of oxygen free radicals in thyroid cells and inhibition of thyroid peroxidase. Exp Biol Med (Maywood). 22: 141-146.

[82] Mizokami T, Wu Li A, El-Kaissi S, Wall J. (2004) Stress and thyroid autoimmunity. Thyroid. 14: 1047–1055.

[83] Klecha A, Barreiro Arcos M, Frick L, Genaro A, Cremaschi G. (2008) Immune-endocrine interactions in autoimmune thyroid diseases. // Neuroimmunomodulation. 15: 68–75.

[84] Kasperlik-Laluska A, Czarnocka B, Czech W (2003) Autoimmunity as the most frequent cause of idiopathic secondary adrenal insufficiency: report of 111 cases. Autoimmunity. 36: 155-159.

[85] Tsatsoulis, A. (2006) The role of stress in the clinical expression of thyroid autoimmunity. Ann. N.Y. Acad. Sci. 1088: 382-395.

[86] Imaizumi M, Akahoshi M, Ichimaru S, Nakashima E, Hida A, Soda M, Usa T, Ashizawa K, Yokoyama N, Maeda R, Nagataki S, Eguchi K (2004) Risk for ischemic heart disease and all-cause mortality in subclinical hypothyroidism. J. Clin. Endocrinol. Metab. 89: 3365-3370.

[87] Crunkhorn S, Patti M (2008) Links between thyroid hormone action, oxidative metabolism, and diabetes risk? Thyroid. 18: 227-237.

[88] Emerson C, Seiler C, Alex S, Fang S, Mori Y, DeVito W (1993) Gene expression and serum thyroxine-binding globulin are regulated by adrenal status and corticosterone in the rat. Endocrinology. 133: 1192-1196.

[89] Tamura M, (1995) Improvement of hypothyroidism after glucocorticoid replacement adrenocorticotropin deficiency. Intern. Med. 34: 559-563.

[90] Nagai Y, Ieki Y, Ohsawa K, Kobayashi K (1997) Simultaneouslly found transient hypothyroidism due to Hashimoto's thyroiditis, autoimmune hepatitis and isolated ACTH deficiency after cessation of glucocorticoid administration. Endocr. J. 44: 453-458.

[91] Yue L, Wang F, Li G (1998) Changes of peripheral tissue thyroid hormone metabolism in rats fed with selenium- and vitamin E-deficient artificial semisynthetic diet. Clin Med. J. 111: 854-857.

[92] Haraguchi K, Onaya T (1991) Autoimmune thyroid dysfunction after treatment for Cushing's syndrome. N. Engl. J. Med. 325: 1708-1712.

[93] Mastorakos G, Ilias I (2000) Maternal hypothalamic–pituitary–adrenal axis in pregnancy and the postpartum period: postpartum–related disorders Ann. N.Y. Acad. Sci. 900: 95-106.

[94] Wick G, Hu Y, Schwarz S, Kroemer G (1993) Immunoendocrine communication via the hypothalamo–pituitary–adrenal axis in autoimmune diseases. Endocr. Rev. 14: 539-563.

Section 4

Prenatal Glucocorticoids and Placental Development

Chapter 13

The Effects of Glucocorticoids on Fetal and Placental Development

Emin Turkay Korgun, Aslı Ozmen, Gozde Unek and Inanc Mendilcioglu

Additional information is available at the end of the chapter

http://dx.doi.org/10.5772/50103

1. Introduction

Glucocorticoids (GCs), steroid hormones produced predominantly by the adrenal gland, are key mediators of stress responses. Whilst the acute and chronic effects of pharmacological glucocorticoid excess are well-recognized (including induction of hyperglycemia, insulin resistance, hyperlipidemia, hypertension and dysphoria, with suppression of immune, inflammatory and cognitive processes), their role in the biology of the response to stress is more nuanced, with balanced homeostatic effects to facilitate short-term survival and recovery from challenge [1, 2]. In addition, glucocorticoids play an essential role in normal fetal development and are important for the development and maturation of various fetal tissues including the liver, lungs, gut, skeletal muscle and adipose tissue in preparation for extrauterine life. Glucocorticoids most notably act during late gestation to stimulate surfactant production by the lung. This action is critical to prepare the fetus for extrauterine life, and it is for this reason that synthetic glucocorticoid treatment is so widely used in preterm pregnancies where lung immaturity threatens neonatal viability. Although these treatments greatly improve survival [3], they are not without adverse effects.

Glucocorticoids regulate many of the processes required for successful embryo implantation, as well as for the subsequent growth and development of the fetus and placenta. In utero, the endometrium, placenta and embryo/fetus are each exposed to physiological glucocorticoids arising from either maternal or fetal adrenal glands. It has been shown that glucocorticoids have several roles in improving the intrauterine environment. For example, in uterus, glucocorticoids regulate the synthesis of prostaglandins that have been implicated to play critical roles during implantation by increasing stromal vascular permeability [4] and in the initiation of parturition [5]. The peri-implantation secretion of human chorionic gonadotrophin (hCG) from human term trophoblasts can be stimulated by up to 10-fold by treatment for 24 to 72 h with synthetic glucocorticoids dexamethasone and triamcinolone [6, 7]. Glucocorticoids have several anti-inflammatory actions required for implantation. In first trimester human cytotrophoblasts, cortisol can suppress the synthesis of the pro-inflammatory interleukin (IL)-1b [8]. Similarly, in term human placental cytotrophoblasts, physiological concentrations of cortisol and numerous synthetic glucocorticoids can inhibit secretion of pro-inflammatory cytokines tumor necrosis factor (TNF)-α, IL-6 and IL-8 without affecting the expression of anti-inflammatory cytokine IL-10 [9-11]. Glucocorticoids contribute to preventing immunological rejection of the fetal semiallograft in the pregnant uterus by inhibiting eosinophil infiltration [12]. Moreover, glucocorticoids profoundly and specifically suppress expression of fibronectin and laminin, two extracellular matrix proteins that are important mediators of uterine–placental adherence [6].

Furthermore, glucocorticoids activate many of the biochemical processes in these tissues such as altering expression of numerous receptors, enzymes, ion channels, transporters, growth factors, cytoskeleton proteins, binding proteins, clotting factors, gap and tight junction proteins and intracellular signaling pathways' components involved in growth. Taken together, these glucocorticoid-induced changes in cell physiology combine to produce functional alterations at the systemic level [13].

In pregnancy, glucocorticoid administration is used mainly in the management of women at risk of preterm labor and in the antenatal treatment of fetuses at risk of congenital adrenal hyperplasia. It is recommended that, for pregnant women who are at risk of preterm delivery within 7 days between 24 weeks and 34 weeks of gestation, a single course of corticosteroid administration should be performed. And a single course of antenatal corticoids should be administered to women with premature rupture of membranes before 32 weeks gestation to reduce the risks of respiratory distress syndrome, perinatal mortality and other morbidities [14]. Numerous evidence indicates that increased exposure of the fetus to glucocorticoids in mid- to late pregnancy may result in adverse outcomes including intrauterine growth restriction (IUGR) [15-18], postnatal hypertension [15, 19], postnatal cardiovascular disease [20], postnatal glucose intolerance [20], increased postnatal activity in the hypothalamo–pituitary–adrenal axis [21-24], effects on fetal brain development [21, 25, 26].

Glucocorticoid actions within the cell are regulated by Glucocorticoid Receptor (GR) [27]. On hormone binding, activated GR translocates from the cytoplasm to the nucleus as a dimer to associate with specific DNA sequences termed glucocorticoid response elements (GREs) and acts as a ligand-dependent transcription factor [28]. GR-mediated transcriptional activation is modulated by phosphorylation [29]. GRs are highly expressed in decidua, chorion, amnion, stromal fibroblasts, vascular smooth muscle cells and endothelial cells of human term placentas, with moderate expression in cytotrophoblasts and negligible expression in syncytiotrophoblast [30-34]. Because the significance of glucocorticoids to the early mammalian embryo is clear and glucocorticoid action within the cell is regulated by GR, we investigated GR expression during the course of rat embryogenesis until day 12 of gestation. The demonstrated ontogenetic pattern of GR expression indicates the potential sites of biological action of the glucocorticoids, providing supportive evidence for its critical importance during the course of embryogenesis in rats [35].

The intracellular enzyme 11β-hydroxysteroid dehydrogenase (11β-HSD) catalyzes the interconversion of bioactive glucocorticoids (cortisol and corticosterone) and their inactive metabolites (cortisone and 11-dehydrocorticosterone). Thus, it is an important modulator of glucocorticoid bioavailability in both glucocorticoid and mineralocorticoid target organs [36]. To date, two 11β-HSD isoenzymes (known as 11β-HSD1 and 11β-HSD2) have been identified, characterized and cloned [37]. The conversion of cortisone to active cortisol is catalyzed by 11β-HSD1, whereas the metabolism of cortisol to cortisone is mediated via both 11β-HSD1 and 11β-HSD2 [38]. In placenta, 11β-HSD1 protein is expressed specifically in the placental villous endothelial cells, amnion, chorionic and extravillous trophoblasts (EVTs). 11β-HSD1 expression increases throughout pregnancy in response to progesterone [39]. As the placenta differentiates, there is an up-regulation in the expression of 11β-HSD2 enzyme that becomes the major placental isoenzyme [40]. 11β-HSD2 protein is localized exclusively in the syncytiotrophoblast and invasive extravillous trophoblasts with no expression in the chorion or amnion [41-43]. The distinct pattern of 11β-HSD1 and -2 localizations may indicate having different physiological functions. In normal pregnancy, maternal glucocorticoid levels are markedly higher than those in the fetal circulation. It has been stated that the role of placental 11β-HSD is to protect the fetus from adverse effects of maternal glucocorticoids. 11β-HSD2 is better suitable for this role because of its location (the site of maternal–fetal exchange) and its enzymatic properties (higher affinity for cortisol). This enzyme acts as a 'barrier' to prevent premature or inappropriate action at glucocorticoid-responsive tissues during fetal development [44]. It has been suggested that a reduction in the expression or activity of placental 11β-HSD2, by leading to increased transplacental passage of active glucocorticoids, reduces fetal growth. 11β-HSD2 knockout (11β-HSD2−/−) mice exhibit reduced birth weight and heightened anxiety in adulthood [45]. Numerous studies have shown that inhibition of 11β-HSD2 during pregnancy leads to a reduction in birth weight and the development of later hypertension and glucose intolerance [46-48], as well as programming increased HPA axis activity and anxiety-related behaviors [49]. Moreover, placentas from 11β-HSD2 knockout mice fetuses have impaired labyrinth zone capillary development accompanied by a decline in vascular endothelial growth factor (VEGF)-A mRNA expression and altered transport of nutrients by system A amino acid transporter (SNAT) [50]. Furthermore, a correlation between decreased activity of 11β-HSD2 in the human placenta and IUGR has been reported [15, 51, 52]. In addition, mutations in the HSD11B2 gene in humans, although rare, markedly reduce birth weight [53]. It was found that while maternal administration of glucocorticoids caused IUGR, glucocorticoid administration directly into the fetal circulation did not restrict fetal growth, which suggests that the growth limiting effects of glucocorticoids are mediated via actions in the utero-placental unit rather than effects on fetal tissues [54]

Placental development is a critical determinant of fetal growth and glucocorticoids affect growth and development of the fetus indirectly by affecting placental development and function. The actions of glucocorticoids on fetal growth are mediated, in part, by changes in the placenta. In sheep, rats, mice and non-human primates, administration of synthetic glucocorticoids during late gestation reduces placental weight. In most of these species, the effect of glucocorticoids on the placenta is greater than that on the fetus [13]. Glucocorticoids have been implicated in the fusion of cytotrophoblast cells to form the syncytiotrophoblast and associated with morphological (accelerated apical microvilli formation, nuclear maturation, and increase in cell organelle number) and functional (elevated hCG secretion and increased 11β-HSD2 mRNA expression) markers of syncytiotrophoblast differentiation. These findings suggest that glucocorticoids stimulate syncytiotrophoblast differentiation and maturation [55-57].

Microarray analysis showed that maternal glucocorticoid administration leads to marked changes in the gene expression profile in the placenta. Dexamethasone (Dex) caused a decrease in expression of genes involved in cell division such as cyclins A2, B1, D2, CDK 2, CDK 4 and M-phase protein kinase along with growth-promoting genes such as epidermal growth factor receptor, bone morphogenetic protein 4 and insulin-like growth factor-binding protein 3. In addition, Dex treatment led to down-regulation of genes involved in protein biosynthesis, skeletal development, and collagen metabolism. There was also decreased expression of genes involved in cell division, DNA replication, chromosome segregation, DNA alkylation, nucleotide and nucleoside biosynthesis, microtubule-based processes, B-cell activation and differentiation processes, innate immune response, antigen processing and presentation, and complement system [58]. Treatment of rats with glucocorticoids restricts placental vascular development via inhibition of the VEGF-A and peroxisome proliferator-activated receptor γ (PPARγ) which is regulated by VEGF-A expression [59, 60]. In addition, in response to glucocorticoid treatment of either the mother or fetus, there are changes in the placental handling of certain amino acids such as alanine, glutamine and glutamate. However, there have been few studies on the effects of glucocorticoids on amino acid transporters in the placenta of any species to date [61, 62]. Additionally, glucocorticoids change the production and metabolism of hormones by the placenta such as prostaglandins, placental lactogen, leptin, corticotrophin-releasing hormone (CRH), estrogens, progesterone and other progestagens [63, 64]. Glucocorticoids also alter the placental activity of various enzymes involved in the synthesis and inactivation of steroids and thyroid hormones such as 17,20-lyase, 17α-hydroxylase, aromatase, renin and endothelial nitric oxide synthase [63].

2. The effects of glucocorticoids on placental cell cycle

Glucocorticoids play a fundamental role in pregnancy with effects on decidualization, implantation, placental development, fetal brain development, lung maturation and parturition but fetal-placental exposure to maternally administered glucocorticoids may lead to abnormalities of fetal and placental growth [15, 19, 65]. The mode of action of glucocorticoids in placental growth inhibition has not been determined.

Human placental development is established by trophoblast invasion into the uterine endometrium and its vasculature. The resulting changes will facilitate an increase in intervillous blood flow and, hence, the exchange of nutrients and molecules between maternal and fetal blood. The transports as well as metabolic and endocrine functions of the placenta reside primarily in the floating villi covered by the syncytiotrophoblast, a tissue that results from terminal differentiation of underlying villous cytotrophoblasts and their subsequent fusion. Anchoring villi establish physical connection of the placenta with the decidua predominantly by a subpopulation of cytotrophoblasts known as EVT. They accumulate at the tips of the anchoring villi and form cell columns. Both villous and extravillous cytotrophoblast subpopulations arise by proliferation and differentiation from stem cells located within the cytotrophoblast layer of the chorionic villi [66].

On the basis of the immunostaining of the Ki67 antigen, a cell cycle regulator with yet unknown role, EVTs have been categorized as the proliferative phenotype, which is primarily located in the proximal part, and the invasive phenotype that is located mainly in the distal part of cell columns [66]. Current understanding assumes that EVT can differentiate, thereby acquiring an invasive phenotype, which eventually enables them to invade the maternal decidua and spiral arteries. Thus placental development involves proliferation and differentiation of the cytotrophoblasts in a manner that is tightly regulated in time and space.

Eukaryotic cell cycle consists of four phases, G1, S, G2 and M. G1 and G2 are preparation phases for DNA synthesis (S) and mitosis (M) phases respectively. During G1 and G2 phases cell growth, doubling of the amount of protein and organelles and preparation for the next phase occurs. If the conditions are not appropriate, cells in G1 phase stop cell cycle progression and enter into a resting state, known as G0 phase, where they continue biological functions but do not go through the rest of the cell cycle. When growth signals are received, cells in G0 phase can continue the cycle through the G1 phase [67, 68].

The eukaryotic cell cycle is regulated by the coordinated activity of a family of cyclin-dependent kinases (CDKs). These are positively and negatively regulated by the cyclin and CDK inhibitor families [69, 70]. Based on the timing of their appearance in the cell cycle, cyclins can be divided into two groups, i.e. the mitotic cyclins A and B and the G1 cyclins of the D and E families [71]. Cyclin A promotes both G1/S and G2/M transitions, whereas cyclin B1 accumulates in the cytosol during late S phase and G2 and enters the nucleus at the onset of mitosis [72].

In mammalian cells, there are at least two distinct families of CDK inhibitors: the INK4 and the Cip/Kip inhibitors (p21, p27, p57). Both families play regulatory roles during the G1/S cell cycle checkpoint [73]. Because of their broader panel of CDKs with which they interact [74], the inhibitors of the Cip/Kip family control other checkpoints as well. p21 plays a role during the G2/M phase transition [75] and may also mediate S phase [76] and G2 arrest [77]. Overall it is correlated with cell cycle arrest before terminal differentiation [78]. Also, p27 has the capacity to arrest cells in G2 [77]. p57 inhibits cyclin A- and E-associated CDKs and therefore regulates G1/S transition and completion of S phase [79] and is primarily expressed in terminally differentiated cells [80].

Despite the importance in understanding the mechanisms controlling proliferation, little is known about how cytotrophoblast proliferation is coordinated with differentiation and what factors determine whether cytotrophoblast cells divide or differentiate and syncytialize. A few studies localized cell cycle regulators that are specifically expressed during key transitions and phases [81-83].

The hypothesis that the coordinated expression of cell cycle progression and inhibition factors will determine whether cytotrophoblasts proliferate or undergo cell cycle arrest or cell cycle exit allowing subsequent differentiation was tested by our team. The cell cycle promoters cyclin A, cyclin B1, proliferating cell nuclear antigen (PCNA), Ki67 and the cell cycle inhibitors p21, p27 and p57 were immunolocalized in tissue sections of first trimester pregnancies (weeks 6 and 9-12). Villous cytotrophoblasts were immunolabelled for Ki67 and cyclin A but only few were stained with anti-cyclin B1. The syncytiotrophoblast was devoid of immunoreactivity for any of the cell cycle progression factors. It expressed especially p21, whereas p27 and p57 were predominantly found in villous cytotrophoblasts. PCNA, Ki67, cyclin A and cyclin B1 were immunolocalized in proximal and distal EVTs of anchoring villi and in EVT which had invaded the upper decidual segments. All EVTs strongly expressed p27 and p57, but not p21. These data clearly suggest different functions for p21, p27 and p57 in placental development with distinct roles for p21 and p57 in syncytiotrophoblast and EVT differentiation, respectively. p27 appears to be involved in both the processes. The results may also challenge the concept of differential mitotic activity in the proximal and distal parts of the first trimester cytotrophoblast cell column, but more functional studies are clearly needed. The presence of p27 and p57 in EVT cells, which invade the deciduas deeply, may account for the loss of mitogenic potential of these cells [84].

Although the architecture of the human and rodent placentas differs, their anatomical structures and molecular mechanisms have been compared [85, 86] and analogies drawn between the various cell types; furthermore, the molecular mechanisms of placental development are thought to be very similar between the two species. Thus, the rodent placenta is increasingly used as a model to study mechanisms underlying placental development [85, 87].

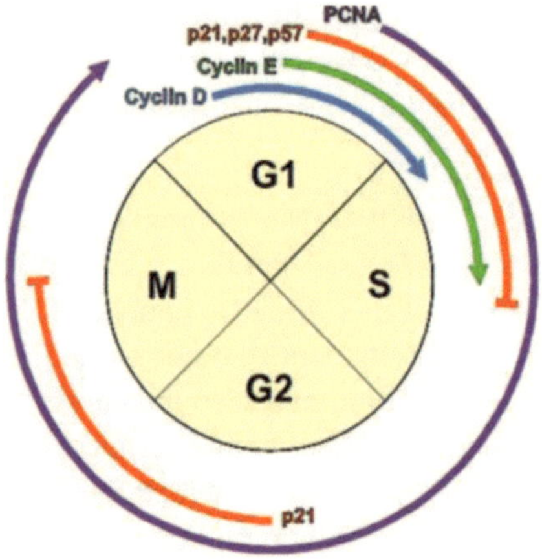

Figure 1. Schematic representation of cell cycle related proteins in rat placenta of our study [88].

We have been used to localize G1 cyclins (D1, D3, E), which are major determinants of proliferation, Cip/Kip inhibitors, p53 as a master regulator and proliferating cell nuclear antigen in all cell types of the rat term placenta. Schematic representation of cell cycle related proteins studied is showed in Figure 1. The proportion of each cell type immunolabeled was counted. Cyclin D1 and cyclin D3 were present mostly in cells of the fetal aspect of the placenta, whereas the G1/S cyclin E was present only in the spongio- and labyrinthine trophoblast populations. Among the Cip/Kip inhibitors, p21 was present only in cells of the fetal aspect whereas p27 and p57 were found in all cell types studied. p53 was only found in a small proportion of cells with no co-localization of p53 and p21 [88]. Schematic representation of our immunohistochemistry results in the rat placenta is showed in Figure 2. The data suggest that the cells of the fetal side of the rat placenta still have some proliferation potential which is kept in check by expression of the Cip/Kip cell cycle inhibitors, whereas cells of the maternal aspect have lost this potential. Apoptosis is only marginal in the term rat placenta. In conclusion, proliferation and apoptosis in rat placental cells appears controlled mostly by the Cip/Kip inhibitors in late pregnancy. It is still not known how coordination mechanisms of proliferation and differentiation are influenced by glucocorticoid induced IUGR in the placenta.

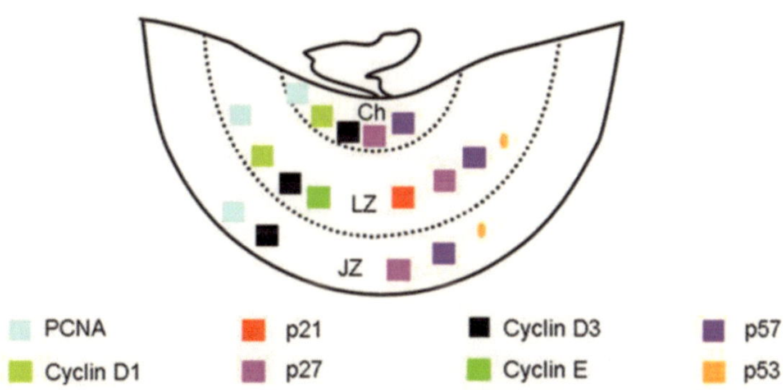

Ch: Chorion, LZ: Labyrinth Zone (fetal placenta), JZ: Junctional Zone (maternal placenta) [88].

Figure 2. Schematic representation of our immunohistochemistry results in the rat placenta.

We aimed to investigate the effects of maternally administered synthetic glucocorticoid Dex on cell proliferation, cell cycle arrest or apoptosis of placental development. We investigated the spatial and temporal immunolocalization of PCNA, Ki67, p27 and p57 in normal and Dex-induced IUGR placental development in pregnant rats. PCNA immunolabeling intensity in placentas of the control group was statistically significantly higher than that in the Dex-induced IUGR group placentas on all days in junctional and labyrinth zones (JZ and LZ, respectively). We observed decreased Ki67 staining intensity in the labyrinth trophoblasts of Dex-induced IUGR placentas compared to controls on day 21. Ki67 immunolabeling intensity was higher in the control group than that in the IUGR group placentas on all days in both zones except for day 21 in the junctional zone. These differences were statistically significant on days 15, 17 and 19 in the junctional zone and on days 13, 15, 17 and 21 in the labyrinth zone. Ki67 staining intensity decreased gradually after day 15 in both zones of control and

IUGR placentas. Ki67 immunostaining intensities were stronger in the labyrinth zone compared to the junctional zone in both groups. Moreover, after day 17, scarcely any Ki67 immunostaining was obtained in the IUGR placentas in the junctional zone. We found stronger p27 immunolabeling intensity in Dex-induced IUGR placentas when compared to control placentas in both junctional and labyrinth zones for all gestational days (Table 1) [89]. In accordance with this, in another study, it was observed that in the Dex-induced human choriocarcinoma JEG-3 cells p27 mRNAs were upregulated [90]. We observed that p57 immunostaining intensities in Dex-induced IUGR placentas were stronger compared to controls in both zones for all gestational days. We found that Dex-induction results in p57 upregulation in rat placental development [89]. In contrast to our results, p57 was not expressed in Dex-induced JEG-3 cells [90]. In another study, we wanted to determine the Ser/Thr protein kinase Akt and a MAPK (Mitogen-Activated Protein Kinase) ERK1/2 related proliferation and apoptosis mechanisms are influenced by Dex-induced IUGR placentas. Thus, we investigated the expression levels and spatio-temporal immunolocalization of Akt, p-Akt, ERK1/2 and p-ERK1/2 proteins in normal and Dex treated placental development of rats. We found that maternal Dex treatment led to a decrease in ERK1/2 and Akt activation during rat placental development together with placental and fetal weight loss. Akt activation was significant at junctional zones of the rat placenta, especially at spongiotrophoblast cells and giant cells, and reduced after dexamethasone treatment. On the other hand, ERK1/2 activation was seen in both junctional and labyrinth zones of the rat placentas and was weaker in labyrinth zones of IUGR group placentas. The decrease in ERK1/2 and Akt activation may result in cell survival inhibition or apoptosis stimulation. Consequently, Dex induced placental and embryonal developmental abnormalities could be associated with reduction of Akt and ERK1/2 activation [91]. In another study, decreased levels of placental Akt phosphorylation was observed after in utero exposure to Dex [92].

Antenatal Dex use is associated with reduction in fetal and placental weight with morphological changes in the placenta. Dex-treated mouse placentas showed swollen trophoblast cells in both the junctional and labyrinth zones and increased apoptosis of trophoblast cells in the junctional zone. Moreover, Dex-treated placentas were hydropic, friable and pale [58]. Increasing antenatal corticosteroid exposure was associated with villous fibrosis, stromal mineralization, and less frequent villous infarction [93]. In addition, treatment with Dex prevented the normal rise in VEGF expression and the associated increase in labyrinthine vascularity over the final third of pregnancy. Therefore, Dex appears to reduce labyrinth zone growth by preventing the normal development of the fetal vasculature within the labyrinth zone [59]. Moreover, microarray analysis showed that Dex caused a decrease in expression of genes involved in cell division such as cyclins A2, B1, D2, CDK 2, CDK 4 and M-phase protein kinase along with growth-promoting genes such as epidermal growth factor receptor, bone morphogenetic protein 4 and insulin-like growth factor-binding protein 3 [58]. In addition, 3H-thymidine incorporation assay revealed that proliferation of trophoblast cell lines JEG-3 and HTR-8/SV neo and human first-trimester primary trophoblasts was time- and dose-dependently inhibited by glucocorticoids [94]. Impaired growth in Dex-treated placentas was also characterized by decreased expression of both prolactin-like protein-B and insulin-like growth factor (IGF)-II, particularly in the junctional zone of the rat placenta [92]. Dex-treatment increased apoptosis of trophoblast cells in mouse and rat placentas. Dex-induced trophoblast apoptosis was mediated through activation of caspases 1 and 3 [58, 95]. Apoptosis was also induced in primary cultures of third trimester human decidual cells when treated with cortisol, cortisone, or dexamethasone [34]. Likewise, Dex was shown to induce both apoptosis and necrosis in primary cultures of term human placental trophoblast, in an in vitro model of syncytialization and in the SGH-PL4 cell line derived from human extravillous trophoblasts by measuring the cytokines TNF-alpha and IFN-gamma using the TUNEL technique, Annexin V binding, fluorescence microscopy and ATP/ADP measurements [96]. In another study, using a human in vitro term placental explant model, Dex treatment was shown to be associated with morphological (accelerated apical microvilli formation, nuclear maturation,

Gestational days	Junctional Zone	Labyrinth Zone	Cell cycle protein
13	↓	↓	PCNA
15	↓	↓	
17	↓	↓	
19	↓	↓	
21	↓	↓	
13	–	↓	Ki67
15	↓	↓	
17	↓	↓	
19	↓	–	
21	–	↓	
13	↑	↑	p27
15	↑	↑	
17	↑	↑	
19	–	↑	
21	↑	↑	
13	↑	–	p57
15	↑	↑	
17	↑	↑	
19	–	–	
21	↑	↑	

Table 1. Immunolabeling intensity changes of PCNA, Ki67, p27 and p57 in the junctional and labyrinth zones of placentas of the IUGR group rat placentas compared to control of given gestational day ($p=<0.05$). –, statistically significantly unchanged; ↑, statistically significantly increased; ↓, statistically significantly decreased.

and increased cell organelle number) and functional (elevated hCG secretion, increased 11β-HSD2 mRNA expression and reduced cytotrophoblast proliferation markers) of syncytiotrophoblast differentiation. These findings suggest that Dex stimulates syncytiotrophoblast differentiation and maturation [57]. In another study, BeWo and JEG-3 choriocarcinoma cell lines used as models for human trophoblast were cultured with another synthetic glucocorticoid triamcinolone acetonide (TA). TA altered the number of viable and dead cells as well as cyclin B1 expression levels shown by Western blotting and to a lesser extent, invasion of BeWo and JEG-3 cell lines determined by Matrigel invasion assay and by measuring the secretion (ELISA) of matrix-metalloproteinases (MMP-2, MMP-9) [97].

3. The effects of glucocorticoids on fetal and placental angiogenesis mechanisms

Angiogenesis is a complex process that may be initiated by a large number of stimuli and that is performed through multiple biologic pathways and a variety of molecules. With the increased understanding of angiogenesis, it has become clear that many of its pathways are parallel and redundant, greatly complicating efforts to interrupt the process. The disruption of one pathway most likely does not abolish completely the formation of new blood vessels, which may explain the less than perfect clinical results achieved when treating neovascular processes with currently available regimens. Combination therapies and drugs that target more than one pathway have become more popular and intensively explored.

Angiogenesis is required for the cyclic processes of endometrial growth, breakdown, and repair during the menstrual cycle, and it provides a richly vascularized tissue receptive for implantation and placentation [98]. Besides, the formation of new blood vessels is essential for organogenesis and successful embryonic and fetal development.

For many years glucocorticoids have been used in pregnant women for several reasons such as risk of premature deliveries or treatment of a variety of medical disorders like bronchial asthma, systemic lupus erythematosous etc.. The dosages and types of glucocorticoids changes depending on the severity of the symptoms and treatment procedure [99].

It is reviewed by Hadoka et al. [100] that endogenous GCs contribute to physiological angiogenesis mechanisms by regulating the new vessel formation processes. Endothelial cells are seem to be a target of glucocorticoid effect as they both express glucocorticoid and mineralocorticoid receptors [101, 102]. But overexposure to glucocorticoids during pregnancy has adverse effects on placental angiogenesis mechanisms. Therefore these steroids should be carefully used in pregnancy.

Hewitt et al. [59] investigated the impact of increased glucocorticoid exposure on the spatial and temporal expression of the endothelial cell-specific mitogen; VEGF and associated placental vascularization over the final third of rat pregnancy. They showed that treatment with dexamethasone prevented the normal rise in VEGF expression as a LZ specific manner. Their data suggest that glucocorticoid induced restriction of fetal and placental growth is mediated, in part, via inhibition of placental VEGF expression and associated reduction in placental vascularization. Therefore, dexamethasone appears to reduce LZ growth by preventing the normal development of the fetal vasculature within the LZ.

As it is mentioned in the study above, GCs have adverse effect on placental angiogenesis mechanisms. This effect would be related with both angiogenic activity of the endothelial cells or maybe related with proliferation or cell survival processes. It was reported in a previous study that GCs inhibit tube formation of cultured endothelial cells [103] but the molecular mechanisms underlying this effect hasn't been clearly understood [104].

Recently, Logie et al. [105] reported that GCs do not affect the endothelial cell viability or proliferation but tube formation capacity. This investigation addressed the hypothesis that the potent antiangiogenic action of glucocorticoids is due to prevention of tube formation by endothelial cells. Cultured human umbilical vein endothelial cells (HUVEC) and aortic endothelial cells (HAoEC) were used to determine the influence of glucocorticoids on tube-like structure (TLS) formation, and on cellular proliferation, viability and migration. Dexamethasone or cortisol (at physiological concentrations) inhibited both basal and prostaglandinF-2α -induced and VEGF stimulated TLS formation in endothelial cells cultured on Matrigel, effects which were blocked with the glucocorticoid receptor antagonist RU38486. Glucocorticoids had no effect on endothelial cell viability, migration or proliferation. Time-lapse imaging showed that cortisol blocked VEGF-stimulated cytoskeletal reorganization and initialization of tube formation. Exposure to glucocorticoids reduced the formation of cell-cell contacts rather than increasing degradation of existing tubes. They concluded that glucocorticoids interact directly with glucocorticoid receptors on vascular endothelial cells (ECs) to inhibit TLS formation. This action, which was conserved in ECs from two distinct vascular territories, was due to alterations in cell morphology rather than inhibition of EC viability, migration or proliferation. These findings provide important insights into the anti angiogenic action of endogenous glucocorticoids in health and disease [105].

According to the results of an ongoing study of us, Triamcinolone treatment decreased VEGF expression in HUVECs. In this study, we tested the hypothesis that IUGR could be observed in fetuses as a result of insufficient nutrient transport depending on the glucocorticoid effect on placental angiogenesis mechanism that leads to inadequate vessel development. HUVECs were cultured at different concentrations (0.5, 5, 50 μmol/L) of the synthetic glucocorticoid triamnicinolone acetonide for 48 and 72 hours. After culture, RT-PCR, ELISA, Western blot and Matrigel experiments were performed. On the other hand, dexamethasone was injected to rats during gestation. Placenta and blood samples were taken from rats on gestational days 14, 16, 18 and 20. RT-PCR and Western blot analyses were performed on placentas while ELISA test was applied to sera and HUVEC culture media. We found that in HUVECs; VEGF, VEGFR1, VEGFR2, Placental Growth Factor (PIGF) and Fibroblast Growth Factor (FGF) gene levels on 48 and 72 hours decreased in 50 mM TA groups compared to control. VEGF protein amount on 48 and 72 hours decreased in TA groups compared to control. VEGFR1 protein quantity decreased and VEGFR2 protein quantity increased in a dose- and time-dependent manner. According to ELISA results, VEGFR1 secreted by HUVEC cells decreased while VEGFR2 and FGF increased. In Matrigel experiments, decreased vessel tube structures were created by HUVEC cells exposed for 72 hours to 50 mM TA. The amount of VEGF in Dex treated rat sera statistically significantly decreased on days 14, 16 and 20, while there is no difference on day 18 compared to control. VEGF protein amount showed a decrease in all gestational days of IUGR group compared to control in rat placentas. VEGFR1 decreased in advancing pregnancy days of control group while increased in parallel to pregnancy days of IUGR group. VEGF and VEGFR1 gene level was lower at term rat placentas compared to control group at gestational day 20. In conclusion our results showed that glucocorticoids had a negative effect on angiogenesis mechanism (Figure 3) via altering the angiogenesis related protein and gene expression, and tube formation capacity and angiogenesis related proteins in sera (A.Ozmen, G.Unek, D.K. Korgun, I.Mendilcioğlu and E.T.Korgun unpublished).

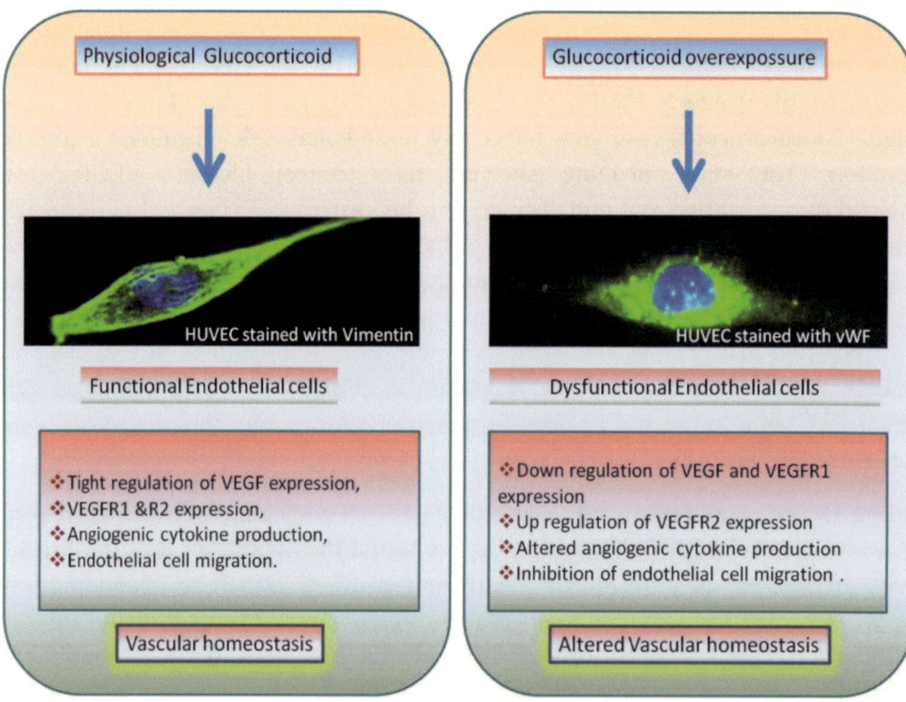

Figure 3. A possible model for glucocorticoid effect on endothelial cells. In physiological conditions; in the case of moderate GC concentrations (left picture), vascular homeostasis is tightly regulated. VEGF, VEGFR1&R2 expression, angiogenic cytokine production, endothelial cell migration, blood flow velocity etc… is maintained in a balance in functional endothelial cells. But when GC concentration is increased (right picture), endothelial cell are subjected to excess GC. And this GC overexposure results with endothelial dysfunction by downregulating VEGF and VEGFR1 expression, upregulating VEGFR2 expression, altering angiogenic cytokine production and by inhibiting endothelial cell migration etc… (vWF: Von Willebrand Factor)

In another study of ours, we investigated the effects of glucocorticoids on rat placental development depending on the PI3K/Akt and MAPK-ERK1/2 pathways [91]. It was observed that, the IUGR group had significantly smaller embryos on day 20 of gestation and had smaller placentas on day 14, 16, 18 and 20 compared with control. Maternal dexamethasone treatment led to a significant decrease in Akt activation on day 16, 18, and 20. Total Akt protein expression was not significantly affected by the treatment. There was a significant decrease in ERK1/2 activation on day 18 in IUGR group; on the other hand there was a significant increase on day 16. Total ERK1/2 protein expression didn't show any significant difference between groups. We observed that phospho-Akt immunolabelings were remarkable in junctional zone in control groups and weaker in IUGR groups. Phospho-ERK1/2 immunolabelings were considerable in the junctional and labyrinth zones in the control groups and weaker in IUGR groups. We found that ERK1/2 activity was decreased in the dexamethasone treated IUGR groups. This decrease was especially seen in the LZ of the rat placenta. Concerning the importance of Erk1/2 on placental vasculature development [106-109], it could be said that the decrease in ERK1/2 activity might be related with vascular failure and this could result with abnormal placental development. Besides it is mentioned in the literature that the PI3K/Akt pathway modulates the expression of some angiogenic factors such as nitric oxide and angiopoietins. Numerous inhibitors targeting the PI3K/Akt pathway have been developed, and these agents have been shown to decrease VEGF secretion and angiogenesis. [110]. Therefore, dexamethasone induced decreased Akt phosphorylation may negatively affect the placental angiogenesis mechanisms. There are some other studies [111, 112] mentioning the effect of GCs on fetal/placental vasculature during pregnancy. These studies report that GCs alter the physiological condition of the vasculature and leads pathological conditions. Aida et al. [111] determined a significant depression of total placental eNOS protein measured by ELISA (betamethasone treated vs control) and immunohistochemistry in both syncytiotrophoblast and vascular endothelium. In conclusion, maternally administered betamethasone produces a consistent decrease in several indices of placental eNOS function that may play a role in the altered cardiovascular dynamics and fetal growth retardation produced by betamethasone administration in late pregnancy.

Angiogenesis is tightly regulated by hormones. Hormones regulate blood vessel growth by controlling the production of local chemical mediators, often other hormones, but also growth factors, cytokines, enzymes, receptors, adhesion molecules, and metabolic factors. As mentioned above, GCs may show their effects directly on endothelial cells or indirectly for example by altering cytokine production that may affect placental vasculature. Xu et al. 2005, [9] studied the effects of GCs on placental cytokine production. Villous explants were cultured with increasing concentrations of glucocorticoids (betamethasone and methyl-prednisolone, 0.0025 mM, 0.25 mM and 25 mM). The dose effect of glucocorticoids on cytokine (TNF-α, IL-6 and IL-10) production was examined using ELISA. There was a stepwise reduction of TNF-α and IL-6 with increasing doses of betamethasone and methyl-prednisolone from placentas of women with preeclampsia and normal pregnancy.

However, IL-10 was not altered in conditioned medium by increasing doses of glucocorticoids. In pregnancy, TNF-α can cause direct damage to endothelial cells, increase endothelial cell permeability, up-regulate endothelial adhesion molecules (ICAM-1, VCAM-1, E-Selectin) and promote vasoconstriction, all of which are identified in the pathogenesis of preeclampsia [113]. IL-10 is an immunosuppressive Th2-type cytokine which is produced by immune cells including T-cells, monocytes, macrophages, granulocytes and NK cells and also trophoblasts. IL-10 has been also shown to be a potent inhibitor of Th1 cell proliferation and the production of Th1-type cytokines such as TNF-α [114].

To observe the influence of maternal betamethasone administration for fetal lung maturation on the arterial, venous and intracardiac blood flow of the fetus and the uterine arteries; twenty-seven women with singleton pregnancies were examined before the first, and 30 min and 8, 24, 48 and 72 h after the second of two single doses of 8 mg of betamethasone. The blood flow velocity waveforms of the umbilical artery (UA), the middle cerebral artery, the uterine arteries, the ductus venosus, the inferior vena cava and the right hepatic vein, the pulmonary trunk, the ductus arteriosus and the right and left intraventricular inflow of the heart was recorded. The resistance index of the UA showed a significant transient decrease 30 min after the second betamethasone dose. The peak systolic velocity of the ductus arteriosus increased significantly 30 min after the 2nd dose and then returned to non-significant values. No significant change was observed in any of the other vessels. So it could be said that Betamethasone causes short-term changes in fetal blood flow. However, this effect seems to be mild and reversible and does not appear to contraindicate the use of corticosteroids to promote fetal lung maturation [115]. Therefore, it could be mentioned that long term dexamethasone usage my result with decreased maternal blood velocity which would negatively affect angiogenesis mechanisms as maternal blood itself contains angiogenesis related proteins.

It is reviewed by Oliver et al. [116] that corticosteroids are believed to act at multiple levels of angiogenesis by regulating growth factors, proteases, and blood cell behavior, and have shown significant promise in clinical studies of neovascularization secondary to diabetes, age-related macular degeneration (AMD), and ocular histoplasmosis syndrome [117-121]. Angiostatic steroids have been proposed to inhibit angiogenesis by altering the capillary basement membrane composition, suppressing its dissolution, and inhibiting endothelial cell migration, in addition to their capacity of regulating the participation of inflammatory cells in the neovascular process [122-124]. There is a growing body of evidence that reports inhibitive effects of glucocorticoids on angiogenesis mechanisms [105, 125-128] but there is limited data about the impact of glucocorticoids on placental angiogenesis mechanisms. Glucocorticoid-mediated inhibition of angiogenesis is important in physiology, pathophysiology and therapy. However, the mechanisms through which glucocorticoids inhibit growth of new blood vessels have not been established. Over-exposure to GCs may alter intracellular signaling pathways such as MAPK/ERK1/2 and PI3K/Akt with a processes mediated by GR and finally expression of angiogenic proteins could be altered (Figure 4).

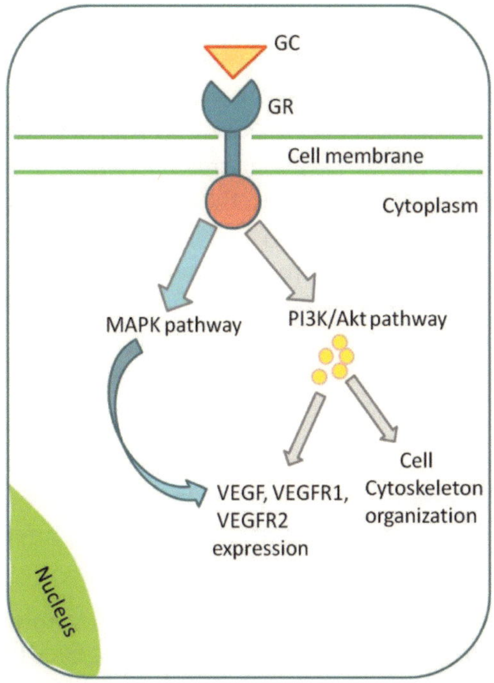

Figure 4. Glucocorticoids might show their effects on angiogenesis mechanisms by altering intracellular signal transduction pathways. GCs affect cellular processes via binding Glucocorticoid receptor. MAPK and PI3K/Akt (by phosphorylation of several downstream molecules; yellow dots in the picture) pathways mediate GC action on placental angiogenesis mechanisms like VEGF, VEGFR1&2 expression and endothelial cell cytoskeleton organization etc... (GC; Glucocorticoid, GR; Glucocorticoid Receptor)

4. The effects of glucocorticoids on placental glucose transporters

The Glut protein family belongs to the Major Facilitator Superfamily (MFS) of membrane transporters [129]. Most Glut proteins catalyze the facilitative (energy-independent) bidirectional transfer of their substrates across membranes. Up to now, 14 functional mammalian-facilitated hexose carriers (GLUTs) have been characterized by molecular cloning [130]. The Glut family members can be grouped into three (Class I, Class II and Class III) different classes based on their sequence similarities [131]. The isoforms GLUT1, 3 and 4 are included in Class I and represent high-affinity transport facilitators.

The existence of glucose transporters in the placenta have been known for many years. GLUT1 protein is present in placental endothelial cells [132, 133] and in the basal [132], or microvillous membranes of the syncytiotrophoblast [133-135]. GLUT3 mRNA is distributed throughout the cells of villous tissue; GLUT3 protein appears to be expressed only in the vascular endothelium and, is not expressed in the syncytiotrophoblast layer of the placenta. A strong GLUT4 signal was observed in intravillous stromal cells, appearing to co-localize with insulin receptors [136], a discovery which complements the observation of GLUT4 in fibroblasts from amnion and chorion [137].

GLUT proteins' cell surface expression level, greatly influences the rate of glucose uptake into the cells [131]. Uptake of glucose by the placenta is facilitated primarily by GLUT1 and in part by GLUT3 transporters [133, 138-140]. A possible major glucose transfer mechanism in the human placental villi may be depicted as follows. Glucose in the maternal bloodstream passes the apical microvillous plasma membrane of syncytiotrophoblast cells by means of GLUT1. Glucose moves through the cytoplasm of the syncytiotrophoblast by simple diffusion and leaves the cytoplasm via GLUT1 in the basal plasma membrane. GLUT1 and GLUT3 proteins contribute to the uptake of glucose by placental endothelial cells, as well as facilitate the transfer of glucose into and out of the fetal blood vessels in the villous core [133, 138-140]. About 25% of glucose entering the placenta is metabolized within this tissue; the majority of glucose is passed to the fetus through placental endothelial cells [141].

Efficient placental (maternal to fetal) transport of glucose is crucial to sustain the normal development and survival of the fetus in utero because its own glucose production is minimal [142]. The factors regulating transplacental glucose transfer are largely unknown.

In our recent study [143], we showed that Triamcinolone administration at doses of 0.5, 5 and 50μmol/L, led to a significant up-regulation of placental GLUT1 and GLUT3 transcripts and protein levels in Human Placental Endothelial Cells (HPECs). After several passages, the endothelial cells were cultured in the presence or absence (controls) of 0.5, 5 and 50μmol/L of TA. The lower (0.5 mmol) dose is a concentration in the lower range of doses generally used in previous cell culture studies [7] and considered comparable to the doses used to promote lung maturation in rats [144]. Other doses (5 and 50 mmol) were used to investigate the potentially detrimental effects of glucocorticoid excess. The highest TA dose administered to the endothelial cell cultures corresponds to the TA concentration in blood resulting after intravenous injection of a dose recommended by the manufacturers for therapy in humans. Our Western blot results showed that GC overexposure significantly increased placental GLUT1 and GLUT3 protein levels in all experimental groups of HPECs. RT-PCR analysis of placental GLUT expressions indicated that both GLUT1 and GLUT3 mRNA levels were affected by the GC induction. It was supposed that GCs caused an increase in placental GLUT proteins and mRNA expression.

The human placenta is a GC responsive organ consisting of multiple cell types including endothelial cells, fibroblasts and trophoblasts that demonstrate changes in gene expression after hormone treatment. However, little is known about the relative expression or activity of the Glucocorticoid Receptor among the various placental cell types. Previous studies have documented that placental endothelial cells expressed GR and Mineralocorticoid Receptor (MR) [101, 102] but the GR regulation of glucose transport have not been studied. We found that GR mRNA and protein expression down-regulated after 24-h cell culture of HPECs. Our results suggest that GC-mediated down-regulation of GR levels occurs through changes in protein and mRNA stability in HPECs after TA treatment. The data from the cell culture strengthens the hypothesis that increased GC levels specifically modulate GLUT expression via the GR.

Collectively, we conclude that TA is a potent regulator of HPECs' GLUT1 and GLUT3 expression (Figure 5). This effect is mediated by GR. We speculate that GC-induced up-regulation of the placental glucose transporter systems contributes to the retarded fetal and placental growth observed with GC treatment.

Similarly in a previous study [18], it is reported that exposure to excess glucocorticoids from day 15 of gestation modified rodent placental glucose transporter protein expression at day 21 of gestation in a concentration-dependent manner.

Dexamethasone treatment from day 15 to day 21 of pregnancy led to fetal hypoglycaemia. GLUT1 and GLUT3 protein expression were detectable in the rat placenta during late gestation, and dexamethasone treatment from day 15 to day 21 of pregnancy significantly decreased placental weight and up-regulated the placental protein expression of both glucose transporters during late gestation in a dose-dependent manner.

Dexamethasone administration at the lower dose (100µg/kg) led to modest up-regulation of placental GLUT1 protein expression, in the absence of any significant change in the protein expression of GLUT3. Dexamethasone at the higher dose (200µg/kg) led to significant up-regulation of the placental expression of both GLUT1 and GLUT3 in rats, with a slightly more marked effect on GLUT3 [18]. It is concluded that, depending on the dose administered, either maturational glucose transporter isoform switching might be accelerated by dexamethasone treatment during late pregnancy or, at a higher dose, placental glucose transporter expression would be down-regulated.

In another study of ours, the glucocorticoid effect on the glucose transporters in the diabetic rat placenta was questioned. It was hypothesized that GCs regulate placental glucose transport in many cell types and tissues and depending on this hypothesis the relationship between glucose transport and the glucocorticoid metabolism in rat placental development of normal and diabetic pregnancy was investigated. The immunohistochemical results indicated that GR and GLUT1 are expressed ubiquitously in the trophoblast and endothelial cells of the labyrinthine zone. Amounts of GR and GLUT1 proteins increased towards the end of gestation both in the control and the diabetic placenta. However, at days 17 and 19 of gestation, only the placental GR protein was significantly increased in the streptozotocin-induced diabetic rats compared to control rats. It is mentioned in this study that there might be a relationship between GR and GLUT1 expressions at the cellular level. GLUT1 does not play a pivotal role in diabetic pregnancies. However, placental growth abnormalities during diabetic pregnancy may be related with the amount of GR [145].

It was previously reported by Hahn et al. for the first time, that both GLUT1 and GLUT3 transcripts and protein were significantly down-regulated in isolated human trophoblast cells and in rat placentas by GCs, suggesting regulation at the transcriptional level [7]. Hyperglycemia is one of the well known systemic effects following GC treatment. Thus, elevated glucose concentrations might have affected placental GLUT expression [146]. However, in the rat model, a single injection of TA resulted in only short term hyperglycemia, followed by hypoglycemia. This hypoglycemia may be the reason for the smaller fetuses and placentas as well as for the markedly reduced weight gain of TA-treated rats during gestational days 16 and 21.The human trophoblast cells were cultured under physiological glucose concentrations, yet their GLUTs were down-regulated similar to those in TA-treated rats. Collectively, the investigators concluded that the synthetic GC Triamcinolone is a potent regulator of human and rodent placental GLUT1 and GLUT3 expression. This effect is mediated by the GR. They speculate that GC-induced down-regulation of the placental glucose transporter systems contributes to the retarded fetal and placental growth observed with GC treatment. This would represent a pathogenetic mechanism different from that leading to intrauterine growth retardation in the absence of GC treatment, in which trophoblast GLUT1 is not altered [134]. However, it is difficult to determine the cause and effect relationships, and the growth restriction could occur first, followed by an appropriate down-regulation of the transporters so as to match fetal size.

Consistent with this study, it was also reported that GLUT1 and GLUT3 mRNA levels were decreased in the dexamethasone treated group in the caruncles of the caw placenta [147]. In this study, plasma glucose concentrations of cows carrying a somatic cell clone fetus during late pregnancy and GLUT mRNA levels at parturition were examined. Parturition was induced by using dexamethasone and some other molecules. Cotyledon and caruncle tissues were removed just after parturition and were used for mRNA extraction. In the caruncules of the Dex induced parturition group GLUT1 and GLUT3 mRNA levels were decreased according to the Clone Pregnancy.

In another rat model, female pregnant rats were subjected to % 50 food restrictions in order to investigate the effect of maternal nutrient on placental GLUTs. In this model fetuses were overexposured to glucocorticoids as maternal protein restriction induces it. At day 21 of pregnancy plasma corticosterone levels were increased. Correspondingly, placental GLUT3 protein was decreased, GLUT1 and GLUT4 protein levels were not affected by maternal feeding regimen and therefore enhanced corticosterone level [148].

Besides placenta, GCs affect glucose transport in a variety of peripheral tissues, such as skeletal muscle, adipocytes, and endothelial cells [149-160]. High affinity low capacity GRs have been identified in the placenta of various species, including man, rat, and mouse [17, 35, 161, 162]. This would have important clinical implications, because GC-induced down-regulation of the placental glucose transport system(s) may contribute to the deleterious side-effects of GC treatment during pregnancy, such as the higher incidence of growth-retarded fetuses [46, 163-165].

Corticosteroids have also been shown to have major effects on fetal glucose homeostasis resulting in long-term persistence of these changes after birth in sheep and rats [166-172]. Prenatal corticosteroid exposure of mice resulted in programming of the fetus such that the adult progeny exhibited glucose intolerance [170, 171]. In addition, repeated courses of maternal corticosteroid administration have been shown to alter fetal glucose homeostasis and hepatic enzyme activity in rats [157, 173].

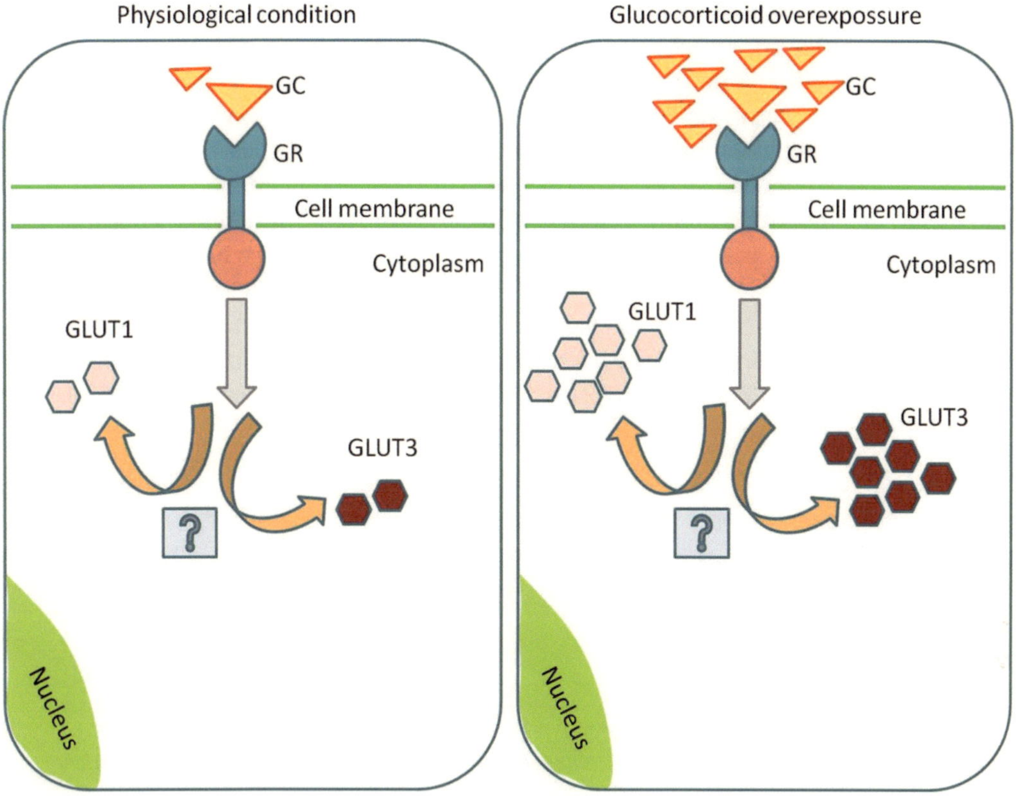

Figure 5. Effect of glucocorticoid overexposure on GLUT1 and GLUT3 expression in placental endothelial cells. GCs bind to GR and activate cellular signal transduction pathways. These molecular mechanisms remain to be unknown. As a result of GC overexposure GLUT1 and GLUT3 mRNA and proteins are increased in placental endothelial cells. Left panel refers possible physiological conditions and right panel refers effects of GC overexposure on GLUTs. (GC; Glucocorticoid, GR; Glucocorticoid Receptor, GLUT; Glucose Transporter)

In summary, the effects of glucocorticoids in placental glucose transport mechanisms in not fully understood. Further studies are needed to explain this issue.

5. Conclusion

Placental and fetal development is effected from glucocorticoids. Physiological glucocorticoid concentrations are necessary for healthy implantation, and pregnancy processes. On the other hand, glucocorticoid overexposure results with fetal and placental defects. Placentas of dexamethasone treated animals are smaller than healthy ones. In IUGR group placentas reduced placental proliferation and induced apoptosis seem to be a reason for decreased placental weigths. Dexamethasone caused a decrease in expression of genes involved in cell division such as cyclins A2, B1, D2, CDK 2, CDK 4 and M-phase protein kinase along with growth-promoting genes such as epidermal growth factor receptor. Moreover, in IUGR placentas cell cycle promoter proteins PCNA, Ki67 is decreased and cell cycle inhibitor proteins p27 and 57 are increased. Altered MAPK and Akt pathways are also unfavorably affected from glucocorticoid treatment. Decreased Akt and MAPK activations would result with reduced proliferation and/or induced apoptosis and reduced angiogenesis. GCs may affect placental angiogenesis by altering VEGF, VEGFR1 and VEGFR2 expression both at protein and gene levels with a direct effect on endothelial cells. Besides, without effecting endothelial cell viability and proliferation, GCs may affect endothelial cell migration and/or capacity of tube formation. The indirect effects of GCs seem to be via altering placental cytokine production processes which have negative effects on angiogenesis mechanisms. Another mechanism by which GCs may alter placental development is glucose transport mechanisms. It seems that GCs affect Glucose transporters via cell type dependent manner. In human endothelial cells GCs will up-regulate GLUT1 and GLUT3 expression but in trophoblast cells GCs adversely down regulates GLUT1 and GLUT3 expression in vitro.

In summary glucocorticoid overexposure may alter fetal development by altering, in part, placental development and function. It is clearly reviewed that placental development, proliferation, angiogenesis and glucose transport mechanisms are negatively affected from excess maternal glucocorticoid.

Author details

Emin Turkay Korgun*, Aslı Ozmen, Gozde Unek
Akdeniz University, Medical Faculty, Histology and Embryology Department, Antalya, Turkey

Inanc Mendilcioglu
Akdeniz University, Medical Faculty, Obstetrics and Gynecology Department, Antalya, Turkey

6. References

[1] Munck A, Naray-Fejes-Toth A (1994) Glucocorticoids and stress: permissive and suppressive actions. Ann N Y Acad Sci 746: 115-30; discussion 131-3.
[2] McEwen BS (2007) Physiology and neurobiology of stress and adaptation: central role of the brain. Physiol Rev 87: 873-904.
[3] Roberts D, Dalziel S (2006) Antenatal corticosteroids for accelerating fetal lung maturation for women at risk of preterm birth. Cochrane Database Syst Rev 3: CD004454.
[4] Kennedy TG (1983) Prostaglandin E2, adenosine 3':5'-cyclic monophosphate and changes in endometrial vascular permeability in rat uteri sensitized for the decidual cell reaction. Biol Reprod 29: 1069-76.
[5] Lopez Bernal A, Rivera J, Europe-Finner GN, Phaneuf S, Asboth G (1995) Parturition: activation of stimulatory pathways or loss of uterine quiescence? Adv Exp Med Biol 395: 435-51.

* Corresponding Author

[6] Guller S, Markiewicz L, Wozniak R, Burnham JM, Wang EY, Kaplan P, Lockwood CJ (1994) Developmental regulation of glucocorticoid-mediated effects on extracellular matrix protein expression in the human placenta. Endocrinology 134: 2064-71.

[7] Hahn T, Barth S, Graf R, Engelmann M, Beslagic D, Reul JM, Holsboer F, Dohr G, Desoye G (1999) Placental glucose transporter expression is regulated by glucocorticoids. J Clin Endocrinol Metab 84: 1445-52.

[8] Librach CL, Feigenbaum SL, Bass KE, Cui TY, Verastas N, Sadovsky Y, Quigley JP, French DL, Fisher SJ (1994) Interleukin-1 beta regulates human cytotrophoblast metalloproteinase activity and invasion in vitro. J Biol Chem 269: 17125-31.

[9] Xu B, Makris A, Thornton C, Hennessy A (2005) Glucocorticoids inhibit placental cytokines from cultured normal and preeclamptic placental explants. Placenta 26: 654-60.

[10] Ma Y, Kadner SS, Guller S (2004) Differential effects of lipopolysaccharide and thrombin on interleukin-8 expression in syncytiotrophoblasts and endothelial cells: implications for fetal survival. Ann N Y Acad Sci 1034: 236-44.

[11] Rosen T, Krikun G, Ma Y, Wang EY, Lockwood CJ, Guller S (1998) Chronic antagonism of nuclear factor-kappaB activity in cytotrophoblasts by dexamethasone: a potential mechanism for antiinflammatory action of glucocorticoids in human placenta. J Clin Endocrinol Metab 83: 3647-52.

[12] Tchernitchin A, Rooryck J, Tchernitchin X, Vandenhende J, Galand P (1975) Effects of cortisol on uterine eosinophilia and other oestrogenic responses. Mol Cell Endocrinol 2: 331-7.

[13] Fowden AL, Li J, Forhead AJ (1998) Glucocorticoids and the preparation for life after birth: are there long-term consequences of the life insurance? Proc Nutr Soc 57: 113-22.

[14] (2011) ACOG Committee Opinion No. 475: Antenatal corticosteroid therapy for fetal maturation. Obstet Gynecol 117: 422-4.

[15] Benediktsson R, Lindsay RS, Noble J, Seckl JR, Edwards CR (1993) Glucocorticoid exposure in utero: new model for adult hypertension. Lancet 341: 339-41.

[16] Levitt NS, Lindsay RS, Holmes MC, Seckl JR (1996) Dexamethasone in the last week of pregnancy attenuates hippocampal glucocorticoid receptor gene expression and elevates blood pressure in the adult offspring in the rat. Neuroendocrinology 64: 412-8.

[17] Bloom SL, Sheffield JS, McIntire DD, Leveno KJ (2001) Antenatal dexamethasone and decreased birth weight. Obstet Gynecol 97: 485-90.

[18] Langdown ML, Sugden MC (2001) Enhanced placental GLUT1 and GLUT3 expression in dexamethasone-induced fetal growth retardation. Mol Cell Endocrinol 185: 109-17.

[19] Sugden MC, Langdown ML, Munns MJ, Holness MJ (2001) Maternal glucocorticoid treatment modulates placental leptin and leptin receptor expression and materno-fetal leptin physiology during late pregnancy, and elicits hypertension associated with hyperleptinaemia in the early-growth-retarded adult offspring. Eur J Endocrinol 145: 529-39.

[20] Barker DJ (1997) Fetal nutrition and cardiovascular disease in later life. Br Med Bull 53: 96-108.

[21] Uno H, Eisele S, Sakai A, Shelton S, Baker E, DeJesus O, Holden J (1994) Neurotoxicity of glucocorticoids in the primate brain. Horm Behav 28: 336-48.

[22] Lesage J, Blondeau B, Grino M, Breant B, Dupouy JP (2001) Maternal undernutrition during late gestation induces fetal overexposure to glucocorticoids and intrauterine growth retardation, and disturbs the hypothalamo-pituitary adrenal axis in the newborn rat. Endocrinology 142: 1692-702.

[23] Bertram CE, Hanson MA (2002) Prenatal programming of postnatal endocrine responses by glucocorticoids. Reproduction 124: 459-67.

[24] de Vries A, Holmes MC, Heijnis A, Seier JV, Heerden J, Louw J, Wolfe-Coote S, Meaney MJ, Levitt NS, Seckl JR (2007) Prenatal dexamethasone exposure induces changes in nonhuman primate offspring cardiometabolic and hypothalamic-pituitary-adrenal axis function. J Clin Invest 117: 1058-67.

[25] Matthews SG (2000) Antenatal glucocorticoids and programming of the developing CNS. Pediatr Res 47: 291-300.

[26] Kranendonk G, Hopster H, Fillerup M, Ekkel ED, Mulder EJ, Taverne MA (2006) Cortisol administration to pregnant sows affects novelty-induced locomotion, aggressive behaviour, and blunts gender differences in their offspring. Horm Behav 49: 663-72.

[27] Funder JW (1997) Glucocorticoid and mineralocorticoid receptors: biology and clinical relevance. Annu Rev Med 48: 231-40.

[28] Li X, Wong J, Tsai SY, Tsai MJ, O'Malley BW (2003) Progesterone and glucocorticoid receptors recruit distinct coactivator complexes and promote distinct patterns of local chromatin modification. Mol Cell Biol 23: 3763-73.

[29] Wang Z, Frederick J, Garabedian MJ (2002) Deciphering the phosphorylation "code" of the glucocorticoid receptor in vivo. J Biol Chem 277: 26573-80.

[30] Yang Z, Guo C, Zhu P, Li W, Myatt L, Sun K (2007) Role of glucocorticoid receptor and CCAAT/enhancer-binding protein alpha in the feed-forward induction of 11beta-hydroxysteroid dehydrogenase type 1 expression by cortisol in human amnion fibroblasts. J Endocrinol 195: 241-53.

[31] Sun K, Myatt L (2003) Enhancement of glucocorticoid-induced 11beta-hydroxysteroid dehydrogenase type 1 expression by proinflammatory cytokines in cultured human amnion fibroblasts. Endocrinology 144: 5568-77.

[32] Sun M, Ramirez M, Challis JR, Gibb W (1996) Immunohistochemical localization of the glucocorticoid receptor in human fetal membranes and decidua at term and preterm delivery. J Endocrinol 149: 243-8.

[33] Chan CC, Lao TT, Ho PC, Sung EO, Cheung AN (2003) The effect of mifepristone on the expression of steroid hormone receptors in human decidua and placenta: a randomized placebo-controlled double-blind study. J Clin Endocrinol Metab 88: 5846-50.

[34] Chan J, Rabbitt EH, Innes BA, Bulmer JN, Stewart PM, Kilby MD, Hewison M (2007) Glucocorticoid-induced apoptosis in human decidua: a novel role for 11beta-hydroxysteroid dehydrogenase in late gestation. J Endocrinol 195: 7-15.

[35] Korgun ET, Dohr G, Desoye G, Demir R, Kayisli UA, Hahn T (2003) Expression of insulin, insulin-like growth factor I and glucocorticoid receptor in rat uterus and

embryo during decidualization, implantation and organogenesis. Reproduction 125: 75-84.

[36] Monder C, Shackleton CH (1984) 11 beta-Hydroxysteroid dehydrogenase: fact or fancy? Steroids 44: 383-417.

[37] Seckl JR (1993) 11 beta-hydroxysteroid dehydrogenase isoforms and their implications for blood pressure regulation. Eur J Clin Invest 23: 589-601.

[38] Seckl JR, Walker BR (2001) Minireview: 11beta-hydroxysteroid dehydrogenase type 1- a tissue-specific amplifier of glucocorticoid action. Endocrinology 142: 1371-6.

[39] Alfaidy N, Li W, MacIntosh T, Yang K, Challis J (2003) Late gestation increase in 11beta-hydroxysteroid dehydrogenase 1 expression in human fetal membranes: a novel intrauterine source of cortisol. J Clin Endocrinol Metab 88: 5033-8.

[40] Hardy DB, Yang K (2002) The expression of 11 beta-hydroxysteroid dehydrogenase type 2 is induced during trophoblast differentiation: effects of hypoxia. J Clin Endocrinol Metab 87: 3696-701.

[41] Krozowski Z, MaGuire JA, Stein-Oakley AN, Dowling J, Smith RE, Andrews RK (1995) Immunohistochemical localization of the 11 beta-hydroxysteroid dehydrogenase type II enzyme in human kidney and placenta. J Clin Endocrinol Metab 80: 2203-9.

[42] Sun K, Yang K, Challis JR (1997) Differential expression of 11 beta-hydroxysteroid dehydrogenase types 1 and 2 in human placenta and fetal membranes. J Clin Endocrinol Metab 82: 300-5.

[43] Driver PM, Kilby MD, Bujalska I, Walker EA, Hewison M, Stewart PM (2001) Expression of 11 beta-hydroxysteroid dehydrogenase isozymes and corticosteroid hormone receptors in primary cultures of human trophoblast and placental bed biopsies. Mol Hum Reprod 7: 357-63.

[44] Alfaidy N, Gupta S, DeMarco C, Caniggia I, Challis JR (2002) Oxygen regulation of placental 11 beta-hydroxysteroid dehydrogenase 2: physiological and pathological implications. J Clin Endocrinol Metab 87: 4797-805.

[45] Holmes MC, Abrahamsen CT, French KL, Paterson JM, Mullins JJ, Seckl JR (2006) The mother or the fetus? 11beta-hydroxysteroid dehydrogenase type 2 null mice provide evidence for direct fetal programming of behavior by endogenous glucocorticoids. J Neurosci 26: 3840-4.

[46] Edwards CR, Benediktsson R, Lindsay RS, Seckl JR (1993) Dysfunction of placental glucocorticoid barrier: link between fetal environment and adult hypertension? Lancet 341: 355-7.

[47] Lindsay RS, Lindsay RM, Waddell BJ, Seckl JR (1996) Prenatal glucocorticoid exposure leads to offspring hyperglycaemia in the rat: studies with the 11 beta-hydroxysteroid dehydrogenase inhibitor carbenoxolone. Diabetologia 39: 1299-305.

[48] Langley-Evans SC (1997) Maternal carbenoxolone treatment lowers birthweight and induces hypertension in the offspring of rats fed a protein-replete diet. Clin Sci (Lond) 93: 423-9.

[49] Welberg LA, Seckl JR, Holmes MC (2000) Inhibition of 11beta-hydroxysteroid dehydrogenase, the foeto-placental barrier to maternal glucocorticoids, permanently

programs amygdala GR mRNA expression and anxiety-like behaviour in the offspring. Eur J Neurosci 12: 1047-54.

[50] Wyrwoll CS, Seckl JR, Holmes MC (2009) Altered placental function of 11beta-hydroxysteroid dehydrogenase 2 knockout mice. Endocrinology 150: 1287-93.

[51] Stewart PM, Rogerson FM, Mason JI (1995) Type 2 11 beta-hydroxysteroid dehydrogenase messenger ribonucleic acid and activity in human placenta and fetal membranes: its relationship to birth weight and putative role in fetal adrenal steroidogenesis. J Clin Endocrinol Metab 80: 885-90.

[52] Kajantie E, Dunkel L, Turpeinen U, Stenman UH, Andersson S (2006) Placental 11beta-HSD2 activity, early postnatal clinical course, and adrenal function in extremely low birth weight infants. Pediatr Res 59: 575-8.

[53] Dave-Sharma S, Wilson RC, Harbison MD, Newfield R, Azar MR, Krozowski ZS, Funder JW, Shackleton CH, Bradlow HL, Wei JQ, Hertecant J, Moran A, Neiberger RE, Balfe JW, Fattah A, Daneman D, Akkurt HI, De Santis C, New MI (1998) Examination of genotype and phenotype relationships in 14 patients with apparent mineralocorticoid excess. J Clin Endocrinol Metab 83: 2244-54.

[54] Newnham JP, Evans SF, Godfrey M, Huang W, Ikegami M, Jobe A (1999) Maternal, but not fetal, administration of corticosteroids restricts fetal growth. J Matern Fetal Med 8: 81-7.

[55] Malassine A, Cronier L (2002) Hormones and human trophoblast differentiation: a review. Endocrine 19: 3-11.

[56] Morrish DW, Dakour J, Li H (1998) Functional regulation of human trophoblast differentiation. J Reprod Immunol 39: 179-95.

[57] Audette MC, Greenwood SL, Sibley CP, Jones CJ, Challis JR, Matthews SG, Jones RL (2010) Dexamethasone stimulates placental system A transport and trophoblast differentiation in term villous explants. Placenta 31: 97-105.

[58] Baisden B, Sonne S, Joshi RM, Ganapathy V, Shekhawat PS (2007) Antenatal dexamethasone treatment leads to changes in gene expression in a murine late placenta. Placenta 28: 1082-90.

[59] Hewitt DP, Mark PJ, Waddell BJ (2006) Glucocorticoids prevent the normal increase in placental vascular endothelial growth factor expression and placental vascularity during late pregnancy in the rat. Endocrinology 147: 5568-74.

[60] Hewitt DP, Mark PJ, Waddell BJ (2006) Placental expression of peroxisome proliferator-activated receptors in rat pregnancy and the effect of increased glucocorticoid exposure. Biol Reprod 74: 23-8.

[61] Timmerman M, Teng C, Wilkening RB, Fennessey P, Battaglia FC, Meschia G (2000) Effect of dexamethasone on fetal hepatic glutamine-glutamate exchange. Am J Physiol Endocrinol Metab 278: E839-45.

[62] Ward JW, Wooding FB, Fowden AL (2004) Ovine feto-placental metabolism. J Physiol 554: 529-41.

[63] Fowden AL, Forhead AJ (2009) Hormones as epigenetic signals in developmental programming. Exp Physiol 94: 607-25.

[64] Fowden AL, Forhead AJ, Coan PM, Burton GJ (2008) The placenta and intrauterine programming. J Neuroendocrinol 20: 439-50.

[65] McDonald TJ, Franko KL, Brown JM, Jenkins SL, Nathanielsz PW, Nijland MJ (2003) Betamethasone in the last week of pregnancy causes fetal growth retardation but not adult hypertension in rats. J Soc Gynecol Investig 10: 469-73.

[66] Kaufmann P, Castelluci M (1997) Extravillous trophoblast in the human placenta: A review. Trophoblast Research 18: 21-65.

[67] Lodish H, Berk A, Kaiser A, Krieger M, Scott P, Bretscher A, Ploegh H, Matsudaira P, *Molecular Cell Biology*. 5th ed. 2002, New York: W H Freeman.

[68] Alberts B, Johnson A, Lewis J, Raff M, Roberts K, Walter P, *Molecular Biology of the Cell*. 4th ed. 2002, New York Garland Science.

[69] Sherr CJ, Roberts JM (1995) Inhibitors of mammalian G1 cyclin-dependent kinases. Genes Dev 9: 1149-63.

[70] Xiong Y (1996) Why are there so many CDK inhibitors? Biochim Biophys Acta 1288: 01-5.

[71] Lew DJ, Dulic V, Reed SI (1991) Isolation of three novel human cyclins by rescue of G1 cyclin (Cln) function in yeast. Cell 66: 1197-206.

[72] Bailly E, Pines J, Hunter T, Bornens M (1992) Cytoplasmic accumulation of cyclin B1 in human cells: association with a detergent-resistant compartment and with the centrosome. J Cell Sci 101 (Pt 3): 529-45.

[73] Hunter T, Pines J (1994) Cyclins and cancer. II: Cyclin D and CDK inhibitors come of age. Cell 79: 573-82.

[74] Harper JW, Elledge SJ (1996) Cdk inhibitors in development and cancer. Curr Opin Genet Dev 6: 56-64.

[75] Dulic V, Stein GH, Far DF, Reed SI (1998) Nuclear accumulation of p21Cip1 at the onset of mitosis: a role at the G2/M-phase transition. Mol Cell Biol 18: 546-57.

[76] Ogryzko VV, Wong P, Howard BH (1997) WAF1 retards S-phase progression primarily by inhibition of cyclin-dependent kinases. Mol Cell Biol 17: 4877-82.

[77] Niculescu AB, 3rd, Chen X, Smeets M, Hengst L, Prives C, Reed SI (1998) Effects of p21(Cip1/Waf1) at both the G1/S and the G2/M cell cycle transitions: pRb is a critical determinant in blocking DNA replication and in preventing endoreduplication. Mol Cell Biol 18: 629-43.

[78] Parker SB, Eichele G, Zhang P, Rawls A, Sands AT, Bradley A, Olson EN, Harper JW, Elledge SJ (1995) p53-independent expression of p21Cip1 in muscle and other terminally differentiating cells. Science 267: 1024-7.

[79] Lee MH, Reynisdottir I, Massague J (1995) Cloning of p57KIP2, a cyclin-dependent kinase inhibitor with unique domain structure and tissue distribution. Genes Dev 9: 639-49.

[80] Yan Y, Frisen J, Lee MH, Massague J, Barbacid M (1997) Ablation of the CDK inhibitor p57Kip2 results in increased apoptosis and delayed differentiation during mouse development. Genes Dev 11: 973-83.

[81] Genbacev O, McMaster MT, Fisher SJ (2000) A repertoire of cell cycle regulators whose expression is coordinated with human cytotrophoblast differentiation. Am J Pathol 157: 1337-51.

[82] DeLoia JA, Burlingame JM, Krasnow JS (1997) Differential expression of G1 cyclins during human placentogenesis. Placenta 18: 9-16.

[83] Ichikawa N, Zhai YL, Shiozawa T, Toki T, Noguchi H, Nikaido T, Fujii S (1998) Immunohistochemical analysis of cell cycle regulatory gene products in normal trophoblast and placental site trophoblastic tumor. Int J Gynecol Pathol 17: 235-40.

[84] Korgun ET, Celik-Ozenci C, Acar N, Cayli S, Desoye G, Demir R (2006) Location of cell cycle regulators cyclin B1, cyclin A, PCNA, Ki67 and cell cycle inhibitors p21, p27 and p57 in human first trimester placenta and deciduas. Histochem Cell Biol 125: 615-24.

[85] Rossant J, Cross JC (2001) Placental development: lessons from mouse mutants. Nat Rev Genet 2: 538-48.

[86] Georgiades P, Ferguson-Smith AC, Burton GJ (2002) Comparative developmental anatomy of the murine and human definitive placentae. Placenta 23: 3-19.

[87] Pijnenborg R, Robertson WB, Brosens I, Dixon G (1981) Review article: trophoblast invasion and the establishment of haemochorial placentation in man and laboratory animals. Placenta 2: 71-91.

[88] Korgun ET, Unek G, Herrera E, Jones CJ, Wadsack C, Kipmen-Korgun D, Desoye G (2011) Mapping of CIP/KIP inhibitors, G1 cyclins D1, D3, E and p53 proteins in the rat term placenta. Histochem Cell Biol 136: 267-78.

[89] Unek G, Ozmen A, Kipmen-Korgun D, Korgun ET (2012) Immunolocalization of PCNA, Ki67, p27 and p57 in normal and dexamethasone-induced intrauterine growth restriction placental development in rat. Acta Histochem 114: 31-40.

[90] Kim ST, Lee SK, Gye MC (2005) The expression of Cdk inhibitors p27kip1 and p57kip2 in mouse placenta and human choriocarcinoma JEG-3 cells. Placenta 26: 73-80.

[91] Ozmen A, Unek G, Kipmen-Korgun D, Korgun ET (2011) The expression of Akt and ERK1/2 proteins decreased in dexamethasone-induced intrauterine growth restricted rat placental development. J Mol Histol 42: 237-49.

[92] Ain R, Canham LN, Soares MJ (2005) Dexamethasone-induced intrauterine growth restriction impacts the placental prolactin family, insulin-like growth factor-II and the Akt signaling pathway. J Endocrinol 185: 253-63.

[93] Ghidini A, Pezzullo JC, Sylvestre G, Lembet A, Salafia CM (2001) Antenatal corticosteroids and placental histology in preterm birth. Placenta 22: 412-7.

[94] Gennari-Moser C, Khankin EV, Schuller S, Escher G, Frey BM, Portmann CB, Baumann MU, Lehmann AD, Surbek D, Karumanchi SA, Frey FJ, Mohaupt MG (2011) Regulation of placental growth by aldosterone and cortisol. Endocrinology 152: 263-71.

[95] Waddell BJ, Hisheh S, Dharmarajan AM, Burton PJ (2000) Apoptosis in rat placenta is zone-dependent and stimulated by glucocorticoids. Biol Reprod 63: 1913-7.

[96] Crocker IP, Barratt S, Kaur M, Baker PN (2001) The in-vitro characterization of induced apoptosis in placental cytotrophoblasts and syncytiotrophoblasts. Placenta 22: 822-30.

[97] Mandl M, Ghaffari-Tabrizi N, Haas J, Nohammer G, Desoye G (2006) Differential glucocorticoid effects on proliferation and invasion of human trophoblast cell lines. Reproduction 132: 159-67.

[98] Clapp C, Thebault S, Jeziorski MC, Martinez De La Escalera G (2009) Peptide hormone regulation of angiogenesis. Physiol Rev 89: 1177-215.

[99] Lunghi L, Pavan B, Biondi C, Paolillo R, Valerio A, Vesce F, Patella A (2010) Use of glucocorticoids in pregnancy. Curr Pharm Des 16: 3616-37.

[100] Hadoke PW, Iqbal J, Walker BR (2009) Therapeutic manipulation of glucocorticoid metabolism in cardiovascular disease. Br J Pharmacol 156: 689-712.

[101] Oberleithner H, Schneider SW, Albermann L, Hillebrand U, Ludwig T, Riethmuller C, Shahin V, Schafer C, Schillers H (2003) Endothelial cell swelling by aldosterone. J Membr Biol 196: 163-72.

[102] Yang S, Zhang L (2004) Glucocorticoids and vascular reactivity. Curr Vasc Pharmacol 2: 1-12.

[103] Rae M, Mohamad A, Price D, Hadoke PW, Walker BR, Mason JI, Hillier SG, Critchley HO (2009) Cortisol inactivation by 11beta-hydroxysteroid dehydrogenase-2 may enhance endometrial angiogenesis via reduced thrombospondin-1 in heavy menstruation. J Clin Endocrinol Metab 94: 1443-50.

[104] Carmeliet P (2000) Mechanisms of angiogenesis and arteriogenesis. Nat Med 6: 389-95.

[105] Logie JJ, Ali S, Marshall KM, Heck MM, Walker BR, Hadoke PW (2010) Glucocorticoid-mediated inhibition of angiogenic changes in human endothelial cells is not caused by reductions in cell proliferation or migration. PLoS One 5: e14476.

[106] Giroux S, Tremblay M, Bernard D, Cardin-Girard JF, Aubry S, Larouche L, Rousseau S, Huot J, Landry J, Jeannotte L, Charron J (1999) Embryonic death of Mek1-deficient mice reveals a role for this kinase in angiogenesis in the labyrinthine region of the placenta. Curr Biol 9: 369-72.

[107] Hatano N, Mori Y, Oh-hora M, Kosugi A, Fujikawa T, Nakai N, Niwa H, Miyazaki J, Hamaoka T, Ogata M (2003) Essential role for ERK2 mitogen-activated protein kinase in placental development. Genes Cells 8: 847-56.

[108] Mikula M, Schreiber M, Husak Z, Kucerova L, Ruth J, Wieser R, Zatloukal K, Beug H, Wagner EF, Baccarini M (2001) Embryonic lethality and fetal liver apoptosis in mice lacking the c-raf-1 gene. EMBO J 20: 1952-62.

[109] Qian X, Esteban L, Vass WC, Upadhyaya C, Papageorge AG, Yienger K, Ward JM, Lowy DR, Santos E (2000) The Sos1 and Sos2 Ras-specific exchange factors: differences in placental expression and signaling properties. EMBO J 19: 642-54.

[110] Karar J, Maity A (2011) PI3K/AKT/mTOR Pathway in Angiogenesis. Front Mol Neurosci 4: 51.

[111] Aida K, Wang XL, Wang J, Li C, McDonald TJ, Nathanielsz PW (2004) Effect of betamethasone administration to the pregnant baboon at 0.75 gestation on placental eNOS distribution and activity. Placenta 25: 780-7.

[112] Schwab M, Coksaygan T, Nathanielsz PW (2006) Betamethasone effects on ovine uterine and umbilical placental perfusion at the dose used to enhance fetal lung maturation. Am J Obstet Gynecol 194: 572-9.

[113] Hunt JS, Chen HL, Miller L (1996) Tumor necrosis factors: pivotal components of pregnancy? Biol Reprod 54: 554-62.
[114] Moore KW, de Waal Malefyt R, Coffman RL, O'Garra A (2001) Interleukin-10 and the interleukin-10 receptor. Annu Rev Immunol 19: 683-765.
[115] Kahler C, Schleussner E, Moller A, Seewald HJ (2004) Doppler measurements in fetoplacental vessels after maternal betamethasone administration. Fetal Diagn Ther 19: 52-7.
[116] Oliver A, Ciulla TA (2006) Corticosteroids as antiangiogenic agents. Ophthalmol Clin North Am 19: 345-51, v.
[117] Challa JK, Gillies MC, Penfold PL, Gyory JF, Hunyor AB, Billson FA (1998) Exudative macular degeneration and intravitreal triamcinolone: 18 month follow up. Aust N Z J Ophthalmol 26: 277-81.
[118] Danis RP, Ciulla TA, Pratt LM, Anliker W (2000) Intravitreal triamcinolone acetonide in exudative age-related macular degeneration. Retina 20: 244-50.
[119] Martidis A, Miller DG, Ciulla TA, Danis RP, Moorthy RS (1999) Corticosteroids as an antiangiogenic agent for histoplasmosis-related subfoveal choroidal neovascularization. J Ocul Pharmacol Ther 15: 425-8.
[120] Penfold PL, Gyory JF, Hunyor AB, Billson FA (1995) Exudative macular degeneration and intravitreal triamcinolone. A pilot study. Aust N Z J Ophthalmol 23: 293-8.
[121] Zein WM, Noureddin BN, Jurdi FA, Schakal A, Bashshur ZF (2006) Panretinal photocoagulation and intravitreal triamcinolone acetonide for the management of proliferative diabetic retinopathy with macular edema. Retina 26: 137-42.
[122] Ingber DE, Madri JA, Folkman J (1986) A possible mechanism for inhibition of angiogenesis by angiostatic steroids: induction of capillary basement membrane dissolution. Endocrinology 119: 1768-75.
[123] Stokes CL, Weisz PB, Williams SK, Lauffenburger DA (1990) Inhibition of microvascular endothelial cell migration by beta-cyclodextrin tetradecasulfate and hydrocortisone. Microvasc Res 40: 279-84.
[124] Tokida Y, Aratani Y, Morita A, Kitagawa Y (1990) Production of two variant laminin forms by endothelial cells and shift of their relative levels by angiostatic steroids. J Biol Chem 265: 18123-9.
[125] Greenberger S, Boscolo E, Adini I, Mulliken JB, Bischoff J (2010) Corticosteroid suppression of VEGF-A in infantile hemangioma-derived stem cells. N Engl J Med 362: 1005-13.
[126] Kluetz PG, Figg WD, Dahut WL (2010) Angiogenesis inhibitors in the treatment of prostate cancer. Expert Opin Pharmacother 11: 233-47.
[127] Weinstein RS, Wan C, Liu Q, Wang Y, Almeida M, O'Brien CA, Thostenson J, Roberson PK, Boskey AL, Clemens TL, Manolagas SC (2010) Endogenous glucocorticoids decrease skeletal angiogenesis, vascularity, hydration, and strength in aged mice. Aging Cell 9: 147-61.
[128] Yano A, Fujii Y, Iwai A, Kageyama Y, Kihara K (2006) Glucocorticoids suppress tumor angiogenesis and in vivo growth of prostate cancer cells. Clin Cancer Res 12: 3003-9.

[129] Pao SS, Paulsen IT, Saier MH, Jr. (1998) Major facilitator superfamily. Microbiol Mol Biol Rev 62: 1-34.

[130] Thorens B, Mueckler M (2010) Glucose transporters in the 21st Century. Am J Physiol Endocrinol Metab 298: E141-5.

[131] Joost HG, Bell GI, Best JD, Birnbaum MJ, Charron MJ, Chen YT, Doege H, James DE, Lodish HF, Moley KH, Moley JF, Mueckler M, Rogers S, Schurmann A, Seino S, Thorens B (2002) Nomenclature of the GLUT/SLC2A family of sugar/polyol transport facilitators. Am J Physiol Endocrinol Metab 282: E974-6.

[132] Farrell CL, Yang J, Pardridge WM (1992) GLUT-1 glucose transporter is present within apical and basolateral membranes of brain epithelial interfaces and in microvascular endothelia with and without tight junctions. J Histochem Cytochem 40: 193-9.

[133] Takata K, Kasahara T, Kasahara M, Ezaki O, Hirano H (1992) Localization of erythrocyte/HepG2-type glucose transporter (GLUT1) in human placental villi. Cell Tissue Res 267: 407-12.

[134] Jansson T, Wennergren M, Illsley NP (1993) Glucose transporter protein expression in human placenta throughout gestation and in intrauterine growth retardation. J Clin Endocrinol Metab 77: 1554-62.

[135] Illsley NP (2000) Glucose transporters in the human placenta. Placenta 21: 14-22.

[136] Xing AY, Challier JC, Lepercq J, Cauzac M, Charron MJ, Girard J, Hauguel-de Mouzon S (1998) Unexpected expression of glucose transporter 4 in villous stromal cells of human placenta. J Clin Endocrinol Metab 83: 4097-101.

[137] Wolf HJ, Desoye G (1993) Immunohistochemical localization of glucose transporters and insulin receptors in human fetal membranes at term. Histochemistry 100: 379-85.

[138] Hahn D, Blaschitz A, Korgun ET, Lang I, Desoye G, Skofitsch G, Dohr G (2001) From maternal glucose to fetal glycogen: expression of key regulators in the human placenta. Mol Hum Reprod 7: 1173-8.

[139] Hauguel-de Mouzon S, Challier JC, Kacemi A, Cauzac M, Malek A, Girard J (1997) The GLUT3 glucose transporter isoform is differentially expressed within human placental cell types. J Clin Endocrinol Metab 82: 2689-94.

[140] Korgun ET, Celik-Ozenci C, Seval Y, Desoye G, Demir R (2005) Do glucose transporters have other roles in addition to placental glucose transport during early pregnancy? Histochem Cell Biol 123: 621-9.

[141] Hauguel-de Mouzon S, Shafrir E (2001) Carbohydrate and fat metabolism and related hormonal regulation in normal and diabetic placenta. Placenta 22: 619-27.

[142] Kalhan SC, D'Angelo LJ, Savin SM, Adam PA (1979) Glucose production in pregnant women at term gestation. Sources of glucose for human fetus. J Clin Invest 63: 388-94.

[143] Kipmen-Korgun D, Ozmen A, Unek G, Simsek M, Demir R, Korgun ET (2011) Triamcinolone up-regulates GLUT 1 and GLUT 3 expression in cultured human placental endothelial cells. Cell Biochem Funct.

[144] Anderson GG, Lamden MP, Cidlowski JA, Ashikaga T (1981) Comparative pulmonary surfactant-inducing effect of three corticosteroids in the near-term rat. Am J Obstet Gynecol 139: 562-4.

[145] Korgun ET, Acar N, Sati L, Kipmen-Korgun D, Ozen A, Unek G, Ustunel I, Demir R (2011) Expression of glucocorticoid receptor and glucose transporter-1 during placental development in the diabetic rat. Folia Histochem Cytobiol 49: 325-34.

[146] Hahn T, Barth S, Weiss U, Mosgoeller W, Desoye G (1998) Sustained hyperglycemia in vitro down-regulates the GLUT1 glucose transport system of cultured human term placental trophoblast: a mechanism to protect fetal development? FASEB J 12: 1221-31.

[147] Hirayama H, Sawai K, Hirayama M, Hirai T, Kageyama S, Onoe S, Minamihashi A, Moriyasu S (2011) Prepartum maternal plasma glucose concentrations and placental glucose transporter mRNA expression in cows carrying somatic cell clone fetuses. J Reprod Dev 57: 57-61.

[148] Lesage J, Hahn D, Leonhardt M, Blondeau B, Breant B, Dupouy JP (2002) Maternal undernutrition during late gestation-induced intrauterine growth restriction in the rat is associated with impaired placental GLUT3 expression, but does not correlate with endogenous corticosterone levels. J Endocrinol 174: 37-43.

[149] Boyett JD, Hofert JF (1972) Studies concerning the inhibition of glucose metabolism in thymus lymphocytes by cortisol and epinephrine. Endocrinology 91: 233-9.

[150] Garvey WT, Huecksteadt TP, Monzon R, Marshall S (1989) Dexamethasone regulates the glucose transport system in primary cultured adipocytes: different mechanisms of insulin resistance after acute and chronic exposure. Endocrinology 124: 2063-73.

[151] Haber RS, Weinstein SP (1992) Role of glucose transporters in glucocorticoid-induced insulin resistance. GLUT4 isoform in rat skeletal muscle is not decreased by dexamethasone. Diabetes 41: 728-35.

[152] Hajduch E, Hainault I, Meunier C, Jardel C, Hainque B, Guerre-Millo M, Lavau M (1995) Regulation of glucose transporters in cultured rat adipocytes: synergistic effect of insulin and dexamethasone on GLUT4 gene expression through promoter activation. Endocrinology 136: 4782-9.

[153] Langdown ML, Holness MJ, Sugden MC (2001) Early growth retardation induced by excessive exposure to glucocorticoids in utero selectively increases cardiac GLUT1 protein expression and Akt/protein kinase B activity in adulthood. J Endocrinol 169: 11-22.

[154] Olgemoller B, Schon J, Wieland OH (1985) Endothelial plasma membrane is a glucocorticoid-regulated barrier for the uptake of glucose into the cell. Mol Cell Endocrinol 43: 165-71.

[155] Weinstein SP, Wilson CM, Pritsker A, Cushman SW (1998) Dexamethasone inhibits insulin-stimulated recruitment of GLUT4 to the cell surface in rat skeletal muscle. Metabolism 47: 3-6.

[156] Ewart HS, Somwar R, Klip A (1998) Dexamethasone stimulates the expression of GLUT1 and GLUT4 proteins via different signalling pathways in L6 skeletal muscle cells. FEBS Lett 421: 120-4.

[157] Gray S, Stonestreet BS, Thamotharan S, Sadowska GB, Daood M, Watchko J, Devaskar SU (2006) Skeletal muscle glucose transporter protein responses to antenatal glucocorticoids in the ovine fetus. J Endocrinol 189: 219-29.

[158] Hernandez R, Teruel T, Lorenzo M (2003) Insulin and dexamethasone induce GLUT4 gene expression in foetal brown adipocytes: synergistic effect through CCAAT/enhancer-binding protein alpha. Biochem J 372: 617-24.

[159] Lundgren M, Buren J, Ruge T, Myrnas T, Eriksson JW (2004) Glucocorticoids down-regulate glucose uptake capacity and insulin-signaling proteins in omental but not subcutaneous human adipocytes. J Clin Endocrinol Metab 89: 2989-97.

[160] Tortorella LL, Pilch PF (2002) C2C12 myocytes lack an insulin-responsive vesicular compartment despite dexamethasone-induced GLUT4 expression. Am J Physiol Endocrinol Metab 283: E514-24.

[161] Costedoat-Chalumeau N, Amoura Z, Le Thi Hong D, Wechsler B, Vauthier D, Ghillani P, Papo T, Fain O, Musset L, Piette JC (2003) Questions about dexamethasone use for the prevention of anti-SSA related congenital heart block. Ann Rheum Dis 62: 1010-2.

[162] Matthews SG, Owen D, Kalabis G, Banjanin S, Setiawan EB, Dunn EA, Andrews MH (2004) Fetal glucocorticoid exposure and hypothalamo-pituitary-adrenal (HPA) function after birth. Endocr Res 30: 827-36.

[163] Garvey D, Scott J (1981) Placental and fetal contraindications of dexamethasone administration to pregnant rats. Experientia 37: 757-9.

[164] Katz VL, Thorp JM, Jr., Bowes WA, Jr. (1990) Severe symmetric intrauterine growth retardation associated with the topical use of triamcinolone. Am J Obstet Gynecol 162: 396-7.

[165] Reinisch JM, Simon NG, Karow WG, Gandelman R (1978) Prenatal exposure to prednisone in humans and animals retards intrauterine growth. Science 202: 436-8.

[166] Gatford KL, Wintour EM, De Blasio MJ, Owens JA, Dodic M (2000) Differential timing for programming of glucose homoeostasis, sensitivity to insulin and blood pressure by in utero exposure to dexamethasone in sheep. Clin Sci (Lond) 98: 553-60.

[167] Gurrin LC, Moss TJ, Sloboda DM, Hazelton ML, Challis JR, Newnham JP (2003) Uising WinBUGS to fit nonlinear mixed models with an application to pharmacokinetic modelling of insulin response to glucose challenge in sheep exposed antenatally to glucocorticoids. J Biopharm Stat 13: 117-39.

[168] Kutzler MA, Molnar J, Schlafer DH, Kuc RE, Davenport AP, Nathanielsz PW (2003) Maternal dexamethasone increases endothelin-1 sensitivity and endothelin a receptor expression in ovine foetal placental arteries. Placenta 24: 392-402.

[169] Moss TJ, Sloboda DM, Gurrin LC, Harding R, Challis JR, Newnham JP (2001) Programming effects in sheep of prenatal growth restriction and glucocorticoid exposure. Am J Physiol Regul Integr Comp Physiol 281: R960-70.

[170] Nyirenda MJ, Lindsay RS, Kenyon CJ, Burchell A, Seckl JR (1998) Glucocorticoid exposure in late gestation permanently programs rat hepatic phosphoenolpyruvate carboxykinase and glucocorticoid receptor expression and causes glucose intolerance in adult offspring. J Clin Invest 101: 2174-81.

[171] Nyirenda MJ, Welberg LA, Seckl JR (2001) Programming hyperglycaemia in the rat through prenatal exposure to glucocorticoids-fetal effect or maternal influence? J Endocrinol 170: 653-60.

[172] Sloboda DM, Newnham JP, Challis JR (2000) Effects of repeated maternal betamethasone administration on growth and hypothalamic-pituitary-adrenal function of the ovine fetus at term. J Endocrinol 165: 79-91.

[173] Drake AJ, Walker BR, Seckl JR (2005) Intergenerational consequences of fetal programming by in utero exposure to glucocorticoids in rats. Am J Physiol Regul Integr Comp Physiol 288: R34-8.

Chapter 14

Prenatal Glucocorticoids: Short-Term Benefits and Long-Term Risks

Milica Manojlović-Stojanoski, Nataša Nestorović and Verica Milošević

Additional information is available at the end of the chapter

http://dx.doi.org/10.5772/51106

1. Introduction

Glucocorticoids are steroid hormones synthesized in the adrenal gland cortex, and most of their physiological effects are mediated by the glucocorticoid receptor (GR), that acts as a ligand-dependent transcription factor. Coordinate changes in metabolism under glucocorticoid influence provide energy that is instantly and selectively available to vital organs, an enables them to deal with immediate environmental demands, at the expense of anabolic pathways, such as bone formation, reproduction, immunological responses and other, that are being blunted or delayed, under glucocorticoid influence [1-3].

During fetal development the synthesis of adrenal glucocorticoids precedes the establishment of a definitive structure of the gland. In rats, secretion of the main glucocorticoid – corticosterone starts as early as on day 13 of development [4] (term=22 days, short gestation period), while in humans secretion of the main glucocorticoid – cortisol starts in the 8th week of pregnancy (term=40 weeks, long gestation period) [5]. Glucocorticoid receptor mRNA is present in the tissue derivatives of all three germ layers from fetal day 13 onwards, and increases gradually during rat fetal development [6]. Human fetal tissues express GR at the gestational age of 6 weeks, meaning that the machinery for hormone action is prepared at the early stages of development [5]. These facts suggest that endogenous glucocorticoids produced by the fetal adrenal glands have a crucial role in fetal growth and the development of individual fetal tissues [7]. In response to the prepartum rise in glucocorticoids a wide variety of changes known as "preparation for birth" occurs, meaning that the maturational changes in many fetal tissues, essential for neonatal survival, are intensified during the last third of gestation. Namely, circulating glucocorticoids induce fetal lung maturation and surfactant production, trigger a variety of physiological effects on brain cell differentiation and synaptogenesis, stimulate the production of hepatic gluconeogenic enzymes, affect pancreatic β-cell development and insulin content, influence renal development and affect the maturation of the immune system [8-10]. Metabolic, cardiovascular and immune adaptations under glucocorticoid influence are fundamental to successfully overcoming birth-related stress and postnatal adaptation of the newborn to environmental challenges [11, 12].

Environmental conditions influence the prevailing nutritional and endocrine status in mothers and fetuses. Numerous animal and human studies have shown that adverse environmental conditions during pregnancy, such as maternal undernutrition [13, 14], stress [15, 16], illness, placental insufficiency [17, 18], as well as prenatal glucocorticoid exposure [19, 20] affect fetal development and postnatal outcome. Changes in the maternal hypothalamic-pituitary-adrenal (HPA) activity, transplacental diffusion of nutrients, hormones and growth factor supply, potently affect the fetal HPA axis influencing glucocorticoid output as well as other developing systems [21, 22]. Gestational age, at which an insult occurs, its nature and intensity, determines the specific tissue or organ which will be affected by the insult. Glucocorticoids are the key mediators between maternal environment and the fetus, and as such are involved in adaptations of the fetus to predicted postnatal environment. Even transient changes in glucocorticoid levels could have long-lasting consequences. The outcome might be growth retardation and change in the developmental trajectory, in the direction that best suited to the expected environment [23, 24]. This phenomenon is known as programming. The adaptations caused by suboptimal intrauterine conditions are appropriate if the predicted and actual postnatal environments match, and lead to survival to reproduce in a deprived environment [25, 26]. If there is a mismatch between the environment predicted and the actual environment experienced postnatally, adaptations are inappropriate and result in the development of disease like hypertension, ischemic heart disease, glucose intolerance, insulin resistance and type 2 diabetes [27-29].

In this chapter the latest findings, with clear statements from the literature, as well as own results regarding the endocrine mechanisms of intrauterine programming mediated by glucocorticoids will be analyzed. The causal relationship between a prenatally programmed endocrine axes and their postnatal functioning that affect growth, stress response, metabolism and reproduction will be discussed. In order to better understand mechanisms of fetal glucocorticoid programming of endocrine axes, special attention will be paid to key points of their development.

2. Development of endocrine axses

2.1. Development of hipothalamic-pituitary-adrenal axis

Functional differentiation of anterior pituitary cells is under the control of transcription factors and their cofactors. The transcription factors expressed in early pituitary development such as Rpx/Hesx1, Ptx1, Ptx2, Lhx3 regulate the formation of Rathke's pouch and maintain the formation of the baseline cellular structure. Signaling between the developing hypothalamus and the Rathe's pouch is also involved in the initial formation of pituitary primordia and further differentiation of the pituitary gland. Hypothalamic BMP 4 and FGF 8 are required for the activation of expression and maintenance of expression of the early transcriptional factors in the pouch. The lineage of adrenocorticotropin (ACTH) producing cells arises first during organogenesis, and thus represents a separate lineage. Pituitary homeobox 1 (Ptx1/Pitx1) was reported as factor for differentiation towards proopiomelanocortin (POMC) cells [30]. In the fetal pituitary the first cells that are immunopositive for ACTH can be found on fetal day 13 in the pars tuberalis anlage, whereas ACTH immunostaining is found 1 day later in the pars distalis [31]. The pars intermedia of the fetal rat pituitary is the last part to display ACTH staining [32]. Although pituitary precursor cells are influenced by spatial cues and extrinsic signals, for the initiation of ACTH synthesis in the fetal pituitary, a certain degree of autonomy exists. Moreover, ACTH immunostaining was found in 11-day-old fetal rat pituitary primordia cultured for 4 days in a serum-free medium, thus without endocrine or neuroendocrine signals [33]. Furthermore, ACTH-containing cells were detected in anencephalic human fetuses [34].

In the next stage of differentiation of ACTH-producing cells, the hypothalamic (corticotropin-releasing hormone) CRH control over ACTH cells has an indispensable role. In rats, the appearance of hypothalamic CRH-containing neurons occurs in lateral hypothalamic areas and in the paraventricular nucleus (PVN) on days 15.5 and 16.5 of gestation, respectively, whereas beaded fibers are visible in the external layer of the median eminence on day 17.5 of gestation [35]. Expression of CRH is correlated with a progressive rise in ACTH in the fetal circulation. A progressive 10-fold increase in ACTH concentration occurs in the pars distalis on days 17–20 of gestation [36], which suggests a crucial role of the developing hypothalamus. From the 20th day of gestation until term, the ACTH concentration remains unchanged. The existence of a mechanism that overcomes the negative feedback effect of elevated glucocorticoid levels on POMC gene expression during late pregnancy was demonstrated [37]. From that period onwards, ACTH is stored in the fetal pituitary gland as a readily releasable pool. Its location near the fenestrated capillary network enables momentary depletion of significant amounts of ACTH, and a subsequent considerable increase in ACTH concentration in the circulation, if physiologically demanded [38].

The cells of the adrenal cortex arise early in development due to the local proliferation of cells from the splanchnic mesoderm. The genes coding the orphan nuclear receptors SF-1 and DAX-1 control the early fetal adrenal cortex development. Knockout mice for these genes manifest adrenal and gonadal agenesis, gonadotropin deficiency and the absence of the hypothalamic ventromedial nucleus [39]. The potential for steroid synthesis occurs early, in 12-day-old rat fetuses [40]. In the later stages of fetal life, ACTH controls growth and development, as well as steroidogenic maturation of the adrenal glands [41]. Histological analysis of a near term rat fetal adrenal glands showed that the main part of the gland is steroidogenic tissue composed of a zona glomerulosa (ZG) and an inner zone (IZ), while the number of migrating chromoblasts is still modest [42]. Both cortical zones are functionally competent and able to produce aldosterone and corticosterone in 19-day-old fetuses [43]. The proliferative activity of adrenocortical cells is most intensive in the outer portion of the glands, in the subcapsular ZG region and outer portion of IZ from where the cells migrated centripetally [44]. A balance between proliferation and cell death enables proper functioning and integrity of the developing adrenal glands. Programmed cell death appears to occur in the inner cortical layers, where many resident macrophages are present [4], as well as in the resorption zones and giant cells [45, 46].

The development of the human adrenal glands exhibits a number of important differences in histological organization and steroidogenic activity in relation to species with a short-term gestation period. The primordium of the human fetal adrenal glands can be recognized by 3–4 weeks of gestation, but by the 8th week of embryonic development the adrenal cortex is clearly identifiable with its characteristic zonal partitioning [47]. The principal steroids of primate fetal adrenal gland, i.e. fetal zone situated in the inner part of the gland, are dehydroepiandrosterone (DHEA) and DHEA sulfate (DHEAS). DHEA serves as a substrate for placental estrone and estradiol production. Rapid growth of the fetal adrenal cortex, especially the fetal zone, with a significant increase in steroidogenic activity begins after week 10 of gestation and continues until term [47]. The definitive zone, positioned at the peripheral part of the gland, is steroidogenically inert, at last until the second trimester of pregnancy. After this period mineralocorticoid production were found, although aldosterone synthesis in the fetal adrenals is in poor correlation with plasma rennin activity. The transitional zone that becomes distinguishable between fetal and definitive zone at the end of the second trimester of pregnancy represents a precursor of the adult zona fasciculata (ZF). The expression of enzymes 3β hydroxysteroid dehydrogenase (3βHSD) and cytochrome P450 17α-hydroxylase/lyase (CYP17) in the transitional zone enables the capacity for cortisol production [48]. In the initial phase, the fetal adrenals begin to produce cortisol between weeks 10 and 20 of gestation, possibly utilizing progesterone as a precursor. However, *de novo* synthesis of cortisol from cholesterol is established fairly late in gestation, leading to a remarkable increase in cortisol concentrations in the third trimester. Immediately after birth, the fetal zone of the adrenal cortex degenerates extensively, whereas the ZF matures in the subsequent period. [48]. Although the presence of ACTH is established in circulation from week 15 of gestation, cortisol and androgen production by the definitive and fetal zone are maximally stimulated by circulating ACTH from midgestation [49].

The functional state of the fetal HPA axis is important for several reasons. Firstly, glucocorticoids play a role in the maturation of numerous organs necessary for intrauterine development and extrauterine existence. Organ systems involved in reaching metabolic homeostasis, stress response and electrolyte balance in outer space are strongly controlled by glucocorticoids [50]. Secondly, the fetal HPA negative feedback mechanism begins to operate between days 15 and 17 of rat gestation [51]. Thus, near term fetuses are able to regulate their own homeostasis and glucocorticoid production in response to different maternal stressors [52] and adverse conditions [37]. Finally, the fetal HPA axis activity strongly affects the timing of parturition [48]. In a number of species at the end of gestation there is an increase in HPA activity, with increased plasma glucocorticoid levels that reflects on the placental trophoblast cells, causing enhanced output of prostaglandins [37]. The effects of prostaglandins on the myometrium associated with increased oxytocin activity represent an important step in the initiation of birth [50].

2.1.1. *Effects of glucocorticoids during fetal development*

Strictly defined spatial and temporal effects of glucocorticoids are actually determined by the previous appearance of the GR. *In situ* hybridization histochemistry revealed GR gene expression in the tissue derivatives of all three germ layers. The facts that intense GR mRNA labeling happened just before the final differentional step for each glucocorticoid target tissue, and that upon differentiation reduced amounts of GR mRNA were found further support the crucial morphogenic role of glucocorticoids during fetal development [6].

Sufficient glucocorticoid levels are essential for the normal maturation of many parts of CNS during the prenatal period. In general, glucocorticoids act on neuronal maturation, replication, differentiation, and programmed cell death [8, 12]. In parallel with reducing the rate of neuronal replication, glucocorticoids promote the differentiation of central noradrenergic, serotonergic and dopaminergic neurons, enhance axonal growth, dendritic arborisation and synaptogenesis in a regionally selective manner, and control programmed cell death [53, 54].

Glucocorticoids promote the differentiation of sympathoadrenal precursors, initially expressed multiple neuronal markers, into endocrine chromaffin cells in the adrenal gland medulla. As sympathoadrenal precursors invade the primordium of the fetal adrenal gland and migrate centripetally, they are exposed to adrenal steroids. The initial adrenaline synthesis occurs in parallel with a sharp rise in the adrenal tissue and plasma glucocorticoid concentrations, and the appearance of GR in the sympathoadrenal precursor cells in 17-day-old rat fetuses [55]. Thus, glucocorticoids represent an important signal for the induction and maintenance of adrenaline synthesis in the adrenal medulla, but initial induction of the adrenaline-synthesizing enzyme, phenylethanolamine-N-methyltransferase is rather determined by a cell-intrinsic timed process in the chromaffin precursors [56].

Glucocorticoids accelerate lung maturation as they speed up the thinning of the double capillary loop to form the thin gas exchanging walls of the alveoli. By enhancing the production of surfactant by type II pneumocytes, glucocorticoids allow the newborn to draw its first breath and enable the start of the breathing process [57].

In the fetal liver, glucocorticoids promote the activity of the key gluconeogenic enzyme systems and hepatic glycogen deposition in preparation for the nutritional transition at birth. Inability of the adrenalectomised sheep fetuses to induce glucogenesis during extreme circumstances such as maternal undernutrition with reductions in hepatic glycogen content was associated with lower circulating concentrations of cortisol [10]. It might be concluded that birth-related stress and subsequent environmental challenges trigger glucocorticoid actions essentially involved in the activation of fetal glucogenesis and glucose availability necessary for maintaining homeostasis after birth.

By combining *in vitro* studies with *in vivo* investigations in mice lacking the GR in the whole organism or in specific pancreatic cell populations, it has been shown that glucocorticoids are important hormones in pancreatic development. Acting before insulin expression onset, glucocorticoids decreased the differentiation of the embryonic pancreas into β-cells favoring acinar cells differentiation. Deletion of the GR in pancreatic precursor cells led to increased β-cell mass. Thus, glucocorticoids unable β-cells mass expansion in later stages, by modifying the balance of specific transcription factors, mostly Pdx-1 [9]. At birth, as the placental source of glucose is lost, tight glycemic control must be established. A prepartum rise in glucocorticoid levels in fetal horse and sheep increases pancreatic β cells sensitivity to glucose and influences the fetal insulin level, enabling active regulation of the glucose level after birth, and thus the transition to enteral supply [10, 22].

The highest expression of the GR mRNA was identified during early kidney development in the developing glomeruli, epithelial cells of the proximal and distal renal tubule, and the central collecting duct. Reduction of GR levels in the fully differentiated glomeruli pointed out the importance of glucocorticoids during a defined period of establishment of the definitive renal structure and function [5].

Effective thermoregulation in response to cold exposure in the extrauterine environment post birth is crucial to prevent hypothermia in newborns. The expression of mitochondrial uncoupling protein (UCP), that catalyzes adaptive thermogenesis in mammalian brown adipose tissue increases dramatically during the final week of gestation in fetal adipose tissue [58]. The late-gestation augment in fetal plasma glucocorticoid levels as well as application of synthetic glucocorticoids enhance mitochondrial UCP expression, suggesting that glucocorticoids are crucially involved in increasing the thermogenic potential of fetal adipose tissue near term [59, 60].

2.2. Development of the somatotropic axis

Growth hormone (GH) is secreted from the anterior pituitary gland under the control of two hypothalamic hormones: the releasing hormone is growth hormone-releasing hormone (GHRH), and the release-inhibiting hormone is somatostatin (SRIH). In addition to these two neurohormones, a number of factors such as free fatty acids, acetylcholine, amino acids, opiates, glucocorticoids and some neuropeptides also have direct or indirect effects on GH release. Most of the metabolic actions of GH are mediated by insulin-like growth factor I (IGF-I), which is produced in many different tissues, with most of the circulating IGF-I being derived from the liver. IGF-I has anabolic as well as metabolic effects in many cell types, acting through autocrine, paracrine and classical endocrine mechanisms. IGF signaling has been recognized as one of the major molecular regulators of cell growth and proliferation [61]. Moreover, it is generally accepted that GH, by controlling important aspects of IGF activity in many tissues and cell types of mammals, is able to coordinate somatic growth in a defined spatio-temporal manner at the whole body level [62]. IGF signaling, however, not only regulates growth but also affects differentiation and may, through epigenetic processes, steer adult cell function as a result of particular conditions during postnatal development [63].

In rat, GHRH neurons are detected at the 16th day of fetal development [64], while SRIH mRNA in the periventricular nucleus of the hypothalamus is expressed on the 14th fetal day [65]. Initial pituitary GH expression is detected on day 15 of gestation using sensitive methods such as the reverse transcriptase-polymerase chain reaction (RT-PCR) [66]. In the following phase of GH cell development the expression of Pit-1 occurs. Pit-1 is a pituitary-specific transcriptional factor that mediates cell proliferation and differentiation into specific hormone-producing cell types – thyrotropes, somatotropes or lactotropes [67]. During this period, the quantity of GH transcripts remains at an extremely low level. A marked increase in cell number and GH production occurs between days 18 and 19 of fetal development [68]. The expression of the GHRH receptor also occurs on fetal day 19 in rats [69, 70].

It has been considered that pituitary GH promotes and controls fetal development and body weight by stimulating the family of hepatic growth factors. Recent investigations showed that extrapituitary GH as well as local production of growth factors had great paracrine/autocrine influence on fetal developmental processes and differentiation. The expression of GH and GH receptor in a wide variety of tissues is established before the pituitary gland and circulatory system become functional [71]. In rats and mice a contribution of the pituitary GH to growth, development and body weight has been demonstrated postnatally, during the second week of life [72]. The influence of pituitary GH on normal growth and body weight in near-term fetuses, immediately after the GH cells become functional, is still difficult to understand and not well defined.

In humans, GH cells are evident at 8 weeks of gestation, with abundant immunoreactive cytoplasmic GH expression. Plasma GH concentrations are highest at midgestation and thereafter fall until term. The pattern of ontogenesis of plasma GH reflects the progressive maturation of hypothalamic–pituitary and forebrain function. The responses of GH to SRIH and GHRH are mature at term in human infants [73].

IGF-1 and IGF-2 mRNA transcripts are present in virtually all fetal tissues [74]. Both IGFs are also detected in the fetal circulation from early gestation, but the plasma concentrations of IGF-II are 3–10 fold higher than those of IGF-I during late gestation [75]. They are present in serum and other extracellular fluids associated with highly specific binding proteins (IGF binding proteins (IGFBPs)). In the fetus, IGFs are predominantly complexed with IGFBP-1 and -2, and the liver is the predominant production site for these IGFBPs [76]. Tissue and plasma IGF-II are higher in the fetus than in newborn or adult animals in most species [77]. In rodents, IGF-II expression disappears from most tissues except the brain by weaning, with the consequence that IGF-II is virtually undetectable in adult plasma [78]. In contrast, plasma IGF-I levels increase rapidly after birth, primarily as a result of the onset of GH stimulated IGF-I production by the liver [79], since IGF regulation is GH-independent during the fetal period [74]. There is, therefore, a shift in IGF predominance from IGF-II before birth to IGF-I after birth, which has led to the concept that IGF-II is the IGF primarily responsible for fetal growth [80].

2.3. Development of hypothalamic-pituitary-thyroid axis

The development of thyroid-stimulating hormone (TSH) cells in the fetal rat pituitary pars distalis is determined by the expression of Pit-1 and TEF transcription factors [67]. Differentiation from precursor cells enables detection of TSH cells mRNA on day 15 of gestation [81], while immunocytochemically recognized TSH cells can be observed in 16.5- to 17.5-day-old fetuses. TSH cells were few in 17.5-day-old rat fetuses, but their number increased thereafter, particularly during the 2nd week after birth [68].

In the rat fetal hypothalamus, thyrotropin-releasing hormone (TRH), which promotes prompt synthesis and secretion of anterior pituitary TSH, is first detected on the 16th day of gestation [82]. The destruction of paraventricular nuclei (PVN), which contain TRH neuronal cell bodies, results in a significant decrease in anterior pituitary TSHβ- and α-subunit mRNA levels, as well as in serum TSH concentrations [83]. During the fetal period a major influence of TSH is to control the morphological and functional maturation of the fetal thyroid gland.

The thyroid gland is derived from the fusion of a medial outpouching from the floor of the primitive pharynx and bilateral evaginations of the fourth pharyngeal pouch, giving rise to the precursors of follicular (thyroxine-producing cells) and parafollicular (calcitonin-producing C cells) cells. Coordinate action of numerous transcription factors is involved in thyroid morphogenesis. Titf1, Hhex, Pax8 and Foxe1 are expressed in the rat just prior to the first appearance of the thyroid diverticulum on fetal day 9.5–10, controlling the proliferation, survival and migration of precursor cells [84]. Targeted disruption of Titf1 in mice results in total absence of the thyroid tissue, while the lack of Pax8 results in follicle agenesis, with the remaining tissue being composed almost exclusively of C-cells [85, 86].

In rats on fetal day 17 significant growth and rapid functional and structural development of the thyroid gland are established. The first appearance of follicles, iodine organification and thyroid hormonogenesis occur in parallel with a marked increase of TSH in fetal circulation and the expression of TSH receptors (TSHR) in thyroid tissue. Thus, upregulation of TSHR gene expression by TSH in fetuses is crucial for further maturation of the thyroid [81].

Deiodinase enzymes provide biologically active triiodothyronine (T3) to developing tissues by activating and/or deactivating systemic serum thyroid hormones (TH). Three types of iodothyronine deiodinases (D1, D2, D3) have been identified, which differ in tissue distribution, substrate specificity and sensitivity to inhibiting compounds [87]. Expression of D1 is low through gestation, while D2 and D3 are the major isoforms in the fetus [88]. D2 is the activating enzyme that catalyzes the removal of one iodide from the outer tyrosine ring of thyroxine (T4) and production of active T3. D3 is the inactivating enzyme that catalyzes the cleaving of one iodide from the inner tyrosine rings of T4 or T3, thus generating reverse T3 (rT3) or T2. Action of D2 and D3 preserves the safe level of T3 in the developing brain and the pituitary [87], while the activity of D3 in the utero-placental unit protects fetal tissues against high maternal T4 concentrations. Local tissue deiodinase activity is essential for compensation and adaption to potential malfunctions in the fetal hypothalamic-pituitary-thyroid (HPT) axis, i.e. in the case of congenital hypothyroidism and normal maternal T4, the transfer of the latter, together with increased brain D2 activity, protects the fetal brain from T3 deficiency [89].

In humans, thyroid gland reaches maturity by the 11th–12th week of gestation, when tiny follicle precursors with thyroglobulin in follicular space can be seen and iodine binding is detected. In this period both T4 and T3 are measurable in fetal serum [90]. At this stage of early development maternal T4 transplacental passage contributes to the fetal hormonal status, which is essential for normal early fetal neurogenesis. In the later stages of development, if fetal thyroid function is normal, placental TH passage is relatively limited due to the presence of D3 [91]. The increase in total T4 and free T4 levels between weeks 18 and 36 of gestation indicates maturation of the HPT axis function, with the establishment of feedback control about midgestation.

2.4. Development of the endocrine pancreas

The embryogenesis of pancreas is mediated by a series of transcription factors involved in morphogenesis. The expression of Pdx1 has been found early in organ formation, in cells that give rise to endocrine and exocrine cells of the mouse neonatal pancreas. In Pdx1 null mice pancreas agenesis occurs. The appearance of insulin and glucose transporter GLUT2 is also regulated by this transcription factor [92]. Transcription factors Hlxb9 and Isl1 are necessary for the initial induction of Pdx1. Hlxb9 is observed during the formation of pancreatic anlage and later during the differentiation of β cells. Neurogenin 3 has been identified as the key regulator of endocrine development, giving rise to all pancreatic endocrine lineages [93].

The pancreas arises from a multipotent endodermal cell population that will produce ductal, exocrine and endocrine cells [94]. The human fetal pancreas develops during the 5th week of gestation, while endocrine cells are identifiable by the 8th or 9th week of gestation. Scattered single endocrine cells are recognized to produce insulin (β-cell), glucagon (α-cells), somatostatin (δ-cells) and pancreatic polypeptide (PP cells). Clusters of epithelial endocrine cells form primitive islets of Langerhans a few weeks later, in parallel with the expression of neural adhesion molecule (N-CAM) [95]. The largest expansion of the β-cell mass has been shown to take place in the second half of prenatal development, from approximately 20 weeks in humans. This developmental period is critical to achieve a β-cell mass required to ensure proper insulin secretion throughout life. It is thought to result from β-cell neogenesis from rapidly dividing undifferentiated progenitor cells [96]. Thereafter, some degree of β-cell expansion persists at least until adolescence due to β-cell neogenesis, mitosis and perhaps to transdifferentiation of α-cells, acinar or ductal cells [97].

During the development of insulin-expressing cells there is a changing phenotype, from progenitor cells to immature β-cells, and finally, to mature adult β-cells. Using gene expression and immunohistochemistry, differences among late-embryonic, neonatal, and adult β-cells were found in a series of markers with transient expression patterns during the perinatal period. Of these, cytokeratin-19, matrix metalloproteinase-2 and surfactant protein-D can be considered as true markers of new and immature β-cells, as their expression is transient and not entirely synchronous, but absent in adults [98]. Sympathetic innervation and vascularization of islets play important roles in normal islet morphogenesis during prenatal life, and have trophic effects on β-cells survival, maturation and insulin secretion [99].

Human and rodent fetal islets are insensitive to glucose, as fetal β-cells do not discriminate between different glucose levels, despite adequate insulin reserves. Relative functional immaturity *in utero* was also recorded in response to circulating amino acids, particularly leucine, catecholamines and neural stimulation, with regard to the capacity to secrete both insulin and glucagon [100]. For blunted capacity for insulin and glucagon secretion several causes are proposed. Firstly, during fetal development in mammals glucose homeostasis is mainly achieved by the mother because of a constant supply of glucose by placental transfer through facilitated diffusion. Secondly, the mechanisms that mediate insulin secretion in adults are immature in fetuses, meaning that the production of cAMP is decreased, expression of glucose transporter GLUT2 is lower and expression of voltage-gated L-type Ca^{2+} channels is diminished in β-cells [100, 101]. Furthermore, generalized immaturity of the metabolic enzyme expression in pancreatic β-cells during the fetal and neonatal period in the rat has been recorded. Lower expression levels of the metabolic enzyme genes such as malate dehydrogenase, glycerol-3-phosphate dehydrogenase, glutamate oxaloacetate transaminase and pyruvate carboxylase were established and confirmed by quantitative PCR during fetal development and several weeks after birth than in adults [102]. During fetal life GH might be involved in the process of β-cell mass expansion and maturation that finally leads to an effective response to hyperglycaemia [103].

2.5. Development of the hypothalamic-pituitary-gonadal axis

Reproductive physiology in mammals is centrally regulated through the hypothalamic–pituitary–gonadal (HPG) axis and depends on gonadotropin-releasing hormone (GnRH). GnRH, a decapeptide, is released into the hypophyseal portal vasculature from axon terminals at the median eminence and binds to the GnRH receptor (GnRHR), which is specifically expressed in gonadotrope cells in the anterior pituitary gland. GnRH signaling controls the biosynthesis and release of luteinizing hormone (LH) and follicle-stimulating hormone (FSH), which in turn regulate the development and activity of the ovaries and testes. LH and FSH, together with TSH, are heterodimeric glycoproteins composed of a common α-subunit (αGSU) and a hormone-specific β-subunit (LHβ, FSHβ).

The crucial maturation events at the hypothalamic–pituitary level are the onset of GnRH synthesis, access of GnRH to the hypothalamic–hypophysial circulation, appearance of GnRH receptors in the pituitary gonadotropes, and the onset of gonadotropin synthesis and secretion. Traces of GnRH in whole rat brain extracts were detected as early as on day 12 of gestation, and by the 17th day of gestation immunoreactive GnRH cells within the brain were distributed in a pattern similar to that of the adult, projecting neurosecretory axons to the median eminence [104].

Although gonadotrope is the last cell type in the anterior pituitary to reach maturation with the expression of terminal differentiation markers LHβ, FSHβ, and GnRHR, αGSU is the first pituitary hormone transcript expressed during development. In mice, it is first detected at fetal day 10.5 in the most ventral region of Rathke's pouch [105]. Gonadotrope specific expression of αGSU is regulated by SF1, which plays essential roles at multiple levels of the reproductive axis, reviewed in [106]. However, no single transcription factor has been demonstrated to be necessary and sufficient for gonadotrope lineage commitment [107]. In the rat pituitary, on fetal day 16 rare LHβ were detected by *in situ* hybridization. Many more cells hybridizing LHβ and FSHβ were observed on day 17. At this stage, the fetal pituitary gland becomes GnRH responsive [104]. Recently, it has been shown that two types of gonadotropes may become responsive to GnRH at different time points during development [108].

In humans, fetal pituitary gonadotropins are secreted as early as at 12 weeks of gestation. Marked rises in the pituitary and plasma concentrations of FSH and LH are observed during the second trimester of gestation, and significantly higher levels of circulating gonadotropins are detected in female than in male fetuses [109].

Gonad development is a unique system in which a single rudimentary tissue can be induced to form one of two different organs, the ovary or the testis. The gonads originate from the thickening of the ventrolateral epithelium along the embryonic mesonephros surface, called the genital ridge, and in mice are visible at fetal day 10. Proliferation of these epithelial cells gives rise to somatic cells of the gonad. By contrast, the germ cell lineage arises outside the urogenital ridge before the formation of gonads. Mouse primordial germ cells (PGCs) are specified in the epiblast, and are first detected at about fetal day 7.25 using alkaline phosphatase as a marker [110]. PGCs proliferate and migrate through the gut mesentery into the urogenital ridge, populating the gonads between the 10th and 11th day of fetal development. The exact trigger that initiates PGCs migration to the genital ridge and the chemoattractants that are required for the directional movement toward the genital ridge are slowly beginning to be understood [111].

In mammals, the choice between the male or the female gonad, is initiated by a single gene on the Y chromosome, Sry (sex-determining region of the Y chromosome). Sry is expressed in the somatic cells of the XY gonad between 10.5 and 12.0 of gestation [112] and encodes a putative transcription factor that acts as a genetic switch for male development. The Sry protein is expressed in each pre-Sertoli cell during a narrow window of several hours in the period of gonadal differentiation, between fetal days 10.5 and 12.5, resulting in up-regulation of Sox9, the major gene transcriptionally downstream of Sry [113]. If Sry is expressed in the rudimentary gonad, either from the Y chromosome or from an ectopic transgene, a testis forms [114]. If Sry is not expressed, as in XX individuals or in cases where Sry is mutated or deleted, an ovary forms [115]. Based on this, it was believed that the presence of Sry actively caused testis development to occur, and that in the absence of Sry the ovary developed passively (i.e. the so-called "default" pathway). Recent discoveries have now made it clear that early ovarian development is an active process that involves the interaction and competition of multiple signaling pathways that specify male or female development. The two alternative sex fates are thought to emerge through the antagonistic activities of sex-specific transcription factors in a restricted number of gonadal cells. This initial cell fate decision is further expanded by extracellular non-cell-autonomous signals that promote one developmental program, while at the same time suppressing the other [116]. Studies have identified two secreted factors, Wnt4 and follistatin, which are required during early gonad development to repress the aspects of testis differentiation in XX gonads, reviewed in [111].

By fetal day 13.5, germ cells in XX and XY gonads have taken different developmental paths. In XY gonads germ cells undergo mitotic arrest as prospermatogonia, whereas in XX gonads the germ cells enter the prophase of the first meiotic division. The fate of germ cells is dependent on the somatic environment, and not on the chromosomal sex of the germ cells [117]. Thus, signals from adjacent somatic cells must direct the differentiation of germ cells in the embryonic gonads, although these signals have not been identified.

The onset of gonadal endocrine activity is very clearly sexually dimorphic. During embryogenesis, male differentiation requires the secretion of three testicular hormones. Anti-Müllerian hormone (AMH), produced by fetal Sertoli cells, induces regression of the Müllerian ducts. Testosterone, produced by Leydig cells, promotes the development of Wolffian duct derivatives and masculinization of the external male genitalia. Finally, insulin-like 3 (Insl3) mediates transabdominal testicular descent into the scrotum [118]. The action of LH and production of testosterone start simultaneously in the rat testis on fetal day 15.5 [119]. In females, differentiation occurs when the absence of AMH allows development of Müllerian structures. The lack of androgens permits degeneration of Wolffian ducts, and the absence of Insl3 maintains the gonads in the abdomen. In the ovary, the responsiveness to LH appears postnatally at the end of the first week of life [120] concomitantly with the onset of steroidogenesis [121]. Functional FSH receptors can be detected some days earlier in the perinatal rat ovary, at the age of 4–5 days [122].

Steroid hormones play a crucial role in fetal gonadal development and ovarian cell wellbeing. Estrogen action is needed for normal ovarian development, follicle survival and the regulation of female reproduction. The role of estrogens in female sexual development has been demonstrated in many studies utilizing mice lacking functional estrogen receptors or estrogen-converting enzymes [123, 124]. However, the developmental role of estrogens in human fetal ovaries is not well known. In contrast, testicular hormones are crucial for testicular formation and function, i.e. induction and maintenance of the male phenotype at all stages of development.

In humans ovarian development starts at around the 5th week of gestation, when primordial germ cells migrate into the undifferentiated gonad. Thereafter, the germ cells undergo multiple mitotic divisions, and the number of oogonia reaches its peak by the 20th week of development. At this time about 7–8 million germ cells are present in the ovary [125]. Simultaneously with mitotic divisions, starting around the fetal age of 11–12 weeks, primordial germ cells begin to enter meiosis [126]. After the 10th week of gestation granulosa cell precursors start to form, and at 24 weeks of development almost all oocytes are enveloped in a primordial follicle structure [127]. The human fetus is exposed to high concentrations of maternal and placental estrogens, and estrogens are produced in several fetal tissues [128, 129]. However, minimal amounts of fetal circulating estrogens are produced in the fetal ovarian follicles [109].

In the human male at 7 weeks of gestation, the presence of germ cells in the embryonic gonadal ridge and of coelomic epithelial cells that give rise to Sertoli cells was observed. This was followed by the appearance of Sertoli cells in the testicular tubules and of Leydig cells at 9 weeks, and also by the appearance of vascular endothelial cells and peritubular myoid cells at 12 weeks [130]. The production of testosterone peaks at around 11 or 12 to 14 weeks of gestation, as determined by measurements in the testis and fetal blood [131]. Between weeks 12 and 20, serum testosterone levels in the male fetus are from 3- to 8-fold higher than in the female [132].

3. Programming

During development, there are critical periods in the course of which a system or an organ has to mature. The critical periods are defined by the epochs of rapid cell division within an organ, and different organs develop at different rates and different times. At these critical periods organs are especially vulnerable to challenges such as decreased oxygenation, nutrient supply, and altered hormone exposure. If adverse conditions are experienced in the window of vulnerability, then the trajectory of development of the responding organ may be changed in ways that result in persistent malfunction. The concepts of "nutritional programming", "fetal programming", "fetal origins of adult disease", "developmental origins of health and disease", "developmental induction", and "developmental programming" [26, 133-135] imply that some stimulus or an insult at these critical, restricted periods in development has long-lasting consequences, setting in train a series of events that culminate in the adult onset of disordered function, while the same environmental stimulus outside that critical period induces only reversible changes. The concept evolved from human epidemiological studies that have shown that impaired intrauterine growth is associated with an increased incidence of metabolic, cardiovascular and other diseases in later life. Low birth weight, in particular, has been linked to hypertension, glucose intolerance, insulin resistance, type 2 diabetes, dyslipidaemia, obesity and reproductive disorders in the adult (Figure 1) [133]. The Dutch famine, a unique "natural experiment" with a well-defined period of food shortage in an otherwise well-nourished population, has shown that maternal undernutrition during gestation compromises health in later life, and that these long-term effects depend on its timing during gestation [136]. Intrauterine growth retardation (IUGR) and/or delays in attaining motor, verbal and social skills were recorded in the offspring of mothers exposed to the influence of a large variety of "stresses" such as loud, unanticipated noise (as experienced by people living under the flight paths of busy airports) and living in a country preparing for and ultimately going to war (e.g. the six-day Israeli war) [137].

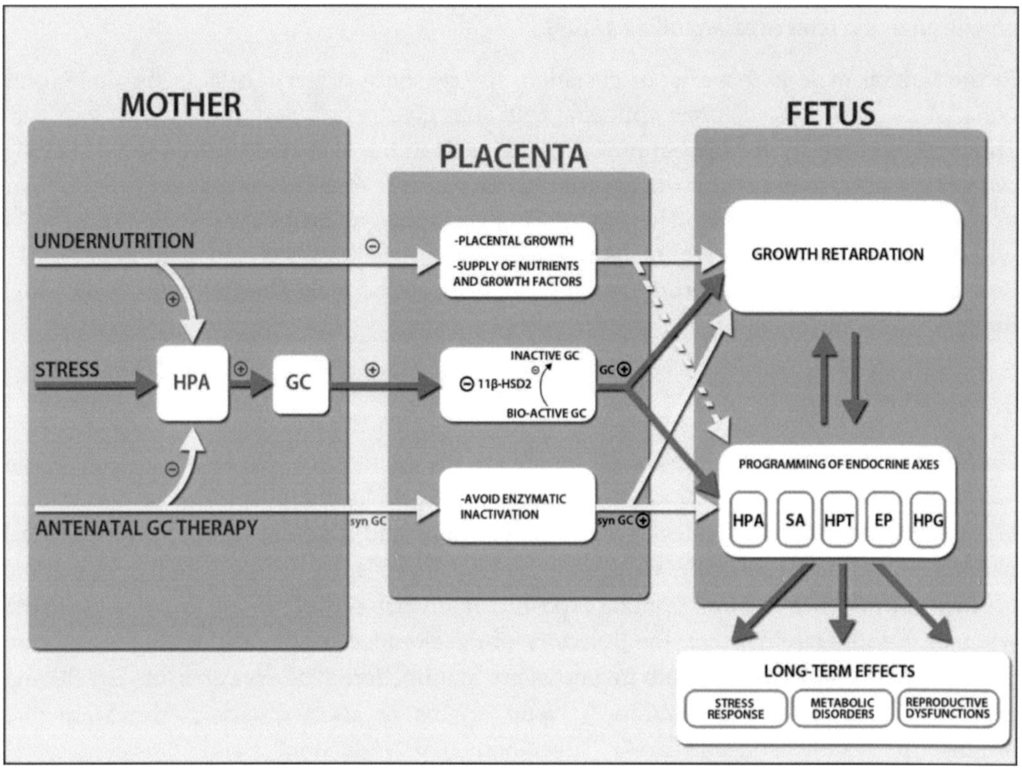

Figure 1. Maternal undernutrition or stress increase maternal glucocoticoid levels and decrease the rate of their inactivation by 11ß-HSD2 in the placenta that results in fetal glucocorticoid overexposure. The synthetic glucocorticoids pass through the enzymatic placental barrier and reach the fetal circulation. Consequences of fetal glucocorticoid overexposure are growth retardation and programming of endocrine axes with long-term effects. HPA-hypothalamic-pituitary-adrenal axis; GC-glucocorticoids; synGC-synthetic glucocorticoids; 11ß-HSD2-11ß-hydroxysteroid dehydrogenase type 2; SA-somatotropic axis; HPT-hypothalamic-pituitary-thyroid axis; EP-endocrine pancreas; HPG-hypothalamic-pituitary-gonadal axis.

The concept of programming has been tested experimentally in numerous species using a wide range of experimental approaches to impair fetal growth. Some of the most commonly used experimental models are maternal undernutrition (calorie restriction, protein deprivation, iron deficiency), placental insufficiency and exposure to glucocorticoids that includes maternal stress, maternal treatment with synthetic glucocorticoids and inhibition of placental 11ß-hydroxysteroid dehydrogenase (11β-HSD2) (Figure 1) [138].

Majority of these experimental models ultimately result in fetal glucocorticoid overexposure, since they mediate the programming effects of nutritional and other environmental challenges during pregnancy [139]. Maternal low-protein diet and placental 11β-HSD2 deficiency cause fetal growth restriction via distinct pathways but with a common component: overexposure of fetoplacental tissues to glucocorticoids. Whatever the source, glucocorticoids play an important role in the regulation of fetal growth, and through this in developmental programming [140]. Glucocorticoids are growth inhibitory and affect development of all the tissues and organ systems that are at increased risk of adult pathophysiology when fetal growth is impaired [11]. Glucocorticoids signal adverse intrauterine conditions and adapt fetal development to ensure the maximum chances of survival both *in utero* and at birth. They act at cellular and molecular levels to induce changes in tissue growth and differentiation by direct and indirect mechanisms. At the cellular level, glucocorticoid exposure *in utero* alters receptors, enzymes, ion channels and transporters in a wide range of different cell types during late gestation. They also change the expression of various growth factors, cytoarchitectural proteins, binding proteins and components of the intracellular signaling pathways [139]. These changes will influence the basal functioning of the cell and its responses to endocrine, metabolic and other stimuli, with consequences for its size, proliferation rate and terminal differentiation. In addition to these direct effects, glucocorticoids can act indirectly on tissue proliferation and differentiation through changes in the cellular secretion of proteins, hormones, growth factors and metabolites [139].

Another major mechanism by which glucocorticoids act on physiological systems is through changes in hormone bioavailability. They alter the production and secretion by the placenta and fetal endocrine glands of a number of hormones, such as estrogen, insulin, gastrin, neuropeptide Y, angiotensin II, T3, noradrenaline and adrenaline. They also regulate hormone receptor densities and the activities of several enzymes involved in activating and inactivating hormones in the fetal tissues. One of the recently proposed mechanisms of programming, with particular emphasis on glucocorticoids, is epigenetic programming. Glucocorticoids act as epigenetic signals that allow transgenerational transmission of non-genomic factors important in developing the optimal phenotype for survival to reproductive age [141]. The consequences of fetal overexposure to either endogenous or exogenous glucocorticoids lead to hypertension, glucose intolerance, insulin resistance, and abnormalities in the HPA function after birth [142].

3.1. Placental 11ß-hydroxysteroid dehydrogenase 2 (11ß-HSD2)

Transcriptional activation of GR is known to be determined by intracellular glucocorticoid availability that is regulated by two distinct isoforms of the enzyme 11ß-HSD. These enzymes control the first critical step for GR activation and target gene expression, while the process has been termed pre-receptor ligand control [2]. 11ß-HSD1 is NADPH-dependent with reductase activity, converting cortisone to the bioactive cortisol in the human, and 11-dehydrocorticosterone to corticosterone in the rat. 11ß-HSD2 is NAD-dependent and catalyzes the rapid metabolism of cortisol and corticosterone to inactive 11-keto forms, cortisone and 11-dehydrocorticosterone, respectively [143]. These enzyme systems function in most fetal gucocorticoid sensitive tissues modulating ligand access to GR. This is especially important for mineralocorticoid sensitive tissues. In the developing kidney, for example, in the presence of 11ß-HSD2, cortisol was efficiently metabolised to inert cortisone, which does not bind to receptors allowing aldosterone action. As a consequence, sodium retention, potassium loss and hypertension are prevented [5].

11ß-HSD2 is highly expressed in the placenta, in the syncytiotrophoblast in humans, and in the labyrinthine zone in rodents, i.e. at the interface between maternal and fetal circulations. Besides the mentioned function, it has an additional role in the placenta: it selectively regulates passage of glucocorticoids from the mother to the fetus, since highly lipophilic glucocorticoid molecules are able to pass freely across the placenta [144, 145]. As glucocorticoid levels are significantly lower in the fetus than in the mother, the 11ß-HSD2 placental enzymatic barrier prevents most of the maternal glucocorticoids from reaching the fetus, protecting the very sensitive fetal tissues from high glucocortivoid levels during development. Although 11ß-HSD2 limits fetal exposure to maternal glucocorticoids, a certain amount avoids enzymatic inactivation and reaches the fetus [146]. 11ß-HSD2 maintains a gradient of glucocorticoids from the maternal to the fetal circulation, although its magnitude varies between species. There is a positive correlation between the materno-fetal gradient and the activity of placental 11ß-HSD2 [139].

Reduced 11ß-HSD2 placental activity results in higher levels of glucocorticoids reaching the fetus, which induces growth retardation and program later disease susceptibility (Figure 1). In rats the lowest placental 11ß-HSD2 activity caused the highest fetal exposure to maternal glucocorticoids is seen in the smallest fetuses with the largest placenta [146]. In addition, low levels of 11ß-HSD2 placental activity decrease birth weight in humans, and can lead to adult hypertension [143]. Furthermore, in 11ß-HSD2 knockout mice fetal weight is significantly reduced in relation to wild type controls, as a consequence, not only of the increased fetal exposure to maternal glucocorticoids, but also altered placental function, i.e. decreased transport of nutrients. Thus, absence of 11β-HSD2 compromises not only fetal but also placental growth, function and morphology, representing an additional mechanism of fetal programming [147]. Since maternal glucocorticoid levels are significantly higher then those in the fetus, even modest perturbations of the placental 11β-HSD2 levels or activity can have a profound impact on fetal glucocorticoid exposure [148]. Inhibition of 11β-HSD2 activity by the application of carbenoxolone to gravid females, a potent inhibitor of 11β-HSD2, reduces birth weight in rats and elevates blood pressure in the adult rat offspring. These effects require the presence of maternal adrenal products, since carbenoxolone given to adrenalectomized pregnant rats had no effect on birth weight or blood pressure [149].

Placental 11ß-HSD2 can be avoided by the application of synthetic glucocorticoids. It has been demonstrated that treatment of pregnant rats with dexamethasone and betamethasone, synthetic glucocorticoids that are poorly metabolized by the enzyme, results in reduced birth weight, higher activity of the HPA axis and elevated blood pressure in the adult offspring (Figure 1) [143]. Synthetic glucocorticoids have been shown to up-regulate the activity of 11ß-HSD2, and, hence, amplify the placental barrier for physiological glucocorticoids [150].

It can be concluded that fetuses are protected from environmental perturbations by an enzymatic placental barrier that, by regulating fetal exposure to maternal glucocorticoids, crucially determines foeto-placental growth. Its deficiency causes programming effects in the offspring.

3.2. Stress during pregnancy and maternal undernutrition

Exposure to stress during pregnancy has been associated with offspring behavior, morphology, physiology, and immunology [151]. Although the mechanisms by which stress during pregnancy can influence the development of the offspring are not entirely known, elevation of the maternal glucocorticoid levels after stress exposure could be the first step in early life programming that predisposes individuals to several illnesses and psychiatric disorders. Maternal exposure to alcohol, repeated restraint stress, electric tail shocks, and undernutrition during pregnancy induced a corticosterone increase [152, 153]. In the offspring of these mothers growth retardation with altered function of the HPA axis and glucocorticoid responses under stress challenge, hyperglycemia and other dysfunctions related to type 2 diabetes, as well as hypertension were established (Figure 1) [14, 15, 153].

Adrenalectomy, as a blockade of the maternal stress-induced corticosterone secretion, suppresses the changes established in the offspring of prenatally stressed dams. The effects of repeated restraint stress during pregnancy on the offspring HPA axis activity and hippocampal mineralocorticoid receptor (MR) level are suppressed by adrenalectomy, while the administration of corticosterone to adrenalectomised mothers reinstates the effects induced by prenatal stress [153]. Furthermore, a pharmacological blockade of the maternal glucocorticoid synthesis with metyrapone also prevented hypertension, which is induced by fetal exposure to maternal low-protein diet [154]. Adrenalectomy carried out during pregnancy (without stress exposure), although it causes the opposite result in relation to stress exposure due to circulating corticosterone levels, also affects offspring development. Maternal adrenalectomy performed during gestation results in a compensatory increase in fetal corticosterone levels [152], decreases body weight in both male and female offspring, while the HPA axis shows a sex-specific pattern of vulnerability. In females, a dramatic increase in hypothalamic CRH and GR mRNA levels was established on day 14 [155]. All this together points out that highly regulated maternal glucocorticoids are indispensable during normal fetal development.

Various types of stress applied during gestation cause a broad spectrum of effects in the offspring at any age. Effects of prenatal stress caused by the restraining of pregnant rats influence the development of fetal hypothalamic PVN neurons in a duration-dependent manner. Long-lasting stress causes neurotoxic changes of the fetal PVN neurons, including CRH neurons that showed significantly shorter total length of the neuronal processes and an increased number of apoptotic cells. On the contrary, short-lasting stress facilitates the development of these fetal PVN neurons that showed enhanced CRH messenger RNA expression, while the varicosities of CRH-containing axons at the median eminence revealed more mature morphology. A greater degree of neuronal differentiation, as manifested by an increase in both the number of branch points and the total length of the processes from the cell body, was also demonstrated [156].

Chronic maternal restraint stress during late gestation decreases placental 11β-HSD2 expression and activity, and reduces body weight in rat fetuses at term. These alterations were associated with reduced pancreatic β-cell mass, growth hormone level, and decreased glucose concentration in fetal plasma [18]. Other results established hyperglycaemia, glucose intolerance and decreased basal leptin levels in prenatally stressed aged male rats as dysfunctions related to type 2 diabetes mellitus [15]. These data suggest that maternal stress and later dysfunctions such as type 2 diabetes could be linked to the restricted fetal growth and the adverse glucocorticoid environment *in utero* as the consequences of decreased placental 11β-HSD2 expression.

Observations from animal and human studies have linked maternal nutritional status and fetal growth retardation with the programming of hypertension and coronary heart disease in later life [27]. In the ewe, undernutrition in early pregnancy leads to placental enlargements, as adaptation to extract more nutrients. There is a correlation between placental weight and systolic blood pressure in adults that tends to rise as placental weight increases [157]. Mild protein restriction during pregnancy attenuates placental 11β-HSD2 expression which leads to overexposure of the fetus to maternal glucocorticoids (Figure 1) [14, 143]. Intrauterine growth retardation and disturbed development of the HPA axis appear as an outcome [15]. In addition, in the adult offspring subjected to maternal undernutrition during pregnancy persistently elevated expression of GR and decreased expression of 11β-HSD2 in the kidney, liver and brain mediated tissue-specific increases in glucocorticoid action. These changes represent potentially important mechanisms contributing to the programming of hypertension *in utero* [158].

As presented, it has so far been established that certain types of stress affect the reduction of placental 11β-HSD2 expression in rats, suggesting that the fetus and placenta are exposed to excessive amounts of glucocorticoids. Thus, deficiency of the placental barrier to maternal glucocorticoids may represent a common pathway between the maternal environment and feto-placental programming of later disease [12, 18]. Secondly, disturbances in placental growth and function, as a consequence of maternal stress exposure, decrease fetal nutrient supply and may further contribute to suboptimal fetal growth [14, 145]. Both changes, i.e. the reduced maternal glucocorticoid inactivation and decreased nutritional supply reflect on the HPA axis activity in fetuses and offspring, although the HPA axis response is differentially affected by the gestational stress procedure (Figure 1) [151]. Thus, the fetal HPA axis is a possible primary target and is intricately involved in early life disturbance caused by maternal stress exposure with far-reaching physiological consequences.

3.3. Antenatal glucocorticoid therapy

Because glucocorticoids have potent influence on maturation of fetal lung and other tissues they have been used for more than 40 years in human pregnancies at risk of preterm delivery. Use of antenatal corticosteroid therapy reduced the complications associated with preterm delivery such as neonatal respiratory distress syndrome (RSD), periventricular hemorrhage, necrotizing enterocolitis and, most importantly, neonatal mortality [159]. According to the National Institute of Health [160] all fetuses between the 24th and 34th week of gestation at risk of preterm delivery should be considered as candidates for the beneficial effects of antenatal glucocorticoid treatment. The recommended treatment consists of two doses of 12 mg betamethasone given 24 h apart, or alternative regimen of four doses of 6 mg dexamethasone given 12 h apart [161]. However, antenatal glucocorticoid therapy may produce growth retardation, affective and cognitive disturbances as well as other disorders in children and adults [162], thus the question of the relative risk and benefit of repetitive courses of prenatal glucocorticoid administration is still open (Figure 1).

Furthermore, the effects of prenatal glucocorticoid administration in cases of congenital adrenal hyperplasia (CAH) that must begin early in the first trimester to be effective in preventing female genital ambiguity are not completely known. CAH is an inherited disease in which a disordered steroidogenic enzyme P450C21 diverts adrenal steroid synthesis away from cortisol toward androgen. As a consequence girls are masculinized, because the adrenal glands secrete large amounts of androgens during prenatal development. Dexamethasone treatment should be introduced very early in pregnancy, before the seventh week of gestation, with the aim to increase fetal glucocorticoid concentrations, thus suppressing the elevated ACTH level that drives adrenal androgen production [146, 163].

In obstetric practice different synthetic glucocorticoids are used: dexamethasone, betamethasone, or prednisolone. Synthetic glucocorticoids are slightly different from their endogenous equivalents in chemical structure. Dexamethasone and bethamethasone both have the additional 9α-fluoro groups, and 16β- or 16α-methyl groups, respectively [164]. Prednisolone differs from cortisol by a 1δ-dehydro configuration (Figure 2). The choice of the concrete drug use will depend on its biological half-life, which represents the time that passes until one half of the initial drug concentration has disappeared from the blood [165]. Physiological and synthetic glucocorticoids have been divided into short-, medium- and long-acting substances dependent on the duration of measurable biological half-life [165]. Cortisol belongs to the short-acting category with the biological half-life of 8–12 h, prednisolone belongs to the medium-acting category with the half-life of 12–36 h, while dexamethasone and betamethasone have long-acting properties, ranging between 36 and 54 h [165].

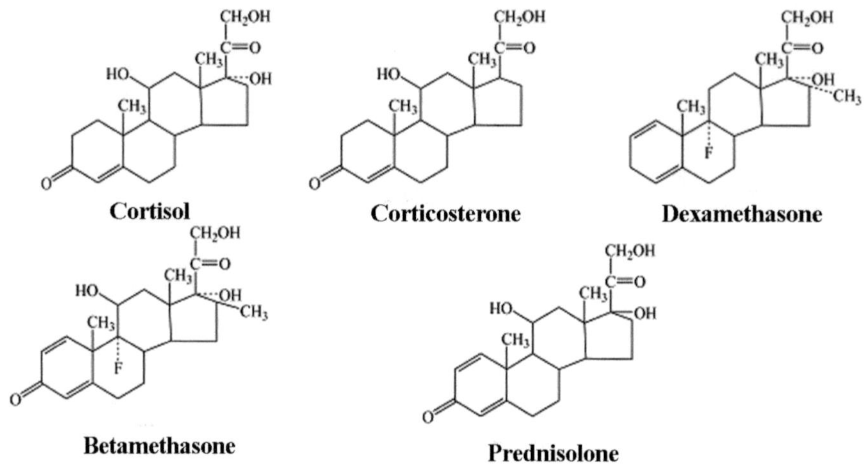

Figure 2. The structural formulas of natural (cortisol, cortocosterone) and synthetic glucocorticoids.

The biological activity of glucocorticoids is partly determined by the rate and selectivity of protein binding, because only the unbound glucocorticoids fraction is biologically active. Gayrard et al. [166] have found that the plasma free cortisol concentrations (6% to 14%), corticosteroid-binding globulin (CBG)-bound (67% to 87%) and albumin-bound (7% to 19%) concentrations are similar within species. Cortisol binding decreases as its concentration increases [167]. In human plasma, betamethasone and dexamethasone bind predominantly to albumin, which has high capacity but low affinity for ligating, while both steroids bind only marginally to CBG [167]. Dexamethasone displays higher protein affinity than betamethasone. The potency of glucocorticoids in a biological system also depends on its affinity for its receptor. Genomic potency of betamethasone was reported to be moderately higher than that of dexamethasone, while both steroids have a 25-fold higher affinity to the GR than cortisol [168].

4. Programming of endocrine axes

4.1. Programming of the fetal hypothalamic-pituitary-adrenal axis

The HPA axis is particularly sensitive to glucocorticoid levels. Fetal exposure to excessive glucocorticoids, natural or synthetic, can occur via a number of mechanisms including maternal stress, undernutrition as well as maternal antenatal treatment. As previously noted, synthetic glucocorticoids such as dexamethasone and betamethasone pass easily through the placental barrier avoiding the placental enzyme 11β-HSD2 [7], while maternal stress and undernutrition affect the same enzyme, resulting in increased fetal exposure to maternal glucocorticoids [18]. As the increased fetal exposure to glucocorticoids occurs during a critical period of the HPA axis development, when its control is just setting up, permanent alterations in the basal and stress induced HPA axis activity and regulation occur in the offspring, and sustain throughout life. Crucial changes that underlie the programming of the HPA axis will be presented below. Additionally, disturbances of the complex maturational process such as HPA axis development that have far-reaching immediate and delayed physiological effects will be discussed later.

The hippocampus represents a major inhibitory input to the HPA axis function. This is the point where glucocorticoid feedback, via GR an MR in the hippocampus and GR in the hypothalamic PVN and anterior pituitary, inhibits further HPA activity [169]. Thus, the balance between GR and MR in the hippocampus is an important factor in determining the HPA axis feedback sensitivity. Prenatal dexamethasone exposure alters GR and MR expression in the developing limbic system of guinea pig fetuses in both a region-specific and a sex-specific manner. After a single dexamethasone dose, female fetuses exhibited a significant increase in MR and GR mRNA levels in the CA1 and CA2 regions of the hippocampus and MR mRNA in the dentate gyrus [170]. Other results showed that multiple dexamethasone administration during pregnancy led to a marked increase in hippocampal GR and MR mRNA levels in male fetuses [171]. In mice, a single course of dexamethasone transiently reduced MR mRNA expression in the fetal hippocampus [172]. In addition, prenatal stress, or dexamethasone exposure are implicated in the development of rat hippocampal GR and MR in the offspring. In rat offspring exposed to glucocorticoid excess during late pregnancy permanently attenuated GR and MR mRNA expression in specific hippocampal regions reduced sensitivity to glucocorticoids [173]. The administration of betamethasone to pregnant sheep resulted in significant increases in MR and 11-βHSD2 gene expression in adult animals, reflecting a possible role for the locally produced glucocorticoids within the hippocampus, and the potential for long term alterations in HPA function [20].

At the level of the hypothalamic PVN, significantly decreased amounts of CRH mRNA were seen in male fetuses and female offspring after treatment of guinea pig mothers with dexamethasone or betamethasone, supporting the idea that synthetic glucocorticoids enter the fetal brain and inhibit central drive to the fetal HPA axis [171]. In addition, it has been shown that prenatal dexamethasone treatment induces a clear delay in increment of CRH in the external zone of the median eminence [174]. Morphometric analyses of rat PVN neurosecretory cells at eight distinct subdivisions indicate that dexamethasone given to pregnant dams causes significant changes in PVN neurosecretory cells in 20-day-old fetuses as well as in neonatal offspring. Significantly decreased neurosecretory cell nuclei volume and number in PVN, due to decreased proliferative activity, were found at the levels were parvocellular neurons are present, i.e. where CRH neurons are dominant [175, 176]. On the other hand, removal of maternal adrenals at day 16 of gestation significantly affected the size of neurosecretory cells in different subgroups of fetal PVN. These effects persisted during the neonatal period [177], confirming that prenatal glucocorticoid exposure alters the development and function of prenatal and neonatal PVN.

Prenatal glucocorticoid application alters the monoaminergic transmitter systems involved in the regulation of GR expression in the brain. Significant differences in the turnovers of serotonin, dopamine and noradrenaline contents between the weeks 3 and 14 of life were found in a wide area in the rat brain [54]. Thus, developmental alterations of monoaminergic neurons, that represent major modulators of the HPA axis function, influence endocrine response in the adult offspring. The data suggest that key targets for programming include GR gene expression and the CRH system [178].

Antenatal treatment with synthetic glucocorticoids affects pituitary development and the differentiation of hormone-producing cell types during the fetal period as well as after birth. A significant reduction in fetal ACTH cell volume and number was demonstrated in 19 and 21-day-old fetuses after multiple prenatal dexamethasone administration (Figure 3) [38, 42]. Dexamethasone decreased the rate of division of both immature cells and the existing fetal ACTH in the period when its proliferation was most intensive, on day 19 of fetal development [179], thus leaving long lasting consequences. Multiple dexamethasone exposure during pregnancy affects the ultrastructure of ACTH cells, which in the Golgi complex show much lower presence of specific granules as well as dilation of the endoplasmatic reticulum [180]. Decreased morphometric parameters of the ACTH cells and their changed ultrastructure resulted in significantly reduced plasma ACTH levels in fetuses and neonatal offspring after multiple dexamethasone administration during pregnancy [180, 181]. On the contrary, a single dose of dexamethasone, given to pregnant rats on day 16 of gestation, suppressed the synthetic activity of fetal ACTH cells, but in the early neonatal period this suppression was followed by stimulation of ACTH secretion and increased circulating ACTH levels [182]. Other results showed that following antenatal exposure to synthetic glucocorticoids in juvenile males POMC mRNA and CRH receptor mRNA on the pituitary level were increased [183].

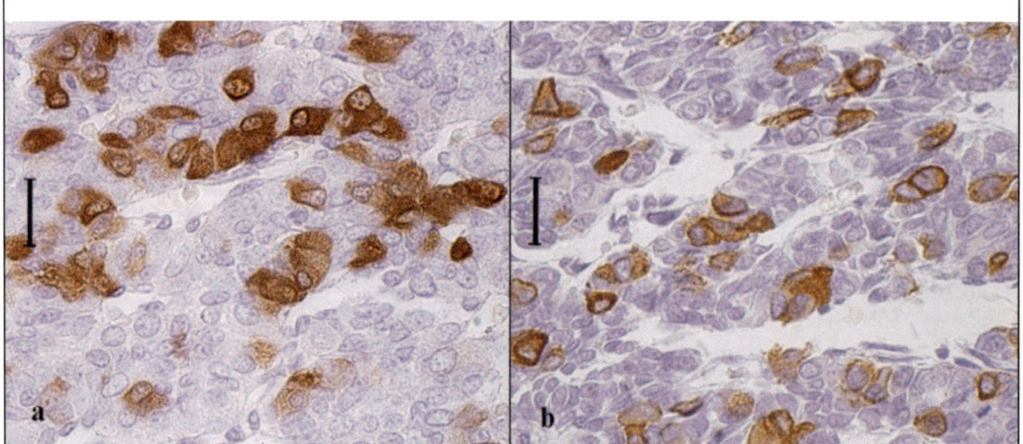

Figure 3. a) Intensive immunopositivity of ACTH cells located near the capillary network is characteristic for 21-day-old fetus. b) Decreased size, immunopositivity and number of ACTH cells in 21-day-old fetuses after maternal dexamethasone administration. Bar - 25 μm.

After maternal glucocorticoid exposure the absence of peaks in ACTH blood concentration in near term (19-day-old) fetuses reduces ACTH-trophic support and reflects on the adrenal glands structure and functional activity [42]. Administration of a single or multiple dexamethasone dose to pregnant rats induced a significant decrease in adrenal glands weight, volume of whole adrenal glands, as well as average volume and total number of cells in near term fetuses and neonatal rat offspring, a consequence of the decreased proliferative activity of adrenocortical cells [45, 46]. Interestingly, in 19-day-old fetuses the proliferative activity of adrenocortical cells that is most intensive in the outer portion of the fetal adrenal glands is markedly reduced in ZG. The proliferation rate of adrenocortical cells in IZ was not affected by prenatal dexamethasone application [42], suggesting that different sensitivity and/or responses of the proliferating cells in ZG and the outer portion of IZ to external stimuli could be a possible mechanism for the formation and maintenance of the zonal structure of the adrenal cortex [184].

In the rat adrenal glands of fetuses and pups of dexamethasone treated dams, during during the early neonatal period adrenocortical cells in various stages of degeneration were abundant, especially near the central part of the gland where zona reticularis (ZR) begins to differentiate. Resorption zones with lymphocytic infiltrations and presence of macrophages and multinuclear giant cells were observed, indicating that remodeling of the adrenal gland

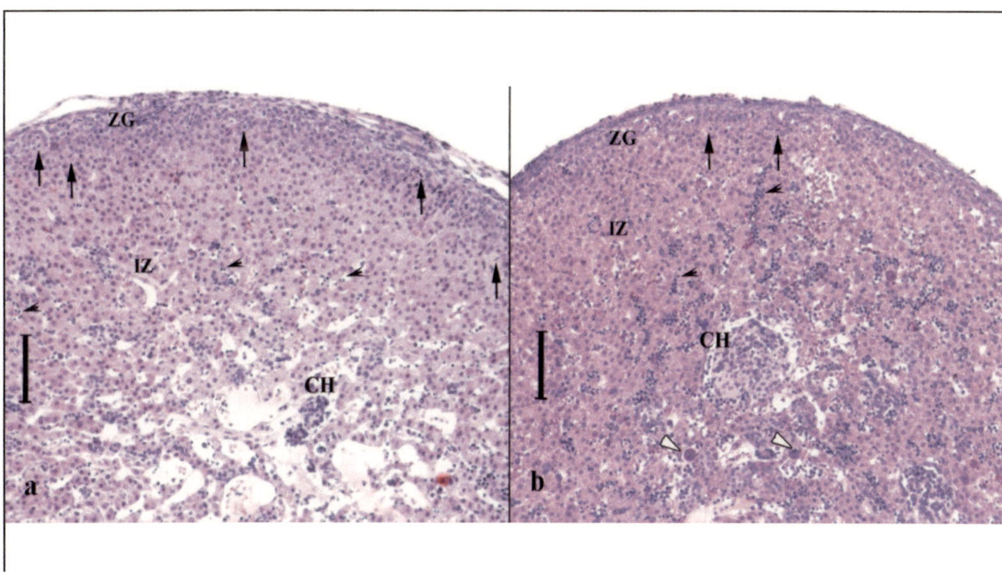

Figure 4. a) Zona glomerulosa (ZG) with numerous dividing cells (→), inner zone (IZ) with lymphocytes (black arrowheads), cellular interspaces, and centrally positioned group of chromoblasts (CH) are seen in adrenal gland of 21-day-old fetus. b) Decreased number of proliferating cells (→) in the adrenal gland of 21-day-old fetuses from gravid females treated with dexamethasone. Infiltration of lymphocytes (black arrowheads) and giant cells (white arrowheads) are indications of intensive tissue remodeling. Bar - 100 μm.

structure is affected by prenatal glucocorticoid exposure (Figure 4) [45, 46]. In the juvenile period, decreased expression of steroidogenic enzyme CYP17 after antenatal exposure to synthetic glucocorticoids has been established, reflecting the persistence of the adrenal glands functional changes [183].

The influence of a single dexamethasone treatment given to gravid females resulted in the decreased volume of adrenal medulla and the number of chromaffin cells that persisted during the fetal and neonatal period. Decreased proliferation of chromaffin cells during the fetal and early neonatal period was followed by significantly higher values in relation to controls during the second neonatal week, indicating the capacity of the adrenal gland medulla to recover [185]. Multiple dexamethasone doses applied during pregnancy exert a more potent inhibitory effect. A reduced number of chromaffin cells and significantly decreased adrenaline content in the adrenals were seen in 14-day-old neonatal offspring [181].

As pointed out, the consequences of fetal glucocorticoid exposure occur at the level of central regulation, pituitary ACTH cells and the adrenal gland, causing programming effects on HPA axis function in later life. In offspring HPA axis activity may be changed in different directions under basal conditions and after stress challenge [186]. Permanently elevated basal plasma glucocorticoid levels [178, 187], greater glucocorticoid response to stress [54] as well as blunted HPA axis response to stress [183] have been established in offspring following antenatal exposure to synthetic glucocorticoids. In addition, antenatal glucocorticoid treatment programs HPA function in the adult offspring in a sex-specific manner [188]. Programming of the fetal HPA axis, although it could have had an adverse postnatal outcome, actually demonstrated the amazing plasticity of the HPA axis.

Exposure to stress or glucocorticoids, exogenous or endogenous, causes fetal growth retardation and low birth weight in parallel with deregulation of the HPA axis during the life cycle [139]. Additionally, there is a correlation between the natural variation in body weight and the HPA axis function in offspring. In adult pigs that were low-weight at birth and remained small after birth altered HPA axis function has been recorded in later life, i.e. elevated adrenal responsiveness to insulin-induced hypoglycaemia [189]. Thus, it can be concluded that growth retardation and programming of the HPA axis are two mutually dependent processes that actually represent the modality by which prenatal environment influences adult stress-related diseases (Figure 1).

It has been shown that in rodents, effects of programming can be induced by insults even in neonatal period of life. One of the striking characteristics of the HPA axis is the stress hypo-responsive period during the first 2 weeks of life for species that are immature at birth, such as rats and mice. During the stress hypo-responsive period there is low basal corticosterone secretion and the inability to increase corticosterone in response to mild stressors, in order to protect the developing nervous system from glucocorticoid excess. Thus, neonatal glucocorticoid exposure and early life experience that activate the HPA axis have programming effects on HPA axis organization and functioning during the life cycle. Postnatal handling attenuated HPA response to stress in adult animals. Most likely this is an indirect effect, caused by altered maternal behavior which results in increased licking and grooming of pups by the dam. It is considered that serotonin plays a crucial role in the persistence of the handling effect through increased hippocampal GR levels [190]. Similarly, as adults, the offspring of mothers that exhibited more licking and grooming of pups during the first 10 days of life showed reduced HPA axis stress response due to increased hippocampal GR mRNA expression and decreased levels of hypothalamic CRH mRNA [191]. On the other hand, maternal separations during the critical periods of hippocampal development can disrupt hippocampal cytoarchitecture and neurogenesis in a stable manner, with stress hyper-responsiveness observed in these animals as adults [192, 193].

4.2. Programming of the somatotropic axis

Programming of the somatotropic axis (GH-IGF axis) is known to be induced by transient events in early postnatal life. The best described example is the effect of transient neonatal manipulation of sex steroids to permanently alter subsequent GH secretion to resemble the pattern of GH secretion of the opposite sex in rodents [194]. Intrauterine programming of the somatotropic (GH-IGF) axis is still not fully understood, despite its importance in postnatal growth and metabolism. Synthetic activity, storage, and proliferation of rat pituitary GH cells, indicated by the significant increase in GH cell immunopositivity, size, and number per volume and unit of area, rise markedly from the 19th till the 21st fetal day [195]. This corresponds with an increase in plasma corticosterone concentration in near term rat fetuses [46]. It has been shown that dexamethasone administered during the last week of pregnancy has a maturational effect on pituitary GH cells in rats [196]. Dexamethasone induced GHRHR mRNA expression and accumulation in the fetal rat pituitary gland [70] and amplified the stimulatory influence of GHRH. As a consequence, dexamethasone induced GH cells to synthesize and release more GH, leading to increases in GH cell size and immunopositivity (Figure 5) [196]. Corticosterone-induced GH cell differentiation involves GH expression in cells not expressing GH mRNA previously [197]. Moreover, dexamethasone can induce GH progenitors to start GH synthesis one day earlier than in normal fetuses. *In vitro* findings suggested that incubation of the pituitary gland with dexamethasone for 24 h increased GH mRNA on fetal day 18 to a level nearly identical to that in intact 19-day-old fetuses [70]. In humans, low-weight babies have high basal GH and low IGF-I concentrations at birth, with an increased GH response to GHRH [198]. These altered concentrations are maintained during early childhood and are accompanied by changes in the pattern of GH secretion. By early adulthood, urinary GH excretion, which reflects GH secretion, is low in men and women with low birth weights, but in old age birth weight is unrelated to either urinary GH excretion or the GH secretory profile [198]. Low birth weight is associated with decreased IGF-I, IGF-II and IGFBP-3, and elevated levels of IGFBP-1 [199].

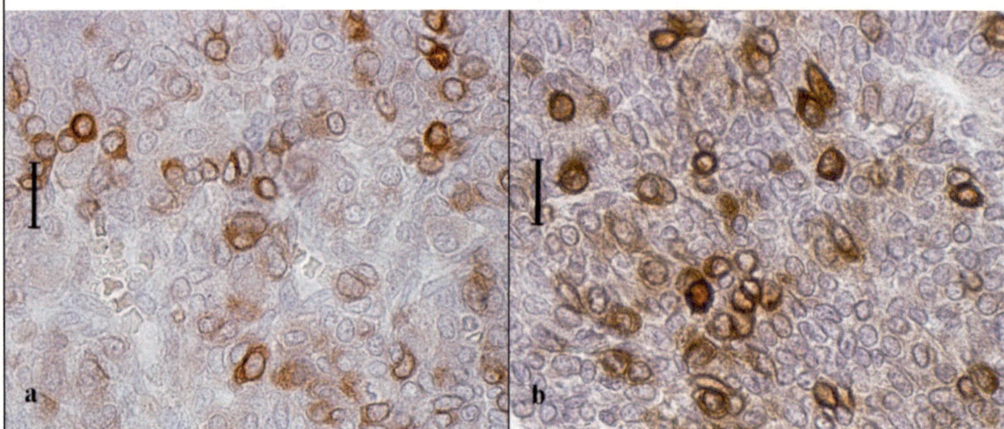

Figure 5. a) Pituitary GH cells of control 21-day-old fetus. b) Intensive immunostaining of GH cells in 21-day-old fetuses after maternal dexamethasone treatment. Bar - 25 μm.

In the fetus, IGF-I together with insulin, acts as a signal of nutrient plenty at the cellular level and promotes tissue growth in line with substrate availability in the fetus [24]. In fetal sheep, concentrations of insulin and IGF-I rise with increasing fetal concentrations of glucose over the normal range of values induced by variations in maternal nutritional state. The rise in fetal plasma IGF-I probably reflects overspill of IGF-I produced by a number of different fetal tissues, since IGF-I is primarily a paracrine growth factor *in utero*. In contrast, the concentrations of cortisol rise as fetal glucose levels decline [200]. Fetal undernutrition induced by maternal dietary manipulation, placental insufficiency and restriction of uterine blood flow, all reduce the circulating levels and tissue expression of IGF-I [200]. Glucocorticoids affect the expression of Igf1 and Igf2 genes, although their effects are tissue and Igf-specific. In fetal sheep, cortisol up- and down-regulates Igf1 gene expression in the liver and skeletal muscle, respectively, whereas it down-regulates Igf2 gene expression in these tissues. These changes in tissue expression occur both in response to exogenous cortisol infusion before term, and when fetal cortisol levels rise endogenously during the immediate prepartum period [200]. The cortisol-induced changes in tissue Igf gene expression are also accompanied by decreases in the fetal growth rate and, close to term, by a fall in plasma IGF-II levels [77, 201]. Cortisol, therefore, appears to initiate the switch from paracrine IGF production *in utero* to the hepatic production of endocrine IGF-I characteristic of the postnatal animal. Glucocorticoids may act on Igf gene expression either directly or indirectly, through changes in the GH receptor gene expression [79] and/or via other transcription factors or cortisol-dependent hormones, such as T3 [202]. This premature transition from IGF-II to

IGF-I production has beneficial effects on tissue differentiation, should delivery occur before full term. However, if delivery is not stimulated prematurely, the glucocorticoid-induced switch from the fetal to the adult mode of somatotrophic regulation may lead to inappropriate changes in cell proliferation and differentiation *in utero* with adverse sequelae both at birth and much later in life [200]. The reduced axial growth and reduced femur and tibia length reported in juvenile rats prenatally exposed to dexamethasone could serve as an illustration [203]. Altogether, the long-term consequences of such fetal changes in the GH-IGF axis are yet not fully understood in terms of functional adaptation or diseases. However, glucocorticoid-induced alterations might appear as potentially beneficial for short-term survival in an environment of shortage of nutritional resources. After birth, normalization of insulin, IGFs and IGFPs occurs. During this period, when suddenly exposed to increased concentrations of insulin and IGF-1, tissues chronically depleted of these two hormones during fetal life may counteract the hike by developing insulin resistance as a metabolic defense against developing hypoglycemia [204]. Therefore, infants with low birth weight who show early and complete growth recovery could be at higher risk for the occurrence of the metabolic syndrome in adulthood. Indeed, recent results in rats have shown permanent and sexually dimorphic changes in the expression of genes involved in the GH-IGF axis in animals that were weaned on to a high fat diet [203].

4.3. Programming of the hypothalamic-pituitary-thyroid axis

Glucocorticoid milieu strongly influences HPT axis activity during critical developmental periods. Prenatal alterations in glucocorticoid levels, caused by the application of synthetic glucocorticoids, maternal undernutrition or adrenalectomy, reflect on the fetal, neonatal and adult HPT axis structure and function.

Unbiased estimation of the cell number applying a design-based modern stereological approach revealed that maternal dexamethasone treatment significantly decreased pituitary TSH cell number in near term fetuses. This result together with the strong immunopositivity of TSH cells, and the fact that the decreased number of TSH cells sustains serum TSH concentrations at the control level, indicates that glucocorticoids exert a maturation-promoting effect on fetal TSH cells enhancing TSH synthesis (Figure 6) [205]. In sheep fetuses, antenatal glucocorticoid administration induced an increase in the circulating T3 concentration. Tissue-specific changes in deiodinase enzyme activities show stimulation of hepatic D1 activity with consequent increases in hepatic T3 production, as well as decreased T3 clearance by suppression of D3 enzymes in the kidney and placenta [206]. In the brain, glucocorticoid application stimulated TH activity during a period between gestational day 20 and neonatal day 12 that largely overlaps with the transient window in time during which brain development is TH sensitive [207]. On the contrary, maternal undernutrition during the gestational period results in lower serum T3 and higher serum reverse T3 concentrations in neonatal pups [208].

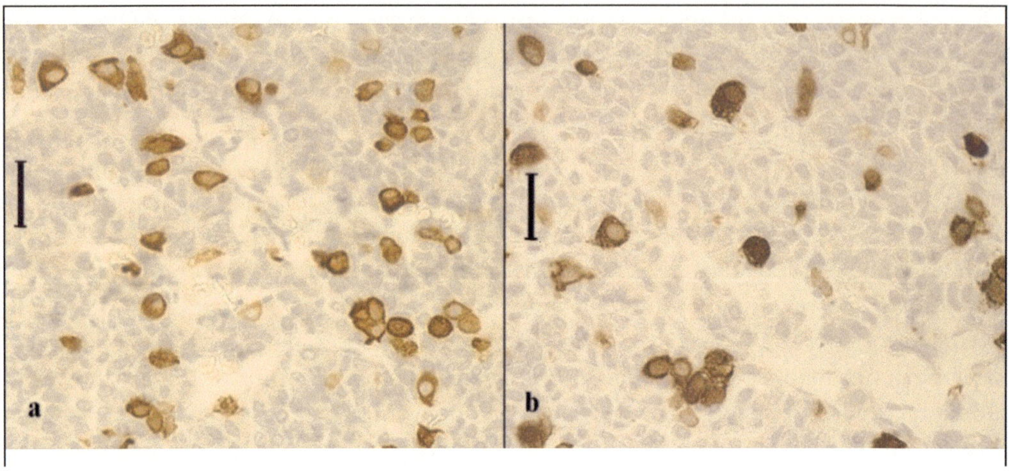

Figure 6. a) Numerous TSH cells characteristic for pituitary of 21-day-old fetus. b) Decreased number of TSH cells, with intense immunopositivity was observed in 21-day-old fetuses after maternal dexamethasone administration. Bar - 25 μm.

Alteration of the glucocorticoid milieu caused by maternal adrenalectomy influences HPT axis functioning in adult offspring. Decreased hypothalamic TRH mRNA levels and increased plasma TSH levels recorded in both male and female adult offspring of adrenalectomized dams were reversed by the administration of corticosterone to the pregnant adrenalectomized dam. The decreased plasma T3 concentrations in female offspring, which were reversed by the administration of higher levels of corticosterone to the adrenalectomized pregnant rats, suggest that the adult HPT axis responded to variations in maternal glucocorticoid milieu in a sex-specific manner [209].

Importantly, TH per se are potent programming factors. Fetal and neonatal hyperthyroidism or hypothyroidism results in programming of the HPT function. During critical periods, TSH secretion is suppressed by an excess of TH, but cannot be increased despite the marked lowering of circulating TH caused by perinatal propylthiouracil administration. More importantly, perinatal thyroid status "programs" its own future reactivity, so that early hypothyroidism results in reduced T4 and T3 levels in adulthood, despite normal levels of TSH [210].

TH influence the accretion, differentiation and metabolism of many tissues and cell types during development in a time-dependent manner. The effects of its deficiency during critical periods, when the tissues still have some plasticity and are in a higher proliferating and differentiating stage, are thus notable, often permanent. Fetal hypothyroidism leads to asymmetrical growth retardation, with reduction in muscle mass [211]. Fetal metabolism and utilization of oxygen, as well as bone tissue growth were adversely affected by TH deficiency in utero [211]. A well known example is that hypothyroidism during the period of thyroid-dependent brain development, in fetuses and during infancy, causes permanent mental retardation [212]. Thus, the structure and function of TH-dependent tissues, determined during critical periods by the striking effects of TH action [139], might be the cause of different (patho)physiological alterations which manifest during the life cycle. The potent influence of glucocorticoids on serum TH concentrations and the TH tissue bioavailability in the same period represents an important additional cause of the programming events recorded in different tissues.

4.4. Programming of endocrine pancreas

A number of epidemiological and clinical studies demonstrate an association between low birth weight and an increased incidence of metabolic, cardiovascular and other diseases in adult life. Adverse intrauterine environment caused by inadequate maternal nutrition status [13], poor placental function [17], maternal stress [15] or treatment with synthetic glucocorticoids [187] is linked with impaired intrauterine growth and increased rates of metabolic diseases such as type 2 diabetes in adulthood.

The increased fetal glucocorticoid exposure observed during and after suboptimal conditions, triggers cell differentiation in many of the tissues, resetting the set points of metabolic homeostasis and endocrine axes and in most individual fetal tissues leads to weight reduction, restricted fetal growth and decreased birth weight [24]. Glucocorticoids therefore switch the cell cycle from tissue accretion to tissue differentiation in preparation for delivery. At the same time, glucocorticoids are involved in the programming of the HPA axis during critical periods, causing structural and functional changes specified in the above section. Alterations in the feedback sensitivity of the fetal HPA axis, as adaptation to suboptimal conditions, mostly result in enhanced HPA axis activity postnatally, under basal conditions or after stress challenge, with elevated glucocorticoid levels [21]. These changes are in close association with the programming of susceptibility in the fetus to develop metabolic syndrome in later life. Indeed, hyperactivity of the HPA axis with chronically elevated glucocorticoids is positively correlated with the metabolic syndrome, which includes a cluster of symptoms such as hyperglycemia, hyperinsulinemia, or insulin resistance. Dyslipidemia, hyperleptinemia, raised serum triglycerides, lowered serum high-density lipoprotein cholesterol, and high blood pressure have also been recorded. All of those risk factors are a prelude to the development of diseases such as type 2 diabetes, atherosclerosis and cardio-vascular complications [28].

Suboptimal conditions *in utero* lead to changes in the endocrine environment which influence fetal development so that its nutrient requirements are decreased and a thrifty phenotype is produced to maximize its chances for survival. These short-term beneficial adaptations may be maladaptive in postnatal life, contributing to poor health outcomes [26]. If postnatal nutrient availability is better than predicted, metabolic dysfunctions occur, as the organism is not adapted to cope with excessive caloric intake in later life. The association of low birth weight with early postnatal catch-up growth, in situations where discrepancies between the pre- and postnatal environment are significant, adversely affects body composition, producing increased susceptibility to non-insulin dependent type 2 diabetes. But if environmental conditions remain unchanged, and the offspring of mothers on a low protein diet continue with the low protein diet during lactation, development of the metabolic phenotype is prevented. The "predictive adaptive response" hypothesis proposes that the degree of mismatch between the pre- and postnatal environments is a major determinant of subsequent disease, and leads to the premise that adult disease arises *in utero* [28, 213].

The thrifty phenotype is not able to respond to unexpected environmental conditions because the changes in metabolic tissues established during critical periods are directed towards low nutritional demands. The fetus adapts to an adverse intrauterine milieu through changes that permanently affect the pancreas, muscles, adipose tissue, and liver structure and function, which are involved in the pathogenesis of obesity and type 2 diabetes [25].

Progressive reduction in insulin-producing β-cell mass is observed in rats with restricted fetal growth [214]. There is evidence that prenatal caloric restriction during pregnancy causes alteration in pancreatic islet neogenesis by decreasing the β-cell precursor pool [215], while maternal protein restriction in rats lowers β-cell proliferation and/or increases apoptosis rates in the fetal endocrine pancreas [215, 216]. Permanent reductions in β-cell mass and its functional efficiency, although achieved by different mechanisms, result in glucose intolerance in adulthood [214]. Nutritional deprivation as severe stress induces a rise in both maternal and fetal corticosterone levels, which in turn are responsible for the observed effects [217].

Prenatal stress that induces a restriction in intrauterine growth in aged male rats causes hyperglycemia, glucose intolerance, and decreased basal leptin levels. Again, an adverse glucocorticoid environment during critical periods might be the underlying mechanism that mediates long-lasting disturbances in feeding behavior and dysfunctions related to type 2 diabetes [15].

Overexposure to exogenous glucocorticoids during different stages of development reduces β-cell mass in the fetal endocrine pancreas: impairment of β-cell commitment is recorded in fetuses exposed to glucocortiocoid during the last week of gestation, while glucocorticoids treatment throughout gestation lowers β-cell proliferation and impairs islet vascularization [218]. Glucocorticoid excess during the last week of gestation leads to lower levels of insulin expression in the β-cells of 3-week-old offspring via a mechanism that involves down-regulation of Pdx-1, the transcription factor that initiates and promotes β-cells development [219]. Programming of the functional capacity of pancreatic β-cell mass by adverse intrauterine conditions increases susceptibility to type 2 diabetes during adulthood that is especially evident if offspring when they are challenged with nutritional abundance. As during adulthood the majority of β-cells are formed through proliferation of the existing cells [220], smaller β-cell mass in the newborn means fewer β-cells will be available for renewal during life, which increases the risk of developing glucose intolerance or diabetes [221].

Impaired insulin action at the major sites of glucose utilization, such as skeletal muscles, liver and adipose tissue, further predisposes to a later diabetic state. Excess prenatal glucocorticoid exposure, uteroplacental insufficiency as well as maternal low protein diet in the perinatal period prepare skeletal muscle metabolism for poor metabolic conditions in later life [22, 25, 213]. These changes include up-regulation of GR expression that determines higher muscle glucocorticoid sensitivity, with the promotion of protein breakdown and blunted protein synthesis in muscles [222]. Prenatal growth restriction caused by adverse intrauterine conditions of different etiology has a long-term influence on adiposity. Redistribution of body fat from the periphery to the central or visceral deposits that have a relatively higher level of GR expression and are thus more sensitive to glucocorticoid action is established in adult rats and sheep prenatally exposed to glucocorticoid excess [223-225], contributing to decreased insulin sensitivity and blunted glucose intake [2]. Adipocytes from 15-month-old low-protein rat offspring are also resistant to the antilipolytic action of insulin and insulin-induced glucose uptake [25]. It can be concluded that adverse conditions during critical periods may program adipocyte metabolism to give rise to later obesity and type 2 diabetes, especially when challenged postnatally with a hypercaloric diet [226]. Suboptimal conditions during fetal development program an increased level of liver GR expression that enables much higher glucocorticoid impact in diabetic animals [227]. Down-regulation of glucokinase activity in parallel with decreased liver glucose uptake, and up-regulation of gluconeogenic enzyme activities, notably phosphoenolpyruvate carboxykinase which catalyzes a rate-limiting step in gluconeogenesis, have been established in rats exposed to excessive glucocorticoids in utero [25, 228]. The programming effects established in glucocorticoid overexposed fetuses with restricted growth are thus directed toward enhanced glucose production and reduced glucose utilization in the liver and other peripheral tissues in adulthood, and represent the structural and physiological basis of the development of type 2 diabetes [19].

4.5. Programming of hipothalamic-pituitary-gonadal axis

Steroid hormone excess during fetal life, including glucocorticoids and sex hormones, is well known to induce permanent alterations in the physiology of the adult HPG axis in both sexes [229]. The majority of data describing the effects of elevated levels of glucocorticoids on the HPG axis and possible mechanisms, come from studies in adults, and there are only limited data on fetal effects. It has been known that the HPA axis, when activated by stress, exerts an inhibitory effect on the female and male reproductive system. Reallocation of resources during the stress response suppresses the reproductive axis, which gives higher priority to an individual's survival rather than the maintenance of species. This effect is responsible for the "hypothalamic amenorrhea of stress" in females, which is observed in anxiety and depression, malnutrition, eating disorders and chronic excessive exercise, and the hypogonadism in Cushing's syndrome [230]. Stressors trigger a rise in glucocorticoids that suppress reproductive functions along the HPG axis [3]. Glucocorticoids decrease expression of GnRH mRNA [231] in the hypothalamus, and are associated with alterations in both FSH and LH cells [232, 233]. Glucocorticoids also affect gonads directly. It has been reported that dexamethasone inhibits ovarian function in immature female rats and the differentiation of granulosa cells by FSH [234]. In the testis, elevated levels of glucocorticoids suppress testosterone biosynthesis [3]. Additionally, dexamethasone induces apoptosis of tubules and germ cells in adult rat testis [235].

Elevation of maternal glucocorticoids induced by maternal stress, undernutrition or exogenously administered dexamethasone or betamethasone, along with IUGR cause alterations in HPG axis function in male and female offspring. The major alterations reported were related to changed sexual behavior, delayed puberty, and delayed development of the gonads. In rats, exposure to prenatal stress demasculinizes and feminizes the behavior of the male offspring. When dams are restrained under bright light from days 14 to 21 of gestation, the male offspring display reduced anogenital distance and lower testis weight at birth compared to controls [18, 236], which could predict impaired sexual activity at adulthood [237]. Prenatal treatment with glucocorticoids caused the disappearance of sexual dimorphism of aromatase activity in the brain preoptic area of rat pups in early postnatal life [238]. Prenatal bethamethasone treatment diminished the testosterone peak in male pups, a peak crucial for brain sexual differentiation. As a consequence, this prenatal treatment may have impaired the hypothalamus–pituitary axis, thus reducing production of testosterone in adulthood and altering the partner preference and sexual behavior [239].

It has been reported that maternal protein restriction altered the key components of pregnant maternal steroid endocrinology, as well as the endocrinology of the offspring. Maternal corticosterone and testosterone levels were elevated, which resulted in an increased anogenital distance in males [240]. In females exposed to protein restriction during development the onset of puberty was delayed and the cycle length was increased [241]. The decrease of LH and slight, but not significant, decrease of FSH levels was detected in adult females that experienced maternal protein restriction at some stage of development. Together with the increases in testosterone levels at 1 year, this presage potential reproductive problems, including changes in the ovarian cycle [241]. Maternal protein restriction leads to similar changes in reproductive hormones in the male offspring [240], indicating that a major effect of the challenge imposed on the developing offspring is to alter hypothalamic–pituitary endocrine function. The reproductive function aged more rapidly in females that had been exposed to protein restriction during development [241]. Testicular and ovarian growth was drastically retarded, and the onset of puberty was delayed in male and female rats prenatally exposed to maternal food restriction [242]. In addition, the ovulation rate in adulthood was reduced in female sheep that experienced undernutrition during the prenatal period [243]. The suggested main mechanism by which maternal calorie restriction induced delay of puberty in the female offspring is that decreased function of the kisspeptin system retards the development of reproductive function and the onset of puberty. Hypothalamic levels of Kiss1 mRNA were decreased in prenatally undernourished rats, and the replacement of kisspeptin normalized the timing of vaginal opening in these females [244]. However, this mechanism is not responsible for delaying puberty in dexamethasone-induced IUGR females, since the levels of Kiss1 mRNA were not altered [245]. On the other hand, alterations of ovarian functions found in dexamethasone-induced IUGR rats, can affect sexual maturation [246]. As ovarian weight in the dexamethasone-induced IUGR rats was lower than in the controls during the prepubertal period (postnatal day 28), but not on the day of vaginal opening, the retardation of ovarian function development might be involved in the delayed onset of puberty [245]. Smith and Waddell [247] have shown that variations in fetal glucocorticoid exposure across the normal physiological range are capable of influencing the timing of subsequent puberty. Puberty was substantially delayed by increased exposure to glucocorticoids, which was most clearly evident in female offspring. Of particular importance were the observations that increased exposure of the fetus to endogenous maternal glucocorticoids (via inhibition of placental 11β-HSD by carbenoxolone treatment) delayed puberty in the female offspring, whereas an experimental reduction in fetal glucocorticoid exposure (by maternal metyrapone treatment) advanced puberty in the male offspring [247].

When higher multiple doses of dexamethasone were administered to dams between the 16th and 18th day of gestation, a significant reduction in body weight was recorded in near-term fetuses that persisted till the peripubertal period of life. The volume of pituitaries of the exposed females were also significanly reduced till the peripubertal period. The absolute number of both types of gonadotropic cells, obtained by design-based stereological methods, was decreased in the pituitaries of exposed females (Figure 7). As the pituitaries, the ovaries of exposed females were smaller than that of controls (Figure 8). Significant decrease in healthy, but an increase in atretic primordial follicles was observed in neonatal period (at 5 days of age) [246]. Alterations in the number of healthy and degenerated germinative cells were evident in fetuses as well, and sustained till the peripubertal period of life. Since the puberty was delayed in females exposed prenatally to dexamethasone, no *corpora lutea* were seen in their ovaries. In contrast, 3-5 *corpora lutea* were present in the ovaries of control females (Figure 8). However, the process of folliculogenesis remained unchanged, since the follicles at all stages of development seen in the ovaries of control females in the neonatal [246], infantile and peripubertal period, were present in the ovaries of females prenatally exposed to high levels of glucocorticoids. Therefore, a clear programming effect of dexamethasone was detected in the female HPG axis. It has been shown that glucocorticoids mediate changes in the dynamic balance between mitosis and apoptosis [248], and may be a mechanism for the control of total cell number in developing tissues and organs [249, 250]. This could be one of the mechanisms by which glucocorticoid overexposure affects the hypothalamic–pituitary–ovarian axis.

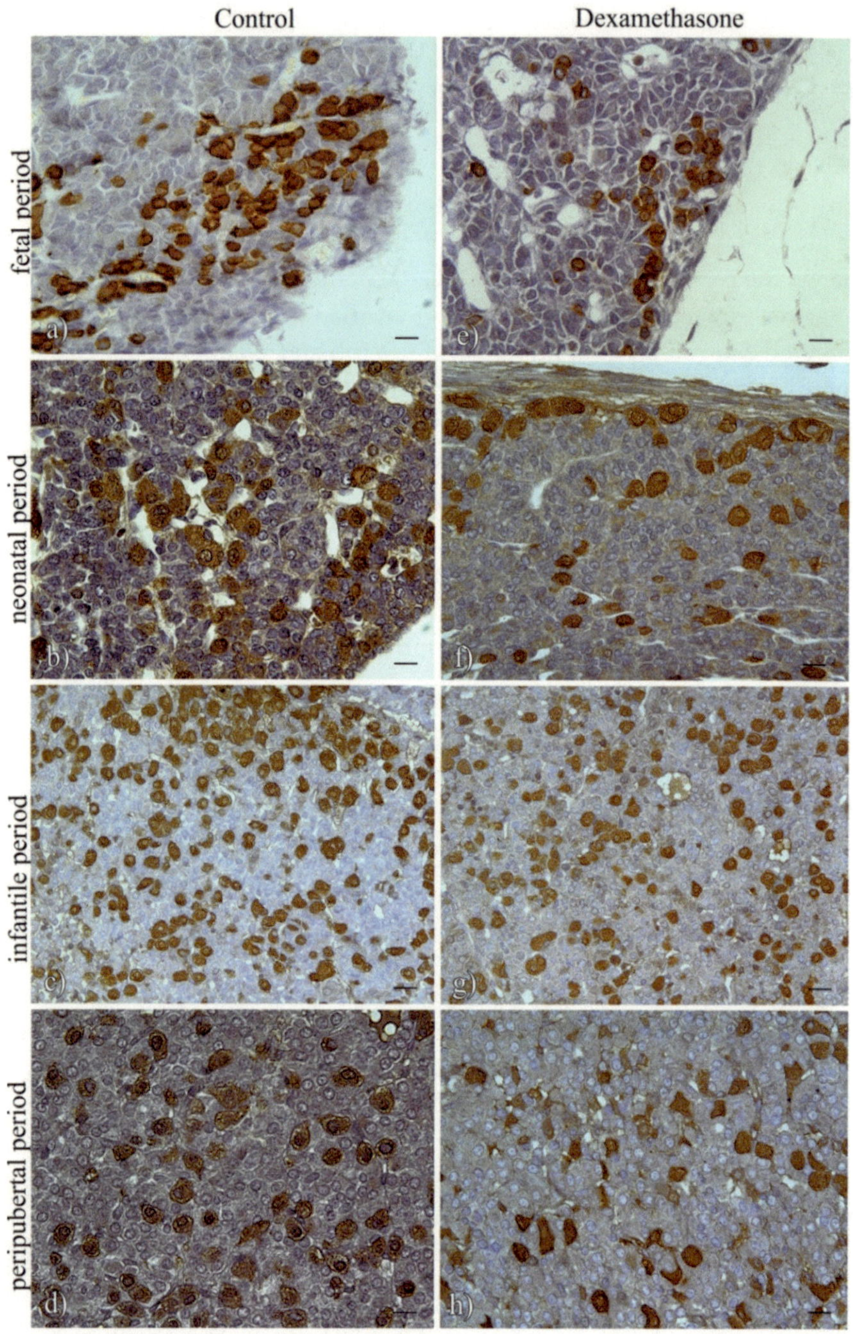

Figure 7. Immunohistochemically stained FSH cells in the pituitaries of control (a-d), and females prenatally exposed to dexamethasone (e-h). FSH cells were examined in different periods of life: in nearm-term fetal period (a, e), neonatal (b, f), infantile (c, g) and peripubertal period (d, h). In all examined periods the number of FSH cells was lower in the pituitaries of dexamethasone exposed females compared to controls. Bar - 20 μm.

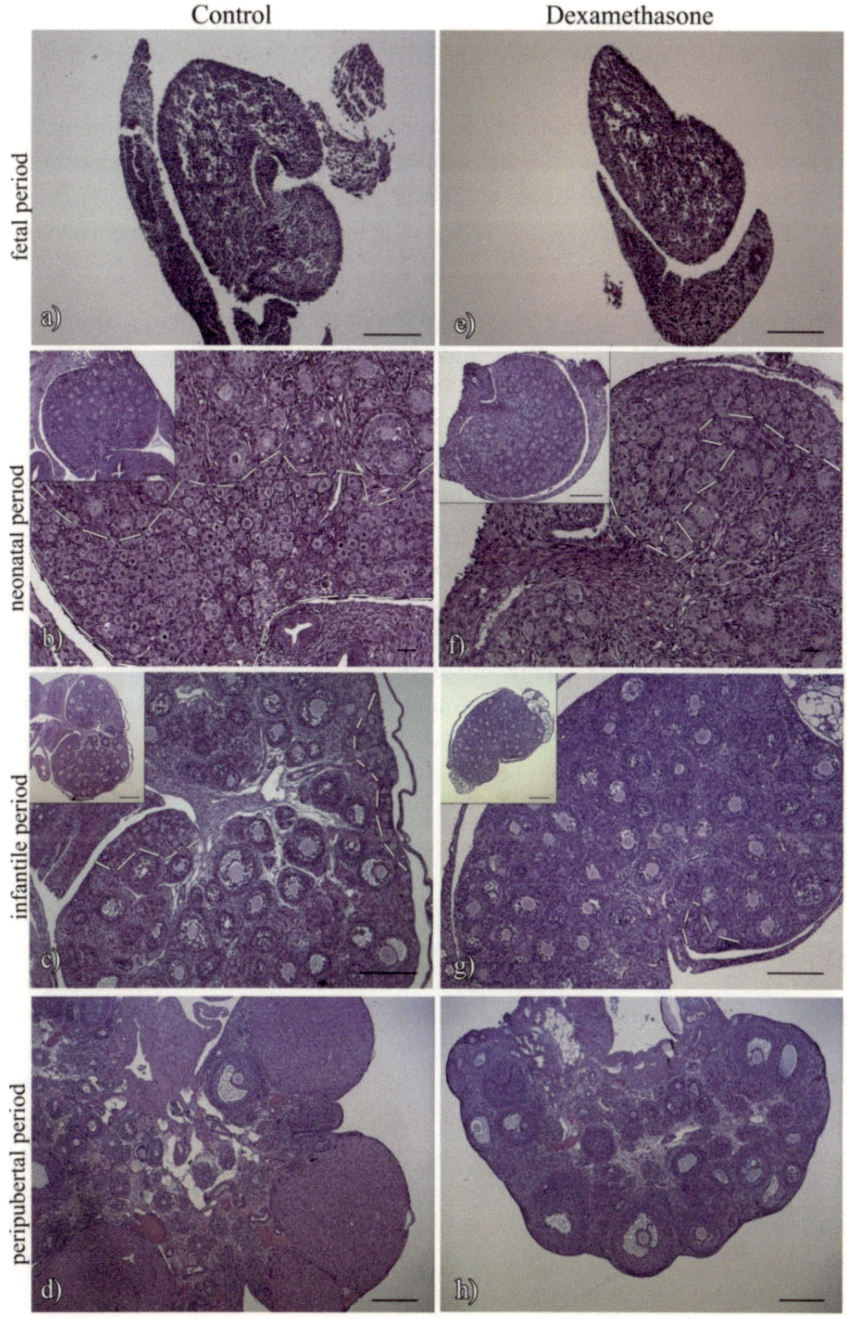

Figure 8. Ovaries of control (a-d), and females prenatally exposed to dexamethasone (e-h). Ovaries were examined in different periods of life: in nearm-term fetal period (a, e), neonatal (b, f), infantile (c, g) and peripubertal period (d, h) and they were smaller in dexamethasone exposed females. Numerous primordial follicles (dashed line) are present in the ovaries of control females, while they were fewer in number in the ovaries of dexamethasone exposed rats in all examined periods of life. Bar - 200 μm. In b) and f) bar - 20 μm.

Maternal bethamethasone administration affected the morphological development of the testes in male sheep fetuses, by reducing the length of testicular cords, the amount of interstitial tissue and testicular weight. Because interstitial tissue is primarily made up of Leydig cells, it is possible that betamethasone altered Leydig cell development. In contrast, there was no inhibitory effect on Sertoli cell number. This could be a result of the direct influence of the glucocorticoid used, since the presence of glucocorticoid receptor was demonstrated in ovine fetal Leydig cells, while the level of glucocorticoid receptor expression in Sertoli cells was low [251].

Fetal overexposure to glucocrticoids without any doubt has programming effects on the HPG axis, and reproduction in later life is thus impaired in both sexes. However, the mechanism of HPG programming is yet to be elucidated. The time interval between the exact insult and a fully functioning HPG axis is long, and prone to influences and interplay with other endocrine axes that are also altered by glucocrticoid overexposure. For example, an impaired somatotropic axis negatively affects reproduction. Somatostatin treatment inhibits pituitary gonadotropic cells and initial folliculogenesis in the ovaries of infant, peripubertal and adult females [252-257]. Polycystic ovary syndrome (PCOS) is of great importance, owing to its prevalence in up to 10% of the women population of reproductive age. Besides being characterized by perturbed gonadotropin secretion and excess production of androgens, PCOS shares a lot of commons with the metabolic syndrome. Metabolic syndrome is also believed to be of fetal origin and the result of programming in which glucocorticoids play a crucial role [213]. The short-term benefits of glucocorticoid exposure are also difficult to establish due to physiological dormancy of the system till puberty. The maturational effect of glucocorticoids is evident in the pituitary and in the ovary, since fetal overexposure induces a decreased volume of these glands, and of the absolute number of gonadotrops and ovarian somatic and germinative cells till puberty (Figure 1).

5. Conclusion

Glucocorticoids have a powerful influence on growth, maturation and tissue remodeling during fetal development. Their use in human pregnancies at risk of preterm delivery reduces neonatal mortality and morbidity. Glucocorticoids are also the key mediators between the maternal environment and the fetus, and their levels rise, in the mother and in the fetus, when the conditions are suboptimal. They reduce fetal growth, force maturational processes and provoke permanent changes in physiological systems in order to adapt the fetus to an adverse postnatal environment and ensure the maximum chances of survival at birth. These short-term beneficial effects of prenatal glucocorticoids are, at the same time, the ones that increase the long-term risks of dysregulation of the metabolic function and endocrine axes, including stress response, growth and reproduction.

Author details

Milica Manojlović-Stojanoski, Nataša Nestorović and Verica Milošević
University of Belgrade, Institute for Biological Research „Siniša Stanković", Serbia

Acknowledgments

This work was supported by the Ministry of Education and Science of the Republic of Serbia, Grant No. 173009

6. References

[1] Hayashi R, Wada H, Ito K, Adcock IM (2004) Effects of Glucocorticoids on Gene Transcription. Eur. j. pharmacol. 500: 51-62.

[2] Rose AJ, Vegiopoulos A, Herzig S (2010) Role of Glucocorticoids and the Glucocorticoid Receptor in Metabolism: Insights from Genetic Manipulations. J. steroid biochem. mol. biol. 122: 10-20.

[3] Whirledge S, Cidlowski JA (2010) Glucocorticoids, Stress, and Fertility. Minerva endocrinol. 35: 109-125.

[4] Mitani F, Mukai K, Miyamoto H, Suematsu M, Ishimura Y (1999) Development of Functional Zonation in the Rat Adrenal Cortex. Endocrinology. 140: 3342-3353.

[5] Condon J, Gosden C, Gardener D, Nickson P, Hewison M, Howie AJ, Stewart PM (1998) Expression of Type 2 11beta-Hydroxysteroid Dehydrogenase and Corticosteroid Hormone Receptors in Early Human Fetal Life. J. clin. endocrinol. metab. 83: 4490-4497.

[6] Kitraki E, Kittas C, Stylianopoulou F (1997) Glucocorticoid Receptor Gene Expression During Rat Embryogenesis. An in Situ Hybridization Study. Differentiation. 62: 21-31.

[7] Miller WL (1998) Steroid Hormone Biosynthesis and Actions in the Materno-Feto-Placental Unit. Clin. perinatol. 25: 799-817.

[8] Flagel SB, Vazquez DM, Watson SJ, Jr., Neal CR, Jr. (2002) Effects of Tapering Neonatal Dexamethasone on Rat Growth, Neurodevelopment, and Stress Response. Am. j. physiol. regul. integr. comp. physiol. 282: R55-63.

[9] Gesina E, Blondeau B, Milet A, Le Nin I, Duchene B, Czernichow P, Scharfmann R, Tronche F, Breant B (2006) Glucocorticoid Signalling Affects Pancreatic Development through Both Direct and Indirect Effects. Diabetologia. 49: 2939-2947.

[10] Fowden AL, Forhead AJ (2011) Adrenal Glands Are Essential for Activation of Glucogenesis During Undernutrition in Fetal Sheep near Term. Am. j. physiol. endocrinol. metab. 300: E94-102.

[11] Fowden AL, Li J, Forhead AJ (1998) Glucocorticoids and the Preparation for Life after Birth: Are There Long-Term Consequences of the Life Insurance? Proc. nutr. soc. 57: 113-122.

[12] Harris A, Seckl J (2011) Glucocorticoids, Prenatal Stress and the Programming of Disease. Horm. behav. 59: 279-289.

[13] Bloomfield FH, Oliver MH, Giannoulias CD, Gluckman PD, Harding JE, Challis JR (2003) Brief Undernutrition in Late-Gestation Sheep Programs the Hypothalamic-Pituitary-Adrenal Axis in Adult Offspring. Endocrinology. 144: 2933-2940.

[14] Belkacemi L, Jelks A, Chen CH, Ross MG, Desai M (2011) Altered Placental Development in Undernourished Rats: Role of Maternal Glucocorticoids. Reprod. biol. endocrinol. 9: 105.

[15] Lesage J, Del-Favero F, Leonhardt M, Louvart H, Maccari S, Vieau D, Darnaudery M (2004) Prenatal Stress Induces Intrauterine Growth Restriction and Programmes Glucose Intolerance and Feeding Behaviour Disturbances in the Aged Rat. J. endocrinol. 181: 291-296.
[16] Kapoor A, Leen J, Matthews SG (2008) Molecular Regulation of the Hypothalamic-Pituitary-Adrenal Axis in Adult Male Guinea Pigs after Prenatal Stress at Different Stages of Gestation. J. physiol. 586: 4317-4326.
[17] Godfrey KM (2002) The Role of the Placenta in Fetal Programming-a Review. Placenta. 23 Suppl A: S20-27.
[18] Mairesse J, Lesage J, Breton C, Breant B, Hahn T, Darnaudery M, Dickson SL, Seckl J, Blondeau B, Vieau D, Maccari S, Viltart O (2007) Maternal Stress Alters Endocrine Function of the Feto-Placental Unit in Rats. Am. j. physiol. endocrinol. metab. 292: E1526-1533.
[19] Seckl JR, Meaney MJ (2004) Glucocorticoid Programming. Ann. NY. acad. sci. 1032: 63-84.
[20] Sloboda DM, Moss TJ, Li S, Matthews SG, Challis JR, Newnham JP (2008) Expression of Glucocorticoid Receptor, Mineralocorticoid Receptor, and 11beta-Hydroxysteroid Dehydrogenase 1 and 2 in the Fetal and Postnatal Ovine Hippocampus: Ontogeny and Effects of Prenatal Glucocorticoid Exposure. J. endocrinol. 197: 213-220.
[21] Matthews SG (2002) Early Programming of the Hypothalamo-Pituitary-Adrenal Axis. Trends. endocrinol. metab. 13: 373-380.
[22] Fowden AL, Gardner DS, Ousey JC, Giussani DA, Forhead AJ (2005) Maturation of Pancreatic Beta-Cell Function in the Fetal Horse During Late Gestation. J. endocrinol. 186: 467-473.
[23] Barker DJ, Eriksson JG, Forsen T, Osmond C (2002) Fetal Origins of Adult Disease: Strength of Effects and Biological Basis. Int. j. epidemiol. 31: 1235-1239.
[24] Fowden AL, Forhead AJ (2009) Endocrine Regulation of Feto-Placental Growth. Horm. res. 72: 257-265.
[25] Ozanne SE, Hales CN (2002) Early Programming of Glucose-Insulin Metabolism. Trends. endocrinol. metab. 13: 368-373.
[26] Hales CN, Barker DJ (1992) Type 2 (Non-Insulin-Dependent) Diabetes Mellitus: The Thrifty Phenotype Hypothesis. Diabetologia. 35: 595-601.
[27] Langley-Evans S, Jackson A (1996) Intrauterine Programming of Hypertension: Nutrient-Hormone Interactions. Nutr. rev. 54: 163-169.
[28] Luo ZC, Xiao L, Nuyt AM (2010) Mechanisms of Developmental Programming of the Metabolic Syndrome and Related Disorders. World. j. diabetes. 1: 89-98.
[29] Vickers MH (2011) Developmental Programming of the Metabolic Syndrome - Critical Windows for Intervention. World. j. diabetes. 2: 137-148.
[30] Osamura RY, Egashira N, Recent Developments in Molecular Embryogenesis and Molecular Biology of the Pituitary, in: Loyd RV (Ed.), Endocrine Pathology Differential

Diagnosis and Molecular Advances, Springer, New York Dordrecht Heidelberg London, 2010. pp. 91-103.

[31] Nemeskeri A, Setalo G, Halasz B (1988) Ontogenesis of the Three Parts of the Fetal Rat Adenohypophysis. A Detailed Immunohistochemical Analysis. Neuroendocrinology. 48: 534-543.

[32] Chatelain A, Dupouy JP, Dubois MP (1979) Ontogenesis of Cells Producing Polypeptide Hormones (Acth, Msh, Lph, Gh, Prolactin) in the Fetal Hypophysis of the Rat: Influence of the Hypothalamus. Cell. tissue. res. 196: 409-427.

[33] Nemeskeri A, Halasz B (1989) Cultured Fetal Rat Pituitaries Kept in Synthetic Medium Are Able to Initiate Synthesis of Trophic Hormones. Cell. tissue. res. 255: 645-650.

[34] Pilavdzic D, Kovacs K, Asa SL (1997) Pituitary Morphology in Anencephalic Human Fetuses. Neuroendocrinology. 65: 164-172.

[35] Daikoku S, Okamura Y, Kawano H, Tsuruo Y, Maegawa M, Shibasaki T (1984) Immunohistochemical Study on the Development of Crf-Containing Neurons in the Hypothalamus of the Rat. Cell. tissue. res. 238: 539-544.

[36] Chatelain A, Dupouy JP (1981) Adrenocorticotrophic Hormone in the Anterior and Neurointermediate Lobes of the Fetal Rat Pituitary Gland. J. endocrinol. 89: 181-186.

[37] Challis JR, Sloboda D, Matthews SG, Holloway A, Alfaidy N, Patel FA, Whittle W, Fraser M, Moss TJ, Newnham J (2001) The Fetal Placental Hypothalamic-Pituitary-Adrenal (Hpa) Axis, Parturition and Post Natal Health. Mol. cell. endocrinol. 185: 135-144.

[38] Stojanoski MM, Nestorovic N, Filipovic B, Milosevic V (2004) Acth-Producing Cells of 21-Day-Old Rat Fetuses after Maternal Dexamethasone Exposure. Acta histochem. 106: 199-205.

[39] Muscatelli F, Strom TM, Walker AP, Zanaria E, Recan D, Meindl A, Bardoni B, Guioli S, Zehetner G, Rabl W, et al. (1994) Mutations in the Dax-1 Gene Give Rise to Both X-Linked Adrenal Hypoplasia Congenita and Hypogonadotropic Hypogonadism. Nature. 372: 672-676.

[40] Rogler LE, Pintar JE (1993) Expression of the P450 Side-Chain Cleavage and Adrenodoxin Genes Begins During Early Stages of Adrenal Cortex Development. Mol. endocrinol. 7: 453-461.

[41] Nussdorfer G, Mazzocchi G, Rebonato L (1971) Long-Term Trophic Effect of Acth on Rat Adrenocortical Cells. An Ultrastructural, Morphometric and Autoradiographic Study. Z. zellforsch. mikrosk. anat. 115: 30-45.

[42] Manolović-Stojanoski M, Nestorović N, Negić N, Filipović B, Šošić-Jurjević B, Milošević V, Sekulić M (2006) The Pituitary-Adrenal Axis of Fetal Rats after Maternal Dedxamethasone Exposure. Anat. embryol. 61-69.

[43] Wotus C, Levay-Young BK, Rogers LM, Gomez-Sanchez CE, Engeland WC (1998) Development of Adrenal Zonation in Fetal Rats Defined by Expression of Aldosterone Synthase and 11beta-Hydroxylase. Endocrinology. 139: 4397-4403.

[44] Mitani F, Mukai K, Ogawa T, Miyamoto H, Ishimura Y (1997) Expression of Cytochromes P450aldo and P45011 Beta in Rat Adrenal Gland During Late Gestational and Neonatal Stages. Steroids. 62: 57-61.

[45] Hristić M, Kalafatić D, Plećaš B, Jovanović V (1995) The Effect of Dexamethasone on the Adrenal Gland in Fetal and Neonatal Rats. J. exp. zool. 272: 281-290.

[46] Hristić M, Kalafatić D, Plećaš B, Manojlović M (1997) The Influence of Prolonged Dexamethasone Treatment of Pregnant Rats on the Perinatal Development of the Adrenal Gland of Their Offspring. J. exp. zool. 279: 54-61.

[47] Bolt RJ, van Weissenbruch MM, Lafeber HN, Delemarre-van de Waal HA (2002) Development of the Hypothalamic-Pituitary-Adrenal Axis in the Fetus and Preterm Infant. J. pediatr. endocrinol. metab. 15: 759-769.

[48] Mesiano S, Jaffe RB (1997) Developmental and Functional Biology of the Primate Fetal Adrenal Cortex. Endocr. rev. 18: 378-403.

[49] Blumenfeld Z, Jaffe RB (1986) Hypophysiotropic and Neuromodulatory Regulation of Adrenocorticotropin in the Human Fetal Pituitary Gland. J. clin. invest. 78: 288-294.

[50] Gluckman PD, Sizonenko SV, Bassett NS (1999) The Transition from Fetus to Neonate--an Endocrine Perspective. Acta. paediatr. suppl. 88: 7-11.

[51] Reichardt HM, Schutz G (1996) Feedback Control of Glucocorticoid Production Is Established During Fetal Development. Mol. med. 2: 735-744.

[52] Ducsay CA (1998) Fetal and Maternal Adaptations to Chronic Hypoxia: Prevention of Premature Labor in Response to Chronic Stress. Comp. biochem. physiol. a mol. integr. physiol. 119: 675-681.

[53] Slotkin TA, Lappi SE, McCook EC, Tayyeb MI, Eylers JP, Seidler FJ (1992) Glucocorticoids and the Development of Neuronal Function: Effects of Prenatal Dexamethasone Exposure on Central Noradrenergic Activity. Biol. neonate. 61: 326-336.

[54] Muneoka K, Mikuni M, Ogawa T, Kitera K, Kamei K, Takigawa M, Takahashi K (1997) Prenatal Dexamethasone Exposure Alters Brain Monoamine Metabolism and Adrenocortical Response in Rat Offspring. Am. j. physiol. 273: R1669-1675.

[55] Seidl K, Unsicker K (1989) The Determination of the Adrenal Medullary Cell Fate During Embryogenesis. Dev. biol. 136: 481-490.

[56] Michelsohn AM, Anderson DJ (1992) Changes in Competence Determine the Timing of Two Sequential Glucocorticoid Effects on Sympathoadrenal Progenitors. Neuron. 8: 589-604.

[57] Pratt L, Magness RR, Phernetton T, Hendricks SK, Abbott DH, Bird IM (1999) Repeated Use of Betamethasone in Rabbits: Effects of Treatment Variation on Adrenal Suppression, Pulmonary Maturation, and Pregnancy Outcome. Am. j. obstet. gynecol. 180: 995-1005.

[58] Pearce S, Mostyn A, Alves-Guerra MC, Pecqueur C, Miroux B, Webb R, Stephenson T, Symond ME (2003) Prolactin, Prolactin Receptor and Uncoupling Proteins During Fetal and Neonatal Development. Proc. nutr. soc. 62: 421-427.

[59] Gnanalingham MG, Mostyn A, Forhead AJ, Fowden AL, Symonds ME, Stephenson T (2005) Increased Uncoupling Protein-2 mRNA Abundance and Glucocorticoid Action in

Adipose Tissue in the Sheep Fetus During Late Gestation Is Dependent on Plasma Cortisol and Triiodothyronine. J. physiol. 567: 283-292.

[60] Myers DA, Hanson K, Mlynarczyk M, Kaushal KM, Ducsay CA (2008) Long-Term Hypoxia Modulates Expression of Key Genes Regulating Adipose Function in the Late-Gestation Ovine Fetus. Am. j. physiol. regul. integr. comp. physiol. 294: R1312-1318.

[61] Nakae J, Kido Y, Accili D (2001) Distinct and Overlapping Functions of Insulin and IGF-I Receptors. Endocr. rev. 22: 818-835.

[62] Lupu F, Terwilliger JD, Lee K, Segre GV, Efstratiadis A (2001) Roles of Growth Hormone and Insulin-Like Growth Factor 1 in Mouse Postnatal Growth. Dev. biol. 229: 141-162.

[63] Murakami S, Salmon A, Miller RA (2003) Multiplex Stress Resistance in Cells from Long-Lived Dwarf Mice. FASEB. J. 17: 1565-1566.

[64] Cella SG, Locatelli V, Broccia ML, Menegola E, Giavini E, De Gennaro Colonna V, Torsello A, Wehrenberg WB, Muller EE (1994) Long-Term Changes of Somatotrophic Function Induced by Deprivation of Growth Hormone-Releasing Hormone During the Fetal Life of the Rat. J. endocrinol. 140: 111-117.

[65] Baram TZ, Lerner SP (1991) Ontogeny of Corticotropin Releasing Hormone Gene Expression in Rat Hypothalamus--Comparison with Somatostatin. Int. j. dev. neurosci. 9: 473-478.

[66] Rodriguez-Garcia M, Jolin T, Santos A, Perez-Castillo A (1995) Effect of Perinatal Hypothyroidism on the Developmental Regulation of Rat Pituitary Growth Hormone and Thyrotropin Genes. Endocrinology. 136: 4339-4350.

[67] Savage JJ, Yaden BC, Kiratipranon P, Rhodes SJ (2003) Transcriptional Control During Mammalian Anterior Pituitary Development. Gene. 319: 1-19.

[68] Taniguchi Y, Yasutaka S, Kominami R, Shinohara H (2001) Proliferation and Differentiation of Thyrotrophs in the Pars Distalis of the Rat Pituitary Gland During the Fetal and Postnatal Period. Anat. embryol. (Berl). 203: 249-253.

[69] Korytko AI, Zeitler P, Cuttler L (1996) Developmental Regulation of Pituitary Growth Hormone-Releasing Hormone Receptor Gene Expression in the Rat. Endocrinology. 137: 1326-1331.

[70] Nogami H, Inoue K, Moriya H, Ishida A, Kobayashi S, Hisano S, Katayama M, Kawamura K (1999) Regulation of Growth Hormone-Releasing Hormone Receptor Messenger Ribonucleic Acid Expression by Glucocorticoids in Mtt-S Cells and in the Pituitary Gland of Fetal Rats. Endocrinology. 140: 2763-2770.

[71] Sanders EJ, Harvey S (2004) Growth Hormone as an Early Embryonic Growth and Differentiation Factor. Anat. embryol. (Berl). 209: 1-9.

[72] Rodier PM, Kates B, White WA, Phelps CJ (1990) Birthdates of the Growth Hormone Releasing Factor Cells of the Rat Hypothalamus: An Autoradiographic Study of Immunocytochemically Identified Neurons. J. comp. neurol. 291: 363-372.

[73] Mulchahey JJ, DiBlasio AM, Martin MC, Blumenfeld Z, Jaffe RB (1987) Hormone Production and Peptide Regulation of the Human Fetal Pituitary Gland. Endocr. rev. 8: 406-425.

[74] Hill DJ, Petrik J, Arany E (1998) Growth Factors and the Regulation of Fetal Growth. Diabetes care. 21 Suppl 2: B60-69.

[75] Daughaday WH, Parker KA, Borowsky S, Trivedi B, Kapadia M (1982) Measurement of Somatomedin-Related Peptides in Fetal, Neonatal, and Maternal Rat Serum by Insulin-Like Growth Factor (IGF) I Radioimmunoassay, IGF-II Radioreceptor Assay (Rra), and Multiplication-Stimulating Activity Rra after Acid-Ethanol Extraction. Endocrinology. 110: 575-581.

[76] Straus DS, Ooi GT, Orlowski CC, Rechler MM (1991) Expression of the Genes for Insulin-Like Growth Factor-I (IGF-I), IGF-II, and IGF-Binding Proteins-1 and -2 in Fetal Rat under Conditions of Intrauterine Growth Retardation Caused by Maternal Fasting. Endocrinology. 128: 518-525.

[77] Gluckman PD, Butler JH (1983) Parturition-Related Changes in Insulin-Like Growth Factors-I and -II in the Perinatal Lamb. J. endocrinol. 99: 223-232.

[78] Lee JE, Pintar J, Efstratiadis A (1990) Pattern of the Insulin-Like Growth Factor II Gene Expression During Early Mouse Embryogenesis. Development. 110: 151-159.

[79] Li J, Gilmour RS, Saunders JC, Dauncey MJ, Fowden AL (1999) Activation of the Adult Mode of Ovine Growth Hormone Receptor Gene Expression by Cortisol During Late Fetal Development. FASEB J. 13: 545-552.

[80] Allan GJ, Flint DJ, Patel K (2001) Insulin-Like Growth Factor Axis During Embryonic Development. Reproduction. 122: 31-39.

[81] Brown RS, Shalhoub V, Coulter S, Alex S, Joris I, De Vito W, Lian J, Stein GS (2000) Developmental Regulation of Thyrotropin Receptor Gene Expression in the Fetal and Neonatal Rat Thyroid: Relation to Thyroid Morphology and to Thyroid-Specific Gene Expression. Endocrinology. 141: 340-345.

[82] Oliver C, Eskay RL, Porter JC (1980) Developmental Changes in Brain Trh and in Plasma and Pituitary Tsh and Prolactin Levels in the Rat. Biol. neonate. 37: 145-152.

[83] Murakami M, Mori M, Kato Y, Kobayashi I (1991) Hypothalamic Thyrotropin-Releasing Hormone Regulates Pituitary Thyrotropin Beta- and Alpha-Subunit mRNA Levels in the Rat. Neuroendocrinology. 53: 276-280.

[84] Parlato R, Rosica A, Rodriguez-Mallon A, Affuso A, Postiglione MP, Arra C, Mansouri A, Kimura S, Di Lauro R, De Felice M (2004) An Integrated Regulatory Network Controlling Survival and Migration in Thyroid Organogenesis. Dev. biol. 276: 464-475.

[85] Kimura S, Hara Y, Pineau T, Fernandez-Salguero P, Fox CH, Ward JM, Gonzalez FJ (1996) The T/Ebp Null Mouse: Thyroid-Specific Enhancer-Binding Protein Is Essential for the Organogenesis of the Thyroid, Lung, Ventral Forebrain, and Pituitary. Genes dev. 10: 60-69.

[86] Mansouri A, Chowdhury K, Gruss P (1998) Follicular Cells of the Thyroid Gland Require Pax8 Gene Function. Nat. genet. 19: 87-90.

[87] Gereben B, Zavacki AM, Ribich S, Kim BW, Huang SA, Simonides WS, Zeold A, Bianco AC (2008) Cellular and Molecular Basis of Deiodinase-Regulated Thyroid Hormone Signaling. Endocr. rev. 29: 898-938.

[88] Kester MH, Martinez de Mena R, Obregon MJ, Marinkovic D, Howatson A, Visser TJ, Hume R, Morreale de Escobar G (2004) Iodothyronine Levels in the Human Developing Brain: Major Regulatory Roles of Iodothyronine Deiodinases in Different Areas. J. clin. endocrinol. metab. 89: 3117-3128.

[89] Obregon MJ, Escobar del Rey F, Morreale de Escobar G (2005) The Effects of Iodine Deficiency on Thyroid Hormone Deiodination. Thyroid. 15: 917-929.

[90] Obregon MJ, Calvo RM, Del Rey FE, de Escobar GM (2007) Ontogenesis of Thyroid Function and Interactions with Maternal Function. Endocr. dev. 10: 86-98.

[91] Patel J, Landers K, Li H, Mortimer RH, Richard K (2011) Thyroid Hormones and Fetal Neurological Development. J. endocrinol. 209: 1-8.

[92] Ashizawa S, Brunicardi FC, Wang XP (2004) Pdx-1 and the Pancreas. Pancreas. 28: 109-120.

[93] Gu G, Dubauskaite J, Melton DA (2002) Direct Evidence for the Pancreatic Lineage: Ngn3+ Cells Are Islet Progenitors and Are Distinct from Duct Progenitors. Development. 129: 2447-2457.

[94] Zaret KS (2008) Genetic Programming of Liver and Pancreas Progenitors: Lessons for Stem-Cell Differentiation. Nat. rev. genet. 9: 329-340.

[95] Lackie PM, Zuber C, Roth J (1994) Polysialic Acid of the Neural Cell Adhesion Molecule (N-Cam) Is Widely Expressed During Organogenesis in Mesodermal and Endodermal Derivatives. Differentiation. 57: 119-131.

[96] Stefan Y, Grasso S, Perrelet A, Orci L (1983) A Quantitative Immunofluorescent Study of the Endocrine Cell Populations in the Developing Human Pancreas. Diabetes. 32: 293-301.

[97] Bonal C, Avril I, Herrera PL (2008) Experimental Models of Beta-Cell Regeneration. Biochem. soc. trans. 36: 286-289.

[98] Aye T, Toschi E, Sharma A, Sgroi D, Bonner-Weir S (2010) Identification of Markers for Newly Formed Beta-Cells in the Perinatal Period: A Time of Recognized Beta-Cell Immaturity. J. histochem. cytochem. 58: 369-376.

[99] Cabrera-Vasquez S, Navarro-Tableros V, Sanchez-Soto C, Gutierrez-Ospina G, Hiriart M (2009) Remodelling Sympathetic Innervation in Rat Pancreatic Islets Ontogeny. BMC dev. biol. 9: 34.

[100] Ammon HP, Glocker C, Waldner RG, Wahl MA (1989) Insulin Release from Pancreatic Islets of Fetal Rats Mediated by Leucine B-Bch, Tolbutamide, Glibenclamide, Arginine, Potassium Chloride, and Theophylline Does Not Require Stimulation of Ca2+ Net Uptake. Cell calcium. 10: 441-450.

[101] Navarro-Tableros V, Fiordelisio T, Hernandez-Cruz A, Hiriart M (2007) Physiological Development of Insulin Secretion, Calcium Channels, and Glut2 Expression of Pancreatic Rat Beta-Cells. Am. j. physiol. endocrinol. metab. 292: E1018-1029.

[102] Jermendy A, Toschi E, Aye T, Koh A, Aguayo-Mazzucato C, Sharma A, Weir GC, Sgroi D, Bonner-Weir S (2011) Rat Neonatal Beta Cells Lack the Specialised Metabolic Phenotype of Mature Beta Cells. Diabetologia. 54: 594-604.

[103] Hoglund E, Mattsson G, Tyrberg B, Andersson A, Carlsson C (2009) Growth Hormone Increases Beta-Cell Proliferation in Transplanted Human and Fetal Rat Islets. JOP. 10: 242-248.

[104] Aubert ML, Begeot M, Winiger BP, Morel G, Sizonenko PC, Dubois PM (1985) Ontogeny of Hypothalamic Luteinizing Hormone-Releasing Hormone (Gnrh) and Pituitary Gnrh Receptors in Fetal and Neonatal Rats. Endocrinology. 116: 1565-1576.

[105] Jorgensen JS, Quirk CC, Nilson JH (2004) Multiple and Overlapping Combinatorial Codes Orchestrate Hormonal Responsiveness and Dictate Cell-Specific Expression of the Genes Encoding Luteinizing Hormone. Endocr. rev. 25: 521-542.

[106] Parker KL, Schimmer BP (1997) Steroidogenic Factor 1: A Key Determinant of Endocrine Development and Function. Endocr. rev. 18: 361-377.

[107] Zhu X, Gleiberman AS, Rosenfeld MG (2007) Molecular Physiology of Pituitary Development: Signaling and Transcriptional Networks. Physiol. rev. 87: 933-963.

[108] Wen S, Ai W, Alim Z, Boehm U (2010) Embryonic Gonadotropin-Releasing Hormone Signaling Is Necessary for Maturation of the Male Reproductive Axis. Proc. natl. acad. sci. U S A. 107: 16372-16377.

[109] Winter JS, Faiman C, Reyes FI (1977) Sex Steroid Production by the Human Fetus: Its Role in Morphogenesis and Control by Gonadotropins. Birth defects. orig. artic. ser. 13: 41-58.

[110] Ginsburg M, Snow MH, McLaren A (1990) Primordial Germ Cells in the Mouse Embryo During Gastrulation. Development. 110: 521-528.

[111] Edson MA, Nagaraja AK, Matzuk MM (2009) The Mammalian Ovary from Genesis to Revelation. Endocr. rev. 30: 624-712.

[112] Gubbay J, Collignon J, Koopman P, Capel B, Economou A, Munsterberg A, Vivian N, Goodfellow P, Lovell-Badge R (1990) A Gene Mapping to the Sex-Determining Region of the Mouse Y Chromosome Is a Member of a Novel Family of Embryonically Expressed Genes. Nature. 346: 245-250.

[113] Sekido R, Bar I, Narvaez V, Penny G, Lovell-Badge R (2004) Sox9 Is up-Regulated by the Transient Expression of Sry Specifically in Sertoli Cell Precursors. Dev. biol. 274: 271-279.

[114] Eicher EM, Shown EP, Washburn LL (1995) Sex Reversal in C57bl/6j-Ypos Mice Corrected by a Sry Transgene. Philos. trans. r. soc. lond. b. biol. sci. 350: 263-268; discussion 268-269.

[115] Lovell-Badge R, Robertson E (1990) Xy Female Mice Resulting from a Heritable Mutation in the Primary Testis-Determining Gene, Tdy. Development. 109: 635-646.

[116] Brennan J, Capel B (2004) One Tissue, Two Fates: Molecular Genetic Events That Underlie Testis Versus Ovary Development. Nat. rev. genet. 5: 509-521.

[117] Adams IR, McLaren A (2002) Sexually Dimorphic Development of Mouse Primordial Germ Cells: Switching from Oogenesis to Spermatogenesis. Development. 129: 1155-1164.

[118] Nef S, Parada LF (1999) Cryptorchidism in Mice Mutant for Insl3. Nat. genet. 22: 295-299.

[119] Warren DW, Huhtaniemi IT, Tapanainen J, Dufau ML, Catt KJ (1984) Ontogeny of Gonadotropin Receptors in the Fetal and Neonatal Rat Testis. Endocrinology. 114: 470-476.

[120] Sokka TA, Hamalainen TM, Kaipia A, Warren DW, Huhtaniemi IT (1996) Development of Luteinizing Hormone Action in the Perinatal Rat Ovary. Biol. reprod. 55: 663-670.

[121] Meijs-Roelofs HM, de Greef WJ, Uilenbroek JT (1975) Plasma Progesterone and Its Relationship to Serum Gonadotrophins in Immature Female Rats. J. endocrinol. 64: 329-336.

[122] Sokka T, Huhtaniemi I (1990) Ontogeny of Gonadotrophin Receptors and Gonadotrophin-Stimulated Cyclic Amp Production in the Neonatal Rat Ovary. J. endocrinol. 127: 297-303.

[123] Couse JF, Hewitt SC, Bunch DO, Sar M, Walker VR, Davis BJ, Korach KS (1999) Postnatal Sex Reversal of the Ovaries in Mice Lacking Estrogen Receptors Alpha and Beta. Science. 286: 2328-2331.

[124] Britt KL, Drummond AE, Dyson M, Wreford NG, Jones ME, Simpson ER, Findlay JK (2001) The Ovarian Phenotype of the Aromatase Knockout (Arko) Mouse. J. steroid. biochem. mol. biol. 79: 181-185.

[125] Baker TG (1963) A Quantitative and Cytological Study of Germ Cells in Human Ovaries. Proc. r. soc. lond. b. biol. sci. 158: 417-433.

[126] Fulton N, Martins da Silva SJ, Bayne RA, Anderson RA (2005) Germ Cell Proliferation and Apoptosis in the Developing Human Ovary. J. clin. endocrinol. metab. 90: 4664-4670.

[127] Hunt PA, Hassold TJ (2008) Human Female Meiosis: What Makes a Good Egg Go Bad? Trends. genet. 24: 86-93.

[128] George FW, Wilson JD (1978) Conversion of Androgen to Estrogen by the Human Fetal Ovary. J. clin. endocrinol. metab. 47: 550-555.

[129] Gurpide E, Schwers J, Welch MT, Vande Wiele RL, Lieberman S (1966) Fetal and Maternal Metabolism of Estradiol During Pregnancy. J. clin. endocrinol. metab. 26: 1355-1365.

[130] Ostrer H, Huang HY, Masch RJ, Shapiro E (2007) A Cellular Study of Human Testis Development. Sex. dev. 1: 286-292.

[131] Reyes FI, Boroditsky RS, Winter JS, Faiman C (1974) Studies on Human Sexual Development. 2. Fetal and Maternal Serum Gonadotropin and Sex Steroid Concentrations. J. clin. endocrinol. metab. 38: 612-617.

[132] Takagi S, Yoshida T, Tsubata K, Ozaki H, Fujii TK, Nomura Y, Sawada M (1977) Sex Differences in Fetal Gonadotropins and Androgens. J. steroid. biochem. 8: 609-620.

[133] Barker DJP, Mothers, Babies and Disease in Later Life, BMJ Publishing, London, 1994.

[134] Gluckman PD, Hanson MA (2004) The Developmental Origins of the Metabolic Syndrome. Trends. endocrinol. metab. 15: 183-187.

[135] Lucas A (1991) Programming by Early Nutrition in Man. Ciba. found. symp. 156: 38-50; discussion 50-35.

[136] Roseboom T, de Rooij S, Painter R (2006) The Dutch Famine and Its Long-Term Consequences for Adult Health. Early hum. dev. 82: 485-491.

[137] Weinstock M, Fride E, Hertzberg R (1988) Prenatal Stress Effects on Functional Development of the Offspring. Prog. brain. res. 73: 319-331.

[138] Nathanielsz PW (2006) Animal Models That Elucidate Basic Principles of the Developmental Origins of Adult Diseases. ILAR J. 47: 73-82.

[139] Fowden AL, Forhead AJ (2004) Endocrine Mechanisms of Intrauterine Programming. Reproduction. 127: 515-526.

[140] Cottrell EC, Holmes MC, Livingstone DE, Kenyon CJ, Seckl JR (2012) Reconciling the Nutritional and Glucocorticoid Hypotheses of Fetal Programming. FASEB J. doi: 10.1096/fj.1012-203489.

[141] Fowden AL, Forhead AJ (2009) Hormones as Epigenetic Signals in Developmental Programming. Exp. physiol. 94: 607-625.

[142] Seckl JR (2004) Prenatal Glucocorticoids and Long-Term Programming. Eur. j. endocrinol. 151 Suppl 3: U49-62.

[143] Edwards CR, Benediktsson R, Lindsay RS, Seckl JR (1996) 11 Beta-Hydroxysteroid Dehydrogenases: Key Enzymes in Determining Tissue-Specific Glucocorticoid Effects. Steroids. 61: 263-269.

[144] Waddell BJ, Benediktsson R, Brown RW, Seckl JR (1998) Tissue-Specific Messenger Ribonucleic Acid Expression of 11beta-Hydroxysteroid Dehydrogenase Types 1 and 2 and the Glucocorticoid Receptor within Rat Placenta Suggests Exquisite Local Control of Glucocorticoid Action. Endocrinology. 139: 1517-1523.

[145] Wyrwoll CS, Holmes MC, Seckl JR (2011) 11beta-Hydroxysteroid Dehydrogenases and the Brain: From Zero to Hero, a Decade of Progress. Front. neuroendocrinol. 32: 265-286.

[146] Seckl JR (1997) Glucocorticoids, Feto-Placental 11 Beta-Hydroxysteroid Dehydrogenase Type 2, and the Early Life Origins of Adult Disease. Steroids. 62: 89-94.

[147] Wyrwoll CS, Seckl JR, Holmes MC (2009) Altered Placental Function of 11beta-Hydroxysteroid Dehydrogenase 2 Knockout Mice. Endocrinology. 150: 1287-1293.

[148] Brown RW, Diaz R, Robson AC, Kotelevtsev YV, Mullins JJ, Kaufman MH, Seckl JR (1996) The Ontogeny of 11 Beta-Hydroxysteroid Dehydrogenase Type 2 and Mineralocorticoid Receptor Gene Expression Reveal Intricate Control of Glucocorticoid Action in Development. Endocrinology. 137: 794-797.

[149] Lindsay RS, Lindsay RM, Edwards CR, Seckl JR (1996) Inhibition of 11-Beta-Hydroxysteroid Dehydrogenase in Pregnant Rats and the Programming of Blood Pressure in the Offspring. Hypertension. 27: 1200-1204.

[150] Kajantie E, Dunkel L, Turpeinen U, Stenman UH, Wood PJ, Nuutila M, Andersson S (2003) Placental 11 Beta-Hydroxysteroid Dehydrogenase-2 and Fetal Cortisol/Cortisone Shuttle in Small Preterm Infants. J. clin. endocrinol. metab. 88: 493-500.

[151] Williams MT, Davis HN, McCrea AE, Hennessy MB (1999) Stress During Pregnancy Alters the Offspring Hypothalamic, Pituitary, Adrenal, and Testicular Response to Isolation on the Day of Weaning. Neurotoxicol. teratol. 21: 653-659.

[152] Sinha P, Halasz I, Choi JF, McGivern RF, Redei E (1997) Maternal Adrenalectomy Eliminates a Surge of Plasma Dehydroepiandrosterone in the Mother and Attenuates the Prenatal Testosterone Surge in the Male Fetus. Endocrinology. 138: 4792-4797.

[153] Barbazanges A, Piazza PV, Le Moal M, Maccari S (1996) Maternal Glucocorticoid Secretion Mediates Long-Term Effects of Prenatal Stress. J. neurosci. 16: 3943-3949.

[154] Langley-Evans SC (1997) Hypertension Induced by Foetal Exposure to a Maternal Low-Protein Diet, in the Rat, Is Prevented by Pharmacological Blockade of Maternal Glucocorticoid Synthesis. J. hypertens. 15: 537-544.

[155] Halasz I, Rittenhouse PA, Zorrilla EP, Redei E (1997) Sexually Dimorphic Effects of Maternal Adrenalectomy on Hypothalamic Corticotrophin-Releasing Factor, Glucocorticoid Receptor and Anterior Pituitary POMC mRNA Levels in Rat Neonates. Brain. res. dev. brain. res. 100: 198-204.

[156] Fujioka T, Sakata Y, Yamaguchi K, Shibasaki T, Kato H, Nakamura S (1999) The Effects of Prenatal Stress on the Development of Hypothalamic Paraventricular Neurons in Fetal Rats. Neuroscience. 92: 1079-1088.

[157] Barker DJ, Bull AR, Osmond C, Simmonds SJ (1990) Fetal and Placental Size and Risk of Hypertension in Adult Life. BMJ. 301: 259-262.

[158] Bertram C, Trowern AR, Copin N, Jackson AA, Whorwood CB (2001) The Maternal Diet During Pregnancy Programs Altered Expression of the Glucocorticoid Receptor and Type 2 11beta-Hydroxysteroid Dehydrogenase: Potential Molecular Mechanisms Underlying the Programming of Hypertension in Utero. Endocrinology. 142: 2841-2853.

[159] Crowley PA (1995) Antenatal Corticosteroid Therapy: A Meta-Analysis of the Randomized Trials, 1972 to 1994. Am. j. obstet. gynecol. 173: 322-335.

[160] NIH (1994) Effect of Corticosteroids for Fetal Maturation on Perinatal Outcomes. NIH Consens Statement. 12: 1-24.

[161] Miracle X, Di Renzo GC, Stark A, Fanaroff A, Carbonell-Estrany X, Saling E (2008) Guideline for the Use of Antenatal Corticosteroids for Fetal Maturation. J. Perinat. Med. 36: 191-196.

[162] Ain R, Canham LN, Soares MJ (2005) Dexamethasone-Induced Intrauterine Growth Restriction Impacts the Placental Prolactin Family, Insulin-Like Growth Factor-Ii and the Akt Signaling Pathway. J. Endocrinol. 185: 253-263.

[163] Lajic S, Nordenstrom A, Ritzen EM, Wedell A (2004) Prenatal Treatment of Congenital Adrenal Hyperplasia. Eur. j. endocrinol. 151 Suppl 3: U63-69.

[164] Diederich S, Eigendorff E, Burkhardt P, Quinkler M, Bumke-Vogt C, Rochel M, Seidelmann D, Esperling P, Oelkers W, Bahr V (2002) 11beta-Hydroxysteroid Dehydrogenase Types 1 and 2: An Important Pharmacokinetic Determinant for the

Activity of Synthetic Mineralo- and Glucocorticoids. J. clin. endocrinol. metab. 87: 5695-5701.

[165] Melby JC (1977) Clinical Pharmacology of Systemic Corticosteroids. Annu. rev. pharmacol. toxicol. 17: 511-527.

[166] Gayrard V, Alvinerie M, Toutain PL (1996) Interspecies Variations of Corticosteroid-Binding Globulin Parameters. Domest anim endocrinol. 13: 35-45.

[167] Peets EA, Staub M, Symchowicz S (1969) Plasma Binding of Betamethasone-3h, Dexamethasone-3h, and Cortisol-14c--a Comparative Study. Biochem. pharmacol. 18: 1655-1663.

[168] Buttgereit F, Burmester GR, Brand MD (2000) Bioenergetics of Immune Functions: Fundamental and Therapeutic Aspects. Immunol. today. 21: 192-199.

[169] de Kloet ER, Reul JM, Sutanto W (1990) Corticosteroids and the Brain. J. steroid. biochem. mol. biol. 37: 387-394.

[170] Dean F, Matthews SG (1999) Maternal Dexamethasone Treatment in Late Gestation Alters Glucocorticoid and Mineralocorticoid Receptor mRNA in the Fetal Guinea Pig Brain. Brain res. 846: 253-259.

[171] McCabe L, Marash D, Li A, Matthews SG (2001) Repeated Antenatal Glucocorticoid Treatment Decreases Hypothalamic Corticotropin Releasing Hormone mRNA but Not Corticosteroid Receptor mRNA Expression in the Fetal Guinea-Pig Brain. J. neuroendocrinol. 13: 425-431.

[172] Noorlander CW, De Graan PN, Middeldorp J, Van Beers JJ, Visser GH (2006) Ontogeny of Hippocampal Corticosteroid Receptors: Effects of Antenatal Glucocorticoids in Human and Mouse. J. comp. neurol. 499: 924-932.

[173] Levitt NS, Lindsay RS, Holmes MC, Seckl JR (1996) Dexamethasone in the Last Week of Pregnancy Attenuates Hippocampal Glucocorticoid Receptor Gene Expression and Elevates Blood Pressure in the Adult Offspring in the Rat. Neuroendocrinology. 64: 412-418.

[174] Bakker JM, Schmidt ED, Kroes H, Kavelaars A, Heijnen CJ, Tilders FJ, van Rees EP (1995) Effects of Short-Term Dexamethasone Treatment During Pregnancy on the Development of the Immune System and the Hypothalamo-Pituitary Adrenal Axis in the Rat. J. neuroimmunol. 63: 183-191.

[175] Hristić M, Kalafatić D, Plećaš B, Mićić Z, Manojlović M (1997) The Paraventricular and Supraoptic Nuclei of Fetal and Neonatal Offspring of Rats Treated with Dexamethasone During Gestation. Acta vet. 47: 95-106.

[176] Kalafatić D, Manojlović-Stojanoski M, Plećaš B, Hristić M (2000) Development and Differentiation of the Nucleus Paraventricularis and Nucleus Supraopticus of the Hypothalamus During the Perinatal Period in Rats. Arch. biol. sci. 52: 19-20.

[177] Kalafatić D, Plećaš B, Hristić M, Manojlović M (1998) Manipulation of Prenatal Blood Glucocorticoid Level Affects Development of the Hipothalamic Paraventricular Nuclei in Rats. Biomed. res. 19: 293-301.

[178] Welberg LA, Seckl JR, Holmes MC (2001) Prenatal Glucocorticoid Programming of Brain Corticosteroid Receptors and Corticotrophin-Releasing Hormone: Possible Implications for Behaviour. Neuroscience. 104: 71-79.

[179] Taniguchi Y, Kominami R, Yasutaka S, Shinohara H (2001) Mitoses of Existing Corticotrophs Contribute to Their Proliferation in the Rat Pituitary During the Late Fetal Period. Anat. embryol. (Berl). 203: 89-93.

[180] Kalafatić D, Plećaš B, Hristić M, Manojlović-Stojanoski M, Čakić M (2000) The Effect of Repeated Maternal Dexamethasone Treatment on Plasma Adrenocorticotropin Concentration and Acth-Cells During the Perinatal Period in Rats. Arch. biol. sci. 52: 159-164.

[181] Manojlović M, Kalafatić D, Hristić M, Plećaš B, Virag A, Čakić M (1998) Treatment of Pregnant Females with Dexamethasone Influences Postnatal Development of the Adrenal Medulla. Ann anat. 180: 131-135.

[182] Kalafatić D, Hristić M, Plećaš B, Manojlović-Stojanoski M (2000) The Effects of Dexamethasone Treatment of Pregnant Rats Neonatal Acth-Cells. Acta vet. 50: 195.

[183] Owen D, Matthews SG (2007) Prenatal Glucocorticoid Exposure Alters Hypothalamic-Pituitary-Adrenal Function in Juvenile Guinea Pigs. J. neuroendocrinol. 19: 172-180.

[184] Miyamoto H, Mitani F, Mukai K, Suematsu M, Ishimura Y (1999) Studies on Cytogenesis in Adult Rat Adrenal Cortex: Circadian and Zonal Variations and Their Modulation by Adrenocorticotropic Hormone. J. biochem. 126: 1175-1183.

[185] Manojlović M, Hristić M, Kalafatić D, Plećaš B, Urešić N (1998) The Influence of Dexamethasone Treatment of Pregnant Rats on the Development of Chromafin Tissue in Their Offspring During the Fetal and Neonatal Period. J. endocrinol. invest. 21: 211-218.

[186] Kapoor A, Petropoulos S, Matthews SG (2008) Fetal Programming of Hypothalamic-Pituitary-Adrenal (Hpa) Axis Function and Behavior by Synthetic Glucocorticoids. Brain. res. rev. 57: 586-595.

[187] Nyirenda MJ, Welberg LA, Seckl JR (2001) Programming Hyperglycaemia in the Rat through Prenatal Exposure to Glucocorticoids-Fetal Effect or Maternal Influence? J. endocrinol. 170: 653-660.

[188] Liu L, Li A, Matthews SG (2001) Maternal Glucocorticoid Treatment Programs Hpa Regulation in Adult Offspring: Sex-Specific Effects. Am. j. physiol. endocrinol. metab. 280: E729-739.

[189] Poore KR, Fowden AL (2003) The Effect of Birth Weight on Hypothalamo-Pituitary-Adrenal Axis Function in Juvenile and Adult Pigs. J physiol. 547: 107-116.

[190] Meaney MJ, Diorio J, Francis D, Weaver S, Yau J, Chapman K, Seckl JR (2000) Postnatal Handling Increases the Expression of Camp-Inducible Transcription Factors in the Rat Hippocampus: The Effects of Thyroid Hormones and Serotonin. J. neurosci. 20: 3926-3935.

[191] Liu D, Diorio J, Tannenbaum B, Caldji C, Francis D, Freedman A, Sharma S, Pearson D, Plotsky PM, Meaney MJ (1997) Maternal Care, Hippocampal Glucocorticoid Receptors, and Hypothalamic-Pituitary-Adrenal Responses to Stress. Science. 277: 1659-1662.

[192] Huot RL, Plotsky PM, Lenox RH, McNamara RK (2002) Neonatal Maternal Separation Reduces Hippocampal Mossy Fiber Density in Adult Long Evans Rats. Brain. res. 950: 52-63.

[193] Lajud N, Roque A, Cajero M, Gutierrez-Ospina G, Torner L (2012) Periodic Maternal Separation Decreases Hippocampal Neurogenesis without Affecting Basal Corticosterone

During the Stress Hyporesponsive Period, but Alters Hpa Axis and Coping Behavior in Adulthood. Psychoneuroendocrinology. 37: 410-420.

[194] Jansson JO, Ekberg S, Isaksson O, Mode A, Gustafsson JA (1985) Imprinting of Growth Hormone Secretion, Body Growth, and Hepatic Steroid Metabolism by Neonatal Testosterone. Endocrinology. 117: 1881-1889.

[195] Manojlović-Stojanoski M, Nestorović N, Negić N, Trifunović S, Sekulić M, Milošević V (2007) Development of Pituitary Acth and Gh Cells in near Term Rat Fetuses. Arch. biol. sci. 59: 37-44.

[196] Manojlović-Stojanoski M, Nestorović N, Negić N, Filipović B, Šošic-Jurjević B, Sekulić M, Milošević V (2007) Influence of Maternal Dexamethasone Treatment on Morphometric Characteristics of Pituitary Gh Cells and Body Weight in near-Term Rat Fetuses. Folia histochem. cytobiol. 45: 51-56.

[197] Porter TE, Dean CE, Piper MM, Medvedev KL, Ghavam S, Sandor J (2001) Somatotroph Recruitment by Glucocorticoids Involves Induction of Growth Hormone Gene Expression and Secretagogue Responsiveness. J. endocrinol. 169: 499-509.

[198] Holt RI (2002) Fetal Programming of the Growth Hormone-Insulin-Like Growth Factor Axis. Trends endocrinol metab. 13: 392-397.

[199] Boyne MS, Thame M, Bennett FI, Osmond C, Miell JP, Forrester TE (2003) The Relationship among Circulating Insulin-Like Growth Factor (IGF)-I, IGF-Binding Proteins-1 and -2, and Birth Anthropometry: A Prospective Study. J. clin. endocrinol. metab. 88: 1687-1691.

[200] Fowden AL (2003) The Insulin-Like Growth Factors and Feto-Placental Growth. Placenta. 24: 803-812.

[201] Fowden AL, Szemere J, Hughes P, Gilmour RS, Forhead AJ (1996) The Effects of Cortisol on the Growth Rate of the Sheep Fetus During Late Gestation. J. endocrinol. 151: 97-105.

[202] Forhead AJ, Li J, Gilmour RS, Fowden AL (1998) Control of Hepatic Insulin-Like Growth Factor Ii Gene Expression by Thyroid Hormones in Fetal Sheep near Term. Am. j. physiol. 275: E149-156.

[203] Carbone DL, Zuloaga DG, Hiroi R, Foradori CD, Legare ME, Handa RJ (2012) Prenatal Dexamethasone Exposure Potentiates Diet-Induced Hepatosteatosis and Decreases Plasma IGF-I in a Sex-Specific Fashion. Endocrinology. 153: 295-306.

[204] Cianfarani S, Germani D, Branca F (1999) Low Birthweight and Adult Insulin Resistance: The "Catch-up Growth" Hypothesis. Arch. dis. child. fetal. neonatal ed. 81: F71-73.

[205] Manojlović-Stojanoski M, Nestorović N, Ristić N, Trifunović S, Filipović B, Šošic-Jurjević B, Sekulić M (2010) Unbiased Stereological Estimation of the Rat Fetal Pituitary Volume and of the Total Number and Volume of Tsh Cells after Maternal Dexamethasone Application. Microsc. res. tech. 73: 1077-1085.

[206] Forhead AJ, Jellyman JK, Gardner DS, Giussani DA, Kaptein E, Visser TJ, Fowden AL (2007) Differential Effects of Maternal Dexamethasone Treatment on Circulating Thyroid Hormone Concentrations and Tissue Deiodinase Activity in the Pregnant Ewe and Fetus. Endocrinology. 148: 800-805.

[207] Van der Geyten S, Darras VM (2005) Developmentally Defined Regulation of Thyroid Hormone Metabolism by Glucocorticoids in the Rat. J. endocrinol. 185: 327-336.

[208] Oberkotter LV, Rasmussen KM (1992) Changes in Plasma Thyroid Hormone Concentrations in Chronically Food-Restricted Female Rats and Their Offspring During Suckling. J. nutr. 122: 435-441.

[209] Slone-Wilcoxon J, Redei EE (2004) Maternal-Fetal Glucocorticoid Milieu Programs Hypothalamic-Pituitary-Thyroid Function of Adult Offspring. Endocrinology. 145: 4068-4072.

[210] Pracyk JB, Seidler FJ, McCook EC, Slotkin TA (1992) Pituitary-Thyroid Axis Reactivity to Hyper- and Hypothyroidism in the Perinatal Period: Ontogeny of Regulation of Regulation and Long-Term Programming of Responses. J. dev. physiol. 18: 105-109.

[211] Fowden AL, Silver M (1995) The Effects of Thyroid Hormones on Oxygen and Glucose Metabolism in the Sheep Fetus During Late Gestation. J. physiol. 482 (Pt 1): 203-213.

[212] Mansourian AR (2011) A Review on the Metabolic Disorders of Iodine Deficiency. Pak. j. biol. sci. 14: 412-424.

[213] Xita N, Tsatsoulis A (2010) Fetal Origins of the Metabolic Syndrome. Ann. NY acad. sci. 1205: 148-155.

[214] Schwitzgebel VM, Somm E, Klee P (2009) Modeling Intrauterine Growth Retardation in Rodents: Impact on Pancreas Development and Glucose Homeostasis. Mol. cell. endocrinol. 304: 78-83.

[215] Dumortier O, Blondeau B, Duvillie B, Reusens B, Breant B, Remacle C (2007) Different Mechanisms Operating During Different Critical Time-Windows Reduce Rat Fetal Beta Cell Mass Due to a Maternal Low-Protein or Low-Energy Diet. Diabetologia. 50: 2495-2503.

[216] Ranta F, Avram D, Berchtold S, Dufer M, Drews G, Lang F, Ullrich S (2006) Dexamethasone Induces Cell Death in Insulin-Secreting Cells, an Effect Reversed by Exendin-4. Diabetes. 55: 1380-1390.

[217] Blondeau B, Lesage J, Czernichow P, Dupouy JP, Breant B (2001) Glucocorticoids Impair Fetal Beta-Cell Development in Rats. Am. j. physiol. endocrinol. metab. 281: E592-599.

[218] Dumortier O, Theys N, Ahn MT, Remacle C, Reusens B (2011) Impairment of Rat Fetal Beta-Cell Development by Maternal Exposure to Dexamethasone During Different Time-Windows. PLoS One. 6: e25576.

[219] Shen CN, Seckl JR, Slack JM, Tosh D (2003) Glucocorticoids Suppress Beta-Cell Development and Induce Hepatic Metaplasia in Embryonic Pancreas. Biochem j. 375: 41-50.

[220] Zhou Q, Brown J, Kanarek A, Rajagopal J, Melton DA (2008) In Vivo Reprogramming of Adult Pancreatic Exocrine Cells to Beta-Cells. Nature. 455: 627-632.

[221] Ackermann AM, Gannon M (2007) Molecular Regulation of Pancreatic Beta-Cell Mass Development, Maintenance, and Expansion. J. mol. endocrinol. 38: 193-206.

[222] Vegiopoulos A, Herzig S (2007) Glucocorticoids, Metabolism and Metabolic Diseases. Mol. cell. endocrinol. 275: 43-61.

[223] Bjorntorp P (1991) Adipose Tissue Distribution and Function. Int. j. obes. 15 Suppl 2: 67-81.

[224] Whorwood CB, Firth KM, Budge H, Symonds ME (2001) Maternal Undernutrition During Early to Midgestation Programs Tissue-Specific Alterations in the Expression of

the Glucocorticoid Receptor, 11beta-Hydroxysteroid Dehydrogenase Isoforms, and Type 1 Angiotensin Ii Receptor in Neonatal Sheep. Endocrinology. 142: 2854-2864.

[225] Cleasby ME, Kelly PA, Walker BR, Seckl JR (2003) Programming of Rat Muscle and Fat Metabolism by in Utero Overexposure to Glucocorticoids. Endocrinology. 144: 999-1007.

[226] Fetita LS, Sobngwi E, Serradas P, Calvo F, Gautier JF (2006) Consequences of Fetal Exposure to Maternal Diabetes in Offspring. J. clin. endocrinol. metab. 91: 3718-3724.

[227] Liu Y, Nakagawa Y, Wang Y, Sakurai R, Tripathi PV, Lutfy K, Friedman TC (2005) Increased Glucocorticoid Receptor and 11{Beta}-Hydroxysteroid Dehydrogenase Type 1 Expression in Hepatocytes May Contribute to the Phenotype of Type 2 Diabetes in Db/Db Mice. Diabetes. 54: 32-40.

[228] Nyirenda MJ, Lindsay RS, Kenyon CJ, Burchell A, Seckl JR (1998) Glucocorticoid Exposure in Late Gestation Permanently Programs Rat Hepatic Phosphoenolpyruvate Carboxykinase and Glucocorticoid Receptor Expression and Causes Glucose Intolerance in Adult Offspring. J. Clin. Invest. 101: 2174-2181.

[229] Davies MJ, Norman RJ (2002) Programming and Reproductive Functioning. Trends. endocrinol. metab. 13: 386-392.

[230] Kalantaridou SN, Makrigiannakis A, Zoumakis E, Chrousos GP (2004) Stress and the Female Reproductive System. J. reprod. immunol. 62: 61-68.

[231] Gore AC, Attardi B, DeFranco DB (2006) Glucocorticoid Repression of the Reproductive Axis: Effects on Gnrh and Gonadotropin Subunit mRNA Levels. Mol. cell. endocrinol. 256: 40-48.

[232] Negić N, Nestorović N, Manojlović-Stojanoski M, Filipović B, Šošić-Jurjević B, Milosević V, Sekulić M (2006) Multiple Dexamethasone Treatment Affects Morphometric Parameters of Gonadotrophic Cells in Adult Female Rats. Folia histochem. cytobiol. 44: 87-92.

[233] Negić N, Nestorović N, Manojlović-Stojanoski M, Filipović B, Šošić-Jurjevic B, Trifunović S, Milosević V, Sekulić M (2007) Pregnancy and Dexamethasone: Effects on Morphometric Parameters of Gonadotropic Cells in Rats. Acta histochem. 109: 185-192.

[234] Tohei A, Kogo H (1999) Dexamethasone Increases Follicle-Stimulating Hormone Secretion Via Suppression of Inhibin in Rats. Eur. j. pharmacol. 386: 69-74.

[235] Yazawa H, Sasagawa I, Nakada T (2000) Apoptosis of Testicular Germ Cells Induced by Exogenous Glucocorticoid in Rats. Hum. reprod. 15: 1917-1920.

[236] Shishkina GT, Bykova TS (1989) [the Postnatal Development of the Genital System in Male Rats Following the Prenatal Administration of Corticosterone]. Ontogenez. 20: 431-434.

[237] Keshet GI, Weinstock M (1995) Maternal Naltrexone Prevents Morphological and Behavioral Alterations Induced in Rats by Prenatal Stress. Pharmacol. biochem. behav. 50: 413-419.

[238] Castellano JM, Bentsen AH, Sanchez-Garrido MA, Ruiz-Pino F, Romero M, Garcia-Galiano D, Aguilar E, Pinilla L, Dieguez C, Mikkelsen JD, Tena-Sempere M (2011) Early Metabolic Programming of Puberty Onset: Impact of Changes in Postnatal Feeding and Rearing Conditions on the Timing of Puberty and Development of the Hypothalamic Kisspeptin System. Endocrinology. 152: 3396-3408.

[239] Piffer RC, Garcia PC, Pereira OC (2009) Adult Partner Preference and Sexual Behavior of Male Rats Exposed Prenatally to Betamethasone. Physiol. behav. 98: 163-167.

[240] Zambrano E, Rodriguez-Gonzalez GL, Guzman C, Garcia-Becerra R, Boeck L, Diaz L, Menjivar M, Larrea F, Nathanielsz PW (2005) A Maternal Low Protein Diet During Pregnancy and Lactation in the Rat Impairs Male Reproductive Development. J. physiol. 563: 275-284.

[241] Guzman C, Cabrera R, Cardenas M, Larrea F, Nathanielsz PW, Zambrano E (2006) Protein Restriction During Fetal and Neonatal Development in the Rat Alters Reproductive Function and Accelerates Reproductive Ageing in Female Progeny. J. physiol. 572: 97-108.

[242] Leonhardt M, Lesage J, Croix D, Dutriez-Casteloot I, Beauvillain JC, Dupouy JP (2003) Effects of Perinatal Maternal Food Restriction on Pituitary-Gonadal Axis and Plasma Leptin Level in Rat Pup at Birth and Weaning and on Timing of Puberty. Biol. reprod. 68: 390-400.

[243] Rae MT, Kyle CE, Miller DW, Hammond AJ, Brooks AN, Rhind SM (2002) The Effects of Undernutrition, in Utero, on Reproductive Function in Adult Male and Female Sheep. Anim. reprod. sci. 72: 63-71.

[244] Iwasa T, Matsuzaki T, Murakami M, Fujisawa S, Kinouchi R, Gereltsetseg G, Kuwahara A, Yasui T, Irahara M (2010) Effects of Intrauterine Undernutrition on Hypothalamic Kiss1 Expression and the Timing of Puberty in Female Rats. J. physiol. 588: 821-829.

[245] Iwasa T, Matsuzaki T, Murakami M, Kinouchi R, Gereltsetseg G, Yamamoto S, Kuwahara A, Yasui T, Irahara M (2011) Delayed Puberty in Prenatally Glucocorticoid Administered Female Rats Occurs Independently of the Hypothalamic Kiss1-Kiss1r-Gnrh System. Int. j. dev. neurosci. 29: 183-188.

[246] Ristić N, Nestorović N, Manojlović-Stojanoski M, Filipović B, Šošić-Jurjević B, Milosević V, Sekulić M (2008) Maternal Dexamethasone Treatment Reduces Ovarian Follicle Number in Neonatal Rat Offspring. J. microsc. 232: 549-557.

[247] Smith JT, Waddell BJ (2000) Increased Fetal Glucocorticoid Exposure Delays Puberty Onset in Postnatal Life. Endocrinology. 141: 2422-2428.

[248] Gao HB, Tong MH, Hu YQ, Guo QS, Ge R, Hardy MP (2002) Glucocorticoid Induces Apoptosis in Rat Leydig Cells. Endocrinology. 143: 130-138.

[249] Evan GI, Brown L, Whyte M, Harrington E (1995) Apoptosis and the Cell Cycle. Curr. opin. cell. biol. 7: 825-834.

[250] King KL, Cidlowski JA (1998) Cell Cycle Regulation and Apoptosis. Annu. rev. physiol. 60: 601-617.

[251] Pedrana G, Sloboda DM, Perez W, Newnham JP, Bielli A, Martin GB (2008) Effects of Pre-Natal Glucocorticoids on Testicular Development in Sheep. Anat. histol. embryol. 37: 352-358.

[252] Nestorović N, Lovren M, Sekulić M, Filipović B, Milošević V (2001) Effects of Multiple Somatostatin Treatment on Rat Gonadotrophic Cells and Ovaries. Histochem. j. 33: 695-702.

[253] Milosević V, Nestorović N, Filipović B, Velkovski S, Startcević V (2004) Centrally Applied Somatostatin Influences Morphology of Pituitary Fsh Cells but Not Fsh Release. Gen physiol biophys. 23: 375-380.

[254] Nestorović N, Lovren M, Sekulić M, Negić N, Šošic-Jurjević B, Filipović B, Milošević V (2004) Chronic Somatostatin Treatment Affects Pituitary Gonadotrophs, Ovaries and Onset of Puberty in Rats. Life sci. 74: 1359-1373.

[255] Nestorović N, Lovren M, Sekulić M, Negić N, Šošić-Jurjević B, Manojlović-Stojanoski M, Filipović B, Milošević V (2004) Effects of Intracerebroventricularly Administered Octreotide on Gonadotrophic Cells in Female Rats. Jugoslov. med. biohem. 23.

[256] Nestorović N, Manojlović-Stojanoski M, Ristić N, Sekulić M, Šošić-Jurjević B, Filipović B, Milošević V (2008) Somatostatin-14 Influences Pituitary-Ovarian Axis in Peripubertal Rats. Histochem. cell. biol. 130: 699-708.

[257] Nestorović N, Ristić N, Manojlović-Stojanoski M, Šošić-Jurjevic B, Trifunović S, Savin S, Milošević V (2011) Somatostatin 14 Affects the Pituitary-Ovarian Axis in Infant Rats. Histol. histopathol. 26: 157-166.

Chapter 15

Sex-Specific Effects of Prenatal Glucocorticoids on Placental Development

Hayley Dickinson, Bree A. O'Connell, David W. Walker and Karen M. Moritz

Additional information is available at the end of the chapter

http://dx.doi.org/10.5772/50200

1. Introduction

The placenta, essential for normal fetal development by providing adequate nutrients to allow appropriate growth and maturation of the fetus in preparation for birth, is also a 'protective' barrier in the sense that it prevents entry into the fetal circulation of substances that are either toxic, or that drive fetal growth at inappropriate rates. An important aspect of this 'filtering' function of the placenta is limiting the entry of glucocorticoids of maternal origin into the fetal compartment. This is achieved by the presence of enzymes, transporters and receptors collectively termed the 'placental glucocorticoid barrier' [1-4].

Antenatal glucocorticoids are routinely administered to the mother for the treatment of a variety of pregnancy and fetal complications. Asthmatic women often experience an increase in severity of their symptoms during pregnancy leading to increased use of glucocorticoids. The threat of preterm birth results in administration of the synthetic glucocorticoid, betamethasone, to rapidly mature fetal organs (especially, the lungs) to promote survival. Further, stressful events during pregnancy such as natural disasters and famines for example, expose fetuses to higher than normal levels of maternally secreted glucocorticoids.

The effects of exposure to high levels of glucocorticoids during fetal development have now been well described [1, 5-9], and the advantages (e.g., maturation of lung surfactant production and increased hepatic glycogen deposition) are offset by effects that limit fetal growth and induce perturbations of brain growth and perfusion [1, 10-11]. However, while fetal/neonatal effects have been intensively investigated, the consequences of glucocorticoid excess on placental structure and function has received little attention to date. The knowledge that male fetuses are more likely to be affected negatively following events that usually increase fetal glucocorticoid exposure, has alerted researchers to the possibility that such sex-related effects could arise in the placenta. This chapter will describe the differences that exist between a male and female placenta with respect to the glucocorticoid barrier, and summarise current human clinical and experimental animal work that has explored the differential response of the placenta of a male and female fetus to glucocorticoid exposure.

2. The placental glucocorticoid barrier

While glucocorticoids are essential for the development of many organs, during pregnancy, the placenta acts as a barrier to prevent excess entry of maternal glucocorticoids into the fetal compartment [12-14]. This placental barrier to glucocorticoids is achieved predominantly by the presence of 11β-hydroxysteriod dehydrogenase type 2 (11βHSD2), which converts the biologically active glucocorticoid (cortisol in humans, corticosterone in mice and rats) to its physiologically inert form [2]. The placental 'barrier' is not complete, and under normal conditions a proportion (~10-15%) of maternal glucocorticoids reaches the fetal circulation [2]. While 11βHSD2 is the major component of the placental glucocorticoid barrier, other proteins contained within the placenta may also help to limit the transfer of maternal glucocorticoid to the fetus. The multi-drug resistance P-glycoprotein (ABCB1) is a membrane-bound protein, which mediates the efflux of glucocorticoids out of the placenta back into the maternal circulation, thus reducing the amount of glucocorticoids able to diffuse down the concentration gradient into the fetal circulation [15-17].

The response of the placenta itself to glucocorticoids is mediated by the glucocorticoid (GR) and mineralocorticoid receptor [18]. The most prominent isoform of the GR, both in the placenta and throughout the whole body, is GRα. This isoform mediates the biological effects of glucocorticoids, which include cell growth, proliferation and differentiation [19]. The placenta has not generally been considered a mineralocorticoid target tissue, however work by Driver et al [20] has suggested that placental trophoblast cells express a functional mineralocorticoid receptor, which is in part responsible for the transport of sodium across the placenta [20]. Because of the limited data on the role of the mineralocorticoid receptor in the placenta, our discussion will focus primarily on GR mediated effects.

3. Causes of elevated glucocorticoids during pregnancy

There are many circumstances during pregnancy in which the circulating levels of maternal glucocorticoids are elevated, resulting in placental and fetal exposure to excess glucocorticoids. The glucocorticoids within the maternal system can either be endogenous, originating from within the mother; or exogenous, where the glucocorticoid has been administered to the mother as a drug or treatment. Exogenous glucocorticoids are generally synthetic, such as betamethasone, dexamethasone or prednisone. The period of time when maternal, and therefore fetal and placental glucocorticoid levels, are elevated will vary considerably depending on the clinical circumstance, and effects arising from either acute or chronic exposures have been identified. Thus, the type of glucocorticoid, duration of exposure, and time in gestation need to be taken into account when determining the consequences for the fetus and placenta.

3.1. Exposure to natural glucocorticoids

Periods of stress, both physical (illness, excess exercise, famine/under nutrition) or psychological (anxiety) in origin, result in the elevation of endogenous glucocorticoids [21]. While cortisol can cross the placenta, it is a good substrate for 11βHSD2, and is readily catalysed by this enzyme under normal levels. However, when levels of cortisol are elevated, the barrier is overwhelmed and more cortisol is able to cross the placenta into the fetal circulation [4]. Deleterious effects of excess endogenous glucocorticoids on the fetus and newborn have been well documented [3, 6, 22-25]. These effects are greater for male fetuses. For example, males have been shown to have greater instances of *in utero* mortality and also increased likelihood of childhood and adult morbidity and mortality [21, 26]. An epidemiology study that examined women who were pregnant at the time of the 2001 terrorist attacks on the World Trade Centre found that there was a higher incidence of low birth weight babies for women who were residing in New York at the time. The greatest proportion of these low birth weight babies came from women who were in their first or second trimester at the time of the attacks [27]. These studies also revealed an increased incidence of male fetal death in New York after September 2001 [28-29]. High maternal stress and thus fetal exposure of cortisol are thought to be the cause of these poor fetal outcomes.

3.2. Exposure to synthetic glucocorticoids

Antenatal glucocorticoids are routinely administered to the mother for the treatment of a variety of pregnancy and fetal complications. Women who suffer from asthma are required to continue their glucocorticoid medication for the ongoing treatment/prevention of their symptoms, which in 33% of cases worsen during pregnancy [30-31]. Women whose babies are at risk of congenital adrenal hyperplasia are administered antenatal glucocorticoid treatment to return fetal adrenal hormone levels to normal and thus virilisation (the abnormal development of male sexual characteristics in a female) and fertility problems are prevented [32]. Further, pregnant mothers threatening preterm birth (~7-10% of all pregnancies), receive antenatal glucocorticoids, to mature the lungs of the fetus prior to birth to reduce neonatal morbidity and mortality [25]. As for cortisol, synthetic glucocorticoids can be catalysed by 11βHSD2, however they are a poor substrate for the enzyme, and more freely cross the placenta than cortisol [33]. The presence of excess maternal glucocorticoids can have positive effects on fetal development and maternal health and in many situations cannot be avoided. The National Institute of Health recommend treatment of all women at risk of preterm delivery, between 24 and 34 weeks of gestation, with synthetic glucocorticoids to prematurely mature fetal organs, primarily the lung, to improve neonatal survival [8]. Therefore a large proportion of this population of babies, are exposed to single, and sometimes multiple courses of synthetic glucocorticoids in the period leading up to birth [25]. While antenatal glucocorticoids are the most effective treatment for improving preterm birth survival rates, the scientific community continues to question whether the use of glucocorticoids to reduce the morbidity and mortality associated with preterm birth, is worth the risk of the potential negative outcomes on metabolism and neurodevelopment seen within these babies during childhood and into adulthood [9]. While the consensus is currently 'yes', the guidelines for women threatening preterm birth state that only a single, and not multiple doses of glucocorticoids, should be given until more convincing data of the benefits of multiple doses are obtained [34]. Much work is examining the outcomes of antenatal glucocorticoids for the fetus, however the effect of glucocorticoids on the placenta, including the potential sex-specific effects, need to be considered as these may contribute to, or compound, the fetal outcomes.

4. Excess glucocorticoids and the programming of disease

The Barker Hypothesis of Developmental Origins of Health and Disease (DoHaD) states that diseases, such as coronary heart disease, hypertension and diabetes, may be consequences of *in utero* 'programming', whereby a stimulus or insult at a critical, sensitive 'window' of fetal life results in long-term changes in structure, physiology or metabolism, leading to diseases later in life [35]. These stimuli are likely to be mediated via a number of different hormones and immune factors, but glucocorticoids have been singled out as one of the most prevalent factors. Epidemiological and experimental animal studies have revealed that excess glucocorticoids *in utero* can be linked to the development of diseases such as hypertension [36-42], depression [43], cardiovascular disease [44], diabetes [45-46] and attention deficit disorders [23, 47]. Further, the outcomes or the severity of these diseases are worse if the offspring affected are male [37-39, 48-51].

Recently, a role for the placenta in mediating developmental programming of excess glucocorticoids and other *in utero* events has been suggested [44, 47, 52-55]. The size (both absolute and relative to fetal size), shape, and vascular development of the placenta have all been identified as potential predictors of adult onset diseases. For instance, a small baby with a large placenta has a relative risk of adult hypertension 3 times that of a large baby with a normal placental size [44]. Further, the abolition of a gene vital for placental, but not cardiac vascular development (*HOXA13*) has been shown to be embryonic lethal in mice, indicating that placental hemodynamics play an important role in the development of the heart, and alterations may lead to the development of cardiovascular problems later in life [56].

5. Susceptibility of the placenta to negative outcomes from glucocorticoid exposure

There are several reasons for the susceptible of the placenta to adverse outcomes caused by excess glucocorticoid exposure. I.) The placenta is in direct contact with the maternal circulation and thus is directly bathed in circulating maternal glucocorticoids. II.) One of the main roles of the placenta, as described above, is as a barrier to prevent fetal exposure to excess glucocorticoids; therefore the placenta may be directly altered by the glucocorticoid exposure *before* 11βHSD2 is able to convert these to their inactive metabolites [57]. III.) The structural development of the placenta occurs through a series of branching events, particularly the placental vasculature. This branching occurs similarly in other organs, such as the lung and kidney, which are particularly vulnerable to excess glucocorticoid exposure during periods of extensive branching [58-60]. Indeed in the evolution of the placenta, the genetic pathways that regulate branching morphogenesis in these other organs has been utilised by the placenta [61-65]. Hence a similar susceptibility could be expected for the placenta.

6. Sex-specific placental regulation of glucocorticoids

The placental is primarily derived from embryonic tissue and therefore has the same genetic content as the fetus. In recent studies examining both human and animal models, a number of fundamental differences between the placenta of a male and female fetus have been uncovered. Differences in placental proportions [66] and surface area [67] have been noted in placentas of males and females. Specifically, females have been shown to have a greater exchange region of the placenta compared to males [66], and within this exchange region, females have been reported to have a larger surface area [67]. Expression of genes and proteins known to have fundamental roles in controlling placental development [66], nutrient transfer, and other placental functions [68-71] differ between a male and female placenta. Specifically, placentas of male fetuses have been reported to have higher levels of the glucose transporter [66], higher levels of epidermal growth factor binding protein at term [68], but lower levels of activity of the sodium-hydrogen exchanger [70]. Levels of pregnancy hormones, produced by the placenta, differ for a male and female. For example, maternal serum human chorionic gonadotrophin levels are significantly higher in pregnancies carrying a female fetus from as early as 3 weeks of pregnancy [72]. Placental levels of progesterone also differ for a male and female fetus in many species, with a study in the gray seal, for example, showing higher levels in females than males [73]. Because progesterone is primarily of placental origin, these differences provide further evidence of the fundamental differences that exist in the placenta of a male and female fetus. Further, the placenta of a male and female fetus have also been shown to respond differently to adverse *in utero* environments including maternal under-nutrition/famine [74] and *in utero* infection [75]. For example, female placentas demonstrated more striking alterations in gene expression in response to restrictions in maternal diet than male placentas when examined by microarray analysis. Further, placentas of male fetuses exhibited a greater immunologicial reaction (greater expression of TNFa, IL-10, and PTGS2) to simulated *in utero* infection. Whether these responses differ because of the fundamental differences that exist between the sexes remains unknown.

Normal physiological glucocorticoid levels: During pregnancy, the term female placenta has significantly higher expression of the GR [31] and 11βHSD2 activity [76] than placentas of male fetuses. Glucocorticoids are known to negatively regulate GR expression [66, 77], therefore the higher GR expression within placentas of female fetuses may be physiological evidence that the female fetal–placental unit is exposed to less bioactive cortisol at term than the male. A downstream consequence of lower glucocorticoid levels may be an enhanced immune response. The activation of the fetal immune system is associated with the activation of the fetal hypothalamic pituitary adrenal axis, which results in the production of glucocorticoids, which in turn modulate the inflammatory response. Glucocorticoids function in a negative feedback loop with the hypothalamic pituitary adrenal axis, such that high glucocorticoid levels suppressing immune function [78]. It has been suggested that this may contribute to the increased viability of female fetuses exposed to a sub-optimal *in utero* environment, compared to males, who are particularly vulnerable to changes in the maternal environment in which increased levels of glucocorticoids are often seen [79] (see above).

Response to excess glucocorticoids: The adverse effects of glucocorticoids during pregnancy on placental weight in the human have been reported as early as 1977 by Koppe and others [80]. Since then, a number of studies, in both humans and animal models, have demonstrated that excess glucocorticoids during gestation have a wide range of consequences for the placenta, which impact its structure and function, ultimately impacting the fetus [22, 81-91]. Recently, these consequences have been shown to occur in a sex-specific manner.

Human evidence

Evidence is beginning to emerge from studies in the clinical setting demonstrating that human placentas are sexually dimorphic in their regulation of normal glucocorticoid levels and these differences are exacerbated in response to excess maternal glucocorticoids. Much of this clinical evidence is arising from the work of Clifton and colleagues, who focus on identifying the effect of glucocorticoids on fetal and placental development, by studying mothers who suffer from asthma and thus use inhaled glucocorticoid treatments throughout their pregnancy. Asthma affects between 3% and 12% of pregnant women worldwide and the prevalence among pregnant women is rising [92]. It is well recognised that women (and their babies) with asthma are at increased risk of poor pregnancy outcomes [93]. Clifton and colleagues have also examined preterm babies and the consequences of excess glucocorticoid exposure on their placentas.

6.1. Effect of glucocorticoids on placental development and other pathways

Female babies born to asthmatic mothers, who utilised inhaled glucocorticoid treatments to manage their symptoms, were found to be growth-reduced unlike male babies born to asthmatic mothers, who were normally grown, despite similar cord blood cortisol levels [76]. Placentas of male and female babies born to these mothers, had reduced vascularisation within the placental villi, resulting in reduced absolute fetal capillary volume [94], although this was most striking in placentas of male fetuses. Further, placentas of glucocorticoid-exposed males also had a reduced fetal capillary length [94], which was not observed in placentas of female fetuses. The authors speculate that glucocorticoid treatment may adversely affect placental vasculogenesis and/or angiogenesis by causing endothelial cell rounding and capillary regression, an observation made in other tissues after glucocorticoid exposure [95-97]. These effects may be mediated by members of the vascular endothelial growth factor family or inflammatory cytokines, both of which play a key role in placental vasculogenesis and angiogenesis [98]. The observed changes in placental morphometry in male placentas would be expected to affect placental heamodynamics, however the absence of these changes in the female placenta do not adequately explain the reduced fetal growth of the female fetus in this high glucocorticoid environment.

A study by Stark et al [99], examined the placental pro-: anti-oxidant balance in response to antenatal betamethasone in placentas of preterm babies. Glucocorticoids have previously been shown to influence fetal reactive oxygen species production and antioxidant defences [100-101]. These pathways are involved in preparing the fetus for the increase in free oxygen radical generation which is experienced during the fetal to neonatal transition [102]. Stark and colleagues observed that a pro-oxidant state was present in placentas of male fetuses, but not females following glucocorticoid exposure. Specifically, they reported that males had higher levels of the oxidative stress marker, protein carbonyl and a decreased level of the anti-oxidant enzyme, glutathione peroxidase. The authors suggested that these findings could contribute to the patho-physiologic processes underlying oxygen radical diseases of the newborn [99]; conditions known to exhibit a male excess [103].

6.2. Sex-specific effects of excess glucocorticoids on the placental glucocorticoid barrier

As the placental glucocorticoid barrier demonstrates sexually dimorphic regulation under normal conditions, and the placental response to glucocorticoids is crucial in determining fetal growth outcomes, the effect of excess maternal glucocorticoids on this barrier have been investigated. The expression of the GR within the placenta of male and female fetuses is reported to be sexually dimorphic under normal conditions (females having higher expression levels), whereas the response of GR to excess glucocorticoids is similar between the sexes [77].

In preterm babies, whose mothers received antenatal betamethasone, the activity of placental 11βHSD2 (predominant component of the glucocorticoid barrier) was reduced in placentas of male fetuses only [104]. This reduction in 11βHSD2 activity would be expected to compound the already increased exposure of the male fetus to cortisol brought about by the decreased term 11βHSD2 activity within male placentas during a normal pregnancy [76]. This may further compound the reduced immune function in male fetuses, thus increasing their susceptibility to disease. Further, glucocorticoids are important for fetal adrenal development [104]. Male preterm babies exposed to excess glucocorticoids *in utero*, have less adrenal activity than female preterm babies exposed to similar levels of glucocorticoids [104], which may explain the increased risk of morbidity and mortality of preterm male babies. We are unaware of any studies that have investigated the other members of the placental glucocorticoid barrier (MR and ABCB1) and their sexually dimorphic response to excess glucocorticoid exposure.

Animal models of glucocorticoid exposure

The effects of excess maternal glucocorticoid exposure, on placental growth and development, has been investigated using a range of animal models including the sheep [105-106], rat [85], mouse [107] and spiny mouse [66]. Most of these studies have utilised synthetic glucocorticoids (namely dexamethasone or betamethasone) and been designed to mimic the level of exposure experienced by the preterm infant. However, there are also a large number of studies using glucocorticoids at other developmental time points including very early in gestation. When considering the data generated from animal models, it is important to take into consideration not only the timing of glucocorticoid exposure but also the timing of placental and fetal development in the species being used, as there is considerable variation in placental development and overall structure between species. Many of these studies, particularly those in the sheep and rat, have not analysed data according to fetal sex. However a couple of recent studies in the mouse and spiny mouse have demonstrated markedly different outcomes in placental development and gene expression in placentas of males and females suggesting that alterations occurring within the placenta, following glucocorticoid exposure, are dependent upon fetal sex.

Sheep

The sheep placenta is made up of 60-70 individual placentomes called cotyledons, which are cup shaped structures with fetal tissue surrounded by maternal tissue. Administration of dexamethasone for 48 hours between 64-66 days of gestation (term=145-150 days) resulted in generally larger cotyledons with overgrowth of the fetal tissue when the placenta was examined at completion of the infusion [105]. However, this was not observed in other studies using betamethasone later in gestation (around 100 days of gestation) [108]. Unfortunately, neither of these studies separated data according to fetal sex. In another study, pregnant ewes received intramuscular injections of dexamethasone on day 40 and 41 of gestation and the placentas were examined at day 50, 100 or 140 days of gestation. In this case, data was analysed separately for males and females and whilst dexamethasone exposure significantly increased placental *11βHSD2* mRNA levels in males compared with controls at 50 and 140 days, in female placentas, levels were not altered by the dexamethasone exposure [106].

Rat

Dexamethasone exposure during late pregnancy has been shown to significantly reduce placental weight in the rat [91, 109]. This was associated with reduced expression of vascular endothelial growth factors (*VEGF*) and placental vascularisation [91] along with altered insulin like growth factor II expression. Neither of these studies looked at sex-specific effects.

Mouse

Given the extensive use of the mouse for development studies, it is somewhat surprising that there has been little research of the effects of glucocorticoids on the mouse placenta. We have recently shown that dexamethasone exposure for 2 days around mid-gestation (day 12.5-14.5 of gestation, term=20 days) caused decreases in fetal body weight at day 14.5, but placental weight was only reduced in placentas from female fetuses [107]. These changes in placental growth were associated with sex-specific changes in placental gene and protein expression: at day 14.5, the placentas from female fetuses had higher mRNA levels of expression of *11βHSD2* and *VEGF*, whilst protein levels of Mitogen-activated protein kinase were significantly reduced. By day 17.5, some 3, days after cessation of the dexamethasone, fetal and placental weights are restored but levels of 11βHSD2 protein are elevated in the placentas of female fetuses. These sex-specific changes in gene and protein levels were not present for nutrient transporters such as glucose transporter 1 and 3 or the major amino acid transports [107].

Spiny mouse

We have also utilised a precocial rodent, the spiny mouse (*Acomys cahirinus*), in which the natural circulating glucocorticoid is cortisol, not corticosterone like other rodents [110], to explore sex-specific effects of glucocorticoids on the placenta. O'Connell et al [66] examined the immediate and long-term consequences of excess maternal glucocorticoids (dexamethasone) administered for a short time (60h) at mid-gestation (day 20, term is 39 days) on placental structure and gene expression. The immediate consequences of glucocorticoid administration were similar between male and female placentas. However, two-weeks post-treatment (day 37), the transcriptional and structural response of the placenta was dependent on the sex of the fetus. Placentas of male fetuses were found to have an increase in the expression of a gene involved in placental patterning, glial cell missing 1 gene; *GCM1*, but also decreases in the expression of the primary placental glucose transporter (solute carrier family 2 (facilitated glucose transporter), member 1; *SLC2A1*). Placentas of male fetuses also had decreased amounts of maternal blood sinusoids, which are involved in the drawing of nutrient poor blood away from the placenta and back into the maternal circulation. Placentas of female fetuses were observed to have increased glucose transporter expression, and an increased amount of maternal blood sinusoids, in other words, the response of a female placenta to excess glucocorticoids was opposite to that of a male. This study highlights that while the immediate response to excess glucocorticoids may be the same for both sexes in this species, these may persist or evolve within the placenta differently, depending on the sex of the fetus [66].

7. Significance

There is now a growing body of evidence to suggest that the placenta of a male and female differs and that this may underlie the greater vulnerability of males to stressors that occur during pregnancy. Here we provided evidence that the placental response to changes in maternal glucocorticoid status differs depending on the sex of the fetus and raises the important question: are differences in fetal outcomes driven by the fetus itself or the placenta. We suggest that the placenta should become an organ of greater interest to clinical obstetrics and perinatology, particularly with respect to how the placenta may function differently for a male and female fetus during periods of high glucocorticoid exposure.

With respect to the clinical use of glucocorticoids, the different response of a male and female to even a small dose of synthetic glucocorticoids must be followed up in a large clinical based study. At least from experimental data, the question has been raised, "Should the sex of the fetus be taken into consideration when synthetic glucocorticoids are administered during pregnancy"?

Author details

Hayley Dickinson*, Bree A. O'Connell and David W. Walker
The Ritchie Centre, Monash Institute of Medical Research, Monash University, Clayton, Australia

Karen M. Moritz
The University of Queensland, School of Biomedical Sciences, St Lucia, Australia

8. References

[1] Harris A, Seckl J (2011) Glucocorticoids, prenatal stress and the programming of disease. Horm Behav; 59:279-89.

[2] Benediktsson R, Calder AA, Edwards CR, Seckl JR (1997) Placental 11 beta-hydroxysteroid dehydrogenase: a key regulator of fetal glucocorticoid exposure. Clin Endocrinol (Oxf); 46:161-6.

[3] Seckl JR (1997) Glucocorticoids, feto-placental 11 beta-hydroxysteroid dehydrogenase type 2, and the early life origins of adult disease. Steroids; 62:89-94.

[4] Seckl JR, Holmes MC (2007) Mechanisms of disease: glucocorticoids, their placental metabolism and fetal 'programming' of adult pathophysiology. Nat Clin Pract Endocrinol Metab; 3:479-88.

[5] Michael AE, Papageorghiou AT (2008) Potential significance of physiological and pharmacological glucocorticoids in early pregnancy. Hum Reprod Update; 14:497-517.

[6] Ortiz LA, Quan A, Weinberg A, Baum M (2001) Effect of prenatal dexamethasone on rat renal development. Kidney Int; 59:1663-9.

[7] Sawady J, Mercer BM, Wapner RJ, Zhao Y, Sorokin Y, Johnson F, et al. (2007) The National Institute of Child Health and Human Development Maternal-Fetal Medicine Units Network Beneficial Effects of Antenatal Repeated Steroids study: impact of repeated doses of antenatal corticosteroids on placental growth and histologic findings. Am J Obstet Gynecol; 197:281 e1-8.

[8] (1995) Effect of corticosteroids for fetal maturation on perinatal outcomes. NIH Consensus Development Panel on the Effect of Corticosteroids for Fetal Maturation on Perinatal Outcomes. JAMA; 273:413-8.

[9] Vos AA, Bruinse HW (2010) Congenital adrenal hyperplasia: do the benefits of prenatal treatment defeat the risks? Obstet Gynecol Surv; 65:196-205.

[10] Wintour EM, Johnson K, Koukoulas I, Moritz K, Tersteeg M, Dodic M (2003) Programming the cardiovascular system, kidney and the brain--a review. Placenta; 24 Suppl A:S65-71.

[11] Uno H, Eisele S, Sakai A, Shelton S, Baker E, DeJesus O, et al. (1994) Neurotoxicity of glucocorticoids in the primate brain. Horm Behav; 28:336-48.

[12] Yang K (1997) Placental 11 beta-hydroxysteroid dehydrogenase: barrier to maternal glucocorticoids. Rev Reprod; 2:129-32.

---

* Corresponding Author

[13] Pepe GJ, Burch MG, Albrecht ED (1999) Expression of the 11beta-hydroxysteroid dehydrogenase types 1 and 2 proteins in human and baboon placental syncytiotrophoblast. Placenta; 20:575-82.

[14] Burton PJ, Waddell BJ (1999) Dual function of 11beta-hydroxysteroid dehydrogenase in placenta: modulating placental glucocorticoid passage and local steroid action. Biol Reprod; 60:234-40.

[15] Parry S, Zhang J (2007) Multidrug resistance proteins affect drug transmission across the placenta. Am J Obstet Gynecol; 196:476 e1-6.

[16] Mark PJ, Waddell BJ (2006) P-glycoprotein restricts access of cortisol and dexamethasone to the glucocorticoid receptor in placental BeWo cells. Endocrinology; 147:5147-52.

[17] Kalabis GM, Kostaki A, Andrews MH, Petropoulos S, Gibb W, Matthews SG (2005) Multidrug resistance phosphoglycoprotein (ABCB1) in the mouse placenta: fetal protection. Biol Reprod; 73:591-7.

[18] Driver PM, Kilby MD, Bujalska I, Walker EA, Hewison M, Stewart PM (2001) Expression of 11 beta-hydroxysteroid dehydrogenase isozymes and corticosteroid hormone receptors in primary cultures of human trophoblast and placental bed biopsies. Mol Hum Reprod; 7:357-63.

[19] Pujols L, Mullol J, Torrego A, Picado C (2004) Glucocorticoid receptors in human airways. Allergy; 59:1042-52.

[20] Driver PM, Rauz S, Walker EA, Hewison M, Kilby MD, Stewart PM (2003) Characterization of human trophoblast as a mineralocorticoid target tissue. Mol Hum Reprod; 9:793-8.

[21] Dickinson H, Wintour EM (2007) Can Life Before Birth Affect Health Ever After? Current Women's Health Reviews; 3:79-88.

[22] Sun K, Yang K, Challis JR (1998) Glucocorticoid actions and metabolism in pregnancy: implications for placental function and fetal cardiovascular activity. Placenta; 19:353-60.

[23] Kapoor A, Petropoulos S, Matthews SG (2008) Fetal programming of hypothalamic-pituitary-adrenal (HPA) axis function and behavior by synthetic glucocorticoids. Brain Res Rev; 57:586-95.

[24] Davis EP, Waffarn F, Sandman CA (2011) Prenatal treatment with glucocorticoids sensitizes the hpa axis response to stress among full-term infants. Dev Psychobiol; 53:175-83.

[25] Matthews SG, Owen D, Kalabis G, Banjanin S, Setiawan EB, Dunn EA, et al. (2004) Fetal glucocorticoid exposure and hypothalamo-pituitary-adrenal (HPA) function after birth. Endocr Res; 30:827-36.

[26] Moritz KM, Cuffe JS, Wilson LB, Dickinson H, Wlodek ME, Simmons DG, et al. (2010) Review: Sex specific programming: a critical role for the renal renin-angiotensin system. Placenta; 31 Suppl:S40-6.

[27] Eskenazi B, Marks AR, Catalano R, Bruckner T, Toniolo PG (2007) Low birthweight in New York City and upstate New York following the events of September 11th. Hum Reprod; 22:3013-20.

[28] Catalano R, Bruckner T, Gould J, Eskenazi B, Anderson E (2005) Sex ratios in California following the terrorist attacks of September 11, 2001. Hum Reprod; 20:1221-7.

[29] Catalano R, Bruckner T, Marks AR, Eskenazi B (2006) Exogenous shocks to the human sex ratio: the case of September 11, 2001 in New York City. Hum Reprod; 21:3127-31.
[30] Murphy VE, Clifton VL, Gibson PG (2006) Asthma exacerbations during pregnancy: incidence and association with adverse pregnancy outcomes. Thorax; 61:169-76.
[31] Clifton VL, Murphy VE (2004) Maternal asthma as a model for examining fetal sex-specific effects on maternal physiology and placental mechanisms that regulate human fetal growth. Placenta; 25 Suppl A:S45-52.
[32] Forest MG (2004) Recent advances in the diagnosis and management of congenital adrenal hyperplasia due to 21-hydroxylase deficiency. Hum Reprod Update; 10:469-85.
[33] Quinkler M, Oelkers W, Diederich S (2001) Clinical implications of glucocorticoid metabolism by 11beta-hydroxysteroid dehydrogenases in target tissues. Eur J Endocrinol; 144:87-97.
[34]Miracle X, Di Renzo GC, Stark A, Fanaroff A, Carbonell-Estrany X, Saling E (2008) Guideline for the use of antenatal corticosteroids for fetal maturation. J Perinat Med; 36:191-6.
[35] Barker DJ, Clark PM (1997) Fetal undernutrition and disease in later life. Rev Reprod; 2:105-12.
[36] Wintour EM, Moritz KM, Johnson K, Ricardo S, Samuel CS, Dodic M (2003) Reduced nephron number in adult sheep, hypertensive as a result of prenatal glucocorticoid treatment. J Physiol (Lond); 549:929-35.
[37] Bertram C, Khan O, Ohri S, Phillips DI, Matthews SG, Hanson MA (2008) Transgenerational effects of prenatal nutrient restriction on cardiovascular and hypothalamic-pituitary-adrenal function. J Physiol; 586:2217-29.
[38] Bertram C, Trowern AR, Copin N, Jackson AA, Whorwood CB (2001) The maternal diet during pregnancy programs altered expression of the glucocorticoid receptor and type 2 11beta-hydroxysteroid dehydrogenase: potential molecular mechanisms underlying the programming of hypertension in utero. Endocrinology; 142:2841-53.
[39] Woods LL, Ingelfinger JR, Nyengaard JR, Rasch R (2001) Maternal protein restriction suppresses the newborn renin-angiotensin system and programs adult hypertension in rats. Pediatr Res; 49:460-7.
[40] Kwong WY, Wild AE, Roberts P, Willis AC, Fleming TP (2000) Maternal undernutrition during the preimplantation period of rat development causes blastocyst abnormalities and programming of postnatal hypertension. Development; 127:4195-202.
[41] Levitt NS, Lindsay RS, Holmes MC, Seckl JR (1996) Dexamethasone in the last week of pregnancy attenuates hippocampal glucocorticoid receptor gene expression and elevates blood pressure in the adult offspring in the rat. Neuroendocrinology; 64:412-8.
[42] Dodic M, Abouantoun T, O'Connor A, Wintour EM, Moritz KM (2002) Programming effects of short prenatal exposure to dexamethasone in sheep. Hypertension; 40:729-34.
[43] Murgatroyd C, Wu Y, Bockmuhl Y, Spengler D (2010) Genes learn from stress: How infantile trauma programs us for depression. Epigenetics; 5.
[44] Thornburg KL, O'Tierney PF, Louey S (2010) Review: The placenta is a programming agent for cardiovascular disease. Placenta; 31 Suppl:S54-9.
[45] Phillips DI, Barker DJ, Fall CH, Seckl JR, Whorwood CB, Wood PJ, et al. (1998) Elevated plasma cortisol concentrations: a link between low birth weight and the insulin resistance syndrome? J Clin Endocrinol Metab; 83:757-60.

[46] De Blasio MJ, Dodic M, Jefferies AJ, Moritz KM, Wintour EM, Owens JA (2007) Maternal exposure to dexamethasone or cortisol in early pregnancy differentially alters insulin secretion and glucose homeostasis in adult male sheep offspring. Am J Physiol Endocrinol Metabol; 293:E75-82.

[47] O'Donnell K, O'Connor TG, Glover V (2009) Prenatal stress and neurodevelopment of the child: focus on the HPA axis and role of the placenta. Dev Neurosci; 31:285-92.

[48] Shoener JA, Baig R, Page KC (2006) Prenatal exposure to dexamethasone alters hippocampal drive on hypothalamic-pituitary-adrenal axis activity in adult male rats. Am J Physiol Regul Integr Comp Physiol; 290:R1366-73.

[49] Mueller BR, Bale TL (2008) Sex-specific programming of offspring emotionality after stress early in pregnancy. J Neurosci; 28:9055-65.

[50] Woods LL, Ingelfinger JR, Rasch R (2005) Modest maternal protein restriction fails to program adult hypertension in female rats. Am J Physiol Regul Integr Comp Physiol; 289:R1131-6.

[51] Rodriguez JS, Zurcher NR, Keenan KE, Bartlett TQ, Nathanielsz PW, Nijland MJ (2011) Prenatal betamethasone exposure has sex specific effects in reversal learning and attention in juvenile baboons. Am J Obstet Gynecol; 204:545 e1- e10.

[52] Burton GJ, Fowden AL (2012) Review: The placenta and developmental programming: Balancing fetal nutrient demands with maternal resource allocation. Placenta; 33 Suppl:S23-7.

[53] Illsley NP, Caniggia I, Zamudio S (2010) Placental metabolic reprogramming: do changes in the mix of energy-generating substrates modulate fetal growth? Int J Dev Biol; 54:409-19.

[54] Godfrey KM (2002) The role of the placenta in fetal programming-a review. Placenta; 23 Suppl A:S20-7.

[55] Fowden AL, Forhead AJ, Coan PM, Burton GJ (2008) The placenta and intrauterine programming. J Neuroendocrinol; 20:439-50.

[56] Shaut CA, Keene DR, Sorensen LK, Li DY, Stadler HS (2008) HOXA13 Is essential for placental vascular patterning and labyrinth endothelial specification. PLoS Genet; 4:e1000073.

[57] Murphy VE, Fittock RJ, Zarzycki PK, Delahunty MM, Smith R, Clifton VL (2007) Metabolism of synthetic steroids by the human placenta. Placenta; 28:39-46.

[58] Dickinson H, Walker DW, Wintour EM, Moritz K (2007) Maternal dexamethasone treatment at midgestation reduces nephron number and alters renal gene expression in the fetal spiny mouse. Am J Physiol Regul Integr Comp Physiol; 292:R453-61.

[59] Oshika E, Liu S, Ung LP, Singh G, Shinozuka H, Michalopoulos GK, et al. (1998) Glucocorticoid-induced effects on pattern formation and epithelial cell differentiation in early embryonic rat lungs. Pediatr Res; 43:305-14.

[60] Bolkenius U, Hahn D, Gressner AM, Breitkopf K, Dooley S, Wickert L (2004) Glucocorticoids decrease the bioavailability of TGF-beta which leads to a reduced TGF-beta signaling in hepatic stellate cells. Biochem Biophys Res Commun; 325:1264-70.

[61] Cross JC, Baczyk D, Dobric N, Hemberger M, Hughes M, Simmons DG, et al. (2003) Genes, development and evolution of the placenta. Placenta; 24:123-30.

[62] Cross JC (2000) Genetic insights into trophoblast differentiation and placental morphogenesis. Semin Cell Dev Biol; 11:105-13.

[63] Rossant J, Cross JC (2001) Placental development: lessons from mouse mutants. Nat Rev Genet; 2:538-48.
[64] Mess A, Carter AM (2007) Evolution of the placenta during the early radiation of placental mammals. Comparative Biochemistry and Physiology - Part A: Molecular & Integrative Physiology; 148:769-79.
[65] Cross JC, Nakano H, Natale DR, Simmons DG, Watson ED (2006) Branching morphogenesis during development of placental villi. Differentiation; 74:393-401.
[66] O'Connell BA, Moritz KM, Roberts CT, Walker DW, Dickinson H (2011) The placental response to excess maternal glucocorticoid exposure differs between the male and female conceptus in spiny mice. Biol Reprod; 85:1040-7.
[67] Grbesa D, Durst-Zivkovic B (1989) The surface of the syncytiotrophoblast in the human placenta at term in relation to the sex of the neonate. Jugosl Ginekol Perinatol; 29:169-71.
[68] Brown MJ, Cook CL, Henry JL, Schultz GS (1987) Levels of epidermal growth factor binding in third-trimester and term human placentas: elevated binding in term placentas of male fetuses. Am J Obstet Gynecol; 156:716-20.
[69] Cleal JK, Day PL, Hanson MA, Lewis RM (2010) Sex differences in the mRNA levels of housekeeping genes in human placenta. Placenta; 31:556-7.
[70] Speake PF, Glazier JD, Greenwood SL, Sibley CP (2010) Aldosterone and cortisol acutely stimulate Na+/H+ exchanger activity in the syncytiotrophoblast of the human placenta: effect of fetal sex. Placenta; 31:289-94.
[71] Haning RV, Jr., Breault PH, DeSilva MV, Hackett RJ, Pouncey CL (1988) Effects of fetal sex, stage of gestation, dibutyryl cyclic adenosine monophosphate, and gonadotropin releasing hormone on secretion of human chorionic gonadotropin by placental explants in vitro. Am J Obstet Gynecol; 159:1332-7.
[72] Yaron Y, Lehavi O, Orr-Urtreger A, Gull I, Lessing JB, Amit A, et al. (2002) Maternal serum HCG is higher in the presence of a female fetus as early as week 3 post-fertilization. Hum Reprod; 17:485-9.
[73] Boyd I (1990) Mass and Hormone Content of Gray Seal Placentae Related to Fetal Sex. J Mammal; 71:101-3.
[74] Mao J, Zhang X, Sieli PT, Falduto MT, Torres KE, Rosenfeld CS (2010) Contrasting effects of different maternal diets on sexually dimorphic gene expression in the murine placenta. Proc Natl Acad Sci U S A; 107:5557-62.
[75] Yeganegi M, Watson CS, Martins A, Kim SO, Reid G, Challis JR, et al. (2009) Effect of Lactobacillus rhamnosus GR-1 supernatant and fetal sex on lipopolysaccharide-induced cytokine and prostaglandin-regulating enzymes in human placental trophoblast cells: implications for treatment of bacterial vaginosis and prevention of preterm labor. Am J Obstet Gynecol; 200:532 e1-8.
[76] Murphy VE, Gibson PG, Giles WB, Zakar T, Smith R, Bisits AM, et al. (2003) Maternal asthma is associated with reduced female fetal growth. Am J Respir Crit Care Med; 168:1317-23.
[77] Hodyl NA, Wyper H, Osei-Kumah A, Scott N, Murphy VE, Gibson P, et al. (2010) Sex-specific associations between cortisol and birth weight in pregnancies complicated by asthma are not due to differential glucocorticoid receptor expression. Thorax; 65:677-83.

[78] Dhabhar FS, McEwen BS (1997) Acute stress enhances while chronic stress suppresses cell-mediated immunity in vivo: a potential role for leukocyte trafficking. Brain Behav Immun; 11:286-306.

[79] Eriksson JG, Kajantie E, Osmond C, Thornburg K, Barker DJ (2010) Boys live dangerously in the womb. Am J Hum Biol; 22:330-5.

[80] Koppe JG, Smolders-de Haas H, Kloosterman GJ (1977) Effects of glucocorticoids during pregnancy on the outcome of the children directly after birth and in the long run. Eur J Obstet Gynecol Reprod Biol; 7:293-9.

[81] Clifton VL, Wallace EM, Smith R (2002) Short-term effects of glucocorticoids in the human fetal-placental circulation in vitro. J Clin Endocrinol Metab; 87:2838-42.

[82] Paakki P, Kirkinen P, Helin H, Pelkonen O, Raunio H, Pasanen M (2000) Antepartum glucocorticoid therapy suppresses human placental xenobiotic and steroid metabolizing enzymes. Placenta; 21:241-6.

[83] Mandl M, Ghaffari-Tabrizi N, Haas J, Nohammer G, Desoye G (2006) Differential glucocorticoid effects on proliferation and invasion of human trophoblast cell lines. Reproduction; 132:159-67.

[84] Matejevic D, Heilmann P, Schuster C, Schoneshofer M, Graf R (1995) Decidua and placenta in mice after treatment with a synthetic glucocorticoid. Reprod Fertil Dev; 7:1551-5.

[85] Waddell BJ, Hisheh S, Dharmarajan AM, Burton PJ (2000) Apoptosis in rat placenta is zone-dependent and stimulated by glucocorticoids. Biol Reprod; 63:1913-7.

[86] Hahn T, Barth S, Graf R, Engelmann M, Beslagic D, Reul JM, et al. (1999) Placental glucose transporter expression is regulated by glucocorticoids. J Clin Endocrinol Metab; 84:1445-52.

[87] Lee MJ, Ma Y, LaChapelle L, Kadner SS, Guller S (2004) Glucocorticoid enhances transforming growth factor-beta effects on extracellular matrix protein expression in human placental mesenchymal cells. Biol Reprod; 70:1246-52.

[88] Siler-Khodr TM, Kang IS, Koong MK, Grayson M (1997) The effect of dexamethasone on CRH and prostanoid production from human term placenta. Prostaglandins; 54:639-53.

[89] Audette MC, Greenwood SL, Sibley CP, Jones CJ, Challis JR, Matthews SG, et al. (2010) Dexamethasone stimulates placental system A transport and trophoblast differentiation in term villous explants. Placenta; 31:97-105.

[90] Jones SA, Brooks AN, Challis JR (1989) Steroids modulate corticotropin-releasing hormone production in human fetal membranes and placenta. J Clin Endocrinol Metab; 68:825-30.

[91] Hewitt DP, Mark PJ, Waddell BJ (2006) Glucocorticoids prevent the normal increase in placental vascular endothelial growth factor expression and placental vascularity during late pregnancy in the rat. Endocrinology; 147:5568-74.

[92] Kurinczuk JJ, Parsons DE, Dawes V, Burton PR (1999) The relationship between asthma and smoking during pregnancy. Women Health; 29:31-47.

[93] Murphy VE, Gibson PG, Smith R, Clifton VL (2005) Asthma during pregnancy: mechanisms and treatment implications. Eur Respir J; 25:731-50.

[94] Mayhew TM, Jenkins H, Todd B, Clifton VL (2008) Maternal asthma and placental morphometry: effects of severity, treatment and fetal sex. Placenta; 29:366-73.

[95] Jung SP, Siegrist B, Wade MR, Anthony CT, Woltering EA (2001) Inhibition of human angiogenesis with heparin and hydrocortisone. Angiogenesis; 4:175-86.

[96] Ingber DE, Madri JA, Folkman J (1986) A possible mechanism for inhibition of angiogenesis by angiostatic steroids: induction of capillary basement membrane dissolution. Endocrinology; 119:1768-75.
[97] Folkman J, Langer R, Linhardt RJ, Haudenschild C, Taylor S (1983) Angiogenesis inhibition and tumor regression caused by heparin or a heparin fragment in the presence of cortisone. Science; 221:719-25.
[98] Charnock-Jones DS, Kaufmann P, Mayhew TM (2004) Aspects of human fetoplacental vasculogenesis and angiogenesis. I. Molecular regulation. Placenta; 25:103-13.
[99] Stark MJ, Hodyl NA, Wright IM, Clifton VL (2011) Influence of sex and glucocorticoid exposure on preterm placental pro-oxidant-antioxidant balance. Placenta; 32:865-70.
[100] Walther FJ, Jobe AH, Ikegami M (1998) Repetitive prenatal glucocorticoid therapy reduces oxidative stress in the lungs of preterm lambs. J Appl Physiol; 85:273-8.
[101] Vento M, Aguar M, Escobar J, Arduini A, Escrig R, Brugada M, et al. (2009) Antenatal steroids and antioxidant enzyme activity in preterm infants: influence of gender and timing. Antioxid Redox Signal; 11:2945-55.
[102] Comporti M, Signorini C, Leoncini S, Buonocore G, Rossi V, Ciccoli L (2004) Plasma F2-isoprostanes are elevated in newborns and inversely correlated to gestational age. Free Radical Biol Med; 37:724-32.
[103] Binet ME, Bujold E, Lefebvre F, Tremblay Y, Piedboeuf B (2012) Role of Gender in Morbidity and Mortality of Extremely Premature Neonates. Am J Perinatol; 29:159-66.
[104] Stark MJ, Wright IM, Clifton VL (2009) Sex-specific alterations in placental 11beta-hydroxysteroid dehydrogenase 2 activity and early postnatal clinical course following antenatal betamethasone. Am J Physiol Regul Integr Comp Physiol; 297:R510-4.
[105] Wintour EM, Alcorn D, McFarlane A, Moritz K, Potocnik SJ, Tangalakis K (1994) Effect of maternal glucocorticoid treatment on fetal fluids in sheep at 0.4 gestation. Am J Physiol; 266:R1174-81.
[106] Braun T, Li S, Sloboda DM, Li W, Audette MC, Moss TJ, et al. (2009) Effects of maternal dexamethasone treatment in early pregnancy on pituitary-adrenal axis in fetal sheep. Endocrinology; 150:5466-77.
[107] Cuffe JS, Dickinson H, Simmons DG, Moritz KM (2011) Sex specific changes in placental growth and MAPK following short term maternal dexamethasone exposure in the mouse. Placenta; 32:981-9.
[108] Braun T, Li S, Moss TJ, Connor KL, Doherty DA, Nitsos I, et al. (2011) Differential appearance of placentomes and expression of prostaglandin H synthase type 2 in placentome subtypes after betamethasone treatment of sheep late in gestation. Placenta; 32:295-303.
[109] Ain R, Canham LN, Soares MJ (2005) Dexamethasone-induced intrauterine growth restriction impacts the placental prolactin family, insulin-like growth factor-II and the Akt signaling pathway. J Endocrinol; 185:253-63.
[110] Dickinson H, O'Connell BA, Quinn T, Cannata D, Moxham A, Walker DW (2010) The spiny mouse - an ideal species to study perinatal biology. Pediatr Res; 68:175.

Chapter 16

The Role of Glucocorticoids in Pregnancy: Four Decades Experience with Use of Betamethasone in the Prevention of Pregnancy Loss

Fortunato Vesce, Emilio Giugliano, Elisa Cagnazzo,
Stefania Bignardi, Elena Mossuto, Tarcisio Servello and Roberto Marci

Additional information is available at the end of the chapter

http://dx.doi.org/10.5772/50797

1. Introduction

'Pregnancy loss' can be defined as the failure by the gestational processes to result in the birth of a viable neonate. Miscarriage is defined as the end of pregnancy before the fetus reaches viability, a condition in turn depending on other variables, among which gestational age, birth weight and maturity, as well as the quality of assistance. Therefore to set, as it is done, at 24 weeks the term before which any birth should be classified as abortion is inadequate, because around this time some fetuses survive. On the other hand, preterm birth, that is strictly related with adverse infant outcome in terms of survival and quality of life, is defined as birth at less than 37 weeks. However it will be recognized that while up to the half of the second trimester no foetus at the moment can survive outside the maternal environment, during the third trimester, rather than from gestational age by itself, pregnancy loss will mainly depend on the pathologic condition leading to premature delivery. Recurrent miscarriage refers to the occurrence of three or even two (von Eye Corleta, 2010) consecutive pregnancy losses. The attempt to distinguish sporadic from repeated abortion stems from the believe that they may have different causes. Nevertheless, although it may be difficult to establish the pathogenic mechanism in single cases, in general it is much better understood today, and it is basically always the same: therefore it appears that separating sporadic from recurrent abortion is no longer needed. Indeed, pregnancy loss can occur at any time throughout gestation and labour as a consequence of a number of pathologic conditions widely recognizing two background pathways, namely the impairment of the blood supply to the foetus and the stimulation of uterine contractions. In the majority of the cases, such complications are triggered by an either pre-existent or acquired inflammatory mechanism. For instance, maternal rheumatic diseases represent a well known condition leading to poor pregnancy outcome (Spinillo et al., 2012), although, as it will be explained ahead, abortion can also represent the only pathologic expression of functional changes resembling inflammation confined at the uterine mucosa level. At this regard, one basic need in approaching the role of glucocorticoids (GCs) in medicine is represented by a reappraisal to the concept itself of inflammation. This, indeed, based on our background medical education, is characterized by classical signs and symptoms (rubor, calor, tumor, dolor and functio laesa) as well as by several hemato-chemical and histological features. However, the cytokines and prostanoids that trigger inflammation are also involved in the regulation of important physiologic functions, among which social behaviour of cells (Biondi et al., 2006), angiogenesis (Suffee et al., 2011), haemostasis (Salgado et al., 1994) and smooth muscle contraction (Shynlova et al., 2009). In obstetrics, processes such as implantation and labour are under the control of these mediators, the **imbalance** of which is able to **deviate a physiological function** towards an inflammatory disease, leading to a wide number of gestational complications, from abortion (Saini et al, 2011) to foetal malformation (Sljivic et al., 2006), intra-uterine growth restriction (Eastabrook et al., 2008), abruptio placentae (Nath et al., 2007), premature delivery (Romero et al., 2002), as well as hyaline membrane disease (Cheah et al., 2005), necrotizing entero-colitis (Xu et al., 2011) and hypoxic ischemic encephalopathy of the newborn (Liu et al., 2010). Such a cytokine and prostanoid **imbalance** may therefore represent the **early change for an eventual, future inflammation**. Surprisingly, instead, implantation and labour themselves are often named as a sort of inflammatory process, thus implying that a pathologic event may be beneficial to human health: such a pointless unsafe concept should be better avoided. Indeed, besides its intrinsic contradiction, it represents an obstacle to the liberal use of some anti-inflammatory drugs, among which GCs, aimed at re-balancing the above mentioned mediators for preventing harmful complications. There is a further point of primary significance to be considered before entering into the specific field of pregnancy regulators, and it deals with the causal relationship between inflammation and infection. At this regard, it is generally accepted that it is the latter to trigger the first, while, based on a number of considerations, at least in some cases the opposite is true. Indeed, most bacteria responsible for infection belong to the saprophytic flora, thus suggesting that their shift to pathogen may be a consequence of an environmental alteration, possibly linked with a cytokine-prostanoid imbalance that leads to the inflammatory response. Such a view is strongly supported in obstetrics, thanks to the fundamental work of professor Romero showing that premature delivery, an ominous condition of pregnancy often complicated by infection, is preceded by an inflammation of gestational tissues: 'the foetal inflammatory response syndrome', that will be explained in a more detailed manner ahead. Being, to the best of our knowledge, the Romero's syndrome the first clinical demonstration of a reversed causal relationship between infection and inflammation, it represents a milestone suggesting to search for similar pathogenic mechanisms in other fields of medicine. In the meantime, it opens to debate upon the role and priority of the drugs currently used in the management of such disease, namely GCs, antibiotics and non steroidal anti-inflammatory compounds.

2. Mediators of physiological pregnancy

Based on the above considerations, we proceed now to analyze the pro- as well as the anti-inflammatory mediators of physiological pregnancy. Cytokines found at the maternal-foetal interface include interferons (IFNs), interleukins (ILs), leukaemia inhibitory factor (LIF), tumour necrosis factors (TNFs), transforming growth factors (TGFs), colony stimulating factors (CSFs), vascular endothelial growth factors (VEGFs) and many others (Chaouat et al., 2007). Although a prevalence of pro-inflammatory cytokines are found during the early stages of pregnancy, the action of the anti-inflammatory is needed as well. For instance, LIF and IL-6 are required for a successful implantation in mice (Robb et al., 1998), but the lack of activity of IL-11 results in reduced fertility (White et al.,2004).

With the aim to shed light upon the complex network of reciprocal influences between cytokines and prostanoids from one side and their trophoblastic target form the other, we provide a more detailed description as regards the macrophage migration inhibitory factor (MIF) system, the interleukin-1 system (IL-1), the Toll-like receptors (TLRs) and the chemicals known as "endocrine disruptors" (EDs). (Figure 1).

2.1. MIF

The need for a balanced action of cytokines, whether or not of the inflammatory type, is confirmed looking at the macrophage migration inhibitory factor (MIF) system. MIF stimulates the production of a large panel of pro-inflammatory molecules, such as TNFα, IFNγ, IL-1β, IL-2, IL-6, IL-8 (Calandra et al., 1995) as well as nitric oxide (NO) (Cunha et al., 1993), matrix metalloproteinases (MMPs) and products of the arachidonic acid pathway (Calandra et al., 2003). MIF protein and mRNA are expressed by first trimester human villous and extra-villous trophoblast, the protein being also found in term placenta, amniotic fluid and maternal serum (Ietta et al. 2002). Their levels are higher at the beginning of first trimester to decline later on. Moreover, they are up-regulated by low oxygen tension, comparable to the values occurring at the very early stage of pregnancy (Ietta et al., 2007). Trophoblast MIF **reduces** the cytotoxicity of decidual natural killer (NK) cells (Arcuri et al., 2006), and intraperitoneal injection of rMIF to pregnant mice induces an increase of endometrial alpha(v),beta-3-integrin subunits and VEGF expression, that are markers of uterine receptivity (Bondza et al., 2008). Accordingly, pregnant MIF-treated mice show an enhanced rate of implanted embryos with respect to controls (Bondza et al., 2008), although fertility is not impaired in MIF knock-out mice (Fingerle-Rowson et al., 2003).

2.2. IL-1

The IL-1 system represents a further regulator of uterine receptivity and embryo implantation At the implantation site, immunoreactive IL-1β was detected in the villous and extravillous trophoblast as well as in the maternal decidual cells (Paulesu et al. 2010). Moreover, interleukin-1 receptor type 1 (IL-1R tI) is expressed by the syncytiotrophoblast, supporting the stimulatory effect of IL-1β on human chorionic gonadotropin (hCG) release (Masuhiro et al., 1991). IL-1 has been reported to stimulate different cytokines in the endometrium, including IL-6, IL-8, LIF and TNF-α, as well as the expression of prostaglandins (PGs)-2 and -2α and their receptor EP1 (Minas et al., 2005). The presence of IL-1α and IL-1β in the embryo culture medium has been correlated with successful implantation after in vitro fertilization (Karagouni et al., 1998). Later studies of endometrial secretions from women before embryo transfer showed the association of lower levels of IL-1β with clinical pregnancy (Boomsma et al., 2009). Since IL-1β and TNFα are significantly related to clinical pregnancy and not embryo implantation, it was suggested that these two cytokines are not associated with the initial apposition and adhesion of the embryo (Boomsma et al., 2009). An inappropriate ratio of IL-1β to IL-α and higher IL-1R tI are involved in the establishment of ectopic pregnancy in the oviduct (Huang et al., 2005). IL-1β mediates the paracrine effect of PG synthesis by inducing COX-2 (Pellicer et al., 2002), and IL-1α induces the production of MMP-1 in stromal fibroblast and raises the activity of MMP-9 in trophoblast (Pellicer et al., 2002). Moreover, it has been shown that trophoblast reduces the secretion of pro-inflammatory cytokines IL-1β, IL-6 and TNFα elicited by low (0.1 μg/mL), but not high, doses lipopolysaccharide (LPS)-activated monocytes (Fest et al., 2007). As the female genital tract is opened to the external environment, cytokine release by gestational tissue can be influenced by external factors. For instance, exposure to seminal plasma factors including TGFβ1 stimulates cytokine production by uterine epithelial cells, with consequent recruitment and activation of macrophages, granulocytes and dendritic cells in the underlying stroma (Gopichandran et al., 2006).

2.3. TLRs

Cytokine release by gestational tissue is further regulated through the action of specific receptors for pathogen-associated molecular patterns, named Toll-like receptors (TLRs). These are present in the epithelial lining as well as in the underlying connective stroma of the human female reproductive tract (Hirata et al., 2007). TLR2 and TLR4 have been detected in villous and extra-villous, but not in syncytial first trimester trophoblast, TLR6, instead, is absent in the first but present in the third trimester trophoblast (Mitsunari et al., 2006). Binding of TLRs with microbial antigens activates the release of pro-inflammatory cytokines, possibly interfering with their physiological gestational balance (Schaefer et al., 2005). In addition to the above mentioned factors, also stress, nutrition, metabolic status, drugs and environmental chemicals (Arck et al., 2008), as well as genetic conditions are known to influence gestational cytokine and prostanoids.

2.4. EDs

Some chemicals defined as "endocrine disruptors" (EDs) are able to act like natural estrogens, interfering with reproductive processes. For instance, it has been recently shown that the ED para-nonylphenol (p-NP) affects trophoblast cytokine secretion as well as cell differentiation and apoptosis (Bechi et al., 2010). In addition to cytokines and prostanoids, also the cellular components of the immune system are involved in the regulation of physiological pregnancy. Among these, NK cells, that are large granular lymphocytes constituting 10-15% of their total circulating number. Even though their main activity is citotoxicity of target cells, in normal pregnancy they provide benefit by secreting cytokines, chemokines and angiogenetic factors which are needed for pregnancy success (Santoni et al., 2008). There is a further class of NK at the decidual level, named uterine NK (uNK), which are provided with phenotypic markers different from peripheral (pNK). uNK cells seem to be necessary for pregnancy success by producing factors that modulate trophoblast invasion and placental vascularization (Saito et al., 1993).

All above evidences outline the concept that there is no single substance, or mediator, or cell type that can be specifically identified as either detrimental or protective towards physiological pregnancy, but rather that it is their imbalance which can lead to an unfavourable outcome.

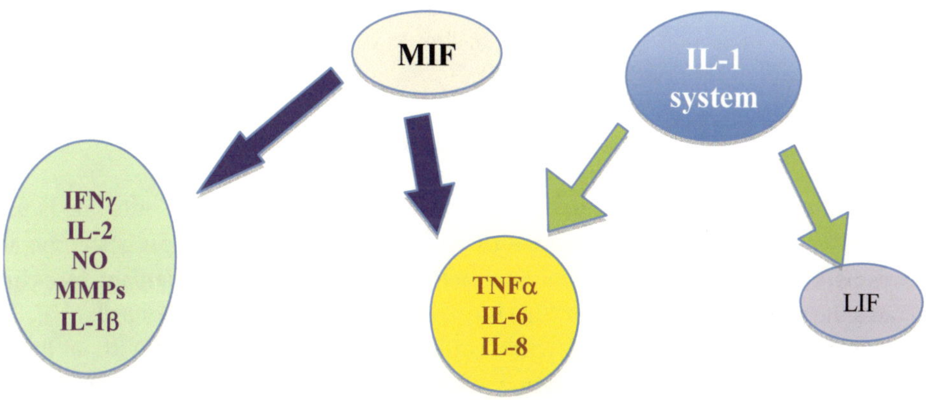

Figure 1. Influences of MIF and IL-1 systems on cytokine network in physiologic pregnancy

3. Hormone regulation of gestational cytokines and prostanoids

Pregnancy can be defined as a vascular phenomenon under the control of steroid hormones. Indeed nearly all above mentioned mediators are directly or indirectly able to interfere with the maternal uterine arteries changes aimed at increasing the foetal blood supply, and they are largely influenced by steroids. Therefore we will look now at the experimental results supporting the specific role of estrogen, progesterone and glucocorticoids in the control of the mediators of gestational functions. In particular, as progesterone and glucocorticoids actions are higly impaired by the abortive drug named mifepristone, we will compare influence of such compounds upon some gestational regulators and functions. Such a comparison should better address to understand the nature of both hormonal protection and drug impairment of pregnancy, provided that their action mechanisms lead to opposite regulatory consequences.

3.1. Estrogen and progesterone

Estradiol and progesterone exert an important role in the regulation of a number of the factors involved in gestational processes thus avoiding harmful inflammatory response (Dekel et al., 2010). By doing so, these hormones also modulate epithelial cells ability to respond to pathogenic microbes. Indeed estradiol suppresses the secretion of MIF, TNFα, IL-6 and IL-8 induced by bacteria in the uterine epithelial cells (EEC-1) (Wira et al., 2010).

Moreover the hormone stimulates IL-1β secretion in LPS-activated human uterine monocytes and down-regulates protein-expression of IL-1RtI, thus inhibiting the IL-1β-mediated inflammatory response. In chorionic explants MIF secretion is dose-dependently modulated by 17β-estradiol (E2) (Ietta et al., 2010). As for progesterone, it favours the secretion of IL-3, IL-4, IL-5 and IL-10, that are reported to inhibit the Th1 response (Pioli et al., 2006). Interestingly, however, dydrogesterone induction of a Th1 to Th2 cytokine shift is also expressed by inhibition of IFN-γ and TNF-α but up-regulation of the production of IL-4 and IL-6. It happens therefore that, given a protective action of progesterone against abortion, IL6, that is able to trigger PG release, thus leading to abortion or premature delivery, being up-regulated by the hormone, should be considered protective in the context of early pregnancy! (Raghupathy et al., 2005).

3.2. Mifepristone

The complexity of the relation between cytokine balance and pregnancy outcome is further expressed by comparison of mifepristone (Ru486), betamethasone and progesterone action mechanisms. As for the antiprogestational action of Ru486, the mechanism by which it inactivates the progesterone receptor (PR) is not completely clarified (Leonhardt et al., 2002). However it appears that its abortive action could be in some way related with an influence on cytokines, as repeated administration of the drug significantly enhances the serum production of TNFα and IFNγ while prolonging LPS-induced depressive-like behaviour in rats (Wang et al., 2011), although it does not exert the same effect in mice (Yang et al., 2008). RU486 also stimulates the expression of IL-6 and LIF protein in human villous trophoblast and stroma cells in early pregnancy, thus questioning the supposed IL6 protective role (Pei et al., 2010). Indeed, while opening to debate the action mechanism of progestogens, GCs and their antagonists at the level of gestational tissues, such contradictory observations do not clarify (whether or not inflammatory) the role of IL6 in pregnancy. RU486 counteracts the hyper-polarization of cell membranes as well as the inhibition of gap-junctions responsible for uterine contraction exerted by the hormone (Garfield et al., 1988). It also stimulates the release of PG and impairs the PG-dehydrogenase activity (Norman et al., 1991). As a consequence, the uterine sensibility to PG is significantly enhanced. Accordingly, the capacity of the drug alone to induce abortion is low, while it raises up to 95% when followed by PG administration (Grimes, 1997). Therefore, once again, it appears that early abortion of an otherwise normal pregnancy is mainly obtained by smooth muscle contraction (and therefore by impairment of utero-placental blood perfusion), rather than by a disturbance of the cellular mechanisms of implantation. However, the antiglucocorticoid nature of RU486 is also well characterized. Indeed, it binds to the glucocorticoid receptor (GR), and oral administration of the drug results in a dose-dependent activation of the hypothalamic-pituitary-adrenal (HPA) axis (Gaillard et al., 1984). Despite the compensatory increase in the serum cortisol concentration, in patients undergoing medical termination of a first trimester pregnancy the net effect of this compound is a profound suppression of circulating GC bioactivity (Heikinheimo et al.; 2003). Given the power of the anti-GC activity of RU486, the question arises whether its abortive action is also due to this property.

Furthermore it is interesting to ascertain whether such an action is to be ascribed to the disturbance of intercellular communication at the earliest stage of blastocyst implantation or to impairment of blood perfusion later on. Indeed, among the potentially positive effects of GC in early pregnancy, promotion of trophoblast growth and invasion have been suggested, along with stimulation of hCG secretion and suppression of NK cells (Michael & Papageorghiou; 2008). By modulating extravillous trophoblast proliferation and invasion, in fact GC may directly influence the capacity of chorionic villi to modify the structure of maternal spiral arteries, a change aimed at meeting the needs of embryo oxygenation and growth. The initial process of invasion belongs to the cross-talk between trophoblast and uterine decidua. Blastocyst attachment appears to be regulated by cell surface signalling molecules among which integrins and fibronectin. At physiological concentrations (100 nmol/l), GCs can suppress the expression of trophoblast integrins while their effects on fibronectin expression are tissue-specific (Burrows et al., 1996). For instance, in human pregnancy at term, dexamethasone suppresses fibronectin expression cytotrophoblasts and amnion while it acts in synergy with transforming growth factor-b towards up-regulation in matched samples of chorion and placental mesenchymal cells (Guller et al., 1995). Moreover, trophoblast functions are regulated by gap-junctional intercellular communication (GJIC) (Malassiné & Cronier, 2005). Gap junctions (GJ) are membrane channels which span the intercellular space, providing a pathway for the exchange of signalling molecules such as second messengers and siRNA. Said channels are constituted by the association of two hemi-channels, termed connexons, each composed of six connexin (Cx) subunits. Trophoblast Cx expression is modulated by hCG and estradiol, and GCs have been shown to enhance trophoblast GJIC in human pregnancy at term (Cronier et al., 1998). We have recently demonstrated that betamethasone selectively modifies trophoblast GR and Cx expression, enhancing the GRα isoform without affecting GRβ, and inhibiting Cx40 expression while increasing that of Cx43 and 45. Furthermore, betamethasone exerts an inhibitory action on cell proliferation. This result could be at least partly due to the inhibitory effect of the reduced expression of Cx40, coupled with an upregulation of Cx43. Indeed, it has been reported that Cx40 is involved in trophoblast proliferation (Winterhager *et al.* 1999; Nishimura *et al.* 2004), and that Cx43 upregulation is associated with an inhibition of JEG-3 cell proliferation (Kibschull *et al.* 2008). By modulating extravillous trophoblast proliferation and invasion, GCs may directly influence the capacity of chorionic villi to modify the structure of maternal spiral arteries, a change aimed at meeting the needs of embryo oxygenation and growth.

RU-486, in spite of its anti-GR property, does not contrast this effect of betamethasone. On the contrary, it induces responses similar to those of the hormone. As for progesterone, it shows the same effect as betamethasone on Cx expression, while it does not affect proliferation. RU-486 does not antagonize the progesterone effect as well. These results, by confirming that neither the abortive action of RU486 nor the protective action of GCs are obtained through their influence on trophoblast Cx expression, along with the other above mentioned evidences, do not exclude that the abortive mechanism of the drug may be also linked to its anti-glucocorticoid action at a level other than Cx (Cervellati et al., 2011).

Moreover, as for the nature of the events leading to pregnancy loss, it appears that it is not to be ascribed to the disturbance of intercellular communication at the earliest stage of blastocyst implantation, but rather to the impairment of blood perfusion and triggering of uterine contractions obtained through an intensive prostaglandin administration later on. If the enhanced responsiveness of myometrium to prostaglandins, that represents the main abortive action of mifepristone, derives from the anti-progesterone or anti-GCs effects, or even both or none of them, remains to be ascertained.

3.3. Influence of GCs on TLR and MIF

Further examples of the regulatory actions of GCs are down-regulation of TLR expression, suppression of pro-inflammatory and up-regulation of anti-inflammatory cytokines by dexamethasone in primary isolated murine liver cells (Broering et al., 2011), as well as inhibition of the human pro-IL-lβ gene by decreasing DNA binding of transactivators to the signal-responsive enhancer (Waterman et al., 2006). It is interesting to observe that the GR can be influenced even independently from GCs. Indeed the unliganded GR attenuates TNF-α stimulated IL-6 transcription by a mechanism involving selective phosphorylation and recruitment of the unliganded GR and GRIP-1 to the IL-6 promoter. It is suggested that such an autoregulatory mechanism may prevent overproduction of IL-6 in the endocervix, possibly protecting against negative effects of excessive inflammation (Verhoog et al., 2011). However GCs are also reported **to induce**, rather than to inhibit, the secretion of MIF (Calandra et al., 1995), thus counteracting the hormone inhibition of pro-inflammatory cytokine production. Such an influence is an example of particular relevance in understanding the nature of a balanced protective action against pregnancy loss.

3.4. Trans-placental passageand action site of GCs

A further matter of debate is represented by the regulation of GCs passage into the foetal circulation by placental 11β-hydroxy-dehydrogenase type 2 (11β-HSD2), the level of expression and activity of which is determined by a delicate balance between stimulatory and inhibitory influences. Studies of human and other primate placentas or derived trophoblast cells have shown that placental 11β-HSD2 activity is **reduced** by progesterone, estrogen, NO, PGs, proinflammatory cytokines and infections, β-adrenoceptor agonists, hypoxia and peroxisome proliferator-activated receptor δ agonists. Conversely, placental 11β-HSD2 activity is **stimulated** by **GCs**, retinoids and activators of the pathway that includes cyclic AMP and protein kinase A (Seckl et al., 2007). Moreover, the exposure of foetal tissues to cortisol may be determined locally by 11β-HSD isoenzymes **within** the foetus, rather than simply by GC metabolism at the materno-fetal interface (McNeil et al., 2007). In the trophoblast cells, (the most abundant site of 11β-HSD1), cortisol up-regulates enzyme expression inducing promoter activity, and the effect is enhanced by IL-1β. This suggests that more biologically active GCs could be generated in the foetal membranes in the presence of infection, which may consequently feed forward in up-regulation of PG synthesis. Intriguingly, foetal membranes are a major site of PG synthesis during pregnancy

(Li et al., 2006), the production of which has been reported to be increased by GCs (Sun et al., 2003). However, such stimulatory actions of GCs on the biosynthetic pathways of PG, rather than simply suggesting adverse clinical outcomes, sharpen the complexity of the hormonal regulatory influence upon the internal homeostasis of organic functions, as they, as it will be said ahead, adequately administrated, ultimately contribute to shift the complicate network of cytokines and prostanoids towards a beneficial direction. All above evidences indicate nothing more than the regulation of gestational processes to rely upon an extremely high number of mediators under physiological hormonal control, that are influenced by both maternal and foetal conditions (either congenital or acquired), as well as by external factors able to modify utero-placental perfusion and myometrial quiescence. As pregnancy loss can occur at any time during gestation and labour, it follows that the outcome of pregnancy will depend on the grade and time of the regulators derangement. In other words, speaking of pregnancy loss, there is no difference between the pathogenic mechanism of abortion and that of premature delivery, other than the first to happen very early, the second at a time when the foetus may have already reached the capacity to survive.

4. Direct and indirect relationship between inflammation and pregnancy loss

Aetiology of pregnancy loss includes chromosomal, anatomical, hormonal, immunological and endocrinological abnormalities, but in most cases the cause remains unexplained. It is frequently claimed that an inflammatory microenvironment is required for adequate tissue remodelling during implantation and the early phase of pregnancy (Challis et al., 2009). On the contrary, the second trimester is characterized by a prevalence of anti-inflammatory signals. An inflammatory pattern is then required near term of pregnancy to induce labour contractions and cervical dilatation (Paulesu et al., 2010). At this regard, for instance, we have demonstrated the presence on human amnion-derived WISH cells of binding sites for formyl-methionyl-leucyl-phenylalanine (fMLP), the classical chemotactic receptor for N-formyl peptides. fMLP induces a significant increase of PGE2 release by these human amnion-derived cells. Such a response in turn is impaired by COX, phospholipase A2, and phospholipase C inhibitors (Biondi et al., 2001). Furthermore we have shown that labouring amniotic membranes express both high- and low-affinity specific receptors for 3H-fMLP, while only the low-affinity are found in non-labouring tissue, and that the peptide is able to significantly increase PG synthesis in perifused amnion fragments from labouring and non-labouring women. (Buzzi et al., 1999). Nevertheless, abnormal inflammatory events may lead to adverse pregnancy outcomes, such as implantation failure, pregnancy loss, preeclampsia, preterm labour, intrauterine growth restriction (IUGR), and foetal inflammatory syndrome (Kwak-Kim et al., 2010). Disregulation of cell function mediators can simply derive from genetic conditions, with no need for infectious or inflammatory external stimuli. Indeed, it has been reported that polymorphisms in immunoregulatory genes IL10, MBL2, TNFRSF6 and TGFB1 may influence susceptibility to chorioamnionitis (Annells et al., 2005), and common genetic variants in proinflammatory cytokine genes, such as some selected TNF/LTA haplotypes, increase the risk for spontaneous preterm birth (Engel et al., 2005).

4.1. The Th1/Th2 paradigm

It has been suggested that a successful pregnancy may be a Th2 type phenomenon, whereas a Th1-type prevalence could be detrimental (Kwak-Kim et al., 2003). Immune regulation of pregnancy is mediated by TH1, TH2 and macrphages throughout the release of a number of cytokines (Table 1). Women with recurrent pregnancy loss have higher peripheral concentrations of certain Th1 cytokines (IL-2, TNF-α, TNF-β, IFN-γ) and lower concentrations of Th2 (IL-4, -5, -6, -10) when compared with successful pregnancy. Th1 cytokines, especially IFN-γ, may activate endothelial cell procoagulants and cause thrombotic and inflammatory reactions at the utero-placental level (Clark et al 1998). As for the mechanism by which thrombotic changes are induced, it has been reported an increased expression of pro-coagulant Fg12 in trophoblast cells from failing pregnancy (Knackstedt et al., 2001). Fg12 is a glycoprotein able to directly cleave prothrombin to thrombin, leading to fibrin deposition. Th1 cytokines up regulate this procoagulant, with consequent activation of the coagulation system and disruption of vascular supply to the placenta. On the contrary, Th2 system can hamper this process, suppressing Th1 response (Saini et al., 2011). Among proinflammatory cytokines, TNF-α is of particular interest. Indeed, even though a low concentration is required for successful implantation, it also causes trophoblast apoptosis in combination with Th1 cytokines such INF-γ. The cytokine could even be involved in pregnancy loss by impairing utero-placental perfusion. A recent study on mouse (Renaud et al., 2011) reported a causal link between maternal inflammation induced by LPS administration and impaired placental perfusion. LPS administration determined a disseminated intravascular coagulation(DIC)-like condition, with clot formation within uterine vessels, decreased diastolic uterine artery flow velocity and evidence of prominent diastolic notches, resulting in placental and foetal hypoxia. Many biological effects of LPS are mediated by TNF-α. Oppositely, IL-10 administration decreased serum level of TNF-α, preventing pregnancy loss after LPS exposure. Cytokines of the IL-1 system (IL-1α, IL-1β and IL-1 receptor antagonist) are an important regulatory element of the Th1/Th2 balance. They have been implicated in implantation, and trophoblastic cells proliferation and invasion (Wang et al., 2002). On the other hand, it is interesting to note that IL-1 system can also function as a co-stimulator for Th2 response. Therefore, altered decidual IL-1β production may cause a reduction in Th2-type cytokine production, contributing to early pregnancy failure. The Th1/Th2 paradigm has recently been expanded into the Th1/Th2/Th17 and Treg (T regulatory cells) one (Peck et Mellins, 2010). Indeed increased peripheral and decidual levels of Th17 cells and their related factors (IL-17, IL-23 and - retinoid orphan nuclear receptor (RORC) have been reported in women with unexplained recurrent spontaneous abortion (RSA) (Wang et al., 2010). In addition, an inverse relationship between Th17 cells and Treg cells in the peripheral blood and decidua lymphocytes in unexplained RSA has been found. Treg cells are defined by secretion of TGF-β and IL10 and the presence of intracellular transcription factor FoxP3. Studies in

Cells	Cytokine	Actions
TH1	IFNγ IL1 IL2 TNFβ TNFα	• Inflammatory reactions • Thrombotic events through up-regulation of Fg12 • Trophoblastic apoptosis, inhibition of trophoblast cell growth and metabolic activity • Promotion of syncytium formation and invasive capacity of trophoblast (TNFα)
TH2	IL4 IL5 IL6 IL10 TGFβ	• Anti-inflammatory action • Enhancement of hCG secretion • Stimulation of growth and differentiation of trophoblast
Macrophage	IL1 system (IL1α, IL1β, IL1ra) LIF	• Stimulation of trophoblast differentiation (LIF)

Table 1. Immune regulation of pregnancy.

animal models (Thuere at al., 2007) have shown that Treg cells are essential for maternal tolerance of the conceptus, and that they exert suppressive actions in the peri-implantation phase. In women, inadequate number of Treg cells or their functional deficiency are linked with infertility, miscarriage and pre-eclampsia (Guerin et al., 2009). It is suggested that impaired Treg function could lead to increased Th1 cytokines (Jin et al., 2009). Nevertheless there are conflicting reports regarding the inflammation state in early pregnancy loss, suggesting adequate balance for Th1/Th2 cytokines, although with a slight shift toward Th2 immunity in successful pregnancy (Saini et al., 2011). A recent study (Calleja-Agius et al., 2012) confirmed an inflammatory state (higher pro-inflammatory cytokines) in normal pregnancy compared with the non pregnant state, which may be disrupted during miscarriage. The study revealed in euploid miscarriage a shift toward Th1 immune response (higher TNF-α/IL-6 ratio) at 6-9 weeks, but a lower TNF-α/IL 10 and IFN-γ/IL10 ratios in the late first trimester compared to normal pregnancy. At this regard it must be noted that the classification of IL-6 remains controversial, as some authors consider it as a Th2 mediator due to its anti-inflammatory properties possibly involved in new vessels generation and tissue remodelling associated with placentation (Jauniaux at al., 1996). A further evidence for an influence of inflammatory mediators in pregnancy is represented by the behaviour of maternal serum MIF (Yamada et al., 2002). Indeed, MIF concentrations in recurrent abortion women with subsequent miscarriage and normal foetal karyotype were lower than those in women with history of RSA with subsequent live birth and those in normal pregnant women. Moreover, MIF acts as an immunosuppressive factor by inhibiting NK cell activity. Since women with RPL and unexplained infertility have increased peripheral blood NK cells and increased NK cytotoxic activity (Yamada et al., 2001), low levels of MIF could lead to insufficient inhibition of NK cell activity and altered cytokines production with impairment of trophoblast proliferation, embryo development, and angiogenesis within placenta. One more pathway leading from inflammation to pregnancy loss acts via the complement system that induces recruitment and activation of inflammatory cells. Antiphospholipid (aPL) antibodies are able to trigger complement system response within decidual tissue, thus inducing inflammation and foetal damage (Salmon & Girardi, 2008). Recruitment of inflammatory cells creates a placental proinflammatory amplification loop, eventually leading to thrombosis, hypoxia, and neutrophil infiltration. Accordingly, increased complement activation is associated with recurrent abortion pre-eclampsia and IUGR (Tincani et al., 2009). A pathogenic mechanism has been postulated for recurrent abortion involving NK cells (Laird et al., 2003). Several studies reported a higher concentration of uNK and pNK as well as a higher proportion of activated pNK in women with history of RSA (Radysh & Chernyshov, 2005).

5. Classical treatment and drugs for preventing pregnancy loss

5.1. Progesterone

Progesterone is secreted by the corpus luteum and the placenta and is necessary for successful implantation and eventually the maintenance of pregnancy. Progesterone is prescribed in 13-40% of women with threatened miscarriage, according to published series because it is expected to support a potentially deficient corpus luteum and induce relaxation of a cramping uterus (Rai & Regan, 2006). This benefit of the hormone could be explained by its immmunomodulatory actions in inducing a pregnancy-protective shift from pro-inflammatoryTh-1 cytokine responses to a more favourable anti-inflammatory Th-2 cytokine response (Raghupathy et al., 2009). The first trial using progesterone for such women was published in the BMJ in 1953 (Swyer & Daley, 1953) and was followed over the decades by several small trials. However, uncertainty remains about the evidence. The latest randomized controlled trial (Haas & Ramsey, 2008) to assess progesterone support for pregnancy showed that it did not reduce the sporadic miscarriage rate. However, in a subgroup analysis of trials involving women with recurrent miscarriage, progesterone treatment appeared to offer a statistically significant decrease in miscarriage rate compared with placebo or no treatment (OR 0.38, 95% CI 0.2–0.7). Nevertheless, in order to understand the limited clinical utility of the conclusions derived from some sort of statistical analysis, it is to be noted that this meta-analysis was based on three small controlled studies, none of which detected a significant improvement in pregnancy outcome! A large multicenter study (PROMISE) is currently under way to assess the benefit of progesterone supplementation in women with unexplained recurrent miscarriage. The trial is expected to report in 2013. At present, progesterone administration is not recommended for unexplained recurrent miscarriage (Coomarasamy et al., 2011).

5.2. Aspirin

Aspirin is largely used in pregnancy because it is believed to increase blood flow to the embryo, act on unrecognized thrombophilias and prevent miscarriage. Pregnancy itself is a hyper-coaguable state associated with increased levels of procoagulant factors and decreased levels of naturally occurring anticoagulants such as protein S (Comp et al., 1986). Microthrombi are a common finding in the placental vasculature of women with recurrent miscarriage (Rushton, 1988). PGs appear to be essential for implantation, although and exogenous administration of high doses induces abortion: the maintenance of pregnancy may be dependent on a mechanism that suppresses prostaglandin synthesis. Aspirin, which suppresses COX, has the potential to support this mechanism. Moreover, the maintenance of pregnancy is said to depend on a shift of pro-inflammatory to anti-inflammatory cytokines. At this regard, aspirin and other antiplatelet agents have been shown to play a role in the inhibition of pro-inflammatory cytokines, such as TNFα and IL-8. In stroke (Al-Bahrani et al., 2007), TNFα induces thrombin generation and IL-8 causes polymorph accumulation (Schraufstatter et al., 2003). Polymorphs react with fibrin and damaged tissues to form clots. However, at present, no report in the medical literature confirms a role for aspirin in preventing recurrent pregnancy loss. Furthermore, it doesn't confer a significant benefit in anti-phospholipid (aPL) syndrome (Pattison et al., 2000) even if the live birth rate increases significantly when heparin is added to treatment. The syndrome is assumed to be responsible for pregnancy loss by causing thrombosis in the small blood vessels of the decidua, leading to subsequent foetal demise. In unexplained pregnancy loss, aspirin had no beneficial effect except for in late pregnancy losses, in cases where hereditary thrombophilias were not excluded. Since there is no study of aspirin in this condition, it's suggested that the positive effects in advanced pregnancy may be due to the action of the drug in such patients (Rai et al., 2000). Nevertheless, the lack of the evidence of any efficacy against RSA, coupled with a reported increased risk of miscarriage and foetal gastroschisis, contraindicate prescribing aspirin in early pregnancy (Carp HJ, 2009).

5.3. COX inhibitors

COX inhibitors impair uterine contractility, are easily administered and have fewer maternal side-effects compared to conventional tocolytics. However, they are not devoid of adverse effects on the foetus and newborn. Indeed, increased neonatal complications including oligohydramnios, renal failure, necrotizing enterocolitis, intraventricular haemorrhage, and closure of the patent ductus arteriosus have been reported with the use of the non-selective COX inhibitor indomethacin (Abou-Ghannam et al. 2011). A recent review includes outcome data from 13 trials for a total of 713 women. with use of indomethacin in 10. When compared with placebo, indomethacin alone resulted in a reduction in birth before 37 weeks gestation, with an increase in gestational age and birth weight. Compared to any other tocolytic, COX inhibition resulted also in reduced maternal drug reaction requiring cessation of treatment. A comparison of non-selective COX inhibitors versus any COX-2 inhibitor did not demonstrate any difference in maternal or neonatal outcomes. However, due to small numbers, all estimates are imprecise and need to be interpreted with caution. Overall, until now there is insufficient information about the role of COX inhibition for women in preterm labour (King et al., 2005).

5.4. Antibiotics

As for antibiotics, their role against infection of the chorioamnionic membranes in preterm labour has been extensively investigated. In these cases, the mechanism by which uterine contractions take place is supposed to be the release of microbial products into the amniotic fluid (Gibbs et al., 1992). There seems to be substantial agreement on the efficacy of antibiotic therapy in the prevention of preterm delivery when there is evidence of infection (Kirshbaum T, 1993), but its utility in idiopathic preterm labour is controversial (Cox et al., 1996). Nevertheless, antibiotics can have beneficial influences not only for their antimicrobial properties but also through a direct tocolytic action on tissues. Indeed, as it will be explained ahead, some among them have the capacity to directly inhibit amniotic IL-6 and PGE2 release, thus offering an explanation for a beneficial response in cases of preterm labour even in the absence of bacterial infection. (Vesce et al., 1998;2004).

5.5. Heparin

Successful pregnancy depending on trophoblast invasion into the uterine vasculature, inadequate placentation and damage to the spiral arteries with impaired flow and prothrombotic changes lead to pregnancy complications that become even more dangerous in hyper-coagulable states. Such complications benefit from prophylactic low molecular weight heparin (LMWH) and unfractionated heparin (UFH), in spite of several drawbacks to their use, including the costs, discomfort of daily injections, risks of bleeding, skin reactions, and thrombocytopenia (Howard, 2009). Indeed, there is general agreement that women with recurrent loss and persistent aPL antibodies positivity should receive antepartum prophylaxis with UFH or LMWH in combination with aspirin (Bates et al., 2008), while, at present, it is claimed that antithrombotic therapy should not be advocated for unexplained recurrent miscarriage in women without an underlying thrombophilia. (Clark et al., 2010). However, although a protective effect in women with heritable thrombophilia is not to be excluded, the British Committee for Standards in Haematology has recently recommended against the antithrombotic therapy in pregnant women with a history of loss based on the results of testing for inherited thrombophilia (Baglin et al., 2010). Low-molecular-weight instead of unfractionated heparin is recommended for the prevention and treatment of venous thromboembolism in pregnant women (Guyatt et al., 2012). In acute cases, anticoagulants should be continued for at least 6 weeks postpartum, for a minimum total duration of the therapy of 3 months. For women who fulfil the laboratory and clinical criteria for aPL antibodies syndrome and history of three or more pregnancy losses, is recommended antepartum administration of prophylactic or intermediate-dose UFH, or prophylactic (LMWH), combined with low-dose aspirin (75-100 mg/d) over no treatment. For women with inherited thrombophilia and a history of pregnancy complications, as well as for those with two or more miscarriages, but without aPL antibodies syndrome or thrombophilia, it is recommended against antithrombotic prophylaxis. (Guyatt et al., 2012).

5.6. Immunotherapy

Idiopathic recurrent miscarriage has traditionally been associated with alloimmune factors, in which uterine CD56+/16 NK cells have been implicated (Quenby et al., 1999). In vitro studies suggest that pregnancy may result in uterine T-cell activation along the Th-2 pathway, resulting in blocking antibodies which mask trophoblast antigens (Wegmann et al., 1993). Activation along the Th-1 pathway, instead, results in the production of abortive cytokines (Raghupathy et al., 2000). Maternal HY-restricting HLA class II alleles are associated with a decreased chance of a live birth in women with secondary recurrent miscarriage with a firstborn boy (Nielsen et al., 2009). Although such mechanisms are intriguing, there is a paucity of validated tests to assess the maternal immune response in pregnancy. Despite this, active and passive immunotherapeutic trials for idiopathic recurrent miscarriage have been reported. Paternal mononuclear cell immunization has been proved not to be effective (Scott, 2003). It is believed that passive immunotherapy with intravenous immunoglobulin (IVIG) may offer benefit in idiopathic secondary (at least one prior ongoing pregnancy), but not idiopathic primary (no prior ongoing pregnancy) recurrent miscarriage (Christiansen et al., 2002). However, such conclusions must be taken with caution because of small heterogeneous sample size. Moreover, IVIG is a highly purified and virally inactivated fractionated blood product made from pooled human plasma, which makes it costly to use and not without risk. Overall, the efficacy of IVIG in women with a history of idiopathic secondary recurrent miscarriage remains controversial, as no significant effect of treatment in these patients was found (Stephenson et al., 2010).

6. Influence of glucocorticoids on foetal development

6.1. Prenatal administration of GCs and HPA function

Several studies in animals have shown that prenatal administration of GCs can cause hormonal changes in the foetus. Epidemiologic research in human even suggested that these may have long-term consequences on health in adult life. This concept is termed 'early life programming' (Seckl, 2004). Great importance is given to the influence of GCs on foetal HPA axis. Several studies assessed basal HPA function in the feto-placental unit by measuring markers of its activity in cord blood and amniotic fluid during gestation and at birth. Compared with unexposed healthy foetuses, cortisol concentrations were significantly lower in otherwise healthy foetuses exposed to synthetic GCs, with values decreasing to the 10% of the controls. These results, however, refer to premature foetuses, which receive 24 mg betamethasone within 24 hours before being delivered (Kajantie et al., 2004). In foetuses of asthmatic mothers who refrained from taking synthetic GCs during pregnancy, cortisol concentrations were even higher compared to those of healthy controls (Murphy et al., 2002). As for placental CRH mRNA, it was slightly higher in asthmatic patients not treated with synthetic GCs. However, treated cases exhibit normal levels irrespective of the treatment dose. Similar to cortisol, ACTH, DHEA and DHEA-S (Parker et al., 1996) concentrations were reduced in treated foetuses.

6.2. Metabolic changes induced by prenatal GCs

The alteration of the HPA activity seems to be closely related to the changes in glucose homeostasis and obesity. In rodent models, administration of dexamethasone leads to permanent hyperglycaemia and hyperinsulinaemia in the offspring (Nyirenda et al., 1998) with life-long elevations in the activity of phosphoenolpyruvate carboxykinase (PEPCK), the enzyme involved in gluconeogenesis. This metabolic effect is correlated with the exposure time, and week 3 of gestation appears to be a critical window for inducing long-term metabolic changes. Similar alterations of glucose homeostasis have been reported in both sheep and non-human primates (de Vries et al., 2007). Although the molecular mechanisms underlying these changes in offspring glucose metabolism have not been fully clarified, the alterations in HPA activity are certainly implicated, as the animals have increased levels of circulating corticosterone, decreased GR expression in the hippocampus, the site of central negative feedback, and increased peripheral GR expression in insulin-sensitive target tissues including liver and muscle in the rat (Nyirenda et al., 1998; Cleasby et al., 2003). The increased PEPCK expression is regulated by transcription factors, including members of the HNF (hepatocyte nuclear factor) and GR that bind to the PEPCK gene promoter. The expression of these factors is increased in liver of rats treated with dexamethasone (Nyirenda et al., 1998), suggesting that the observed increase in PEPCK may be a secondary effect. Thus, changes in key transcription factors may underlie permanent changes in glucose metabolism. The influence of prenatal GCs is also expressed in the foetal pancreas. GC signalling is important in pancreatic beta cell development, with potential underlying mechanisms including their interaction with the transcription factors that control proliferation and differentiation of the Langerhans islets cells (Gesina et al., 2006). Among these, IGF (insulin-like growth factor) 2, the IGF receptor, and several IGF binding proteins (Hill et al., 2000) may lead to a decreased insulin secretion, with consequent hyperglycaemia in adult life. Prenatal GC exposure is also associated with alterations in fat distribution and function. Offspring of rats treated with dexamethasone during days 8, 10 and 12 of pregnancy have increased intra-abdominal fat depots, and a parallel increase in circulating leptin levels (Dahlgren et al., 2001). Moreover, treatment of rats with dexamethasone in the last week of pregnancy leads to an increase in GR expression in visceral adipose tissue and alterations in fat metabolism which may contribute to insulin resistance (Cleasby et al., 2003). Recent evidence also shows that the activity of 11β-HSD type 1 may be 'programmed' by prenatal GC therapy. Indeed, a brief antenatal exposure to GCs in pregnant marmosets resulted in up-regulation of 11β-HSD1 mRNA expression and activity in subcutaneous, but not visceral, fat of the offspring (Nyirenda et al., 2009). The increase in 11β-HSD1 occurred before the animals developed obesity or overt features of the metabolic syndrome. This up-regulation of 11β-HSD1 suggests a novel mechanism underlying the foetal origins of obesity.

6.3. The impact of GCs on foetal bone

Another interesting field of research is represented by the influence of prenatal GCs on foetal bone. Indeed, GCs are known to affect skeletal growth and adult bone metabolism, but their impact on foetal bone remains to be elucidated. Some Authors (Swolin-Eide et al.,

2002) reported prenatal dexamethasone exposure to affect skeletal growth in rats. Dexamethasone-exposed male but not female rat offspring showed transient increases in crown–rump length and tibia and femur lengths at 3–6 weeks of age. In contrast, the cortical bone dimensions were altered in 12-week-old female but not male, and the areal bone mineral densities of the long bones and the spine were unchanged in both male and female suggesting a gender specific effect. Following these results, research was addressed to investigate some biochemical markers of bone turnover such as 4,5 carboxy-terminal propeptide of type I procollagen (PICP) and cross-linked carboxy-terminal telopeptide of type I collagen (ICTP). A single course of antenatal corticosteroids reduced umbilical cord levels of PICP without influence on ICTP (Korakaki et al., 2007). Instead, according to other Authors (Fonseca et al., 2009), umbilical cord serum levels of ICTP, the marker for foetal bone resorption, decreased only when the doses were ≥ 4.

6.4. Conclusion

Overall, it appears that, in animals, programming effects of GCs exposure during gestation involve:

- hyperglycaemia throughout a gluconeogenesis enzyme modulation coupled with a decreased growth of pancreatic islets;
- increased deposition of visceral fat related with an increase in circulating levels of leptin and expression of GR in the fat tissue;
- gender-specific manner stimulation of bone growth without influence on mineralization.

However, the results of these experimental studies, performed on a variety of animal species, using high doses and different types of GC, cannot be extended to human pregnancy, that is provided with distinct metabolising capacity at the utero-placental level. Indeed, GCs are largely prescribed for a variety of maternal and foetal conditions during human pregnancy, where none of the above reported complications and side effects have been confirmed. The absolute indications for using these compounds are Addison syndrome and hypopituarism. Furthermore, they are largely utilized for maternal asthma, collagen disease, ulcerative colitis, regional enteritis, and need of immunosuppression. Moreover, there is a number of specific indications to early administration for pregnancy-induced pathology. Among these foetal atrio-ventricular block, congenital adrenal hyperplasia, cystic adenomatoid malformation of the lung, alloimune thrombocytopenia, recurrent pregnancy loss and antiphospholipid antibody syndrome. In addition, clinical conditions that benefit from use of GCs in advanced pregnancy are related with premature delivery, aimed at the prevention of neonatal respiratory distress syndrome, intraventricular haemorrhage and necrotizing enterocolitis (Lunghi et al., 2010). All above conditions provide evidence for substantial advantages in foetal and maternal prognosis of prenatal administration of GCs, compared to feared, but unproved, side effects such as malformation and intrauterine growth restriction. At this regard, it has been reported that triamcinolone acetonide, a synthetic glucocorticoid, induces cleft palate resulting from poor development of palatal shelves in mice (Furukawa et al., 2004). Nevertheless, direct extrapolation to humans of teratogenic effects of GCs in animals is tenuous. Indeed, a prospective controlled cohort study, based on self-reported drug exposure and maternal interview as a source, collected 311 pregnancies receiving systemic use of different GCs in the first trimester. The rate of major congenital anomalies was compared to that of 790 controls that were counselled for non-teratogenic exposure. There was no case of oral cleft and no pattern of anomalies among the GCs exposed group, supporting the opinion that these hormones do not represent a major teratogenic risk in humans (Gur et al.,2004). A survey of the literature concerning 468 pregnant women treated with corticosteroids outside the transplant setting demonstrated an overall malformation rate of 3.5%, thus within the expected incidence in the general population (Danesi & Del Tacca, 2004). Moreover, a study on more than 6600 infants reported that maternal exposure to orally inhaled budesonide during pregnancy is not associated with an increased risk of congenital malformations or other adverse foetal outcomes (Rahimi et al., 2006). As for foetal growth, a systematic review of animal studies examining the association of GCs on birth outcome reported a reduction in birth weight (Aghajafari, 2002). However, it should be considered that animal experiments demonstrating negative effects employed doses equivalent to 20-100 times a 'replacement' dose of steroids for a human patient. Nevertheless studies in human were addressed to assess both the effect of early exposure protracted for a long time and that of late administration for preventing the complications of premature delivery. Interestingly, although a recent study suggests that foetal growth becomes sensitive to GCs when the treatment starts early and is prolonged for a long time (Gur et al., 2004), dexamethasone given from the 10th week throughout pregnancy in the presence of female foetuses affected by 21-hydroxylase deficiency did not influence weight, length and head circumference of the newborns (Carlson et al., 1999). As for advanced pregnancy, randomized controlled studies have shown that treatment for preventing respiratory distress syndrome of the neonate leads to birth weight reduction only after four or more courses, and that these parameters normalized by the time of hospital discharge (Bonanno et al., 2007). Moreover, a meta-analysis of five trials in which 2028 pregnant women were treated with GCs in late pregnancy found no significant effect on birth weight (Crowther et al., 2007). Two main exceptions can be raised towards human clinical studies: first, the time elapsing between administration of the drug and delivery appears to be too short to influence foetal growth; second, obstetrical diseases affecting foetal growth are necessarily included in the study sample, and therefore it is not possible to discriminate their influence from that of the hormone. The only way to avoid such a bias should be to administrate GC to healthy volunteers along the course of physiological pregnancy, something that happened to us in some way to do, in our long experience with low dose betamethasone therapy throughout gestation (see ahead). Based on our results, there is no persuasive evidence for any adverse effect neither of long duration low dose (see ahead), nor of short duration high dose GC on foetal growth.

7. Need and rules for antibiotic and glucocorticoid therapy in advanced pregnancy: The foetal inflammatory response syndrome.

We have previously treated in a more detailed manner the main indications to glucocorticoid therapy in human pregnancy (Lunghi et al., 2010). Nevertheless, for the purposes of the present chapter, it is necessary to stress the concepts dealing with the "Foetal Inflammatory Response Syndrome" (FIRS) (Romero et al., 1998). Indeed, being paradigmatic of the negative effects of inflammation on pregnancy, it offers the chance to clarify the rationale for the appropriate use of GCs and antibiotics for preventing harmful complications. FIRS is defined as a systemic inflammation characterized by an elevation of foetal plasma IL-6. In this syndrome a foetal plasma IL-6 level above 11 pg/ml is a major independent risk factor for the subsequent development of severe neonatal morbidity. Such a condition can be found even in the absence of microbial invasion of the amniotic cavity and any other sign of infection, as a foetal immune reaction characterized by increase in monocyte and neutrophil activation, and without correlation with maternal plasma or amniotic fluid concentration of the cytokine. It has been suggested that the foetus uses the effector limb of the immune response via the secretion of pro-inflammatory cytokines to signal the onset of labour and exit a hostile intrauterine environment (Romero et al., 1998). Whatever its teleological meaning, FIRS, also expressed by increased concentrations of foetal MMP-9, an enzyme involved in the digestion of type IV collagen and in the pathophysiology of preterm premature rupture of the membranes, can progress towards multiple organ dysfunction. (Romero et al., 2002). A further enzyme involved in such inflammatory process is MMP-8. Indeed an elevated MMP-8 concentration (>23 ng/mL), is present in 81% of the cases with cervical insufficiency, while a positive microbial culture is found only in 8%. These results indicate that, regardless of the eventual microbial involvement, inflammation is a risk factor for impending preterm delivery (Lee et al., 2008). Overall, the evidences above speak in favour of a leading role of inflammation in the pathogenesis not only of premature birth, but also of ominous perinatal complications such as respiratory distress syndrome (RDS), cerebral haemorrhage and necrotizing enterocolitis (NEC). Evidently, in this perspective, the causal role of infection appears substantially scaled. Accordingly, there is no evidence for a clear benefit of antibiotic treatment in infectious conditions that are associated with premature delivery, such as bacterial vaginosis and urinary infections (McDonald et al., 2007). In addition, treating women at risk with antibiotics does not reduce the incidence of subsequent of preterm delivery (Simcox et al., 2007), and among women with Group B streptococcal bacteriuria, exposure to additional antibiotics even increases the risk (Anderson et al., 2008). Conflicting reports do not clarify the role of prophylactic antibiotic therapy for inhibiting preterm labour. For instance, one meta-analysis including 11 trials on 7428 women with intact membranes showed a reduction in maternal infection, but failed to demonstrate benefit or harm for the neonatal outcome (King et al., 2002). On the contrary routine antibiotic prophylaxis during the second or third trimester of pregnancy reduces the risk of pre-labour rupture of the membranes, with beneficial effects on birth weight and the risk of postpartum endometritis in high risk women, according to a further meta-analysis (Thinkhamrop et al., 2002). As regards to the conflicting results of clinical studies about the administration of antibiotics in the prevention and cure of preterm delivery, it must be said that their Authors did not take into account the direct anti-inflammatory capacity that some of them are able to exert on gestational tissues. Indeed, we have demonstrated that ampicillin inhibits PGE release from amnion tissue in vitro, either in basal condition or upon addition of arachidonic acid or oxytocin to the medium (Vesce et al., 1998). Furthermore, it strongly reduces IL-6 level in amniotic fluid of patients sampled 4 hours after drug administration (Vesce et al., 2004). Ceftriaxone and gentamycin significantly and reversibly inhibit both basal and arachidonic acid- or oxytocin-stimulated PGE release from amnion, although to a lesser extent compared with ampicillin. On the contrary tetracycline and erythromycin do not influence the PG output. Of key importance from a clinical standpoint, the inhibitory effect of ampicillin is enhanced in an additive manner by ceftriaxone, reduced by gentamycin, and abolished by tetracycline and erythromycin (Vesce F et al., 1999). The above evidences indicate that, at least in pregnancy, the inhibitory action of β-lactamines on amniotic IL-6 and PGE release could be of value independently from their antibacterial action. Conversely, the classes of antibiotics that do not exert any inhibition on PGE release should not be used when preterm labour is not induced through a bacterial mediation. Furthermore, in cases of premature labour of inflammatory origin subsequently complicated by superimposed infection, macrolides addition to β-lactamines may eradicate infection, but it does not counteract the triggering pathogenic mechanism. In other words, in interpreting the efficacy of antibiotics in the management of premature labour, it is mandatory to know whether or not they directly inhibit inflammatory cytokines and prostanoids. It has been claimed that antibiotic therapy of premature labour in the presence of infection leads to the release of microbial products which may exacerbate the cytokine response and worsen the clinical picture. It has been also hypothesized that a similar scenario may occur in patients with microbial invasion of decidua and amniotic cavity. Such an initial worsening of the inflammatory response may accelerate the process of premature parturition and foetal damage. Nevertheless, it has been also suggested that transient down-regulation of the effects of the inflammatory response would permit the time that is required to eradicate the infectious process, without injury to the foetus. Indeed, anti-inflammatory cytokines, antibody to macrophage migration inhibitory factor and antioxidants, may also play a role in preventing delivery, neonatal injury, and long-term perinatal morbidity. Accordingly, a combination of antibiotics and immunomodulators (dexamethasone and indomethacin), in experimental premature labour induced by intra-amniotic inoculation with group B streptococci. in non human pregnant primates, was effective to eradicate infection, suppress the inflammatory response, and prolong gestation (Tsuzuki et al., 2009). One more aspect needs to be clarified before reporting our experience with use of low dose betamethasone for the prevention of pregnancy loss, and it deals with the necessity to discriminate the pathogenic role of prematurity from inflammation and hypoxia. Indeed, prematurity is still reported everywhere as the leading cause of perinatal morbidity and mortality (Mwaniki et al., 2012). Such a concept is obviously provided with some validity, but in the general contest of pregnancy complications it needs to be adequately scaled. Basically, it appears to stem from the link between prematurity and hyaline membrane disease (HMD) of the lung, an ominous disease that is ascribed to the failure of immature type II alveolar cells to produce sufficient surfactant (i. e. lecithin). As betamethasone was historically recognized to be able to prevent HMD, its efficacy was intended as a sort of "maturational promotion". However, there are good reasons to believe that the main pathogenic mechanism is rather of a hypoxic-inflammatory type. Indeed, premature foetuses express RDS of diverse intensity at the same gestational age, in relation with the grade of the pathology causing premature birth. Pregnancy complications leading to premature birth are largely a consequence of an inflammatory mechanism. Accordingly, prematurity is characterized by two other complications, i. e. NEC and encephalopathy, marked by high levels of inflammatory cytokines that also benefit from the action of betamethasone. Finally, the drug efficacy is limited to its timely prenatal administration, as it lacks when the hormone is given after birth, suggesting that it stimulates the production of an extra amount surfactant at a level other than the foetal alveoli that is subsequently delivered to the lung before birth thru gasping efforts a typical feature of foetal hypoxia. As we have demonstrated, the site of lecithin release in the foetal compartment is represented by amnion tissue (Vesce F et al., 1992). Based on these considerations, chronic intrauterine distress appears to play a major role compared to gestational age in the pathogenic mechanism of the 'prematurity' syndrome. Indeed, all above evidences indicates that FIRS proceeds from inflammatory processes endowed themselves with the capacity to lead to all above mentioned dangerous perinatal complications, infection included. Timely addition of GCs addressed to rebalance cytokines and prostanoids regulating the inflammatory response, represents therefore an unavoidable therapeutic approach.

8. Personal experience with low-dose betamethasone administration throughout pregnancy for prevention of pregnancy loss

The clinical observations by the corresponding author of the present chapter regarding pregnancy loss begun during the early seventies, when progesterone therapy was the main choice in cases of either threatened or recurrent abortion at the Department of Obstetrics and Gynaecology of Ferrara University. However, as ultrasounds became available, it clearly appeared to the echographers that, based on the above mentioned theoretical benefits, the drug was given blindly, even to patient with missed abortion as well as to those who never would have needed it. Indeed, there was no practical way (as it still substantially lacks today) to investigate the causes of abortion in single cases, and the explanation given to the patient dealt almost invariably with either corpus luteum deficiency or aneuploidy. Soon after we were informed that corticosteroids had been occasionally used successfully in patients with recurrent abortion when an "immunological basis" for rejection of the conceptus was hypothesized (Professor Denis Hawkins, of London, personal communication). In addition, administration of cortisone 25-75 mg/day up to 64 days during the first trimester for the treatment of hyperemesis had already been reported long before (Wells, 1953). At that stage, after observing many more cases of recurrent abortion, all treated with various regimens of progesterone, we concluded that there was no reason for further giving this drug to such women. The first case of recurrent abortion occasionally treated with betamethasone was 34 years ago a patient with bronchial asthma that, in spite of progesterone therapy, had experienced three early pregnancy losses. Subsequently she had gone through two years of anovulatory sterility, followed by several attempts to medical induction of ovulation, all ended in ovarian hyperstimulation syndrome. This patient was therefore counselled to assume 0.5 mg betamethasone daily for the next three months for treating asthma, and she started a spontaneous pregnancy one month later. Once adequately informed of a possible protective action of the hormone, she accepted to continue with the same regimen up to the end of pregnancy, when she delivered a normal foetus. Such a successful outcome encouraged us to cautiously adopt over the years low dose betamethasone therapy in all our patients with history of recurrent abortion previously unsuccessfully treated with progesterone. Furthermore, as we became aware of the high efficacy of the hormone, we extended its use to some other cases where protection of the first pregnancy was advisable even in the absence of previous pregnancy loss. These included, for instance, women of advanced age with or without previous sterility. We may say that there are several reasons for such a policy. The first one is represented by the lack of efficacy of progesterone in our experience, coupled with the tenuous and controversial evidence of a protective role in the above reported literature. A further point in favour of preventive GCs administration is that there are women who will not have the chance of a second pregnancy, and therefore they are suitable for prevention of possible inflammatory complications, for the timely diagnosis of which there are no available tests in the clinical practice. Indeed, as it became clear later on, GCs regulate the inflammatory process by modulating cytokine production (IL-6 and TNFα) (Thum et al., 2008) and decreasing maternal NK population (Quenby et al., 2005), two among the good reasons to adopt them in the clinical management of these cases. The study of this particular mechanism of GC in early pregnancy has been enhanced in the last years the focus being directed on prednisolone, the role of which in the prevention of recurrent pregnancy loss is currently under trial (Thang et al., 2009). However, its pharmacokinetic characteristics require a high dose to obtain the therapeutic effect. For instance, in the case reported by Quenby et al. (2003), a patient with history of 14 consecutive abortions between the 8th and 10th week of gestation, first received 5 mg/day preconceptual prednisolone, leading to 5 further abortions. Only when the dose was raised up to 20 mg/day she became able to deliver a preterm viable baby. Indeed, as it has been explained above, the trans-placental passage of the drug is highly impaired by 11-β-HSD isoenzymes. By contrast, compared to prednisolone, betamethasone is little metabolized by the placenta and it is ten times more effective (Burton & Waddell, 1999). Therefore, we decided to focus on betamethasone that is extensively used in advanced pregnancy for prevention of neonatal respiratory distress syndrome (Sotiriadis et al., 2009) but it is not adopted in early pregnancy, due to all above mentioned possible negative influences in animals, although they have not been confirmed in humans. Taking into account all these evidences, we choose to administer a low dose betamethasone, in order to obtain a better protective effect on pregnancy, avoiding at the same time significant maternal dose-dependent side effects. In our experience this therapeutic approach proved to be coupled with great efficacy and lack of significant complications. We treated over 200 cases until today, as other pregnancies are going on at the moment, the main indication being a history of recurrent pregnancy loss. There were cases in which the usual dose of 0.5 mg/day was ineffective to prevent abortion, and it was doubled during the subsequent pregnancy, to be increased up to 2 mg/day month by month, due to heavy bleeding around the time of the expected menstrual flow. These cases, not included in the sample below, ultimately ended with the birth of healthy babies around term. As expected, there were cases of pregnancy complications, such as premature delivery, IUGR, preeclampsia, abruptio placentae, gestational diabetes, that were handled with the standard obstetric care. Indeed, betamethasone does not represent the panacea for every adverse gestational condition. Overall, besides the high effectiveness of the therapy in preventing pregnancy loss, we can testify that neither foetal malformations nor significant maternal or foetal adverse effect of betamethasone were observed. No chance of a prospective randomized case-control study was offered at our Institution, in order to statistically prove the greater efficacy of betamethasone compared to other therapies. However we were able to analyze retrospectively a total of 101 treated patients as regards to some foetal biometric parameters and birth weight. Furthermore we performed two prospective studies aimed at verify two relevant end-points provided with physio-pathologic and clinical implications:

- the possible positive correlation of foetal growth restriction with maternal **peripheral** NK cells concentration;
- the possible efficacy of low-dose betamethasone therapy in decreasing the maternal **peripheral** NK cells concentration.

Our retrospective analysis includes 166 patients admitted to the Section of Obstetrics and Gynaecology of Ferrara University from the late seventies to 2010. The population was divided into three groups:

- (Group A): 80 patients treated by low dose betamethasone (0, 5 mg/daily) throughout pregnancy for previous history of recurrent miscarriage;
- (Group B): 65 patients with physiological pregnancy;
- (Group C): 21 patients affected by rheumatologic disease treated by prednisone (4-16 mg/daily).

Foetal growth was assessed by measuring the weight, head circumference and length at the birth. First data evaluation revealed neonatal weight and length significantly lower in the treated groups (2843,5 g and 48,14 cm in group A; 3262,92 g and 49,93 cm in group B; 2901,90 g and 49,67 in group C (Figure 2). Instead the head circumference was not statistically different among three groups (respectively 33.6 cm, 34.03 cm and 34.3 cm).

However in evaluating biometric parameters of the newborns, the pathological conditions of pregnancy that may lead to foetal growth restriction must be considered (Grivell et al., 2009). Among these, premature delivery, pre-eclampsia, gestational diabetes, hypothyroidism and bronchial asthma (Murphy & Gibson, 2011; Mitanchez, 2010; Krassas et al., 2010). Therefore, to get a more accurate evidence of the effect of betamethasone alone on foetal growth, we normalized the study population by excluding 26 patients suffering from the above mentioned diseases. By doing so, as expected, the differences among the neonatal biometric parameters were no more significant in the three groups (3144 g, 3262 g and 3171 g respectively for the birth weight; 49.73 cm, 49.3 cm and 49.63 cm for the neonatal length; 34.25 cm, 34.03 cm and 34.53 cm for the head circumference) (Figure 3).

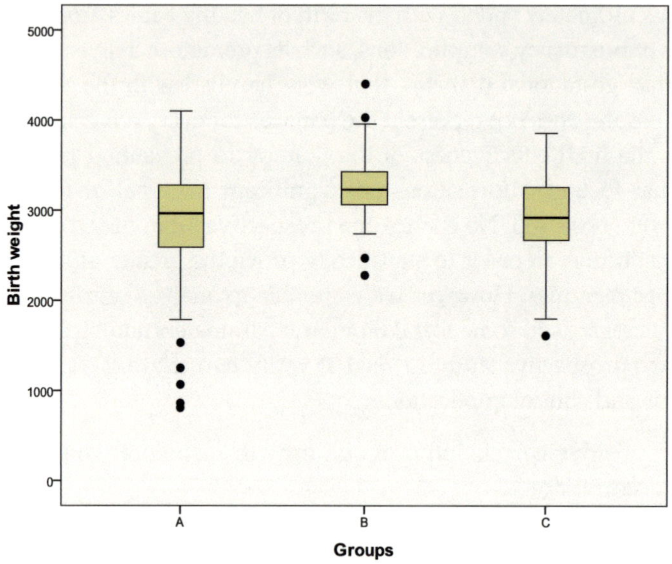

Figure 2. Distribution of birth weight in three groups. Group A (treated by betamethasone): 2843,5 g; Group B (physiologic pregnancy): 3262,92 g; Group C (rheumatologic diseases): 2901,90 g.

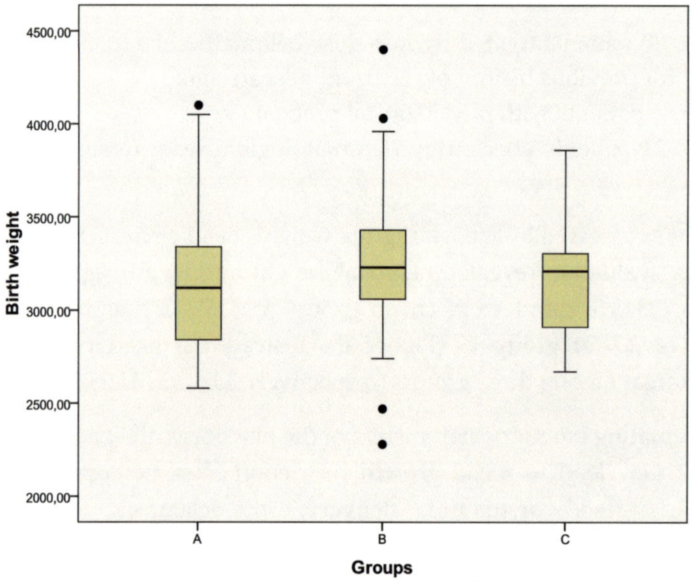

Figure 3. Distribution of birth weight in three groups after normalization of the study population. Group A (treated by betamethasone): 3144 g; Group B (physiologic pregnancy) 3262 g; Group C (rheumatologic diseases): 3171 g.

Moreover, by analyzing the distribution of birth weight values, we observed that one third of the newborns reached a weight higher than the fiftieth percentile in the treated group. Being all the patients upon the same betamethasone regimen, such an observation confirms that the cause of decreased neonatal weight should be ascribed to factors other than the hormone. The result of our attempt to homogenize the study sample highlights the need to take with caution the conclusions of other reports where different classes of patients were accidentally mixed up. As a matter of fact, most cases of GCs administration reported in the literature belong to pathologic conditions leading by themselves to foetal growth restriction (Davis et al., 2009; Kumar & Seshadri, et al., 2005). Coming to our first prospective study, we must recall that impairment of foetal oxygenation and growth, besides being linked with the above mentioned influences of unbalanced cytokines on utero-placental perfusion, is also reflected in the correlation between high values of uNK and IUGR (Williams et al., 2009). Therefore we decided to analyze the circulating lymphocyte subsets, mainly to search for a correlation between **peripheral** maternal NK concentration and foetal growth restriction. Such a possible link, to our knowledge never investigated before, could open the way to a practical test for the early diagnosis of a harmful complication. We selected ten pregnant women with a history of a successful pregnancy as a control group (group 1), plus ten with a diagnosis of IUGR, i.e. with foetal ultrasound biometric parameters below the 10th percentile (group 2). The course of pregnancy was normal in both groups, ending in spontaneous or elective caesarean delivery at term. Fresh blood samples drawn during the third trimester were analyzed at the Laboratory of the Haematological Unit of Ferrara University. Our study demonstrates that the number of peripheral leukocytes, the number of lymphocytes and their percentage were constant ($p<0,75$; $p<0,93$; $p<0,49$) while significant changes are observed for the NK cells. In particular:

- Significantly higher NK percentage (% $CD56^+$ cells) in group 2 (20,9) compared to group 1 (15,1) ($p<0,01$) (Figure 4);
- No significant increase in NK total number ($CD56^+$ U/μl cells) (419,6) in group 2 compared to group 1 (341,4) ($p< 0,10$);
- Significantly higher percentage NK subset ($CD2^+CD56^+$ cells) in group 2 (18,8) compared to group 1 (13,4) ($p<0.02$) (Figure 5).

By analyzing the other lymphocyte subsets, we observed a non significant $CD4^+$ T decrease along with a $CD8^+$ T increase, with a consequent decrease of their ratio. Moreover, there were no differences in the absolute count and percentage of the following lymphocyte subsets: T($CD3^+$) lymphocytes, T activated lymphocytes ($CD3^+$ HLA-DR^+), CD45 leukocytes, HLA-DR cells and B lymphocytes ($CD19^+$ e $CD19^+CD5^+$).

Therefore, increased peripheral NK percentage was the only significant feature of lymphocyte subset linked with IUGR in our study sample. Subsequently, with the aim to contribute to a better knowledge of the basic mechanisms of GCs protection, we evaluated the influence of betamethasone on the percentage of maternal pNK and other components of the lymphocyte subset in women with history of RSA. The patients with known anatomical, hormonal, genetic, infectious, autoimmune causes of abortion, as well as those with psychiatric disease were excluded from the study. Ten pregnant women with history of RSA

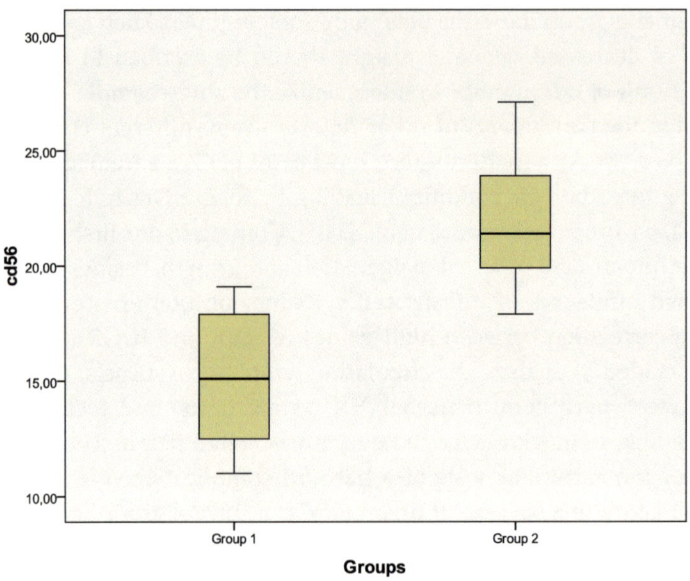

Figure 4. Comparison of pNK percentage (% CD56 +) between patients with adequate foetal growth (Group 1) and those with growth restriction (Group 2)

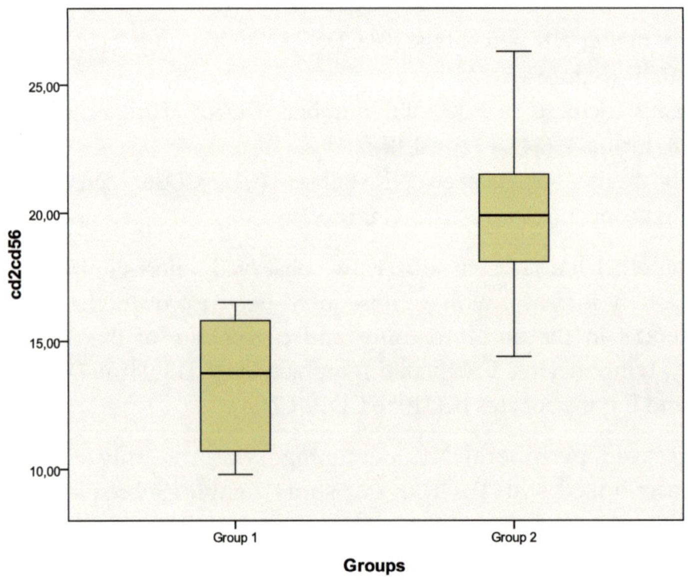

Figure 5. Comparison of the mean value of the CD2 + CD56 + subset percentage between patients with adequate foetal growth (Group 1) and those with growth restriction (Group 2).

were consecutively recruited (group 1). They were given oral betamethasone 0.5mg/daily from the fifth week of pregnancy until delivery. Ten normal pregnant women with previous history of successful pregnancies served as a control group (group 2). Blood samples were drawn at each one of the three trimesters (t1-first trimester, t2-second, t3-third). Fresh samples were analyzed at the Laboratory of the Haematology Unit of Ferrara University. The comparison between the two groups showed that lymphocytes percentage was significantly lower upon betamethasone therapy only in the third trimester (p-value =0,035). The percentage of T CD4+ cells in the third trimester was higher in treated women (46,4%) compared with controls (42,2%) (p-value =0,031), while that of T CD8+ cells was significantly lower in RSA in the second and in the third trimester. Comparison of CD2+, CD3+, CD5+, CD19+, CD45+, CD3+HLA-DR+ and CD19+CD5+ cells percentage between groups revealed no difference. As for NK, during the first trimester their percentage in RSA did not differ from that of the controls (gr1=15,0%, gr2=15,3%). However in the second trimester it became significantly lower (gr1=15,2%, gr2=17,6%, p-value=0,045). In the third trimester, despite a drop of their percentage (reaching 12,0%), only the absolute NK count decrease reached statistical significance. The percentage of NK subset CD2+CD56+ in the second and third trimester was significantly lower in group 1 (Figure 6). Our data on controls show the absence of significant changes in leukocyte and NK count and percentage throughout pregnancy. Coming to leukocyte subsets, we registered a lymphocytes decrease in the second trimester and a subsequent raise in the third, and a T CD4+ lymphocytes decrease with a T CD8+ increase throughout pregnancy. All together, these results substantially agree with the previous studies on physiologic pregnancy (Radysh et al., 2005).

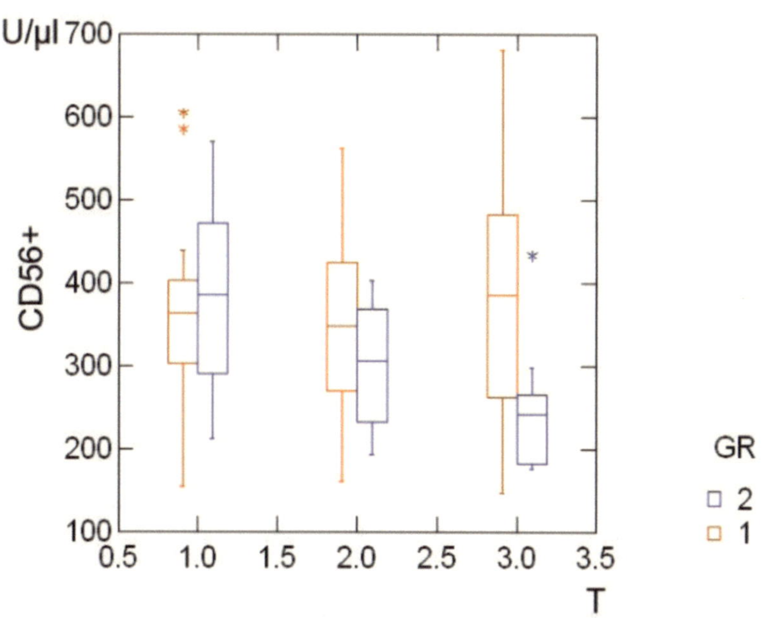

Figure 6. Trend of CD56 + cells U / l in group 1 and group 2 in the three trimesters. Time = 1.0 1^ trimester, 2.0 = 2^ trimester, 3.0 = 3^ trimester. Gr1 = normal pregnancy, Gr.2 = pregnancy with history of RSA treated with betamethasone

In the present study, moreover, we found that chronic low dose betamethasone administration leads to a significant decrease of leukocyte total number. Such behaviour is opposite to the well known leukocyte increase that follows 24 mg betamethasone administration during the third trimester for the prevention of hyaline membrane disease of the newborn. In addition, the lymphocytes percentage decrease caused by betamethasone reached statistical significance compared with controls in the third trimester. Such a result is likely to be related to the reduction of pNK. In treated cases NK percentage and number during the second and third trimester respectively reached lower values compared to controls. However, their values during the first trimester did not differ. Since it has been reported that women with history of RSA have a higher peripheral NK percentage, the absence of a difference between treated cases and physiological pregnancies during the first trimester in our data can be interpreted as an effect of betamethasone administration. In other words, betamethasone in RSA was able to decrease NK to values equal to (first trimester) and lower than (second and third) those in physiological pregnancy. With regard to the other lymphocyte subsets, it had been reported that women with RSA have a higher T cytotoxic CD8+ and T activated cells (CD3+HLA-DR+) percentage as compared to physiological pregnancy. Our work showed that betamethasone is able to decrease T CD8+ percentage to the same or even lower values compared to physiological pregnancy. In addition, we found no differences for T activated cells, between physiological pregnancy and treated RSA group, probably due to a suppressive action of the hormone. Previous studies demonstrated a CD19+CD5+ decrease in normal pregnancy. These are B lymphocytes producing auto-antibodies, and their percentage typically raises in RSA and in ANA positive women. Indeed, their percentage is reported to fall from 4,17% in the first trimester to 1,92% in the third. In contrast, we did not find any difference in CD19+CD5+ percentage between the 2 groups. In conclusion, our research shows that 0.5 mg/day betamethasone therapy throughout pregnancy in RSA women reduces pNK cells, CD19+CD5+ and CD3+HLA-DR+ lymphocytes. Such a finding, based on the above reported data in the literature, suggests that, besides the possible rebalancing effect of the drug upon the inflammatory cytokines at the implantation site, successful outcome probably derives also from an action on the cellular components of the immune system. It is noteworthy that the clinical result is obtained with use of a low dose that proved to be harmless for the foetus and devoid of maternal side effects.

9. Conclusive remarks

We have reported in the present chapter the regulation of the gestational processes as it appears from the data in the literature. Pregnancy can be essentially interpreted as a vascular phenomenon resulting from a balanced activation and release of a great number of mediators upon hormonal control. Corpus luteum progesterone is required before conception in order to adapt the uterine decidua to the subsequent early phase of implantation. However it was shown long ago that from the seventh week onward the corpus luteum is no more needed, as at this stage castration becomes unable to interrupt pregnancy. In spite of such evidence, the hormone is extensively used for prevention of abortion, and it keeps on being advocated even later on (Lucovnik et al., 2011), mainly based on its immuno-modulatory and myometrial relaxing effects. Recent research shed light on a more relevant cause of pregnancy loss than progesterone deficiency that is represented by inflammation at any stage of the gestational process. It can be triggered along a number of pathways, infection included. Nevertheless, infection, although accounting for ominous complications, has been found in some cases to represent a consequence rather than the cause of gestational inflammation. Inflammatory changes appear quite often to derive from a derangement of cytokines and prostanoids involved in the regulation of gestational physiological processes. A great number of cell function mediators has been found to be linked either with favourable outcome or with pregnancy loss, depending on the experimental model as well as on the gestational stage, but none can be identified alone as the keystone, successful pregnancy appearing the result of a balanced action of all mediators together. On the contrary, their imbalance leads to the activation of blood coagulation and stimulation of uterine contraction, the basic mechanisms for any pregnancy loss, aneuploid included (Vesce et al., 1996; Vesce et al., 2001; Vesce 2002). Myometrial activity is triggered by the release of prostanoids, mainly PGs of the E type, upon the action of many unbalanced cytokines. During the first trimester such abnormalities are confined to the feto-placental unit, while from late second to the third they can involve the maternal organism as well, leading to the variable clinical signs of preeclampsia. Outcome of pregnancy depends on the time of onset, the grade and the duration of cytokine imbalance. Moreover it must be considered that the maternal vascular adaptation is induced by the foetus itself, through the action of mediators released by trophoblastic cells on the uterine spiral arteries, and that even apparently late complications, such as preeclampsia, derive their origin from early foetal inadequacy (Vesce et al., 1997) Derangement of such mediators largely recognizing an inflammatory pathogenic mechanism, and low dose betamethasone being devoid of significant foetal side effects, there is no reason for administrating the glucocorticoids whose transfer to the foetus is highly impaired by 11β-HSD iso-enzymes. Indeed two possible scenarios can be identified:

- the trophoblast is able to modify the uterine vessels, but the unfavourable decidual environment impairs such a potential capacity;
- the maternal environment is favourable, but the trophoblast is unable to correctly operate.

In either one of the cases, there are several possible treatments that, like in any other disease, can be classified as symptomatic or etiological: the first are addressed to counteract uterine contractions and blood clotting, the second aimed at rebalancing maternal, as well as foetal, cytokine derangement that leads to abnormal prostanoids release. However, none of the available therapeutic options is able to reverse endothelial damage, once it is already established. Moreover, only etiological therapies are provided with the capacity to prevent the clinical pictures of pregnancy loss in high risk cases. Therefore, once the risk identified, etiological prevention and cure must start as early as possible, in some cases even before conception, and last enough to ensure foetal survival. In our opinion, GCs are the best preventive choice, as they represent the natural controller of the cross-talk that trophoblast entertains with maternal cells, throughout their entangled cytokine network. In this perspective, their efficacy is not to be intended simply as the result of a mere anti-inflammatory action, but rather as a complex direct and indirect regulatory influence on the mediators of cell functions. For instance, betamethasone, from one hand directly down-regulates the synthesis of inflammatory cytokines, while from the other it indirectly does the opposite by stimulating the MIF system. Unfortunately, in spite of the clinical evidence of the lack of significant maternal and foetal side effects of appropriate doses extensively reported in the literature, coupled with the great therapeutic benefits in life-threatening pregnancy complications, the concern for a negative impact on foetal morphogenesis and growth, mainly derived from experiments in animals with use of high doses, still impairs the correct adoption of GCs in the prevention of gestational risk. In the present chapter we reported some data from our long term use of low dose betamethasone throughout gestation for the prevention of pregnancy loss. Basically it is justified by the concept that pregnancy loss is the results of a cytokine imbalance possibly leading to inflammation, a derangement for which the use of progesterone is clinically proved to be either unsuitable or ineffective. In our experience, low dose betamethasone therapy is provided with great efficacy and devoid of significant foetal and maternal side effects. It will keep on representing the first choice therapy for protection of pregnancy in our practice.

Author details

Fortunato Vesce, Emilio Giugliano, Elisa Cagnazzo,
Stefania Bignardi, Elena Mossuto, Tarcisio Servello and Roberto Marci
Department of Biomedical Sciences and Advanced Therapy,
Section of Obstetrics and Gynecology, University of Ferrara, Italy

10. References

Abou-Ghannam G, Usta IM, Nassar AH (2011) Indomethacin in Pregnancy: Applications and Safety Am J Perinatol In press

Aghajafari F (2002) Repeated doses of antenatal corticosteroids in animals: a systematic review. American Journal of Obstetrics and Gynecology 186:843

Al-Bahrani A, Taha S, Shaath H & Bakhiet M (2007) TNF-alpha and IL-8 in acute stroke and the modulation of these cytokines by antiplatelet agents. Curr Neurovasc Res 4:31-7

Anderson BL, Simhan HN, Simons K & Wiesenfeld HC (2008) Additional antibiotic use and preterm birth among bacteriuric and nonbacteriuric pregnant women. Int J Gynaecol Obstet 102:141-5

Annells MF, Hart PH, Mullighan CG, Heatley SL, Robinson JS & McDonald HM (2005) Polymorphisms in immunoregulatory genes and the risk of histologic chorioamnionitis in Caucasoid women: a case control study. BMC Pregnancy Childbirth.5:4

Arck PC, Gilhar A, Bienenstock J & Paus R (2008) The alchemy of immune privilege explored from a neuroimmunological perspective. Curr Opin Pharmacol 8: 480-9.

Arcuri, F., Ricci, C., Ietta, F., Cintorino, M., Tripodi, S.A., Cetin, I., Garzia, E., Schatz, F., Klemi, P., Santopietro, R. et al. (2001) Macrophage migration inhibitory factor in the human endometrium: expression and localization during the menstrual cycle and early pregnancy. Biol. Reprod., 64, 1200–1205.

Arcuri F, Cintorino M, Carducci A, Papa S, Riparbelli MG, Mangioni S, Di Blasio AM, Tosi P & Viganò P (2006) Human decidual natural killer cells as a source and target of macrophage migration inhibitory factor. Reproduction. 131:175-82.

Baglin T, Gray E, Greaves M, Hunt BJ, Keeling D, Machin S, Mackie I, Makris M, Nokes T, Perry D, Tait RC, Walker I & Watson H (2010) Clinical guidelines for testing for heritable thrombophilia. Br J Haematol 149: 209–220

Bates SM, Greer AI, Pabinger I, Sofaer S & Hirsh J (2008) Venous thromboembolism, thrombophilia, antithrombotic therapy, and pregnancy: American College of Chest Physicians Evidence- Based Clinical Practice Guidelines (8th edition). Chest. 133: 844S-88

Bechi N, Ietta F, Romagnoli R, Jantra S, Cencini M, Galassi G,Serchi T, Corsi I, Focardi S & Paulesu L (2010) Environmental levels of para-nonylphenol are able to affect cytokine secretion in human placenta. Environ Health Perspect 118: 427-31

Biondi C, Pavan B, Ferretti ME, Corradini FG, Neri LM & Vesce F (2001) Formyl-methionyl-leucyl-phenylalanine induces prostaglandin E2 release from human amnion-derived WISH cells by phospholipase C-mediated [Ca+]i rise. Biol Reprod. 64:865-70.

Biondi C, Ferretti ME, Pavan B, Lunghi L, Gravina B, Nicoloso MS, Vesce F & Baldassarre G (2006) Prostaglandin E2 inhibits proliferation and migration of HTR-8/SVneo cells, a human trophoblast-derived cell line. Placenta 27:592-601.

Bonanno C, Fuchs K & Wapner RJ (2007) Single versus repeat courses of antenatal steroids to improve neonatal outcomes: risks and benefits. Obstet Gynecol Surv 62:261-71

Bondza PK, Metz CN & Akoum A (2008) Postgestational effects of macrophage migration inhibitory factor on embryonic implantation in mice. Fertil Steril.90:1433-43

Boomsma CM, Kavelaars A, Eijkemans MJ, Lentjes EG, Fauser BC, Heijnen CJ & Macklon NS (2009) Endometrial secretion analysis identifies a cytokine profile predictive of pregnancy in IVF. Hum Reprod. 24:1427-35.

Broering R, Montag M, Jiang M, Lu M, Sowa JP, Kleinehr K, Gerken G & Schlaak JF (2011) Corticosteroids shift the Toll-like receptor response pattern of primary-isolated murine liver cells from an inflammatory to an anti-inflammatory state.Int Immunol 23:537-44

Burrows TD, King A & Loke YW (1996) Trophoblast migration during human placental implantation. Hum Reprod Update 2:307-21.

Burton PJ & Waddell BJ (1999) Dual function of 11beta-hydroxysteroid dehydrogenase in placenta: modulating placental glucocorticoid passage and local steroid action. Biol Reprod. 60:234-40

Buzzi M, Vesce F, Ferretti ME, Fabbri E & Biondi C (1999) Does formyl-methionyl-leucyl-phenylalanine exert a physiological role in labor in women? Biol Reprod. 60:1211-6.

Calandra T, Bernhagen J, Metz CN, Spiegel LA, Bacher M, Donnelly T, Cerami A & Bucala R (1995) MIF as a glucocorticoid-induced modulator of cytokine production. Nature 377: 68-71.

Calandra T & Roger T (2003) Macrophage migration inhibitory factor: a regulator of innate immunity. Nat Rev Immunol 3: 791-800

Calleja-Agius J, Jauniaux E, Pizzey AR & Muttukrishna S (2012) Investigation of systemic inflammatory response in first trimester pregnancy failure. Hum Reprod. 27:349-57.

Cardaropoli S, Paulesu L, Romagnoli R, Ietta F, Marzioni D, Castellucci M, Rolfo A, Vasario E, Piccoli E, Todros T. Macrophage migration inhibitory factor in fetoplacental tissues from preeclamptic pregnancies with or without fetal growth restriction. Clin Dev Immunol. 2012;2012:639342.

Carlson AD, Obeid JS, Kanellopoulou N, Wilson RC & New MI (1999) Congenital adrenal hyperplasia: update on prenatal diagnosis and treatment. J Steroid Biochem Mol Biol. 69:19-29.

Carp HJ (2009) Aspirin in Recurrent Miscarriage: Is There an Indication? Isr Med Assoc J 11:178-82

Cervellati F, Pavan B, Lunghi L, Manni E, Fabbri E, Mascoli C, Biondi C, Patella A & Vesce F (2011) Betamethasone, progesterone and RU-486 exert similar effects on connexin expression in trophoblast-derived HTR-8/SVneo cells. Reprod Fertil Dev. 23:319-28

Challis JR, Lockwood CJ, Myatt L, Norman JE, Strauss JF 3rd, Petraglia F. Inflammation and pregnancy. Reprod Sci. 16:206-15

Chaouat G, Dubanchet S & Ledée N (2007) Cytokines: important for implantation? J Assist Reprod Genet 24: 491-505

Cheah FC, Winterbourn CC, Darlow BA, Mocatta TJ & Vissers MC (2005) Nuclear factor kappaB activation in pulmonary leukocytes from infants with hyaline membrane disease: associations with chorioamnionitis and Ureaplasma urealyticum colonization. Pediatr Res. 57:616-23.

Christiansen OB, Pedersen B, Rosgaard A & Husth M (2002) A randomized, double-blind, placebo-controlled trial of intravenous immunoglobulin in the prevention of recurrent miscarriage: evidence for a therapeutic effect in women with secondary recurrent miscarriage. Hum Reprod 17:809–816

Clark DA, Chaouat G, Arck PC, Mittruecker HW & Levy GA (1998) Cytokine-dependent abortion in CBA x DBA/2 mice is mediated by the procoagulant fgl2 prothrombinase. J Immunol. 160:545-9.

Clark P, Walker ID, Langhorne P,Crichton L, Thomson A, Greaves M, Whyte S & Greer IA (2010) The Scottish Pregnancy Intervention Study: a multicenter randomized controlled trial of low molecular weight heparin and low dose aspirin in women with recurrent miscarriage. Blood 115:4162–4167

Cleasby ME, Kelly PA, Walker BR & Seckl JR (2003) Programming of rat muscle and fat metabolism by in utero overexposure to glucocorticoids, Endocrinology 144:999–1007

Comp PC, Thurnau GR, Welsh J & Esmon CT (1986) Functional and immunologic protein S levels are decreased during pregnancy. Blood 68: 881-5

Coomarasamy A, Truchanowicz EG & Rai R (2011) Does first trimester progesterone prophylaxis increase the live birth rate in women with unexplained recurrent miscarriages? BMJ. 342:d1914.

Cox SM,Bohman VR,Sherman ML & Leveno KJ (1996) Randomized investigation of antimicrobials for the prevention of preterm birth. Am J Obstet Gynecol 174: 296-10

Cowchock S & Reece EA (1997) Do low-risk pregnant women with antiphospholipid antibodies need to be treated? Organizing Group of the Antiphospholipid Antibody Treatment Trial. Am J Obstet Gynecol 176: 1099-100

Cronier L, Alsat E, Harve` JC, De´le´ze J & Malassine` A (1998) Dexamethasone stimulates gap-junctional communication, peptide hormone production and differentiation in human term trophoblast. Placenta 19(Suppl. 1), 35–49

Crowther CA & Harding JE (2007) Repeat doses of prenatal corticosteroids for women at risk of preterm birth for preventing neonatal respiratory disease. Cochrane Database Syst Rev 3:CD003935

Cunha FQ, Weiser WY, David JR, Moss DW, Moncada S & Liew FY (1993) Recombinant migration inhibitory factor induces nitric oxide synthase in murine macrophages. J Immunol 150: 1908-12.

Dahlgren J, Nilsson C, Jennische E, Ho HP, Eriksson E, Niklasson A, Björntorp P, Albertsson Wikland K & Holmäng A. (2001) Prenatal cytokine exposure results in obesity and gender-specific programming, Am. J. Physiol. Endocrinol. Metab. 281:E326–E334

Danesi R & Del Tacca M (2004) Teratogenesis and immunosuppressive treatment. Transplant Proc 36:705-7

Davis EP, Waffarn F, Uy C, Hobel CJ, Glynn LM & Sandman CA (2009) Effect of prenatal glucocorticoid treatment on size at birth among infants born at term gestation. J Perinatol 29:731-7

de Vries A, Holmes MC, Heijnis A, Seier JV, Heerden J, Louw J, Wolfe-Coote S, Meaney MJ, Levitt NS & Seckl JR (2007) Prenatal dexamethasone exposure induces changes in nonhuman primate offspring cardiometabolic and hypothalamic–pituitary–adrenal axis function. J. Clin. Invest. 117:1058–1067

Dekel N, Gnainsky Y, Granot I & Mor G (2010) Inflammation and implantation. Am J Reprod Immunol 63: 17-21

Eastabrook G, Hu Y & von Dadelszen P (2008) The role of decidual natural killer cells in normal placentation and in the pathogenesis of preeclampsia. J Obstet Gynaecol Can. 30:467-76.

Engel SA, Erichsen HC, Savitz DA, Thorp J, Chanock SJ & Olshan AF (2005) Risk of spontaneous preterm birth is associated with common proinflammatory cytokine polymorphisms. Epidemiology 16:469-77.

Fest S, Aldo PB, Abrahams VM, Visintin I, Alvero A, Chen R, Chavez SL, Romero R & Mor G (2007) Trophoblast-macrophage interactions: a regulatory network for the protection of pregnancy. Am J Reprod Immunol.57:55-66.

Fingerle-Rowson G, Petrenko O, Metz CN, Forsthuber TG, Mitchell R, Huss R, Moll U, Müller W & Bucala R (2003) The p53-dependent effects of macrophage migration inhibitory factor revealed by gene targeting. Proc Natl Acad Sci U S A. 100:9354-9

Fonseca L, Ramin SM, Mele L, Wapner RJ, Johnson F, Peaceman AM, Sorokin Y, Dudley DJ, Spong CY, Leveno KJ, Caritis SN, Miodovnik M, Mercer B, Thorp JM, O'sullivan MJ, Carpenter MW, Rouse DJ & Sibai B; Eunice Kennedy Shriver National Institute of Child

Health and Human Development (NICHD) Maternal Fetal Medicine Units Network (MFMU) (2009) Bone metabolism in fetuses of pregnant women exposed to single and multiple courses of corticosteroids. Obstet Gynecol. 114:38-44

Furukawa S, Usuda K, Abe M & Ogawa I (2004) Histopathological findings of cleft palate in rat embryos induced by triamcinolone acetonide. J Vet Med Sci 66:397-402

Gaillard R, Riondel A, Muller A, Herrmann W & Baulieu EE (1984) RU 486: A steroid with antiglucocorticosteroid activity that only disinhibits the human pituitary-adrenal system at a specific time of day. Proc Natl Acad Sci USA 81:3879–3882

Garfield RE, Blennerhasset MG & Miller SM (1988) Control of myometrial contractility: role and regulation of gap-junctions. Oxf Rev Reprod Biol 10:436-90

Gesina E, Blondeau B, Milet A, Le Nin I, Duchene B, Czernichow P, Scharfmann R, Tronche F & Breant B (2006) Glucocorticoid signalling affects pancreatic development through both direct and indirect effects, Diabetologia 49:2939–2947

Gibbs RS, Romero R, Hiller SL, Eschenbach DA, Sweet RL (1992) A review of premature birth and subclinical infection. Am J obstet Gynecol 166. 1515-28

Gopichandran N, Ekbote UV, Walker JJ, Brooke D & Orsi NM (2006) Multiplex determination of murine seminal fluid cytokine profiles. Reproduction 131: 613-21

Grimes DA (1997) Medical abortion in early pregnancy: a review of the evidence. Obstet Gynecol 89:790-6

Grivell R, Dodd J & Robinson J (2009) The prevention and treatment of intrauterine growth restriction. Best Pract Res Clin Obstet Gynaecol. 2009 23:795-807

Guerin LR, Prins JR & Robertson SA (2009) Regulatory T-cells and immune tolerance in pregnancy: a new target for infertility treatment? Hum Reprod Update 15:517-35.

Guller S, Kong L, Wozniak R & Lockwood CJ (1995) Reduction of extracellular matrix protein expression in human amnion epithelial cells by glucocorticoids: a potential role in preterm rupture of the fetal membranes. J Clin Endocrinol Metab. 80:2244-50.

Gur C, Diav-Citrin O, Shechtman S, Arnon J & Ornoy A (2004) Pregnancy outcome after first trimester exposure to corticosteroids: a prospective controlled study. Reprod Toxicol 18: 93-101

Guyatt GH, Akl EA, Crowther M, Gutterman DD & Schuünemann HJ; American College of Chest Physicians Antithrombotic Therapy and Prevention of Thrombosis Panel. (2012) Executive summary: Antithrombotic Therapy and Prevention of Thrombosis, 9th ed: American College of Chest Physicians Evidence-Based Clinical Practice Guidelines. Chest 141(2 Suppl):7S-47S

Haas DM & Ramsey PS (2008) Progestogen for preventing miscarriage. Cochrane Database Syst Rev (2):CD003511

Heikinheimo O, Raivio T, Honkanen H, Ranta S & Jänne OA.Termination of pregnancy with mifepristone and prostaglandin suppresses transiently circulating glucocorticoid bioactivity. J Clin Endocrinol Metab. 88:323-6

Hill DJ & Duvillie B (2000) Pancreatic development and adult diabetes. Pediatr. Res.48:269–274

Hirata T, Osuga Y, Hamasaki K, Hirota Y, Nose E, Morimoto C, Harada M, Takemura Y, Koga K, Yoshino O, Tajima T, Hasegawa A, Yano T & Taketani Y (2007) Expression of toll-like receptors 2, 3, 4, and 9 genes in the human endometrium during the menstrual cycle. J Reprod Immunol. 74: 53-60

Huang HY, Chan SH, Wu CH, Wang CW, Lai CH & Soong YK (2005) Interleukin-1 system messenger ribonucleic acid and protein expression in human fallopian tube may be associated with ectopic pregnancy. Fertil Steril.84:1484-92.

Ietta F, Todros T, Ticconi C, Piccoli E, Zicari A, Piccione E & Paulesu L (2002) Macrophage migration inhibitory factor in human pregnancy and labor. Am J Reprod Immunol. 48:404-9.

Ietta F, Wu Y, Romagnoli R, Soleymanlou N, Orsini B, Zamudio S, Paulesu L & Caniggia I (2007) Oxygen regulation of macrophage migration inhibitory factor in human placenta. Am J Physiol Endocrinol Metab. 292:E272-80.

Ietta F, Bechi N, Romagnoli R, Bhattacharjee J, Realacci M, Di Vito M, Ferretti C & Paulesu L (2010) 17β-Estradiol modulates the macrophage migration inhibitory factor secretory pathway by regulating ABCA1 expression in human first-trimester placenta.Am J Physiol Endocrinol Metab. 298:E411-8

Jauniaux E, Gulbis B, Schandene L, Collette J & Hustin J (1996) Distribution of interleukin-6 in maternal and embryonic tissues during the first trimester. Mol Hum Reprod 2:239-43.

Jin LP, Chen QY, Zhang T, Guo PF, Li DJ. The CD4+CD25 bright regulatory T cells and CTLA-4 expression in peripheral and decidual lymphocytes are down-regulated in human miscarriage. Clin Immunol. 2009 Dec;133(3):402-10.

Kajantie E, Raivio T, Janne OA, Hovi P, Dunkel L & Andersson S (2004) Circulating glucocorticoid bioactivity in the preterm newborn after antenatal betamethasone treatment. J Clin Endocrinol Metab 89:3999–4003

Karagouni EE, Chryssikopoulos A, Mantzavinos T, Kanakas N & Dotsika EN (1998) Interleukin-1beta and interleukin-1alpha may affect the implantation rate of patients undergoing in vitro fertilization-embryo transfer. Fertil Steril. 70:553-9.

Kibschull M, Gellhaus A & Winterhager E. (2008). Analogous and unique functions of connexins in mouse and human placental development. *Placenta* 29, 848–854. doi:10.1016/J.PLACENTA.2008.07.013

King J & Flenady V (2002) Prophylactic antibiotics for inhibiting preterm labour with intact membranes. Cochrane Database Syst Rev 4:CD000246

King J, Flenady V, Cole S, Thornton S (2005) Cyclo-oxygenase (COX) inhibitors for treating preterm labour. Cochrane Database Syst Rev (2):CD001992.

Kirshbaum T (1993)Antibiotics in the treatment of preterm labor. Am J Obstet Gynecol 16 1239-46

Knackstedt M, Ding JW, Arck PC, Hertwig K, Coulam CB, August C, Lea R, Dudenhausen JW, Gorczynski RM, Levy GA & Clark DA (2001) Activation of the novel prothrombinase, fg12, as a basis for the pregnancy complications spontaneous abortion and pre-eclampsia. Am J Reprod Immunol. 46:196-210.

Korakaki E, Gourgiotis D, Aligizakis A, Manoura A, Hatzidaki E, Giahnakis E, Marmarinos A, Kalmanti M & Giannakopoulou C (2007) Levels of bone collagen markers in preterm infants: relation to antenatal glucocorticoid treatment. J Bone Miner Metab 25:172–178

Krassas GE, Poppe K & Glinoer D (2010) Thyroid function and human reproductive health.Endocr Rev 31:702-55

Kumar P & Seshadri R. Neonatal morbidity and growth in very low birth-weight infants after multiple courses of antenatal steroids. J Perinatol 25:698–702.

Kwak-Kim JY, Chung-Bang HS, Ng SC, Ntrivalas EI, Mangubat CP, Beaman KD, Beer AE & Gilman-Sachs A (2003) Increased T helper 1 cytokine responses by circulating T cells are present in women with recurrent pregnancy losses and in infertile women with multiple implantation failures after IVF. Hum Reprod.18:767-73.

Kwak-Kim J, Park JC, Ahn HK, Kim JW & Gilman-Sachs A (2010) Immunological modes of pregnancy loss. Am J Reprod Immunol. 63:611-23.

Laird SM, Tuckerman EM, Cork BA, Linjawi S, Blakemore AI & Li TC (2003) A review of immune cells and molecules in women with recurrent miscarriage. Hum Reprod Update 9:163-74

Lee SE, Romero R, Park CW, Jun JK & Yoon BH (2008) The frequency and significance of intraamniotic inflammation in patients with cervical insufficiency. Am J Obstet Gynecol 198:633.e1-8

Leonhardt SA & Edwards DP (2002) Mechanism of action of progesterone antagonists. Exp Biol Med 227:969-80

Li W, Gao L, Wang Y, Duan T, Myatt L & Sun K (2006) Enhancement of cortisol-induced 11beta-hydroxysteroid dehydrogenase type 1 expression by interleukin 1beta in cultured human chorionic trophoblast cells. Endocrinology 147: 2490-5.

Liu J & Feng ZC (2010) Increased umbilical cord plasma interleukin-1 beta levels was correlated with adverse outcomes of neonatal hypoxic-ischemic encephalopathy. J Trop Pediatr. 56:178-82

Lucovnik M, Kuon RJ, Chambliss LR, Maner WL, Shi SQ, Shi L, Balducci J & Garfield RE (2011) Progestin treatment for the prevention of preterm birth. Acta Obstet Gynecol Scand. 90:1057-69

Lunghi L, Pavan B, Biondi C, Paolillo R, Valerio A, Vesce F & Patella A (2010) Use of glucocorticoids in pregnancy. Curr Pharm Des. 16:3616-37.

Malassine′ A & Cronier L. (2005). Involvement of gap junctions in placental functions and development. Biochim. Biophys. Acta 1719:117–124.

Masuhiro K, Matsuzaki N, Nishino E, Taniguchi T, Kameda T, Li Y, Saji F & Tanizawa O (1991) Trophoblast-derived interleukin-1 (IL-1) stimulates the release of human chorionic gonadotropin by activating IL-6 and IL-6-receptor system in first trimester human trophoblasts. J Clin Endocrinol Metab.72:594-601.

McDonald HM, Brocklehurst P & Gordon A (2007) Antibiotics for treating bacterial vaginosis in pregnancy. Cochrane Database Syst Rev 1:CD000262;

McNeil CJ, Nwagwu MO, Finch AM, Page KR, Thain A, McArdle HJ & Ashworth CJ. (2007) Glucocorticoid exposure and tissue gene expression of 11beta HSD-1, 11beta HSD-2, and glucocorticoid receptor in a porcine model of differential fetal growth. Reproduction 133: 653-61

Michael AE & Papageorghiou AT (2008) Potential significance of physiological and pharmacological glucocorticoids in early pregnancy. Hum Reprod Update 14:497-517

Minas V, Loutradis D & Makrigiannakis A (2005) Factors controlling blastocyst implantation. Reprod Biomed Online. 10:205-16.

Mitanchez D (2010) Fetal and neonatal complications of gestational diabetes: perinatal mortality, congenital malformations, macrosomia, shoulder dystocia, birth injuries, neonatal outcomes. J Gynecol Obstet Biol Reprod (Paris). 39:S189-99

Mitsunari M, Yoshida S, Shoji T, Tsukihara S, Iwabe T, Harada T & Terakawa N (2006) Macrophage-activating lipopeptide-2 induces cyclooxygenase-2 and prostaglandin E(2) via toll-like receptor 2 in human placental trophoblast cells. J Reprod Immunol 72:46-59

Murphy VE, Zakar T, Smith R, Giles WB, Gibson PG & Clifton VL (2002) Reduced 11β-hydroxysteroid dehydrogenase type 2 activity is associated with decreased birth weight centile in pregnancies complicated by asthma. J Clin Endocrinol Metab 87:1660–1668

Murphy VE & Gibson PG (2011) Asthma in pregnancy. Clin Chest Med.32:93-110

Mwaniki MK, Atieno M, Lawn JE & Newton CR (2012) Long-term neurodevelopmental outcomes after intrauterine and neonatal insults: a systematic review. Lancet. 379:445-52

Nath CA, Ananth CV, Smulian JC, Shen-Schwarz S & Kaminsky L (2007) Histologic evidence of inflammation and risk of placental abruption. Am J Obstet Gynecol.197:319.e1-6.

Nielsen HS, Steffensen R, Varming K, Van Halteren AG, Spierings E, Ryder LP, Goulmy E & Christiansen OB (2009) Association of HY-restricting HLA class II alleles with pregnancy outcome in patients with recurrent miscarriage subsequent to a firstborn boy. Hum Mol Genet 18:1684–1691

Nishimura T, Dunk C, Lu Y, Feng X, Gellhaus A, Winterhager E, Rossant J & Lye SJ. (2004). Gap junctions are required for trophoblast proliferation in early human placental development. *Placenta* 25, 595–607. doi:10.1016/J.PLACENTA.2004.01.002

Norman JE, Kelly RW & Baird DT (1991) Uterine activity and decidual prostaglandin production in women in early pregnancy in response to mifepristone with or without indomethacin in vivo. Hum Reprod 6:740-4

Nyirenda MJ, Lindsay RS, Kenyon, Burchell A & Seckl JR (1998) Glucocorticoid exposure in late gestation permanently programs rat hepatic phosphoenolpyruvate carboxykinase and glucocorticoid receptor expression and causes glucose intolerance in adult offspring, J. Clin. Invest. 101:2174–2181

Nyirenda MJ, Carter R, Tang JI, de Vries A, Schlumbohm C, Hillier SG, Streit F, Oellerich M, Armstrong VW, Fuchs E & Seckl JR. (2009) Prenatal programming of metabolic syndrome in the common marmoset is associated with increased expression of 11beta-hydroxysteroid dehydrogenase type 1, Diabetes 58:2873–2879

Parker Jr CR, AtkinsonMW,Owen J & AndrewsWW (1996) Dynamics of the fetal adrenal, cholesterol, and apolipoprotein B responses to antenatal betamethasone therapy. Am J Obstet Gynecol 174:562–565

Pattison NS, Chamley LW, Birdsall M, Zanderigo AM, Liddell HS & McDougall J (2000) Does aspirin have a role in improving pregnancy outcome for women with the antiphospholipid syndrome? A randomized controlled trial. Am J Obstet Gynecol 183: 1008-12

Paulesu L, Bhattacharjee J, Bechi N, Romagnoli R, Jantra S & Ietta F (2010) Pro-inflammatory cytokines in animal and human gestation. Curr Pharm Des. 16:3601-15

Peck A & Mellins ED (2010) Plasticity of T-cell phenotype and function: the T helper type 17 example. Immunology. 129:147-53.

Pei K, Yu C, Shi X & Jia M (2010) The effects of mifepristone on the expressions of osteopontin, interleukin-6 and leukemia inhibitory factor in the villi of early pregnant women. Contraception. 82:379-84

Pellicer A, Dominguez F, Remohi J & Simón C (2002) Molecular basis of implantation. Reprod Biomed Online. 5:44-51. J Reprod Immunol. 72:46-59.

Pioli PA, Weaver LK, Schaefer TM, Wright JA, Wira CR & Guyre PM (2006) Lipopolysaccharide-induced IL-1 beta production by human uterine macrophages up-regulates uterine epithelial cell expression of human beta-defensin 2. J Immunol 176: 6647-55

Quenby S, Bates M, Doig T, Brewster J, Lewis-Jones DI, Johnson PM & Vince G (1999) Pre-implantation endometrial leukocytes in women with recurrent miscarriage. Hum Reprod 14:2386–2391

Quenby S, Farquharson R, Young M & Vince G (2003) Successful pregnancy outcome following 19 consecutive miscarriages: case report. Hum Reprod. 18:2562-4.

Quenby S, Kalumbi C, Bates M, Farquharson R & Vince G (2005) Prednisolone reduces preconceptual endometrial natural killer cells in women with recurrent miscarriage. Fertil Steril. 84:980-4.

Radysh TV & Chernyshov VP (2005) Immunopathophysiologic characteristics of early pregnancy in women with recurrent miscarriage. Fiziol Zh. 51:65-72.

Raghupathy R, Makhseed M, Azizieh F, Omu A, Gupta M & Farhat R (2000) Cytokine production by maternal lymphocytes during normal human pregnancy and in unexplained recurrent spontaneous abortion. Hum Reprod 15:713–718

Raghupathy R, Al Mutawa E, Makhseed M, Azizieh F & Szekeres-Bartho J (2005) Modulation of cytokine production by dydrogesterone in lymphocytes from women with recurrent miscarriage. BJOG. 112:1096-101.

Raghupathy R, Al-Mutawa E, Al-Azemi M, Makhseed M, Azizieh F & Szekeres-Bartho J (2009) Progesterone-induced blocking factor (PIBF) modulates cytokine production by lymphocytes from women with recurrent miscarriage or preterm delivery. JReprod Immunol 80:91–9

Rahimi R, Nikfar S & Abdollahi M (2006) Meta-analysis finds use of inhaled corticosteroids during pregnancy safe: a systematic meta-analysis review. Hum Exp Toxicol. 25:447-52.

Rai R, Backos M, Baxter N, Chilcott I, Regan L. Recurrent miscarriage – an aspirin a day? Hum Reprod 2000; 15: 2220-3

Rai R & Regan L (2006) Recurrent miscarriage. Lancet 368:601-1

Renaud SJ, Cotechini T, Quirt JS, Macdonald-Goodfellow SK, Othman M, Graham CH. Spontaneous pregnancy loss mediated by abnormal maternal inflammation in rats is linked to deficient uteroplacental perfusion. J Immunol. 2011 Feb 1;186(3):1799-808.

Robb L, Li R, Hartley L, Nandurkar HH, Koentgen F & Begley CG (1998) Infertility in female mice lacking the receptor for interleukin 11 is due to a defective uterine response to implantation. Nat Med 4: 303-8

Romero R, Gomez R, Ghezzi F, Bo Hyun Yoon, Mazor M, Edwin SS & Berry SM (1998) A fetal systemic inflammatory response is followed by the spontaneous onset of preterm parturition. Am J Obstet Gynecol 179:186-93.

Romero R, Chaiworapongsa T, Espinoza J, Gomez R, Yoon BH, Edwin S, Mazor M, Maymon E & Berry S (2002) Fetal plasma MMP-9 concentrations are elevated in preterm premature rupture of the membranes. Am J Obstet Gynecol 187:1125-30

Ryu JS, Majeska RJ, Ma Y, LaChapelle L & Guller S (1999) Steroid regulation of human placental integrins: suppression of alpha2 integrin expression in cytotrophoblasts by glucocorticoids. Endocrinology. 140:3904-8

Rushton DI (1988) Placental pathology in spontaneous miscarriage. In: Beard RW, Sharp F, eds. Early Pregnancy Loss: Mechanisms and Treatment. London: Royal College of Obstetricians and Gynaecologists : 149-58

Saini V, Arora S, Yadav A & Bhattacharjee J (2011) Cytokines in recurrent pregnancy loss. Clin Chim Acta.412:702-8

Saito S, Nishikawa K, Morii T, Enomoto M, Narita N, Motoyoshi K & Ichijo M (1993) Cytokine production by CD16-CD56bright natural killer cells in the human early pregnancy decidua. Int Immunol. 5:559-63

Salgado A, Bóveda JL, Monasterio J, Segura RM, Mourelle M, Gómez-Jiménez J & Peracaula R (1994) Inflammatory mediators and their influence on haemostasis. Haemostasis 24:132-8

Salmon JE & Girardi G (2008) Antiphospholipid antibodies and pregnancy loss: a disorder of inflammation. J Reprod Immunol. 77:51-6.

Santoni A, Carlino C & Gismondi A (2008) Uterine NK cell development, migration and function. Reprod Biomed Online 16:202-10

Schaefer TM, Fahey JV, Wright JA & Wira CR (2005) Innate immunity in the human female reproductive tract: antiviral response of uterine epithelial cells to the TLR3 agonist poly (I:C). J Immunol 174: 992-1002

Schraufstatter IU, Trieu K, Zhao M, Rose DM, Terkeltaub RA & Burger M (2003) IL- 8-mediated cell migration in endothelial cells depends on cathepsin B activity and transactivation of the epidermal growth factor receptor. J Immunol 171: 6714-22

Scott JR (2003) Immunotherapy for recurrent miscarriage. Cochrane Database Syst Rev 1:CD000112

Seckl JR (2004) Prenatal glucocorticoids and long-term programming, Eur. J. Endocrinol 151:49–62

Seckl JR & Holmes MC (2007)Mechanisms of Disease: glucocorticoids, their placental metabolism and fetal 'programming' of adult pathophysiology. Nature Clinical Practice Endocrinology & Metabolism 3:479-88.

Shynlova O, Tsui P, Jaffer S & Lye SJ (2009) Integration of endocrine and mechanical signals in the regulation of myometrial functions during pregnancy and labour. Eur J Obstet Gynecol Reprod Biol 144 Suppl 1:S2-10

Simcox R, Sin WT, Seed PT, Briley A & Shennan AH (2007) Prophylactic antibiotics for the prevention of preterm birth in women at risk: a meta-analysis. Aust N Z J Obstet Gynaecol 47:368-77.

Sljivic S, Kamenov B, Maglajlic S, Djordjevic V, Stojkovic-Eferica I, Stojanovic M, Stefanovic M, Mihailovic D, Mrkaic L & Tasic G (2006) Possible interactions of genetic and immuno-neuro-endocrine regulatory mechanisms in pathogenesis of congenital anomalies. Med Hypotheses. 67:57-64.

Sotiriadis A, Makrydimas G, Papatheodorou S & Ioannidis JP (2009) Corticosteroids for preventing neonatal respiratory morbidity after elective caesarean section at term. Cochrane Database Syst Rev. CD006614

Spinillo A, Beneventi F, Ramoni V, Caporali R, Locatelli E, Simonetta M, Cavagnoli C, Alpini C, Albonico G, Prisco E & Montecucco C. (2012) Prevalence and significance of previously undiagnosed rheumatic diseases in pregnancy. Ann Rheum Dis. In press

Stephenson MD, Kutte WH, Purkiss S, Librach C, Schultz P, Houlihan E & Liao C (2010) Intravenous immunoglobulin and idiopathic secondary recurrent miscarriage: a multicentered randomized placebo-controlled trial, Human Reproduction 25:2203–2209

Suffee N, Richard B, Hlawaty H, Oudar O, Charnaux N & Sutton A (2011) Angiogenic properties of the chemokine RANTES/CCL5. Biochem Soc Trans 39:1649-53.

Sun K, Ma R, Cui X, Campos B, Webster R, Brockman D & Myatt L (2003) Glucocorticoids induce cytosolic phospholipase A2 and prostaglandin H synthase type 2 but not microsomal and cytosolic prostaglandin E synthase (PGES) expression in cultured primary human amnion cells. J Clin Endocrinol Metab 88: 5564–71.

Swolin-Eide D, Dahlgren J, Nilsson C, Albertsson Wikland K, Holmäng A & Ohlsson C. Affected skeletal growth but normal bone mineralization in rat offspring after prenatal dexamethasone exposure. J Endocrinol. 174:411-8.

Swyer GI, Daley D. Progesterone implantation in habitual abortion. BMJ 1953;1:1073-7

Tang AW, Alfirevic Z, Turner MA, Drury J & Quenby S. (2009) Prednisolone Trial: Study protocol for a randomised controlled trial of prednisolone for women with idiopathic recurrent miscarriage and raised levels of uterine natural killer (uNK) cells in the endometrium. Trials. 10;10:102

Thinkhamrop J, Hofmeyr GJ, Adetoro O & Lumbiganon P (2002) Prophylactic antibiotic administration in pregnancy to prevent infectious morbidity and mortality. Cochrane Database Syst Rev 4:CD002250

Thuere C, Zenclussen ML, Schumacher A, Langwisch S, Schulte-Wrede U, Teles A, Paeschke S, Volk HD & Zenclussen AC (2007) Kinetics of regulatory T cells during murine pregnancy. Am J Reprod Immunol. 58:514-23

Thum MY, Bhaskaran S, Abdalla HI, Ford B, Sumar N & Bansa (2008) Prednisolone suppresses NK cell cytotoxicity in vitro in women with a history of infertility and elevated NK cell cytotoxicity. l A.Am J Reprod Immunol. 59:259-65

Tincani A, Cavazzana I, Ziglioli T, Lojacono A, De Angelis V & Meroni P (2010) Complement activation and pregnancy failure. Clin Rev Allergy Immunol. 39:153-9

Tsuzuki Y, Takeba Y, Kumai T, Matsumoto N, Mizuno M, Murano K, Asoh K, Takagi M, Yamamoto H & Kobayashi S (2009) Antenatal glucocorticoid therapy increase cardiac alpha-enolase levels in fetus and neonate rats. Life Sci 85:609-16.

Verhoog NJ, Du Toit A, Avenant C & Hapgood JP (2011) Glucocorticoid-independent repression of tumor necrosis factor (TNF) alpha-stimulated interleukin (IL)-6 expression by the glucocorticoid receptor: a potential mechanism for protection against an excessive inflammatory response. J Biol Chem 286:19297-310.

Vesce F, Pareschi MC, Travagli S, Tarabbia C, Pansini F, Salvatorelli G, Gulinati AM, Grandi E & Biondi C (1992) Betamethasone-induced lecithin release in vitro from the fetal membranes. Gynecol Obstet Invest. 33:134-7

Vesce F, Farina A, Jorizzo G, Tarabbia C, Calabrese O, Pelizzola D & Giovannini G, Piffanelli A (1996) Raised level of amniotic endothelin in pregnancies with fetal aneuploidy. Fetal Diagn Ther. 11:94-8.

Vesce F, Farina A, Giorgetti M, Jorizzo G, Bianciotto A, Calabrese O & Mollica G (1997) Increased incidence of preeclampsia in pregnancies complicated by fetal malformation. Gynecol Obstet Invest. 44:107-11.

Vesce F, Buzzi M, Ferretti ME, Pavan B, Bianciotto A, Jorizzo G & Biondi C (1998) Inhibition of amniotic prostaglandin E release by ampicillin. Am J Obstet Gynecol 178: 759-64

Vesce F, Pavan B, Buzzi M, Pareschi MC, Bianciotto A, Iorizzo G & Biondi C (1999) Effect of different classes of antibiotics on amniotic prostaglandin E release. Prostaglandins Other Lipid Mediat. 57:207-18

Vesce F, Scapoli C, Giovannini G, Piffanelli A, Geurts-Moespot A & Sweep FC (2001) Plasminogen activator system in serum and amniotic fluid of euploid and aneuploid pregnancies. Obstet Gynecol. 97:404-8.

Vesce F, Scapoli C, Giovannini G, Tralli L, Gotti G, Valerio A & Piffanelli A (2002) Cytokine imbalance in pregnancies with fetal chromosomal abnormalities. Hum Reprod. 17:803-8

Vesce F, Pavan B, Lunghi L, Giovannini G, Scapoli C, Piffanelli A &Biondi C (2004) Inhibition of amniotic Interleukin-6 and Prostaglandin E2 release by ampicillin Obstet Gynecol 103: 108-113

von Eye Corleta H (2010) It is time to respect the American Society for Reproductive Medicine definition of recurrent pregnancy loss. Fertil Steril 94(4):e61

Wang ZC, Yunis EJ, De los Santos MJ, Xiao L, Anderson DJ & Hill JA (2002) T helper 1-type immunity to trophoblast antigens in women with a history of recurrent pregnancy loss is associated with polymorphism of the IL1B promoter region. Genes Immun. 3:38-42

Wang WJ, Hao CF, Yi-Lin, Yin GJ, Bao SH, Qiu LH & Lin QD (2010) Increased prevalence of T helper 17 (Th17) cells in peripheral blood and decidua in unexplained recurrent spontaneous abortion patients. J Reprod Immunol. 84:164-70.

Wang D, Lin W, Pan Y, Kuang X, Qi X & Sun H (2011) Chronic blockade of glucocorticoid receptors by RU486 enhances lipopolysaccharide-induced depressive-like behaviour and cytokine production in rats. Brain Behav Immun. 25:706-14

Waterman WR, Xu LL, Tetradis S, Motyckova G, Tsukada J, Saito K, Webb AC, Robinson DR & Auron PE (2006) Glucocorticoid inhibits the human pro-interleukin lbeta gene

(ILIB) by decreasing DNA binding of transactivators to the signal-responsive enhancer. Mol Immunol 43:773-82

Wegmann TG, Lin H, Guilbert L & Mosmann TR (1993) Bidirectional cytokine interactions in the maternal-fetal relationship: is successful pregnancy a TH2 phenomenon? Immunol Today 14:353–356

Wells C N (1953) Treatment of hyperemesis gravidarum with cortisone. Am J Obstet Gynecol 66:598-601

White CA, Robb L & Salamonsen LA (2004) Uterine extracellular matrix components are altered during defective decidualization in interleukin-11 receptor alpha deficient mice. Reprod Biol Endocrinol 2: 76

Williams PJ, Bulmer JN, Searle RF, Innes BA & Robson SC (2009) Altered decidual leucocyte populations in the placental bed in pre-eclampsia and foetal growth restriction: a comparison with late normal pregnancy. Reproduction. 138:177-84

Wira CR, Fahey JV, Ghosh M, Patel MV, Hickey DK & Ochiel DO (2010) Sex hormone regulation of innate immunity in the female reproductive tract: the role of epithelial cells in balancing reproductive potential with protection against sexually transmitted pathogens. Am J Reprod Immunol 63: 544-65

Winterhager E, Von Ostau C, Gerke M, Gruemmer R, Traub O & Kaufmann P. (1999). Connexin expression patterns in human trophoblast cells during placental development. *Placenta* 20, 627–638. doi:10.1053/PLAC.1999.0434

Xu J, Treem WR, Roman C, Anderson V, Rubenstein R & Schwarz SM (2011) Ileal immune dysregulation in necrotizing enterocolitis: role of CD40/CD40L in the pathogenesis of disease. J Pediatr Gastroenterol Nutr. 52:140-6.

Yamada H, Kato EH, Kobashi G, Ebina Y, Shimada S, Morikawa M, Sakuragi N & Fujimoto S (2001) High NK cell activity in early pregnancy correlates with subsequent abortion with normal chromosomes in women with recurrent abortion. Am J Reprod Immunol. 46:132-6.

Yamada H, Kato EH, Morikawa M, Shimada S, Saito H, Watari M, Minakami H & Nishihira J (2003) Decreased serum levels of macrophage migration inhibition factor in miscarriages with normal chromosome karyotype. Hum Reprod. 18:616-20.

Yang B, Trump RP, Shen Y, McNulty JA, Clifton LG, Stimpson SA, Lin P & Pahel GL (2008) RU486 did not exacerbate cytokine release in mice challenged with LPS nor in db/db mice. BMC Pharmacol.8:7

Chapter 17

Glucocorticoids: Biochemical Group That Play Key Role in Fetal Programming of Adult Disease

Aml Mohammed Erhuma

Additional information is available at the end of the chapter

http://dx.doi.org/10.5772/50798

1. Introduction

1.1. Glucocorticoids discovery started 160 years ago

Glucocorticoids are subclass from corticosteroids. The other subclass of corticosteroids is mineralocorticoids. Historically, the discovery of glucocorticoids has been commenced during the early of last century. In fact, glucocorticoids have revealed themselves by their absence. In 1849, Thomas Addison, who was a physician at Guy`s Hospital in London, had noticed that certain patients were presenting with a cluster of characteristic clinical picture including anemia, weakness, peculiar dark skin color and eventually death (1). He presented his observation on 11 cases at the South London medical society meeting. In 1855 he published monograph entitled (On the Constitutional and Local Effects of Disease of the Supra-Renal capsules), (2, 3). 100 years later, Dr Philip Hench with a collaborated work with Edward Kendall, Professor of Physiological Chemistry, were both at Mayo Clinic which was first rheumatic disease service, had extracted "substance X" and in 21 September 1948 first injection of substance X was given to 29 years old lady who was suffering from severe, erosive arthropathies and became able to walk out of the hospital after 4 days of treatment. Dr Hench then named substance X Cortisone and shared the Nobel prize with professor Kendall in 1950 (4).

1.2. Glucocorticoids characteristics

Glucocorticoids (GCs) are belonging to the steroid group of the hormones that bind to the glucocorticoid receptor, which is present in almost all cells (5). This is the reason why the GCs play wide range of vital physiological roles in the human and other vertebrate bodies (6, 7). They play pivotal role in modulation and regulation of metabolism (8), immune system reaction (9, 10) and more significantly they are essential for normal development and cognition (11).

1.2.1. Biochemical characteristics

To know how GCs exerts their wide range effects, it is crucial to know about their structure and the synthesis pathway. GCs are one of the steroid hormones group. All steroid hormones are derived from cholesterol. These include: sex hormones (Testosterone, estrone (E1), estradiol (E2), estriol (E3), and progesterone) adrenal cortex hormones (Cortisone, the main glucocorticoid and Aldosterone, the main mineralocorticoid) in addition to vitamin D. It is essential to know that androgens are the synthetic precursors of estrogens which mediated mainly by a specific cytochrome P 450 enzyme named aromatase. Each one of these steroid hormones can be a product and precursor in the same time. This is the reason why any defect in the synthesis of one steroid hormone will lead to derangement in the synthesis of the other hormones. For instance, in congenital adrenal hyperplasia (CAH), an autosomal recessive gene defect of the enzyme 21-hydroxylase, there will be blocked synthesis of aldosterone and cortisol pathways. Subsequently, all precursors will be directed toward androgenic pathway which does not involve 21-hydroxylation and eventually lead to excess production of androgens (Figure 1). Fetus with this congenital disease will be exposed to high levels of androgens as early as 3 months of gestation and hence during a critical window of sexual differentiation. As a result a female fetus will develop an ambiguous genitalia or male external genitalia under the influences of adrenal androgens. However, this is associated with varying degrees of GCs and mineralocorticoids deficiencies. In severe cases there will be salt wasting with low sodium and potassium in serum due to aldosterone deficiency (12). Currently, all neonates in the most of world are screened for CAH by measuring 17-Hydroxyprogesteron (17-OHP) in filter-paper blood samples at week one of life. An elevated 17-OHP indicated affected baby. Recently, there are promising clinical trials in prenatal diagnosis and treatments of such condition by giving the mother dexamethasone injections to prevent increased secretion of Adreno-Cortico-Tropic Hormone (ACTH) and subsequently adrenal androgens(13-17).

1.2.2. Physiological characteristics

GCs are needed mainly for energy where as mineralocorticoids are needed for mineral balance. GCs regulates wide range of cellular, molecular and the physiological processes in human body that are crucial for life such as growth, reproduction, essential metabolism, immune responses and inflammatory reactions, as well as central nervous system and cardiovascular functions (19-22). For all these roles to be achieved, adrenal GCs is considered as a ring which coupled with many other rings to form an integrated chain that acts in coordination, this chain is the hypothalamus-pituitary- adrenal axis.

1.2.2.1. Hypothalamus-pituitary-adrenal axis (HPA axis)

HPA axis serves as a master that controls major body systems and is considered as a main connecting pathway between central nervous system and endocrine system. It regulates majority of physiological function as well as it maintains homeostasis in acute stress. In the later situation, the brain will signal the stress to the paraventricular nucleus (PVN) in the hypothalamus which eventually secretes corticotrophin releasing hormone (CRH). CRH is then transported through hypophyseal portal system to the pituitary gland and induces the conversion of pro-opiomelanocortin into ACTH as well as its secretion from anterior pituitary to the systemic circulation. ACTH is the primary regulator of adrenal cortical steroidogenesis. ACTH will induce the synthesis of adrenal steroids (GCs and androgens) in zonae fasciculate and reticularis of adrenal cortex (Figure 1). The ACTH itself is under the influences of negative feedback inhibition which exerted by the plasma levels of circulating free GCs (Figure 2).

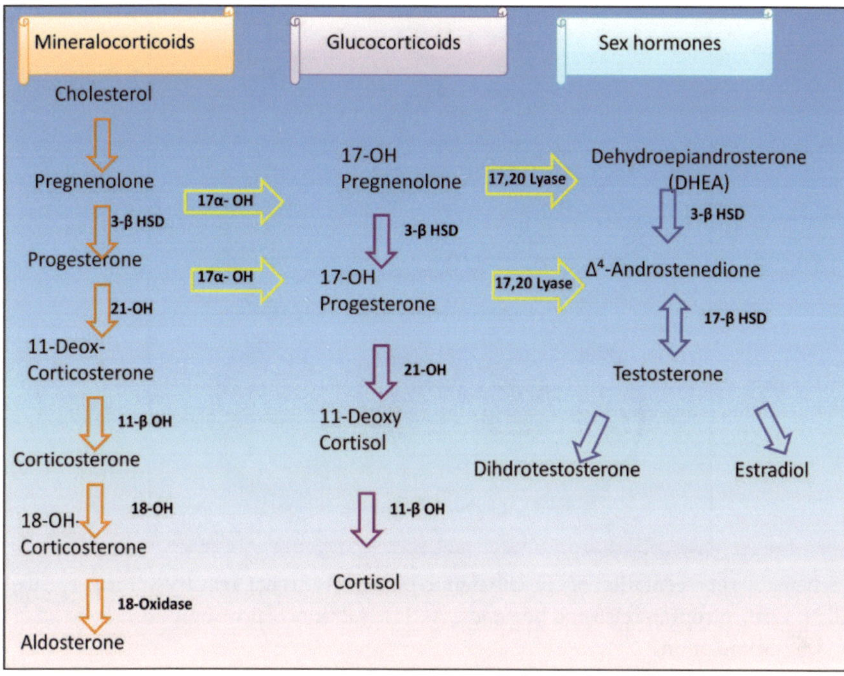

Figure 1. Adrenal gland steroidogenesis. The synthesis of adrenal steroids is started by transfer of cholesterol either from blood or from adrenal gland lipid droplets into mitochondria where it will be converted to pregnenolone. In zona glomerulosa pregnenolone will be hydroxylated to corticosterone and further oxidized to aldosterone where as in zona fasciculate and zona reticularis it will be hydoxylated to cortisol or undergoes cleavage to form the main adrenal androgen (DHEA). HSD: Hydroxysteroid Dehydrogenase, OH: Hydroxylase, (18). Adrenal androgen synthesis is increased about age of 8 years, independent of gonads and puberty, and responsible for pubic and axillary hair growth and termed adrenarche.

1.2.2.2. Molecular mechanisms of GCs action

GCs secretion from zona fasciculata up on ACTH stimulation is not a continuance process but rather in a specific pattern known as circadian rhythm. Once GCs in circulation, 95% of them will be bound to a carrier proteins: 80–90% to corticosteroid binding globulin (CBG) and 10–15% to albumin, leaving only about 5% as active unbound cortisol (23). The free cortisol is the one which mediates the biological effect of GCs since it is able to diffuse through the cell membrane freely. The GCs are metabolized in liver by reduction followed by conjugation rendering them water soluble and ready for renal excretion in urine. Both liver and kidney contain the enzyme 11 β-Hydroxysteroid dehydrogenase (11 β-HSD).There is two isoforms of this enzyme which catalyzes the opposite reactions. 11 β-Hydroxysteroid Dehydrogenase-2 (11 β-HSD 2) will inactivate the cortisol by converting it into cortisone. The 11 β-Hydroxysteroid dehydrogenase-1 (11 β-HSD 1) will convert inactive cortisone into cortisol. The net result will determine the plasma level of active cortisol in the body (24).

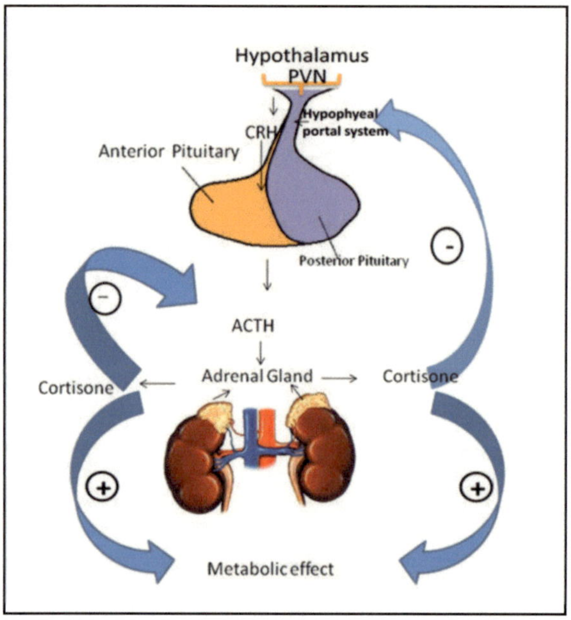

Figure 2. Schematic representation of Hypothalamic-pituitary-adrenal axis. PVN: Paraventricular nucleus, CRH: Corticotrophin releasing hormone, ACTH: Adrenocorticotropic hormone, ⊖: Inhibition, ⊕:Stimulation

Once free GCs defused through the plasma membrane of the target cell they will bind to intra-cytoplasmic receptors called glucocorticoids receptor (GR). GR-GCs complex will be now translocated to the nucleus and bind to glucocorticoids responsive elements (GRE) in the promoter of the target gene (Figure 3).

Human GR is 94 kDa protein which belongs to nuclear receptors known as Steroid/Thyroid/Retinoic acid superfamily and characterizing by being a ligand-dependent transcription factors that induce or suppress target gene expression (25). GCs are also able to alter gene expression of target genes independently to DNA-binding, but through interaction with other transcription factors, such as nuclear factor- κB, activator protein-1, p53 and signal transducers and activators of transcription (25).

Interestingly, there are two isoforms of GR, alpha (α) and beta (β) (26, 27). The GR-α is the one which is able to bind with glucocorticoids and subsequently to the GCs responsive element (GRE) of the DNA promoter region on the target gene. However, GR-β has no such ability to bind to GCs but its main role thought to be inhibitory to GR-α action by competitive interference on the GRE target sites (28). It has been found that the variations in expression of GR-β is responsible for tissue sensitivity and resistance to GCs. Clinically, pathological conditions such as hypertension, rheumatoid arthritis, systemic lupus erythmatosis, ischemic heart disease and nasal carriage of Staphylococcus aureus are all associated with GR-β protein over-expression (29).

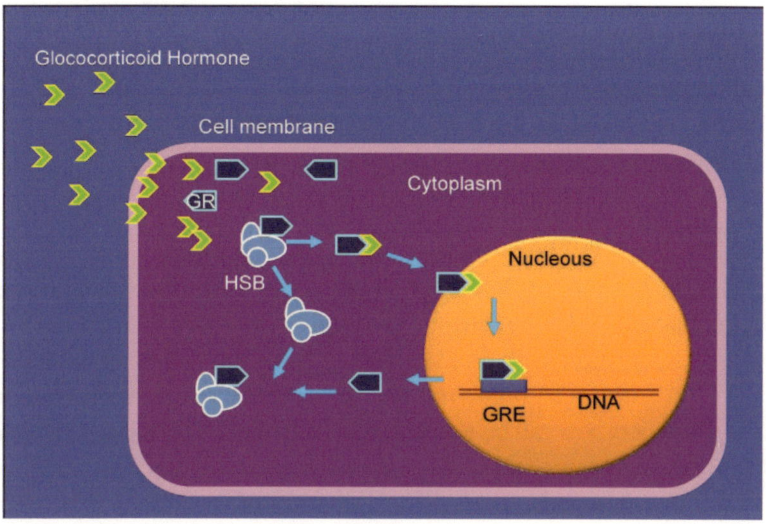

Figure 3. Representation of how glucocorticoid hormone enters to the cell and bind to intracellular glucocorticoids receptors (GR). Up on binding to GR they dissociate from heat shock proteins (HSP). The glucocorticoids-receptor complex enters the nucleus and bind to glucocorticoids responsive element (GRE) in the promoter of the responsive gene (25). Lastly, GR exit nucleus and recycled along with the HSP in the cytoplasm.

2. Tissue responses to glucocorticoids

As mentioned earlier that GR exist in almost every human cell, then we should not get surprised to observe the profound molecular, cellular, metabolic and other known biological events modulation in response to GCs excess or deficiency. Notwithstanding, for more understanding of these complex relationship and the huge difference in the treatment-response equation we categorized the human tissue into adult or mature human tissue and fetal or immature human tissue.

2.1. Adult (mature) tissue response to glucocorticoids

Adult cells and tissue characterized by being fully differentiated and mature. Therefore, influences will mainly affect their function.

2.1.1. Immune system

It is well established that the first medical use of GCs 60 years ago was for inflammation and autoimmune disease (30). GCs have significant influences on both cellular and humeral immunity. They induce plasma cell immunoglobuline production and secretion and hence enhance humeral immunity (31). With regard to cellular immunity, GCs induce T-cell lymphocytosis (32), basophil apoptosis and neutrophilia by increasing bone marrow release of polymorphic neutrophils and decrease their migration to the inflammatory site (33, 34). Moreover, GCs enhances the phagocytosis and hence maximize the tissue clearance ability of the microorganisms and foreign antigens (35). It has been recently revealed that GCs can exert their immune-function manipulation at gene expression level. Galon and colleagues found that GCs significantly suppress the proinflamatory cytokines (IL1b, TNFa, IL-6, IL-8, IL- 12, IL-18) and chemokines gene expression where as the gene expression of anti-inflammatory cytokines (IL-10 and TGFb) are up-regulated (22).

2.1.2. Musculoskeletal system

It is known, from long history of GCs use, that prolonged high doses of GCs results in bone mineralization depletion with subsequent osteoporosis (36). As a result bone formation will be decreased and resorption will be increased (37-41). Bone loss occur in the first few months of treatment and can be improved after cessation of treatment (42-44). Importantly, the GCs induced-osteoporosis can be prevented by calcium and vitamin D supplementation along with GCs treatment course (45). GCs will also cause proximal myopathy which is dose dependent and again improves with discontinuation of treatment (46). GCs treatment increases the risk of femoral head avascular necrosis through a not well established mechanism, although some preliminary evidence pointing to venous endothelial injury (47, 48).

2.1.3. Vascular system

Use of GCs is associated with increased risk of ischemic heart disease and heart failure by increasing the occurrence of hypertension, hyperglycemia, dyslipideamia and obesity (49, 50). Rapid GCs infusion especially in patients with renal and cardiac co-morbidity was associated with sudden death (51).

2.1.4. Serum lipid levels

There are conflicting results from different studies regarding GCs induced hyperlipideamia. Berg and Nilsson-Ehle found that GCs may induce hyperlipideamia through ACTH suppression (52). Whereas others found that GCs may induce favorable lipid profiles in patients aged 60 years or more (53).

2.1.5. Serum glucose levels

GCs are considered diabetogenic hormones. Patients receiving therapeutic doses of GCs will have deranged plasma glucose level and even frank diabetes in glucose intolerant individuals (54, 55). The GCs-induced hyperglycemia is mainly due to reduced glucose peripheral disposal along with increased hepatic gluconeogenesis (56).

2.1.6. Central nervous system

Prolonged use of high doses of GCs is associated with marked behavioral and cognitive deficits. These disorders are more prevalent in those who have risk factors such as pre-existing psychiatric disorders, family history of depression or alcoholism (57). These disturbances are ranging from sleeping disturbances, insomnia, to hypomania, depression and psychosis (58) as well as memory disturbances (59). Recently, more evidences are accumulated to affirm the relationship between exposure to high GCs and impaired cognition. Ioannis and others found that chronic stress, through high endogenous GCs, precipitate cognitive impairment and Alzheimer's like disease (60).

2.1.7. Gastrointestinal system

Gastritis, peptic ulceration, and gastrointestinal hemorrhage all have been found to complicate GCs therapy especially if non-steroidal anti-inflammatory drugs are used concomitantly (61). Although, Chrousos and collegues indicated that GCs therapy could be related to acute pancreatitis in GCs user (62), but more recent studies have proven the opposite that GCs are not an etiological factor (63).

2.2. Fetal (Immature) tissue responses to glucocorticoids

Human intrauterine development is divided mainly into three stages: Zygote, from fertilization to implantation, embryo, from implantation to 8 weeks and fetus, from 8 weeks till term. The embryo and fetal tissues are characterized by rapid division and growth rendering them very susceptible to environmental influences and easily adaptive.

2.2.1. Short term effects of GCs over exposure in fetal life

2.2.1.1. Fetal over exposure to endogenous GCS

Fetal plasma GCs are mainly of maternal adrenal origin (64). This is essentially because of the biochemical, "partial" barrier role played by the placenta. The placenta contains the enzyme 11 β-HSD 2 which is responsible for inactivation of maternal cortisol into cortisone (Section 1.2.2) and hence maintains a normal feto-maternal concentration gradient of the hormone (65). This concentration gradient is species specific where it reaches 180 ng/ml in human; it is only 2 and 15 ng/ml in sheep and pig respectively (66). Therefore, we can assume that fetal exposure to maternal GCs is, at least partly, dependent on the placental activity of this enzyme. This is supported by the finding that in human umbilical cord blood cortisone/cortisol ratio, as a marker of placental 11 β-HSD 2, and the enzyme activity itself and its mRNA expression were lower in human pregnancies which complicated by intrauterine growth restriction (IUGR) (67) and each unit increase in cortisol/cortisone ratio was found to be associated with 1.6 mm Hg higher systolic blood pressure at 3 years of age (68).

GCs are essential for optimal fetal tissue maturation. GR are expressed in brain (69) where it is essential for development of neurons, the building unit in CNS, as well as the formation of synapses by facilitating cortisone-induced axons and dendrites remodeling and neurons myelination (70). Human nervous system development during fetal life is a complex process where extensive proliferation of neurons occurs after initial migration between week 8 and 16 of gestation (71) to reach, at 28 weeks, approximately 40 % higher than total number of neurons in adult (72). These enormous numbers of neurons start to be connected by an extensive network of synapses where between 24 and 34 weeks of gestation more that 10,000 new synapses per second are formed (73). Therefore, exposure to altered plasma level of cortisone during these stages of development and vulnerability is able to alter the basic structure and subsequently the function of the CNS (74). The Maternal and fetal HPA axis are independent (Figure 4) where maternal cortisol is prevented to enter fetal compartment by placental 11 β-HSD 2 until late gestation where placental enzyme drops sharply and allow high levels of maternal free cortisol to enhance fetal lung, CNS and other tissue maturation (75). However, the placenta secretes placental corticotrophin releasing hormone (P-CRH) which is the major, if not the only, mean of cross talk between maternal and fetal HPA axis. As mentioned earlier (Section 1.2.2) that maternal cortisol is exerting negative feedback inhibition on her hypothalamus release of CRH, on contrast, it induces P-CRH secretion as pregnancy advances (76) which in turn will increase maternal and fetal adrenal cortisol secretion (77, 78).

Therefore, maternal either biological stress, like nutritional deprivation, immune reaction, hypertension, or psychological stress will be associated with high maternal cortisol and P-CRH which disrupt fetal nervous system development and affect postnatal cognitive and neuromuscular function. High P-CRH, as a marker of maternal stress, during third trimester associated with weak fetal responsiveness to noval stimuli (79). Postnataly, there is significant reduction in physical and neuromuscular development in neonates who exposed to higher maternal cortisol as well as P-CRH during second and third trimester respectively (80). Those neonates also express prolonged cortisol response to stress, which similar to the effect of synthetic prenatal GCs (81). Interestingly, these behavioral, cognitive and neuromuscular deficiency of offspring exposed to endogenous maternal GCs were accompanied by reduction in the volume of the areas responsible for these functions (82, 83).

Immune system disorder also noted in offspring exposed to maternal prenatal stress with higher incidence of childhood skin, respiratory and other general infections and increased antibiotics use (84). In addition, they have increased body weight which was significantly apparent at age of 10 years (85). More specifically, maternal high CRH during second trimester was found to be associated with offspring adiposity at age of 3 years (86).

2.2.1.2. Antenatal synthetic steroid (dexamethasone and betamethsone) exposure

Maternal administration of synthetic GCs such as dexamethasone and betamethasone, which are poor substrates for 11 β-HSD 2 (87), during pregnancy can cross the placenta (88) in quantities sufficient to induce immediate fetal changes such as reduction in umbilical artery pulsatility index and improved velocity (89) along with transient suppression of fetal breathing and fetal movement resulting in lowering the score of biophysical profile (90). 11 β-HSD 2 is expressed mainly in placental cytotrophoblasts, the progenitors, only upon syncytialization into syncytiotrophoblasts (91). Li and colleagues found that up on syncytialization the expressions of SP1 transcription factor as well as the cAMP pathway are markedly activated (91).

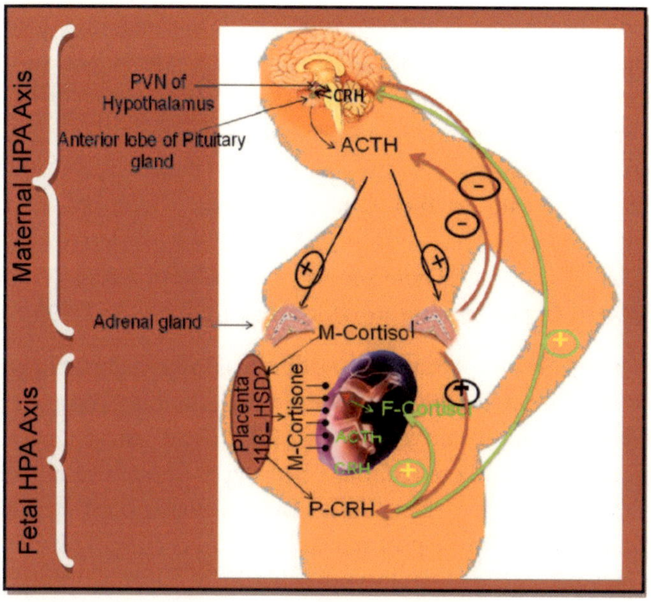

Figure 4. Fetal and maternal HPA axes are two independent systems. The P-CRH stimulates the production of both maternal and fetal cortisol. Maternal cortisol has negative feedback inhibition on her CRH and ACTH but exerts positive feedback stimulation on P-CRH. Placental 11 β-HSD 2 inactivates maternal cortisol into cortisone and hence partially protects the fetus from endogenous maternal GCs over exposure. H: Hypothalamus, P: Pituitary, HPA: Hypothalamo-Pituitary-Adrenal, P-CRH: Placental Corticotrophin Releasing Hormone, ACTH: Adreno-Corticotrophic Hormone, 11 β-HSD 2:11-β-Hydroxysteroid dehydrogenase-2, GCs:Glucocorticoids, M-Cortisol: Maternal cortisol, M-Cortisone: Maternal cortisone, PVN: Paraventricular nucleus, (-): Inhibition, (+): Stimulation.

GCs are strong inducers of HLA-G gene expression in choriocarcinoma JEG-3 cell lines. The HLA-G molecules play a pivotal role in regulating feto-maternal interface and essential for protecting the allogenic fetus from maternal immune attack (92).

After the finding that surfactant deficiency in premature infants (less than 37 weeks of gestation) is the leading cause of respiratory distress syndrome (RDS) in 1959 (93) and high mortality rate among preterm infants because of this lung immaturity (94, 95) a continuous work was done to prevent such fatal condition. Clinically, GCs has been used to prevent neonatal respiratory distress syndrome successfully (96). Thereafter, many studies found that maternal treatment of GCs will significantly decrease neonatal death due to reduction of intraventricular haemorrhage and necrotising enterocolitis beside reduction in RDS (97, 98). However, randomized controlled trials shown that no differences in the effectiveness of both dexamethasone and betamethasone in reducing the rate of respiratory distress syndrome, need for vasopressor therapy, necrotizing enterocolitis, retinopathy of prematurity, patent ductus arteriosus, neonatal sepsis, and neonatal mortality but reduction in the frequency of intraventricular haemorrhage was more with dexamethasone compared to betamethasone (99).

When synthetic GCs administered during pregnancy they can cross placenta freely since they are not a good substrates to 11 β-HSD 2 (88) and is not bound by CBP (100). Although, the mechanism by which GCs enhance fetal lung maturity is not well established, the administration of antenatal GCs in threatened preterm labour was widely recommended by many institutes. For instance, the National Institutes of Health (NIH) published a Consensus Development Conference Statement in 1994 on the use of antenatal GCs (101) and in 2002, the American College of Obstetricians and Gynecologists' Committee on Obstetric Practice (ACOG) supported the conclusions of the NIH consensus conference (102), whereas, the Royal College of Obstetricians and Gynecologists (RCOG) published guideline in 1996 (103) about antenatal GCs use in preterm labour which then up dated in 1999 and further in 2004.

Recently, there are many evidences that GCs induce fetal lung maturity at both transcriptional and post transcriptional levels (104-106). Pulmonary surfactant is a complex lipoprotein which main action is to reduce surface tension in the alveoli, and subsequently prevent alveolar collapse upon expiration (107). There are four major types of surfactant proteins (SP) A, B, C and D (108). GCs act mainly by increasing the surfactant protein-B (SP-B) mRNA expression at transcription level and its stability at post transcription level (109). Treatment consists of two doses of 12 mg of betamethasone given intramuscularly 24 hours apart or four doses of 6 mg of dexamethasone given intramuscularly 12 hours apart. Optimal benefit begins 24 hours after initiation of therapy and lasts 7 days (101). It has been recently established the use of repeated GCs courses every 14 days for those who still not delivered after the first course. Studies on animal models and also on human showed no additional benefits from repeated courses compared with single GCs course (110-112) and even can be harmful (113-116).

In fact, multiple courses of antenatal GCs have been found to be associated with reduction in ponderal measurements including birth weight, height (116-120) and birth head circumference (117, 119, 121) and higher infant blood pressure and myocardial wall thickness (122, 123) also with maternal infection such as chorioamnionitis and endometritis (116, 121, 124). Rodríguez-Pinilla also reported that antenatal exposure to single steroid course is able to produce similar effects of multiple courses on birth weight and height but not head circumference (117).

With regard to fetal bone metabolism, there were few studies addressing this subject. However, the available data do suggest that both single as well as multiple antenatal steroid courses have no detrimental effects on fetal bone metabolism as evidenced by umbilical cord serum levels of carboxy-terminal propeptide of type I procollagen, a marker for bone formation, and cross-linked carboxy-terminal telopeptide of type I procollagen, a marker of bone resorption (125-127).

The impact of maternal GCs administration antenataly on neonatal hypothalamic-pituitary-adrenal (HPA) axis has been examined extensively but data are controversy. Sandesh Kiran and coworkers found that multiple courses of antenatal dexamethasone causing a significant decrease in RDS without adrenal suppression, decreased growth or impaired neuro-development (128). However, Schäffer and colleagues found that single course of antenatal GCs can lead to absence of stress-induced plasma cortisone and cortisol elevation in neonates at 4 days of life (129). On the other hand, Davis reported that antenatal GCs administration in threatened preterm labour was associated with higher pain-induced plasma cortisol elevation despite no difference in baseline levels than non-treated matched infants at 24 hr after birth (81). Others have assessed the impact of antenatal corticosteroid courses on HPA axis by measuring neonatal 17-OHP in filter-paper blood spots collected between 72 and 96 hr after birth, which usually used for screening the neonates for CAH (Section 1.2.1) (130). These studies revealed a significant reduction of blood 17-OHP in those received multiple courses compared to non-treated matched neonates (130). This fact raise the suspicion in the effectiveness of this screening test in this particular group of neonates as prenatal steroid-induced reduction in 17-OHP could be interpreted falsely as negative test in affected newborns. Ng et al found that at postnatal day 7 and 14 neonatal plasma ACTH and cortisone levels measured after human corticotrophin releasing hormone (hCRH) stimulation test was mildly lower in those exposed to multiple dexamethasone injections antenataly than none treated neonates. Interestingly, there was a negative correlation between plasma cortisone and the number of dexamethasone injections antenataly (131). These finding strongly indicate that antenatal steroid therapy, multiple courses in particular, has impact, which could be transient, on HPA axis harmony and neonatal observation during the first few days is warranted. Animal model of prenatal betamethasone using guinea pigs reported same finding that ACTH and plasma cortisol both suppressed by prenatal betamethasone treatment. This was assosiated with significant reduction in hippocampal mineralococrticoids receptor mRNA and protein expression especially in male offspring with no much difference among GR mRNA and protein expression (132).

It has been found that multiple prenatal steroid courses are not associated with a deleterious effect on auditory neural maturation when assessed at 24 hr after birth (133). However, the use of multiple dexamethasone but not betamethasone are associated with persistent increases in brain parenchymal echogenicity in preterm infants (134) as well as cystic leukomalacia and neurodevelopmental delay at 2 years of age (135). Animal models of prenatal steroid therapy presented some evidence regarding possible mechanism by which antenatal glucocorticoids prevent intraventricular haemorrhage in preterm infants. In mice, prenatal steroid therapy can induce choroid plexus capillary stability and maturation by increasing basement membrane thickness and integrity with subsequent reduction in both peri and intraventricular haemorrhage (136). The frequency and severity of periventricular and intraventricular haemorrhage were even less if vitamin K injection administered antenataly along with steroid course (137).

More recent data comparing the efficacy of single steroid course with multiple courses stated that there were no significant differences in the frequency of respiratory distress syndrome, intraventricular hemorrhage, necrotizing enterocolitis, sepsis and neonatal mortality in neonates receiving either single betamethasone course or multiple courses (138).

According to the same study, the use of multiple courses is not superior to single course. Similar beneficial effect was noted from the use of single and multiple antenatal steroid courses in decreasing the need for postnatal blood pressure support in extreme preterm infants born between 24 to 28 weeks of age (139).

On the same bases, the ACOG Committee on Obstetric Practice (2011) has published its opinion regarding the use of multiple courses. The committee recommended the use of single corticosteroids course to all pregnant women at risk of preterm delivery at 24 to 34 weeks gestation. Another single rescue course of antenatal corticosteroids may be considered if the initial steroid course was given more than 2 weeks earlier (140).

2.2.2. Long term effects of prenatal GCs overexposure

There are accumulating evidence about solid role played by fetal overexposure to both endogenous or synthetic GCs and the risk of developing metabolic and cardiovascular disease in adulthood (141, 142). This remote response to an intrauterine insult has been termed (fetal programming of adult disease).

3. Fetal programming of adult disease

Programming refers to physiological, metabolic, or behavioral adaptation resulting from exposure to or lack of hormones, nutrients, stress, and other agents at critical period during embryonic and fetal development. These insults may encode the function of organs and systems and manifested later as elevated risk for disease in adult life (143, 144). The concept of programming was emerged from many epidemiological studies. For instant, follow up study of a cohort of men who were born during Duch famine in 1944-45 found that exposure to undernutrition during the first half of pregnancy were significantly associated with obesity at adulthood (145). subsequent studies have linked the low birth weight with developing of hypertension, ischaemic heart disease, glucose intolerance, insulin resistance, type 2 diabetes, hyperlipidaemia, hypercortisolaemia, obesity, obstructive pulmonary disease, renal failure and reproductive disorders in the adult (146).

The factors that can programme disease risk in later life are multiple but interact together and include undernutrition (147), stress(148) and endocrine disturbances (149). It has been found that maternal undernutrition leads to decreased placental and fetal birth weight associated with elevated maternal plasma GCs and reduced placental expression of 11 β-Hydroxysteroid Dehydrogenase-2 and subsequently fetal over exposure to maternal corticosterone in rat (150). Maternal low protein diet, for instance, programmed the development of hypertension (151, 152), glucose intolerance (153, 154) and even feeding behavioral abnormalities (155). In human, fetal over exposure to endogenous maternal GCs, such as in maternal psychological stress, programmed the development of metabolic syndrome with higher BMI and body fat percentage, insulin resistance, and atherogenic lipid profile in the offspring at adult life (156). Moreover, adult offspring exposed to prenatal maternal stress, and hence high endogenous GCs, have altered T-helper 1 and 2 balance and abnormal cytokines and ultimately become more prone to develop autoimmune disorders and asthma (157). Similarly, there was impaired cognitive performance as well as memory in the offspring who exposed to maternal stress and higher endogenous GCs. This disturbances in mental function was associated with altered HPA axis in later life where ACTH was increased and plasma cortisol level was decreased (158).

Interestingly, the same programming effect was observed using synthetic GCs such as dexamethasone, which is poor substrate to 11 β-Hydroxysteroid Dehydrogenase-2 (142, 159). Prenatal exposure to synthetic GCs resulted in anxiety and depressive-like behavior in adult offspring. There was altered brain structure with significant increase in volume of the bed nucleus of the stria terminalis and on the other hand decrease amygdala volume due to dendritic atrophy. Dopamin was reduced and dopamin receptor 2 was up regulated in this area (160, 161).

Dexamethasone exposure during late gestation is also able to alter the hepatic and adipose tissue activity and mRNA expression of β-HSD 1 in marmoset monkey with subsequent development of obesity and overt metabolic syndrome (162). It is clear from these data that both fetal exposure to undernutrition, as stress event that lead to fetal over exposure to endogenous maternal GCs, as well as overexposure to synthetic GCs, which are poor substrates to placental 11 β-HSD 2, share common mechanistic pathway in the programming of metabolic syndrome in the offspring at adult life.

3.1. Proposed mechanism of fetal programming of adult disease

The concept of the programming has its roots since 50 years ago (163) and proven by both animal (152, 164) and human studies (119, 149), however, the mechanism that events during intrauterine life are carried in the memory of every molecule, gene, cell, tissue and systems` organs of the body still not completely revealed. Many hypotheses have been proposed with their inherited power and weakness. These include epigenetic modifications of DNA, altered gene expression and regulation, disruption of organ structure by variation in cell number and differentiation and apoptotic remodeling (165, 166). "Hormonal imprinting" where exposure to abnormal levels of a particular hormone during specific window of tissue plasticity is able to exert lifelong abnormal metabolism is another proposed mechanism (167).

3.1.1. Tissue remodeling

In maternal undernutrition model, programming was found to be associated with decreased organ size and total cell mass. Programming of diabetes, in this model, was accompanied by altered pancreatic structure, with predominantly a decrease in β-cell mass (153) due, primarily, to decreased proliferation and increased apoptosis (168). In this model, last week of rat pregnancy was identified as the critical window of programming. Similarly, programming of hypertension was linked to decreased number of nephrons and impaired renal electrolytes and fluid balance (169). GCs, both synthetic one and endogenous, are mediating their programming effects through similar mechanism. As mentioned previously that the observed psychological, behavioral and neuromuscular disturbances were all associated with decreased volume of brain area responsible on that particular function. Moreover, dexamethasone prenatally caused marked reduction in thymus (170). Therefore, antenatal exposure to glucocorticoids above the physiological limit will perturb the growth and ultimate size of the developing fetal organs and eventually their functional capacity which then manifested as disease in adult life.

3.1.2. Epigenetic DNA modification

Epigenetic phenomenon refers to altered heritable genomic function without change in DNA sequence (171). Epigenetic modification involves mainly DNA methylation, histone modification, and miRNA effects (172). DNA methylation has been well explored. In this case there is methylation of cytosine residues within CpG dinucleotides. When this abnormal methylation of CpG islands occur in the promoter region of genes it will result in silencing of genetic information and subsequently to altered biological function (171). Methylation status is a dynamic status and changes are observed since fertilization where both maternal and paternal genomes undergo extensive demethylation followed by selective methylation just prior to implantation (173). This alteration in methylation status has been suggested to play role in cell differentiation and organ development (174). DNA methylation blocks the binding of transcription factors to the promoter of the target gene (Figure 5) and hence prevent gene expression or it promote the binding of the methyl CpG binding protein (MeCP2) which recruits other protein complexes to bind to DNA resulting in a closed chromatin structure and transcriptional silencing (174).

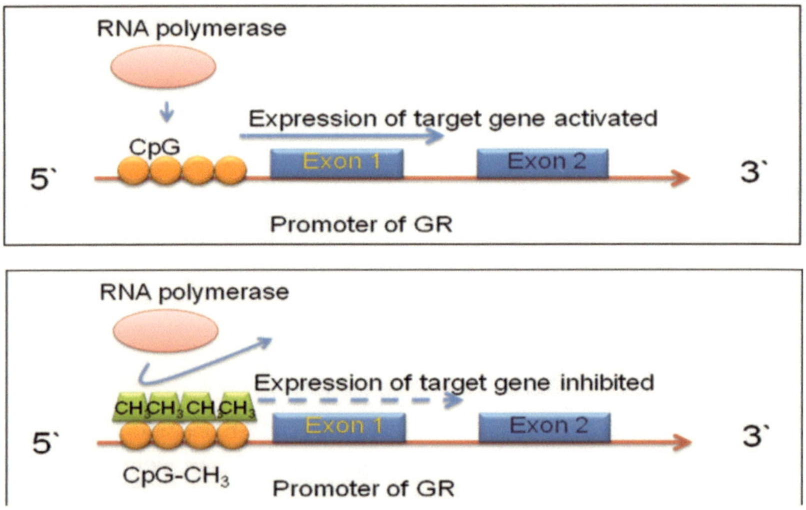

Figure 5. Epigenetic modification of GR promoter by CpG altered methylation.

Maternal low protein diet during pregnancy as experimental model of programming of metabolic syndrome like phenotype has been found to be associated with altered DNA methylation in key genes. For instance, maternal low protein diet resulted in GR over expression and 11 β-HSD 2 decreased expressions in liver, lung, kidney and brain of the offspring (175). GCs induce the hepatic expression and activity of phosphoenolpyruvate carboxykinase (PEPCK) the key enzyme responsible for gluconeogenesis and subsequently produce insulin resistance in this model (176). Interestingly, these changes in expression of target genes were associated with altered methylation status in their promoter area. Namely, GR promoter was found to be hypomethylated in liver tissue of 5 weeks old offspring (177). Some preliminary evidence suggest that hypomethylation of GR occur during early embryogenesis even before cell line differentiation, this was because of finding that GR hypomethylation found in all examined tissue of the offspring in this model (174). GR promoter hypomethylation was associated with histone modification, due to decreased acetylation, in way facilitating transcription (178). Supplementation of maternal low protein diet with glycine or folic acid prevented the development of metabolic syndrome like phenotype as well as GR promoter hypomethylation. Similarly, perinatal stress exposure resulted in altered stress response in the offspring which found to be accompanied with GR promoter hypermethylation at specific CpG dinucleotides in the hippocampus of the offspring. These changes were reversed in adult brain with intra-cranial histone deacetylase inhibitor administration (179). Similarly, in human fetal exposure to maternal stress during second and third trimesters was associated with increased methylation in specific CpG sequence in axon 1F of the GR gene analyzed in cord blood mononuclear cells and at 3 months of offspring age there was significant association between higher CpG methylation in GR gene and higher plasma cortisol response to stress (180). These epigenetic DNA modification seen in antenatal malnutrition or dexamethasone exposure are transmitted to the second generation (181), however, in human it needs to be further explored. It has been suggested that GCs exposure, either endogenous as in maternal psychological stress or in food deprivation or due to antenatal synthetic GCs administration, lead to altered DNA methylation via reduce folic acid availability (182). N5- methyltetrahydrofolate is folic acid derivative and it is considered one of the important methyl donors, therefore, any constrain on folic acid availability will affect methyl donors availability as well.

All these valuable data gave strong evidence that intrauterine life environment has crucial role in human health during adulthood and that the unfavorable conditions will act on the basic unit in the body, that is DNA. Therefore, altered DNA function via epigenetic modification will constrain the functional capacity of key organs when needed to work with their full capacity at adult life and ultimately expressed as disease. The understanding of the mechanism of disease can open the door for discovering early markers for the risk of developing disease and importantly more targeted therapeutic strategies.

3.1.3. Glucocorticoids over exposure

Most of animal models of disease programming and human studies including epidemiological data indicated that glucocorticoids have crucial role in the development of cardio-metabolic and neouro-psychological disease at adulthood. This deleterious effect of glucocorticoids can be exerted directly up on maternal administration of synthetic glucocorticoids and by stress induced endogenous maternal glucocorticoids hypersecretion or indirectly through other types of stress such as food restriction. The development of low birth weight, hypertension, glucose intolerance and insulin resistance in offspring of rat dams fed low protein diet during pregnancy were linked to decreased placental 11 β-HSD 2 expression and activity which resulted in high influx of maternal glucocorticoids to fetal compartment in addition to increased sensitivity of key metabolic organs such as liver, kidney and adipose tissue to glucocorticoids secondary to increased GR expression in these organs (175, 183). The development of metabolic syndrome like phenotype in this animal model has been replicated in human offspring who were exposed to prenatal synthetic glucocorticoids due to threatened preterm delivery to induce lung maturity and also in human offspring who were exposed to high maternal glucocorticoids secondary to maternal stress during pregnancy. Therefore, fetal glucocorticoids over exposure is the main programming pathway despite the variation in the prenatal insult. This hypothesis has many supporting evidence from low protein diet model and other human studies. In rodent, treatment of pregnant dams with placental 11 β-HSD 2 inhibitor, carbenoxolone, resulted in low birth weight and hypertension at adulthood (141). Hypertension in low protein model also was glucocorticoid dependent as maternal adrenalectomy significantly reduced the blood pressure to control levels and corticosterone replacement restored the hypertensive state seen these exposed offspring (151). In human, the placental 11 β-HSD 2 activity correlated with birth weight (184) and reduced in pre-eclampsia (185) and in intrauterine growth restricted fetuses (186). Moreover, 11 β-HSD 2 gene mutation constantly resulted in lower fetal birth weight compared to normal human fetus (187). High maternal GCs associated with decreased placental 11 β-HSD 2, elevated fetal plasma GCs, lower hepatic 11 β-HSD 2 protein expression and enzyme activity which cause over expression and activity of key hepatic gluconeogenesis enzyme, phosphoenolpyruvate kinase (PEPCK), which is linked to insulin resistance and glucose intolerance. In the kidney, the main role of 11 β-HSD 2 is to prevent GCs occupying and activating mineralocorticoid receptor (MR) (188), see figure 6.

GCs-exposed offspring has decreased 11 β-HSD 2 expression and increased GR expression as well as GR promoter hypomethylation in kidney (189). Cortisol will then exert mineralocorticoid activity through MR binding in kidney and resulted in sodium and water retention, hypokalaemia, low plasma renin and aldosterone concentrations, and eventually hypertension in adult life (190). In brain the observed cognitive deficit, altered memory and psychological disturbances in GCs exposed offspring was associated with decreased GR expression in hippocampus (191), which could block the negative feedback regulation of HPA axis by plasma cortisol and hence resulted in abnormal regulation of this crucial nuerohormonal axis. GCs induce the expression of key lipogenic transcription factor, Sterol regulatory element binding protein-1c (SREBP-1c) in liver (192). SREBP-1c transgenic mice, with mRNA and protein over expression of this nuclear factor, developed hyperinsulinaemia, hyperglycaemia, and hepatic steatosis (193, 194).

Interestingly, the metabolic syndrome like phenotype seen in low-protein diet exposed offspring was associated with abnormal expression of SREBP-1c. SREBP-1c mRNA and protein expression were both suppressed from birth until age 9 months in the rat offspring. At 18 months, however, marked over expression seen specially in hepatic tissue with development of non-alcoholic fatty liver, hypercholestreamia, hpertriglycerideamia, hyperglycemia and insulin resistance (147).

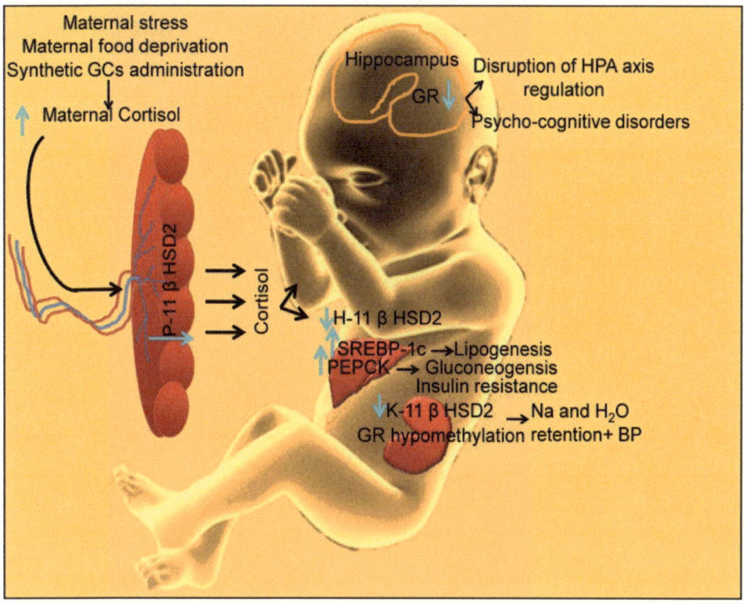

Figure 6. Glucocorticoids central role in the programming of the adult disease. Prenatal exposure to high maternal or synthetic glucocorticoids associated with decreased P-11βHSD2, K-11βHSD2 and H-11βHSD2 expression and activity. In liver this will induce SREBP-1c and lipogenesis and PEPCK and hepatic gluconeogenesis. In kidney, GR hypomethylation and decreased K-11βHSD2 activity associated with more Na and H_2O retention and eventually high BP. P-11βHSD2: Placental 11β Hydroxysteroid dehydrogenase 2, K: Kidney, H: Hepatic, SREBP-1c: Sterol Regulatory Element Binding Protein-1c, PEPK: Phosphoenolpyruvate kinase, Na: Sodium, BP: Blood pressure.

4. Conclusions

The understanding of pathogenesis of adult cardio-metabolic and psycho-cognitive disorders is now advanced beyond the idea that such diseases are result of current behavioral and environmental factors. It is well established that adult health originated from wellbeing during fetal life or even at gametes stage. Grandparents' environmental challenges can have impact on human health many generations later. In fact, factors which operate at early life will increase the individual`s susceptibility and vulnerability to adverse environmental events in later life. It is obvious now that different early life environmental events share common programming pathway. The mechanism of programming started to be revealed which include epigenetic DNA modification and promoter methylation status resulting in altered gene expression as well as glucocorticoids over exposure as a primary mechanism where as tissue remodeling and decreased organ and body size as a secondary mechanism. Glucocrticoids over exposure is the main triggering stimulus in this programming, therefore the widely clinical use of prenatal glucocorticoids such as betamethasone and dexamethasone to induce lung maturity in preterm fetus need to be carefully evaluated since they access fetal compartment very easily. Introduction of multiple courses of glucocorticoids as a routine should be discouraged and instead it should be restricted to wisely selected cases. The maximum number of safest courses and lowest therapeutic dose of each subsequent course should be standardized. However, prenatal glucocorticoids have provided the suitable model to study the effects of direct maternal administration of this programming hormone in human candidates. Notwithstanding, these studies still in their neonatal stage and extensive research in this particular area is warranted. The identification of how early life unfavorable environment still able to express pathogenesis at adulthood is crucial to set up pre-disease markers which can be applied clinically in health screening even before the disease itself develops. This will lead to early behavioral and life style interventions which may postponed the onset of disease for many years or even freeze the pathogenesis at its pre-disease stage. Obviously this will lead to decrease financial burden on the health authorities and will markedly cuts the expenses of medical and surgical treatment of the resulted complications.

Author details

Aml Mohammed Erhuma
School of Biomedical Sciences, Nottingham University, Queen`s Medical Centre, Nottingham, UK

Acknowledgement

I would like to express my thanks to Professor Simon Langley-Evans for his valuable advises. My thanks also to my husband and children: Bushra, Tasneem, Lina and Abdul-Rahman for continuance support.

5. References

[1] Addison T. Anemia-disease of supra renal capsule. Med Gazette 1849;43:517-518.
[2] Addison T. On the constitutional and local Effects of Disease of the Supra-Renal Capsules. Samuel Highley, London 1855.
[3] Graner JL. Addison, pernicious anemia and adrenal insufficiency. CMAJ. 1985;133(9):855-7.
[4] Lloyd M. Philip Showalter Hench, 1896-1965. Rheumatology (Oxford) 2002;41(5):582-4.
[5] Nørgaard P, Poulsen H. Glucocorticoid receptors in human malignancies: a review. Ann Oncol. 1991;2(8):541-57.
[6] Chrousos GP, Kino T. Glucocorticoid signaling in the cell. Expanding clinical implications to complex human behavioral and somatic disorders. Ann N Y Acad Sci 2009;1179:153-66.
[7] Zanchi NE, Filho MrAdS, Felitti V, Nicastro H, Lorenzeti FbM, Lancha AH. Glucocorticoids: Extensive physiological actions modulated through multiple mechanisms of gene regulation. Journal of Cellular Physiology 2010;224(2):311-315.

[8] Dallman MF, Strack AM, Akana SF, Bradbury MJ, Hanson ES, Scribner KA, et al. Feast and Famine: Critical Role of Glucocorticoids with Insulin in Daily Energy Flow. Frontiers in Neuroendocrinology 1993;14(4):303-347.

[9] Gaillard R. Interaction between the hypothalamo-pituitary-adrenal axis and the immunological system. Ann Endocrinol (Paris). 2001;62(2):155-63.

[10] Da Silva JA. Sex hormones and glucocorticoids: interactions with the immune system. Ann N Y Acad Sci 1999;876:102-17; discussion 117-8.

[11] Giannopoulos G. Early events in the action of glucocorticoids in developing tissues. J Steroid Biochem 1975;6(5):623-31.

[12] Iavazzo C, Myriokefalitaki E, Ntziora F, Bozemberg T, Baskozos I, Papargyriou T, et al. Classic congenital adrenal hyperplasia with virilisation and salt-wasting: from birth to the adult life. Bratisl Lek Listy 2011;112(11):651-2.

[13] Speiser PW, Laforgia N, Kato K, Pareira J, Khan R, Yang SY, et al. First trimester prenatal treatment and molecular genetic diagnosis of congenital adrenal hyperplasia (21-hydroxylase deficiency). J Clin Endocrinol Metab 1990;70(4):838-48.

[14] Forest MG, David M. Antenatal diagnosis and treatment of congenital adrenal hyperplasia due to 21-hydroxylase deficiency. Rev Prat 1991;41(13):1183-7.

[15] Dorr H, Sippell W, Haack D, Bidlingmaier F, Knorr D. Pitfalls of Prenatal treatment of Congenital Adrenal Hyperplasia due to 21-Hydroxylase Deficiency. Program and Abstract. In: 25th Annual meeting of the European Society for Paediatric Endocrinology; 1986; Zurich; 1986.

[16] Evans MI, Chrousos GP, Mann DW, Larsen JW, Jr., Green I, McCluskey J, et al. Pharmacologic suppression of the fetal adrenal gland in utero. Attempted prevention of abnormal external genital masculinization in suspected congenital adrenal hyperplasia. Jama 1985;253(7):1015-20.

[17] Mercado AB, Wilson RC, Cheng KC, Wei JQ, New MI. Prenatal treatment and diagnosis of congenital adrenal hyperplasia owing to steroid 21-hydroxylase deficiency. Journal of Clinical Endocrinology & Metabolism 1995;80(7):2014-20.

[18] Charmandari E, Brook CG, Hindmarsh PC. Why is management of patients with classical congenital adrenal hyperplasia more difficult at puberty? Arch Dis Child 2002;86(4):266-9.

[19] Kino T, Chrousos G. Glucocorticoid effects on gene expression. In: Steckler T KN, Reul JMHM, editor. Handbook of Stress and the Brain. Amsterdam: Elsevier; 2005. p. 295-311.

[20] Chrousos GP. The glucocorticoid receptor gene, longevity, and the complex disorders of Western societies. Am J Med 2004;117(3):204-7.

[21] Chrousos GP, Charmandari E, Kino T. Glucocorticoid action networks--an introduction to systems biology. J Clin Endocrinol Metab 2004;89(2):563-4.

[22] Galon J, Franchimont D, Hiroi N, Frey G, Boettner A, Ehrhart-Bornstein M, et al. Gene profiling reveals unknown enhancing and suppressive actions of glucocorticoids on immune cells. Faseb J 2002;16(1):61-71.

[23] Cameron A, Henley D, Carrell R, Zhou A, Clarke A, Lightman S. Temperature-responsive release of cortisol from its binding globulin: a protein thermocouple. J Clin Endocrinol Metab 2010;95(10):4689-95.

[24] David EG, Armen H, Tashjian J, Ehrin JA, April WA. Pharmacology of the Adrenal Cortex. In: David EG, editor. Principles of pharmacology: the pathophysiologic basis of drug therapy. second ed. USA: Lippincott Williams & Wilkins; 2008. p. 493-508.
[25] Nicolaides NC, Galata Z, Kino T, Chrousos GP, Charmandari E. The human glucocorticoid receptor: molecular basis of biologic function. Steroids 2010;75(1):1-12.
[26] Hollenberg SM, Weinberger C, Ong ES, Cerelli G, Oro A, Lebo R, et al. Primary structure and expression of a functional human glucocorticoid receptor cDNA. Nature 1985;318(6047):635-41.
[27] Duma D, Jewell CM, Cidlowski JA. Multiple glucocorticoid receptor isoforms and mechanisms of post-translational modification. J Steroid Biochem Mol Biol 2006;102(1-5):11-21.
[28] Bamberger CM, Bamberger AM, de Castro M, Chrousos GP. Glucocorticoid receptor beta, a potential endogenous inhibitor of glucocorticoid action in humans. J Clin Invest 1995;95(6):2435-41.
[29] Chung CC, Shimmin L, Natarajan S, Hanis CL, Boerwinkle E, Hixson JE. Glucocorticoid receptor gene variant in the 3' untranslated region is associated with multiple measures of blood pressure. J Clin Endocrinol Metab 2009;94(1):268-76.
[30] Hench P. Effects of cortisone in the rheumatic diseases. Lancet 1950;2(6634):483-4.
[31] Cupps TR, Edgar LC, Thomas CA, Fauci AS. Multiple mechanisms of B cell immunoregulation in man after administration of in vivo corticosteroids. J Immunol 1984;132(1):170-5.
[32] Sbiera S, Dexneit T, Reichardt SD, Michel KD, van den Brandt J, Schmull S, et al. Influence of short-term glucocorticoid therapy on regulatory T cells in vivo. PLoS One 2011;6(9):e24345.
[33] Cox G. Glucocorticoid treatment inhibits apoptosis in human neutrophils. Separation of survival and activation outcomes. J Immunol 1995;154(9):4719-25.
[34] Nakagawa M, Bondy GP, Waisman D, Minshall D, Hogg JC, van Eeden SF. The effect of glucocorticoids on the expression of L-selectin on polymorphonuclear leukocyte. Blood 1999;93(8):2730-7.
[35] van der Goes A, Hoekstra K, van den Berg TK, Dijkstra CD. Dexamethasone promotes phagocytosis and bacterial killing by human monocytes/macrophages in vitro. J Leukoc Biol 2000;67(6):801-7.
[36] Curtiss PH, Jr., Clark WS, Herndon CH. Vertebral fractures resulting from prolonged cortisone and corticotropin therapy. J Am Med Assoc 1954;156(5):467-9.
[37] Lukert BP, Raisz LG. Glucocorticoid-induced osteoporosis: pathogenesis and management. Ann Intern Med 1990;112(5):352-64.
[38] Adler RA, Rosen CJ. Glucocorticoids and osteoporosis. Endocrinol Metab Clin North Am 1994;23(3):641-54.
[39] Canalis E. Clinical review 83: Mechanisms of glucocorticoid action in bone: implications to glucocorticoid-induced osteoporosis. J Clin Endocrinol Metab 1996;81(10):3441-7.
[40] Lane NE, Lukert B. The science and therapy of glucocorticoid-induced bone loss. Endocrinol Metab Clin North Am 1998;27(2):465-83.
[41] Manolagas SC, Weinstein RS. New developments in the pathogenesis and treatment of steroid-induced osteoporosis. J Bone Miner Res 1999;14(7):1061-6.

[42] Pocock NA, Eisman JA, Dunstan CR, Evans RA, Thomas DH, Huq NL. Recovery from steroid-induced osteoporosis. Ann Intern Med 1987;107(3):319-23.
[43] Reid IR, Heap SW. Determinants of vertebral mineral density in patients receiving long-term glucocorticoid therapy. Arch Intern Med 1990;150(12):2545-8.
[44] Reid DM, Hughes RA, Laan RF, Sacco-Gibson NA, Wenderoth DH, Adami S, et al. Efficacy and safety of daily risedronate in the treatment of corticosteroid-induced osteoporosis in men and women: a randomized trial. European Corticosteroid-Induced Osteoporosis Treatment Study. J Bone Miner Res 2000;15(6):1006-13.
[45] Vermaat H, Kirtschig G. Prevention and treatment of glucocorticoid-induced osteoporosis in daily dermatologic practice. Int J Dermatol 2008;47(7):737-42.
[46] Sun L, Trausch-Azar JS, Muglia LJ, Schwartz AL. Glucocorticoids differentially regulate degradation of MyoD and Id1 by N-terminal ubiquitination to promote muscle protein catabolism. Proc Natl Acad Sci U S A 2008;105(9):3339-44.
[47] Nishimura T, Matsumoto T, Nishino M, Tomita K. Histopathologic study of veins in steroid treated rabbits. Clin Orthop Relat Res 1997(334):37-42.
[48] Weinstein RS, Nicholas RW, Manolagas SC. Apoptosis of osteocytes in glucocorticoid-induced osteonecrosis of the hip. J Clin Endocrinol Metab 2000;85(8):2907-12.
[49] Souverein PC, Berard A, Van Staa TP, Cooper C, Egberts AC, Leufkens HG, et al. Use of oral glucocorticoids and risk of cardiovascular and cerebrovascular disease in a population based case-control study. Heart 2004;90(8):859-65.
[50] Wei L, MacDonald TM, Walker BR. Taking glucocorticoids by prescription is associated with subsequent cardiovascular disease. Ann Intern Med 2004;141(10):764-70.
[51] White KP, Driscoll MS, Rothe MJ, Grant-Kels JM. Severe adverse cardiovascular effects of pulse steroid therapy: is continuous cardiac monitoring necessary? J Am Acad Dermatol 1994;30(5 Pt 1):768-73.
[52] Berg AL, Nilsson-Ehle P. ACTH lowers serum lipids in steroid-treated hyperlipemic patients with kidney disease. Kidney Int 1996;50(2):538-42.
[53] Choi HK, Seeger JD. Glucocorticoid use and serum lipid levels in US adults: the Third National Health and Nutrition Examination Survey. Arthritis Rheum 2005;53(4):528-35.
[54] Miller SE, Neilson JM. Clinical Features of the Diabetic Syndrome Appearing after Steroid Therapy. Postgrad Med J 1964;40:660-9.
[55] Gurwitz JH, Bohn RL, Glynn RJ, Monane M, Mogun H, Avorn J. Glucocorticoids and the risk for initiation of hypoglycemic therapy. Arch Intern Med 1994;154(1):97-101.
[56] Olefsky JM, Kimmerling G. Effects of glucocorticoids on carbohydrate metabolism. Am J Med Sci 1976;271(2):202-10.
[57] Minden SL, Orav J, Schildkraut JJ. Hypomanic reactions to ACTH and prednisone treatment for multiple sclerosis. Neurology 1988;38(10):1631-4.
[58] Naber D, Sand P, Heigl B. Psychopathological and neuropsychological effects of 8-days' corticosteroid treatment. A prospective study. Psychoneuroendocrinology 1996;21(1):25-31.
[59] Keenan PA, Jacobson MW, Soleymani RM, Mayes MD, Stress ME, Yaldoo DT. The effect on memory of chronic prednisone treatment in patients with systemic disease. Neurology 1996;47(6):1396-402.

[60] Souza-Talarico JNd, Marin M-F, Sindi S, Lupien SJ. Effects of stress hormones on the brain and cognition Evidence from normal to pathological aging. Dement Neuropsychol 2011;5(1):8-16.

[61] Gabriel SE, Jaakkimainen L, Bombardier C. Risk for serious gastrointestinal complications related to use of nonsteroidal anti-inflammatory drugs. A meta-analysis. Ann Intern Med 1991;115(10):787-96.

[62] Chrousos GA, Kattah JC, Beck RW, Cleary PA. Side effects of glucocorticoid treatment. Experience of the Optic Neuritis Treatment Trial. Jama 1993;269(16):2110-2.

[63] Derk CT, DeHoratius RJ. Systemic lupus erythematosus and acute pancreatitis: a case series. Clin Rheumatol 2004;23(2):147-51.

[64] Mastorakos G, Ilias I. Maternal and fetal hypothalamic-pituitary-adrenal axes during pregnancy and postpartum. Ann N Y Acad Sci 2003;997:136-49.

[65] Seckl JR. Glucocorticoid programming of the fetus; adult phenotypes and molecular mechanisms. Mol Cell Endocrinol 2001;185(1-2):61-71.

[66] Fowden AL, Forhead AJ. Endocrine mechanisms of intrauterine programming. Reproduction 2004;127(5):515-26.

[67] Dy J, Guan H, Sampath-Kumar R, Richardson BS, Yang K. Placental 11beta-hydroxysteroid dehydrogenase type 2 is reduced in pregnancies complicated with idiopathic intrauterine growth Restriction: evidence that this is associated with an attenuated ratio of cortisone to cortisol in the umbilical artery. Placenta 2008;29(2):193-200.

[68] Huh SY, Andrew R, Rich-Edwards JW, Kleinman KP, Seckl JR, Gillman MW. Association between umbilical cord glucocorticoids and blood pressure at age 3 years. BMC Med 2008;6:25.

[69] Sanchez MM, Young LJ, Plotsky PM, Insel TR. Distribution of corticosteroid receptors in the rhesus brain: relative absence of glucocorticoid receptors in the hippocampal formation. J Neurosci 2000;20(12):4657-68.

[70] Raschke C, Schmidt S, Schwab M, Jirikowski G. Effects of betamethasone treatment on central myelination in fetal sheep: an electron microscopical study. Anat Histol Embryol 2008;37(2):95-100.

[71] Kostovic I, Judas M, Rados M, Hrabac P. Laminar organization of the human fetal cerebrum revealed by histochemical markers and magnetic resonance imaging. Cereb Cortex 2002;12(5):536-44.

[72] Huttenlocher PR, Dabholkar AS. Regional differences in synaptogenesis in human cerebral cortex. J Comp Neurol 1997;387(2):167-78.

[73] Levitt P. Structural and functional maturation of the developing primate brain. J Pediatr 2003;143(4 Suppl):S35-45.

[74] Seckl JR, Meaney MJ. Glucocorticoid "programming" and PTSD risk. Ann N Y Acad Sci 2006;1071:351-78.

[75] Murphy VE, Clifton VL. Alterations in human placental 11beta-hydroxysteroid dehydrogenase type 1 and 2 with gestational age and labour. Placenta 2003;24(7):739-44.

[76] Lowry PJ. Corticotropin-releasing factor and its binding protein in human plasma. Ciba Found Symp 1993;172:108-15; discussion 115-28.

[77] Cheng YH, Nicholson RC, King B, Chan EC, Fitter JT, Smith R. Corticotropin-releasing hormone gene expression in primary placental cells is modulated by cyclic adenosine 3',5'-monophosphate. J Clin Endocrinol Metab 2000;85(3):1239-44.

[78] Sandman CA, Davis EP, Buss C, Glynn LM. Prenatal programming of human neurological function. Int J Pept 2011;2011:837596.

[79] Sandman CA, Wadhwa PD, Chicz-DeMet A, Porto M, Garite TJ. Maternal corticotropin-releasing hormone and habituation in the human fetus. Dev Psychobiol 1999;34(3):163-73.

[80] Ellman LM, Schetter CD, Hobel CJ, Chicz-Demet A, Glynn LM, Sandman CA. Timing of fetal exposure to stress hormones: effects on newborn physical and neuromuscular maturation. Dev Psychobiol 2008;50(3):232-41.

[81] Davis EP, Waffarn F, Sandman CA. Prenatal treatment with glucocorticoids sensitizes the hpa axis response to stress among full-term infants. Developmental Psychobiology 2011;53(2):175-183.

[82] Buss C, Davis EP, Muftuler LT, Head K, Sandman CA. High pregnancy anxiety during mid-gestation is associated with decreased gray matter density in 6-9-year-old children. Psychoneuroendocrinology 2010;35(1):141-53.

[83] Connolly JD, Goodale MA, Menon RS, Munoz DP. Human fMRI evidence for the neural correlates of preparatory set. Nat Neurosci 2002;5(12):1345-52.

[84] Beijers R, Jansen J, Riksen-Walraven M, de Weerth C. Maternal prenatal anxiety and stress predict infant illnesses and health complaints. Pediatrics 2010;126(2):e401-9.

[85] Li J, Olsen J, Vestergaard M, Obel C, Baker JL, Sorensen TI. Prenatal stress exposure related to maternal bereavement and risk of childhood overweight. PLoS One 2010;5(7):e11896.

[86] Gillman MW, Rich-Edwards JW, Huh S, Majzoub JA, Oken E, Taveras EM, et al. Maternal corticotropin-releasing hormone levels during pregnancy and offspring adiposity. Obesity (Silver Spring) 2006;14(9):1647-53.

[87] Diederich S, Eigendorff E, Burkhardt P, Quinkler M, Bumke-Vogt C, Rochel M, et al. 11beta-hydroxysteroid dehydrogenase types 1 and 2: an important pharmacokinetic determinant for the activity of synthetic mineralo- and glucocorticoids. J Clin Endocrinol Metab 2002;87(12):5695-701.

[88] Anderson AB, Gennser G, Jeremy JY, Ohrlander S, Sayers L, Turnbull AC. Placental transfer and metabolism of betamethasone in human pregnancy. Obstet Gynecol 1977;49(4):471-4.

[89] Thuring A, Malcus P, Marsal K. Effect of maternal betamethasone on fetal and uteroplacental blood flow velocity waveforms. Ultrasound Obstet Gynecol 2011;37(6):668-72.

[90] Rotmensch S, Liberati M, Celentano C, Efrat Z, Bar-Hava I, Kovo M, et al. The effect of betamethasone on fetal biophysical activities and Doppler velocimetry of umbilical and middle cerebral arteries. Acta Obstet Gynecol Scand 1999;78(9):768-73.

[91] Li JN, Ge YC, Yang Z, Guo CM, Duan T, Myatt L, et al. The Sp1 Transcription Factor Is Crucial for the Expression of 11Î²-Hydroxysteroid Dehydrogenase Type 2 in Human Placental Trophoblasts. Journal of Clinical Endocrinology & Metabolism 2011;96(6):E899-E907.

[92] Akhter A, Das V, Naik S, Faridi RM, Pandey A, Agrawal S. Upregulation of HLA-G in JEG-3 cells by dexamethasone and hydrocortisone. Arch Gynecol Obstet 2012;285(1):7-14.

[93] Avery ME, Mead J. Surface properties in relation to atelectasis and hyaline membrane disease. AMA J Dis Child 1959;97(5, Part 1):517-23.

[94] Dollfus C, Patetta M, Siegel E, Cross AW. Infant mortality: a practical approach to the analysis of the leading causes of death and risk factors. Pediatrics 1990;86(2):176-83.

[95] Wang ML, Dorer DJ, Fleming MP, Catlin EA. Clinical outcomes of near-term infants. Pediatrics 2004;114(2):372-6.

[96] Liggins GC, Howie RN. A controlled trial of antepartum glucocorticoid treatment for prevention of the respiratory distress syndrome in premature infants. Pediatrics 1972;50(4):515-25.

[97] Roberts D, Dalziel S. Antenatal corticosteroids for accelerating fetal lung maturation for women at risk of preterm birth. Cochrane Database Syst Rev 2006;3:CD004454.

[98] Elimian A, Verma U, Canterino J, Shah J, Visintainer P, Tejani N. Effectiveness of antenatal steroids in obstetric subgroups. Obstet Gynecol 1999;93(2):174-9.

[99] Elimian A, Garry D, Figueroa R, Spitzer A, Wiencek V, Quirk JG. Antenatal betamethasone compared with dexamethasone (betacode trial): a randomized controlled trial. Obstet Gynecol 2007;110(1):26-30.

[100] Hughes I, Cutfield W. The adrenal cortex. In: Gluckman P, Heymann M, editors. Pediatrics, perinatology, the scientific basis. London: Arnold; 1996. p. 500- 514.

[101] NIH. ACOG committee opinion. Antenatal corticosteroid therapy for fetal maturation. Number 147--December 1994. Committee on Obstetric Practice. American College of Obstetricians and Gynecologists. Int J Gynaecol Obstet 1995;48(3):340-2.

[102] ACOG. ACOG committee opinion. Antenatal corticosteroid therapy for fetal maturation. American College of Obstetricians and Gynecologists; 2002 Jul.

[103] RCOG. RCOG Guidelines Number 7 ACS to prevent respiratory distress syndrome. London: RCOG; 1996.

[104] Tillis CC, Huang HW, Bi W, Pan S, Bruce SR, Alcorn JL. Glucocorticoid regulation of human pulmonary surfactant protein-B (SP-B) mRNA stability is independent of activated glucocorticocorticoid receptor. American Journal of Physiology - Lung Cellular and Molecular Physiology 2011;300(6):L940-L950.

[105] Whitsett JA, Matsuzaki Y. Transcriptional Regulation of Perinatal Lung Maturation. Pediatric clinics of North America 2006;53(5):873-887.

[106] Venkatesh VC, Iannuzzi DM, Ertsey R, Ballard PL. Differential glucocorticoid regulation of the pulmonary hydrophobic surfactant proteins SP-B and SP-C. Am J Respir Cell Mol Biol 1993;8(2):222-8.

[107] Clements J, King R. Composition of the surface active material. In: RG C, editor. The biochemical basis of pulmonary function. New York: Marcel Dekker; 1976. p. 363-387.

[108] Liley HG, White RT, Warr RG, Benson BJ, Hawgood S, Ballard PL. Regulation of messenger RNAs for the hydrophobic surfactant proteins in human lung. J Clin Invest 1989;83(4):1191-7.

[109] Huang HW, Bi W, Jenkins GN, Alcorn JL. Glucocorticoid regulation of human pulmonary surfactant protein-B mRNA stability involves the 3'-untranslated region. Am J Respir Cell Mol Biol 2008;38(4):473-82.

[110] Smith LM, Qureshi N, Chao CR. Effects of single and multiple courses of antenatal glucocorticoids in preterm newborns less than 30 weeks' gestation. J Matern Fetal Med 2000;9(2):131-5.

[111] Guinn DA, Atkinson MW, Sullivan L, Lee M, MacGregor S, Parilla BV, et al. Single vs weekly courses of antenatal corticosteroids for women at risk of preterm delivery: A randomized controlled trial. Jama 2001;286(13):1581-7.

[112] Wijnberger LD, Mostert JM, van Dam KI, Mol BW, Brouwers H, Visser GH. Comparison of single and repeated antenatal corticosteroid therapy to prevent neonatal death and morbidity in the preterm infant. Early Hum Dev 2002;67(1-2):29-36.

[113] Uno H, Lohmiller L, Thieme C, Kemnitz JW, Engle MJ, Roecker EB, et al. Brain damage induced by prenatal exposure to dexamethasone in fetal rhesus macaques. I. Hippocampus. Brain Res Dev Brain Res 1990;53(2):157-67.

[114] Dunlop SA, Archer MA, Quinlivan JA, Beazley LD, Newnham JP. Repeated prenatal corticosteroids delay myelination in the ovine central nervous system. J Matern Fetal Med 1997;6(6):309-13.

[115] Stewart JD, Gonzalez CL, Christensen HD, Rayburn WF. Impact of multiple antenatal doses of betamethasone on growth and development of mice offspring. Am J Obstet Gynecol 1997;177(5):1138-44.

[116] Ogunyemi D. A comparison of the effectiveness of single-dose vs multi-dose antenatal corticosteroids in pre-term neonates. J Obstet Gynaecol 2005;25(8):756-60.

[117] Rodriguez-Pinilla E, Prieto-Merino D, Dequino G, Mejias C, Fernandez P, Martinez-Frias ML. Antenatal exposure to corticosteroids for fetal lung maturation and its repercussion on weight, length and head circumference in the newborn infant. Med Clin (Barc) 2006;127(10):361-7.

[118] Mazumder P, Dutta S, Kaur J, Narang A. Single versus multiple courses of antenatal betamethasone and neonatal outcome: a randomized controlled trial. Indian Pediatr 2008;45(8):661-7.

[119] Norberg H, Stalnacke J, Heijtz RD, Smedler AC, Nyman M, Forssberg H, et al. Antenatal corticosteroids for preterm birth: dose-dependent reduction in birthweight, length and head circumference. Acta Paediatr 2011;100(3):364-9.

[120] Peltoniemi OM, Kari MA, Hallman M. Repeated antenatal corticosteroid treatment: a systematic review and meta-analysis. Acta Obstet Gynecol Scand 2011;90(7):719-27.

[121] Abbasi S, Hirsch D, Davis J, Tolosa J, Stouffer N, Debbs R, et al. Effect of single versus multiple courses of antenatal corticosteroids on maternal and neonatal outcome. Am J Obstet Gynecol 2000;182(5):1243-9.

[122] Bloomfield F, Knight D, Harding J. Side effects of 2 different dexamethasone courses for preterm infants at risk of chronic lung disease: a randomized trial. J Pediatr. 1998;133(3):395-400.

[123] Mildenhall LF, Battin MR, Morton SM, Bevan C, Kuschel CA, Harding JE. Exposure to repeat doses of antenatal glucocorticoids is associated with altered cardiovascular status after birth. Arch Dis Child Fetal Neonatal Ed 2006;91(1):F56-60.

[124] Mariotti V, Marconi AM, Pardi G. Undesired effects of steroids during pregnancy. J Matern Fetal Neonatal Med 2004;16 Suppl 2:5-7.

[125] Lindahl K, Rubin CJ, Brandstrom H, Karlsson MK, Holmberg A, Ohlsson C, et al. Heterozygosity for a coding SNP in COL1A2 confers a lower BMD and an increased stroke risk. Biochem Biophys Res Commun 2009;384(4):501-5.

[126] Saarela T, Risteli J, Kauppila A, Koivisto M. Effect of short-term antenatal dexamethasone administration on type I collagen synthesis and degradation in preterm infants at birth. Acta PÃ¦diatrica 2001;90(8):921-925.

[127] Korakaki E, Gourgiotis D, Aligizakis A, Manoura A, Hatzidaki E, Giahnakis E, et al. Levels of bone collagen markers in preterm infants: relation to antenatal glucocorticoid treatment. J Bone Miner Metab 2007;25(3):172-8.

[128] Sandesh Kiran PS, Dutta S, Narang A, Bhansali A, Malhi P. Multiple courses of antenatal steroids. Indian J Pediatr 2007;74(5):463-9.

[129] Schaffer L, Luzi F, Burkhardt T, Rauh M, Beinder E. Antenatal betamethasone administration alters stress physiology in healthy neonates. Obstet Gynecol 2009;113(5):1082-8.

[130] Gatelais F, Berthelot J, Beringue F, Descamps P, Bonneau D, Limal JM, et al. Effect of single and multiple courses of prenatal corticosteroids on 17-hydroxyprogesterone levels: implication for neonatal screening of congenital adrenal hyperplasia. Pediatr Res 2004;56(5):701-5.

[131] Ng PC, Wong GW, Lam CW, Lee CH, Fok TF, Wong MY, et al. Effect of multiple courses of antenatal corticosteroids on pituitary-adrenal function in preterm infants. Arch Dis Child Fetal Neonatal Ed 1999;80(3):F213-6.

[132] Owen D, Matthews SG. Glucocorticoids and sex-dependent development of brain glucocorticoid and mineralocorticoid receptors. Endocrinology 2003;144(7):2775-84.

[133] Amin SB, Guillet R. Auditory neural maturation after exposure to multiple courses of antenatal betamethasone in premature infants as evaluated by auditory brainstem response. Pediatrics 2007;119(3):502-8.

[134] Spinillo A, Chiara A, Bergante C, Biancheri D, Fabiana D, Fazzi E. Obstetric risk factors and persistent increases in brain parenchymal echogenicity in preterm infants. Bjog 2004;111(9):913-8.

[135] Spinillo A, Viazzo F, Colleoni R, Chiara A, Maria Cerbo R, Fazzi E. Two-year infant neurodevelopmental outcome after single or multiple antenatal courses of corticosteroids to prevent complications of prematurity. Am J Obstet Gynecol 2004;191(1):217-24.

[136] Liu J, Feng ZC, Yin XJ, Chen H, Lu J, Qiao X. The role of antenatal corticosteroids for improving the maturation of choroid plexus capillaries in fetal mice. Eur J Pediatr 2008;167(10):1209-12.

[137] Liu J, Wang Q, Zhao JH, Chen YH, Qin GL. The combined antenatal corticosteroids and vitamin K therapy for preventing periventricular-intraventricular hemorrhage in premature newborns less than 35 weeks gestation. J Trop Pediatr 2006;52(5):355-9.

[138] Bontis N, Vavilis D, Tsolakidis D, Goulis DG, Tzevelekis P, Kellartzis D, et al. Comparison of single versus multiple courses of antenatal betamethasone in patients with threatened preterm labor. Clin Exp Obstet Gynecol 2011;38(2):165-7.

[139] Nair GV, Omar SA. Blood pressure support in extremely premature infants is affected by different courses of antenatal steroids. Acta Paediatr 2009;98(9):1437-43.

[140] ACOG. ACOG Committee Opinion No. 475: Antenatal corticosteroid therapy for fetal maturation. Obstet Gynecol 2011;117(2 Pt 1):422-4.

[141] Benediktsson R, Lindsay RS, Noble J, Seckl JR, Edwards CR. Glucocorticoid exposure in utero: new model for adult hypertension. Lancet 1993;341(8841):339-41.

[142] Nyirenda MJ, Lindsay RS, Kenyon CJ, Burchell A, Seckl JR. Glucocorticoid exposure in late gestation permanently programs rat hepatic phosphoenolpyruvate carboxykinase and glucocorticoid receptor expression and causes glucose intolerance in adult offspring. J Clin Invest 1998;101(10):2174-81.

[143] Seckl JR. Physiologic programming of the fetus. Clin Perinatol 1998;25(4):939-62, vii.

[144] Barker DJ. In utero programming of chronic disease. Clin Sci (Lond) 1998;95(2):115-28.

[145] Ravelli GP, Stein ZA, Susser MW. Obesity in young men after famine exposure in utero and early infancy. N Engl J Med 1976;295(7):349-53.

[146] Barker D. Mothers, Babies and Disease in Later Life. London: BMJ Publishing.; 1994.

[147] Erhuma A, Salter AM, Sculley DV, Langley-Evans SC, Bennett AJ. Prenatal exposure to a low-protein diet programs disordered regulation of lipid metabolism in the aging rat. Am J Physiol Endocrinol Metab 2007;292(6):E1702-14.

[148] Lazinski MJ, Shea AK, Steiner M. Effects of maternal prenatal stress on offspring development: a commentary. Arch Womens Ment Health 2008;11(5-6):363-75.

[149] Seckl JR. Prenatal glucocorticoids and long-term programming. Eur J Endocrinol 2004;151 Suppl 3:U49-62.

[150] Belkacemi L, Jelks A, Chen CH, Ross MG, Desai M. Altered placental development in undernourished rats: role of maternal glucocorticoids. Reprod Biol Endocrinol 2011;9:105.

[151] Gardner DS, Jackson AA, Langley-Evans SC. Maintenance of maternal diet-induced hypertension in the rat is dependent on glucocorticoids. Hypertension 1997;30(6):1525-30.

[152] Langley-Evans SC. Hypertension induced by foetal exposure to a maternal low-protein diet, in the rat, is prevented by pharmacological blockade of maternal glucocorticoid synthesis. J Hypertens 1997;15(5):537-44.

[153] Dahri S, Snoeck A, Reusens-Billen B, Remacle C, Hoet JJ. Islet function in offspring of mothers on low-protein diet during gestation. Diabetes 1991;40 Suppl 2:115-20.

[154] Pinheiro AR, Salvucci ID, Aguila MB, Mandarim-de-Lacerda CA. Protein restriction during gestation and/or lactation causes adverse transgenerational effects on biometry and glucose metabolism in F1 and F2 progenies of rats. Clin Sci (Lond) 2008;114(5):381-92.

[155] Bellinger L, Langley-Evans SC. Fetal programming of appetite by exposure to a maternal low-protein diet in the rat. Clin Sci (Lond) 2005;109(4):413-20.

[156] Entringer S, Wust S, Kumsta R, Layes IM, Nelson EL, Hellhammer DH, et al. Prenatal psychosocial stress exposure is associated with insulin resistance in young adults. Am J Obstet Gynecol 2008;199(5):498 e1-7.

[157] Entringer S, Kumsta R, Nelson EL, Hellhammer DH, Wadhwa PD, Wust S. Influence of prenatal psychosocial stress on cytokine production in adult women. Dev Psychobiol 2008;50(6):579-87.
[158] Entringer S, Buss C, Kumsta R, Hellhammer DH, Wadhwa PD, Wust S. Prenatal psychosocial stress exposure is associated with subsequent working memory performance in young women. Behav Neurosci 2009;123(4):886-93.
[159] Tang JI, Kenyon CJ, Seckl JR, Nyirenda MJ. Prenatal overexposure to glucocorticoids programs renal 11beta-hydroxysteroid dehydrogenase type 2 expression and salt-sensitive hypertension in the rat. J Hypertens 2011;29(2):282-9.
[160] McArthur S, McHale E, Dalley JW, Buckingham JC, Gillies GE. Altered Mesencephalic Dopaminergic Populations in Adulthood as a Consequence of Brief Perinatal Glucocorticoid Exposure. Journal of Neuroendocrinology 2005;17(8):475-482.
[161] Oliveira Mr, Rodrigues A-Jo, LeÃ£o P, Cardona D, PÃªgo J, Sousa N. The bed nucleus of stria terminalis and the amygdala as targets of antenatal glucocorticoids: implications for fear and anxiety responses. In: Psychopharmacology: Springer Berlin / Heidelberg; 2012. p. 443-453.
[162] Nyirenda MJ, Carter R, Tang JI, de Vries A, Schlumbohm C, Hillier SG, et al. Prenatal programming of metabolic syndrome in the common marmoset is associated with increased expression of 11beta-hydroxysteroid dehydrogenase type 1. Diabetes 2009;58(12):2873-9.
[163] Neel JV. Diabetes mellitus: a "thrifty" genotype rendered detrimental by "progress"? Am J Hum Genet 1962;14:353-62.
[164] Erhuma A, Bellinger L, Langley-Evans SC, Bennett AJ. Prenatal exposure to undernutrition and programming of responses to high-fat feeding in the rat. Br J Nutr 2007;98(3):517-24.
[165] Waterland RA, Garza C. Potential mechanisms of metabolic imprinting that lead to chronic disease. Am J Clin Nutr 1999;69(2):179-97.
[166] Waterland RA, Jirtle RL. Early nutrition, epigenetic changes at transposons and imprinted genes, and enhanced susceptibility to adult chronic diseases. Nutrition 2004;20(1):63-8.
[167] Csaba G. Phylogeny and ontogeny of hormone receptors: the selection theory of receptor formation and hormonal imprinting. Biol Rev Camb Philos Soc 1980;55(1):47-63.
[168] Berney DM, Desai M, Palmer DJ, Greenwald S, Brown A, Hales CN, et al. The effects of maternal protein deprivation on the fetal rat pancreas: major structural changes and their recuperation. The Journal of Pathology 1997;183(1):109-115.
[169] Langley-Evans SC, Welham SJ, Jackson AA. Fetal exposure to a maternal low protein diet impairs nephrogenesis and promotes hypertension in the rat. Life Sciences 1999;64(11):965-974.
[170] Dietert RR, Lee JE, Olsen J, Fitch K, Marsh JA. Developmental immunotoxicity of dexamethasone: comparison of fetal versus adult exposures. Toxicology 2003;194(1-2):163-76.
[171] Lorenzen JM, Martino F, Thum T. Epigenetic modifications in cardiovascular disease. Basic Res Cardiol 2012;107(2):1-10.

[172] Hussain N. Epigenetic Influences That Modulate Infant Growth, Development, and Disease. Antioxid Redox Signal 2012.
[173] Bird A. DNA methylation patterns and epigenetic memory. Genes Dev 2002;16(1):6-21.
[174] Burdge GC, Hanson MA, Slater-Jefferies JL, Lillycrop KA. Epigenetic regulation of transcription: a mechanism for inducing variations in phenotype (fetal programming) by differences in nutrition during early life? Br J Nutr 2007;97(6):1036-46.
[175] Bertram C, Trowern AR, Copin N, Jackson AA, Whorwood CB. The maternal diet during pregnancy programs altered expression of the glucocorticoid receptor and type 2 11beta-hydroxysteroid dehydrogenase: potential molecular mechanisms underlying the programming of hypertension in utero. Endocrinology 2001;142(7):2841-53.
[176] Burns SP, Desai M, Cohen RD, Hales CN, Iles RA, Germain JP, et al. Gluconeogenesis, glucose handling, and structural changes in livers of the adult offspring of rats partially deprived of protein during pregnancy and lactation. J Clin Invest 1997;100(7):1768-74.
[177] Lillycrop KA, Phillips ES, Jackson AA, Hanson MA, Burdge GC. Dietary protein restriction of pregnant rats induces and folic acid supplementation prevents epigenetic modification of hepatic gene expression in the offspring. J Nutr 2005;135(6):1382-6.
[178] Lillycrop KA, Slater-Jefferies JL, Hanson MA, Godfrey KM, Jackson AA, Burdge GC. Induction of altered epigenetic regulation of the hepatic glucocorticoid receptor in the offspring of rats fed a protein-restricted diet during pregnancy suggests that reduced DNA methyltransferase-1 expression is involved in impaired DNA methylation and changes in histone modifications. Br J Nutr 2007;97(6):1064-73.
[179] Weaver IC, Meaney MJ, Szyf M. Maternal care effects on the hippocampal transcriptome and anxiety-mediated behaviors in the offspring that are reversible in adulthood. Proc Natl Acad Sci U S A 2006;103(9):3480-5.
[180] Oberlander TF, Weinberg J, Papsdorf M, Grunau R, Misri S, Devlin AM. Prenatal exposure to maternal depression, neonatal methylation of human glucocorticoid receptor gene (NR3C1) and infant cortisol stress responses. Epigenetics 2008;3(2):97-106.
[181] Drake AJ, Walker BR, Seckl JR. Intergenerational consequences of fetal programming by in utero exposure to glucocorticoids in rats. Am J Physiol Regul Integr Comp Physiol 2005;288(1):R34-8.
[182] Terzolo M, Allasino B, Bosio S, Brusa E, Daffara F, Ventura M, et al. Hyperhomocysteinemia in patients with Cushing's syndrome. J Clin Endocrinol Metab 2004;89(8):3745-51.
[183] Langley-Evans SC, Phillips GJ, Benediktsson R, Gardner DS, Edwards CR, Jackson AA, et al. Protein intake in pregnancy, placental glucocorticoid metabolism and the programming of hypertension in the rat. Placenta 1996;17(2-3):169-72.
[184] Stewart PM, Rogerson FM, Mason JI. Type 2 11 beta-hydroxysteroid dehydrogenase messenger ribonucleic acid and activity in human placenta and fetal membranes: its relationship to birth weight and putative role in fetal adrenal steroidogenesis. Journal of Clinical Endocrinology & Metabolism 1995;80(3):885-90.
[185] McCalla CO, Nacharaju VL, Muneyyirci-Delale O, Glasgow S, Feldman JG. Placental 11 beta-hydroxysteroid dehydrogenase activity in normotensive and pre-eclamptic pregnancies. Steroids 1998;63(10):511-5.

[186] McTernan CL, Draper N, Nicholson H, Chalder SM, Driver P, Hewison M, et al. Reduced Placental 11 Beta-Hydroxysteroid Dehydrogenase Type 2 mRNA Levels in Human Pregnancies Complicated by Intrauterine Growth Restriction: An Analysis of Possible Mechanisms. Journal of Clinical Endocrinology & Metabolism 2001;86(10):4979-4983.

[187] Kitanaka S, Tanae A, Hibi I. Apparent mineralocorticoid excess due to 11 beta-hydroxysteroid dehydrogenase deficiency: a possible cause of intrauterine growth retardation. Clin Endocrinol (Oxf) 1996;44(3):353-9.

[188] Martinerie L, Pussard E, Meduri G, Delezoide AL, Boileau P, Lombes M. Lack of renal 11 Beta-hydroxysteroid dehydrogenase type 2 at birth, a targeted temporal window for neonatal glucocorticoid action in human and mice. PLoS One 2012;7(2):e31949.

[189] Wyrwoll CS, Mark PJ, Waddell BJ. Developmental programming of renal glucocorticoid sensitivity and the renin-angiotensin system. Hypertension 2007;50(3):579-84.

[190] Ferrari P, Lovati E, Frey FJ. The role of the 11beta-hydroxysteroid dehydrogenase type 2 in human hypertension. J Hypertens 2000;18(3):241-8.

[191] Basta-Kaim A, Budziszewska B, Leskiewicz M, Fijal K, Regulska M, Kubera M, et al. Hyperactivity of the hypothalamus-pituitary-adrenal axis in lipopolysaccharide-induced neurodevelopmental model of schizophrenia in rats: effects of antipsychotic drugs. Eur J Pharmacol 2011;650(2-3):586-95.

[192] Erhuma A, McMullen S, Langley-Evans SC, Bennett AJ. Feeding pregnant rats a low-protein diet alters the hepatic expression of SREBP-1c in their offspring via a glucocorticoid-related mechanism. Endocrine 2009;36(2):333-8.

[193] Shimomura I, Hammer RE, Richardson JA, Ikemoto S, Bashmakov Y, Goldstein JL, et al. Insulin resistance and diabetes mellitus in transgenic mice expressing nuclear SREBP-1c in adipose tissue: model for congenital generalized lipodystrophy. Genes & Development 1998;12(20):3182-3194.

[194] Horton JD, Shimomura I, Ikemoto S, Bashmakov Y, Hammer RE. Overexpression of sterol regulatory element-binding protein-1a in mouse adipose tissue produces adipocyte hypertrophy, increased fatty acid secretion, and fatty liver. J Biol Chem 2003;278(38):36652-60.

Section 5

Glucocorticoids in Modern Clinical Therapy

Chapter 18

Glucocorticoid Therapy in Systemic Lupus Erythematosus – Clinical Analysis of 1,125 Patients with SLE

Hiroshi Hashimoto

Additional information is available at the end of the chapter

http://dx.doi.org/10.5772/52044

1. Introduction

Systemic lupus erythematosus (SLE), which is an inflammatory disease of unknown cause, is a representative autoimmune disease. Although SLE has multisystem organ involvement with a predilection for females, the disease varies from mild to severe and/or from active to inactive. The severity and activity of the disease affect SLE prognosis [1]. Glucocorticosteroids (steroids) have anti-inflammatory and immunosuppressive effects, although the biological effects of steroids are multiple. The anti-inflammatory effect of steroids is powerful and acts rapidly, and the immunosuppressive effect after administration of large doses of steroids is also strong. Therefore, steroids play a major and essential role in the treatment and management of SLE patients, especially those having severe and active SLE. However, the effectiveness and usefulness of steroids are limited because of their severe side effects, unresponsiveness and resistance to steroids. In these situations, additional therapies such as immunosuppressive agents or plasmapheresis, etc. are usually used in conjunction with steroids.

This paper will present clinical data related to steroid therapy from 1,125 patients with SLE who were examined and treated in Juntendo University Hospital between 1955 and 2002. It will show the benefits and risks of treatment with steroids and/or combined therapy with steroids and immunosuppressants.

2. Clinical presentation of 1,125 patients with SLE

2.1. Clinical findings

One thousand one hundred and twenty-five SLE patients fulfilling four or more of the revised ACR (American College of Rheumatology) criteria [2] were examined and treated at the Department of Internal Medicine and Rheumatology in Juntendo University School of Medicine between 1955 and 2002. In all patients, the diagnosis and treatment procedures were conducted during a period when the use of steroids and immunosuppressive agents was common. Computerized analysis of clinical manifestations, laboratory and immunological findings, treatments, complications, causes of death and prognosis was conducted.

The distribution of age at diagnosis and the difference in gender, showing that mean age at diagnosis was 27.1 years old and the male to female ratio was 1:9. In children and adults over the age of 50, the incidence of SLE demonstrated only a slight female predominance, however, for those in their twenties, thirties and forties, close to 90% of patients were women. The frequencies of major clinical manifestations and laboratory findings from observations together with the data from other investigators [3-6] are shown in Table 1.

Manifestations	Harvey, et al. [4] 105 cases 1954	Dubois, et al. [5] 520 cases 1964	Pistiner, et al. [6] 464 cases 1991	Hashimoto, et al. 1125 cases 2002
I. Systemic				
fever	86	84	41	79
weight loss	71	51	-	-
adenopathy	34	59	10	28
II. Musculoskeletal				
arthritis/arthralgia	90	92	91	89
myalgias	-	48	79	31
aseptic bone necrosis	-	5	5	10
III. Cutaneous-vascular				
butterfly area lesions	39	57	34	70
alopecia	3	21	31	48
photosensitivity	11	33	37	40
discoid lesion	-	29	23	17
urticaria	7	7	4	25
oral/nasal ulcer	14	9	19	42
subcutaneous nodules	10	5	-	5
Raynaud's phenomenon	10	18	25	48
IV. Renal				
proteinuria/abnormal sediment	65	46	31	95
nephrotic syndrome	-	23	14	17
V. Cardiopulmonary				
cardiomagaly	15	16	-	-
pericarditis	45	31	2	7
myocarditis	40	8	12	2
heart murmur	44	20	12	14
Libman-Sacks valvlitis	32	-	1	(10/45) 22
hypertension	14	25	25	38
pleurisy	56	45	31	11
lupus pneumonitis	22	1	6	4
pulmonary hypertension	-	-	-	(11/487) 2
VI. Nervous system				
psychosis	19	12	5	21
seizures	17	14	6	8
peripheral neuritis	-	12	5	7
cytoid bodies	24	10	4	(8/63) 13
VII. Gastrointestinal				
abdominal pain	10	19	1	5
ascitis	-	11	-	2
peritonitis	-	-	-	1
hepatomegaly	-	-	-	11
splenomegaly	-	-	-	4
VIII. Laboratory findings				
anemia	78	57	30	63
hemolytic anemia	-	-	8	11
leukopenia	-	43	51	62
thrombocytopenia	26	7	16	34
elevated IgG	-	-	-	(634/1011) 63
elevated IgM	-	-	-	(438/1010) 43
elevated IgA	-	-	-	(154/1010) 15
low CH50	-	-	-	(660/1025) 64
low C3	-	-	39	(712/ 940) 76
low C4	-	-	-	(659/ 939) 70
false positive STS	15	11	-	(78/ 510) 15
anti-cardiolipin antibody	-	-	38	(177/ 349) 51
lupus anticoagulant	-	-	-	(151/349) 43
LE cell	82	82	42	(448/957) 47
antinuclear antibody	-	-	96	97
anti-DNA antibody	-	-	40	(645/935) 69
anti-U1RNP antibody	-	-	14	(314/876) 36
anti-Sm antibody	-	-	6	(645/935) 20
anti-SSA antibody	-	-	19	(371/814) 46
RAHA test	-	-	-	(308/739) 42
RAPA test	-	-	-	(195/557) 35
RA test	-	-	-	(352/908) 39

Table 1. Cumulative percentage incidence of clinical and laboratory manifestations in SLE

2.2. Treatment according to disease severity

Clinical subsets of SLE were divided into three groups according to disease severity that related to prognosis [7]. They were severe, moderate and mild diseases. Severe disease included organ-threatening conditions: lupus nephritis; rapidly progressive glomerulonephritis (RPGN), diffuse proliferative glomerulonephritis (DPGN), nephrotic syndrome, neuropsychiatric lupus (NPLE); acute confusional state or organ brain syndrome, while pulmonary manifestations included acute lupus pneumonitis, alveolar hemorrhage, etc. Moderate disease: lupus nephritis without renal failure, pleuritis, pericarditis, meningitis, hemolytic anemia, thrombocytopenic purpura, etc. Mild disease: arthralgia/arthritis, myopathy, skin rash, etc.

Nonsteroidal anti-inflammatory drugs	800/1125 (71%)
Steroids (initial dose of steroids) (n=1125)	
no	99 (9%)
PSL ≦ 39mg/day	769 (68%)
PSL 40-59mg/day	133 (12%)
PSL ≧ 60mg/day	124 (11%)
Pulse therapy	171 (15%)
Immunosuppressants	300/1125 (27%)
azathioprine	160 (53%)
6-mercaptoprine	26 (9%)
cyclophosphamide	70 (23%)
mizoribin	32 (11%)
others	12 (4%)
Plasmapheresis	105/953 (11%)
Hemodialysis	25/1125 (2%)

PSL:prednisolone

PSL ≦39mg/day was used for patients with mild or moderate diseases.
PSL 40-59mg/day was used for patients with moderate or severe diseases.
PSL ≧60mg/day was used for patients with severe diseases. Pulse therapy was used for patients with severe diseases followed by large doses of steroids.

Table 2. Treatments of 1125 SLE patients

Treatments including steroids and immunosuppressive agents are shown in Table 2. Steroids were a mainstay of treatment for SLE. Although there are several kinds of steroids, prednisolone (PSL) is commonly used to treat SLE. The initial dose of steroids was usually determined according to the severity and activity of the disease. The above severe diseases required large doses of steroids usually of 1 mg/kg/day of PSL or more. Sometimes steroid pulse therapy (methylprednisolone 0.5-1g/day, intravenously administration, for 3days) was used followed by large doses of steroids. The above moderate to mild diseases usually required 0.5-1mg/kg/day and less than 0.5mg/kg/day of PSL, respectively. When a satisfactory response was achieved, the daily dose was reduced by 5 to 10% over 2 or 3 weeks until reaching a maintenance dose of 0.2 to 0.3mg/kg/day.

Steroids have sometimes little or no effect because of impaired bioavailability due to reduced steroid absorption, increased steroid metabolism, induction of activating protein 1(AP-1) which is mutually antagonistic with steroid receptors for trans-activation effects [8], and insensitive steroid-mediated apoptosis of T cells [9], etc. Furthermore, steroids characteristically have a high risk of serious side effects such as infection, gastric ulcer, diabetes mellitus, osteoporosis, etc. Therefore, the effectiveness and usefulness of steroids were limited because of severe side effects, unresponsiveness and resistance to steroids. In these situations, immunosuppressive agents such as cyclophosphamide, azathioprine, mizoribine, tacrolimus and/or plasmapheresis or other innovative therapies were usually used in conjunction with steroids. Recently, belimumab (anti-BLyS antibody), the first targeted biological drug, was approved for treatment of SLE by the FDA [10]. Targeted biological and small-molecule therapies in SLE are going to begin to take the place of steroids that have been used as the major drug in SLE for more than 50 years.

2.3. Prognosis and causes of death

In this paper, the survival rate was 93% at 5years, 89% at 10years and 69% at 20years after diagnosis. One hundred and fifty-one out of 1,125 patients (13%) died. The causes of death were renal failure (30%), cerebrovascular diseases (23%), infection (19%), and others. Infections which led to causes of death included sepsis or bacteremia due to E. coli, methicillin resistant Staphylococcus aureus (MRSA), candidiasis, asprgilosis, Klebsiella, Pseudomonas, etc., and tuberculosis, pneumocyctis carini pneumonia, Cryptococcus meningitis, listeria meningitis, cytomegalovirus infection, etc. In the last 2 or 3 decades it has been noted that the prognosis of SLE has improved [11-13]. Changes in the mortality rate in accordance with the cause of death in SLE patients were also observed, showing a significant reduction in death due to renal failure.

3. Steroid therapy in principal organ involvement in SLE

3.1. Lupus nephritis (LN)

3.1.1. Clinical analysis of LN

LN is one of the diseases influencing the prognosis of SLE. The diseases of LN vary from mild to severe and from active to inactive. The clinical pictures of LN and the types of the World Health Organization (WHO) classification according to histopathological findings [14] in this study are shown in Table 3.

Persistent proteinuria of more than 0.2g/day and less than 3.5g/day was observed in approximately 37% of cases and profuse proteinuria of more than 3.5g per day was observed in approximately 17% of cases. Patients without proteinuria accounted for 16%. Abnormal urinary sediments including erythrocytes, leukocytes and casts were observed frequently. An increasing serum creatinine level was observed in 41% of cases. The WHO classification according to histopahological findings of LN by renal biopsy was used in this study, although the classification of LN by the International Nephrology/Renal Pathology Society (ISN/RPS) was proposed in 2003[15]. Diffuse proliferative glomerulonephritis (DPGN) of Type IV, which has a poor prognosis, could be seen in 55 of 216 cases (25%), which underwent renal biopsy. Membranous glomerulonephritis (MGN) of Type V characteristic of nephrotic syndrome, was observed in 18% of cases. Types I and II, which are thought to have better prognosis, were observed in 23% and 16% of cases, respectively. Advanced Type VI, which indicates end stage GN, could be seen in 12% of cases.

A. Urinalysis, Renal function	n=1125 (%)
No proteinuria	176 (16)
Proteinuria	949 (84)
Intermittent	431 (45)
Persistent	354 (37)
Profuse (>3.5g/day)	164 (17)
Microhematuria	1066 (95)
Urine casts	838 (74)
Elevated BUN	659/1063 (62)
Elevated S-creatinine	429/1047 (41)
B. Histopathological findings (WHO classification)	n=216 (%)
I. Minimal change (MC) or Normal	49 (23)
II. Mesagial alteration	34 (16)
III. Focal segmental glomerulonephritis (FGN)	35 (16)
IV. Diffuse proliferative glomerulonephritis (DPGN)	55 (25)
V. Membranous glomerulonephritis (MGN)	39 (18)
VI. Advanced	4 (12)

Table 3. Lupus nephritis in 1125 cases

3.1.2. Treatment of LN

The available therapeutic procedures include steroids, immunosuppressive agents, plasmapheresis, anticoagulants and hemodialysis, etc. Steroids were the first choice for treatment of LN. However, doses of steroids were determined according to urinary findings, renal function and renal histopathological findings evaluating the activity and severity of LN. The patients with active and /or severe LN, including persistent or profuse proteinuria, renal dysfunction, DPGN of type IV, rapidly progressive glomerulonephritis (RPGN) or MGN of Type V in conjunction with low serum complement levels and high titers of anti-dsDNA antibodies, were initially treated with large doses of steroids (PSL 1-1.5mg/kg/day) as induction therapy for remission. Steroid pulse therapy was often administered at first. It led to more rapid recovery which might be result of a rapid nongenomic physicochemical effect. The patients with intermittent proteinuria, abnormal urine sediments, and Type II or III, were initially treated with PSL less than 0.5-1mg/kg/day. After PSL administration for 3-6 weeks, the dosage of PSL was then reduced by nearly 10% every 2–3 weeks according to the improvement in proteinuria, urinary sediments, abnormal renal function, low serum complement levels and high titers of anti-dsDNA antibodies. If PSL had no or incomplete response, the dosage was increased by 20% or steroid pulse therapy was conducted again. In the patients with DPGN or RPGN, intravenous pulse therapy of cyclophosphamide (IVCY) (500-750mg, monthly for 3 to 6 months), as immunosuppressive agent, was used. Alternative induction therapies included combined therapies with steroids and immunosuppressive agents such as daily oral cyclophosphamide, azathioprine, tacrorimus, mizoribine, and cyclosporine, etc. If an incomplete response after 2 months treatment with

PSL alone was also observed, immunosuppressant agents were administered in addition to PSL. If the patients had high titers of anti-dsDNA antibodies and/or immune complexes, plasmapheresis was conducted in conjunction with the above steroid and immunosuppressant agent treatment. In patients who achieved remission showing less than 0.5g/day of proteinuria, inactive urine sediment, normal complement levels and /or quiescent extrarenal lupus activity, they continued maintenance treatment with a maintenance dosage of steroids of PSL 5–15mg/day. Thereafter, the PSL dosage was tapered to discontinuance in an extremely gradual manner.

3.1.3. Outcome and prognosis of LN

During the past half century, the prognosis of SLE has significantly improved. One of the major factors in this improvement is the significant reduction in renal death. This is assumed to be partially due to early diagnosis and early treatment with the development of diagnostic procedures, as well as the development of treatments including the implementation of hemodialysis [1,11-13]. However, the remission rate of lupus nephritis was not so high.

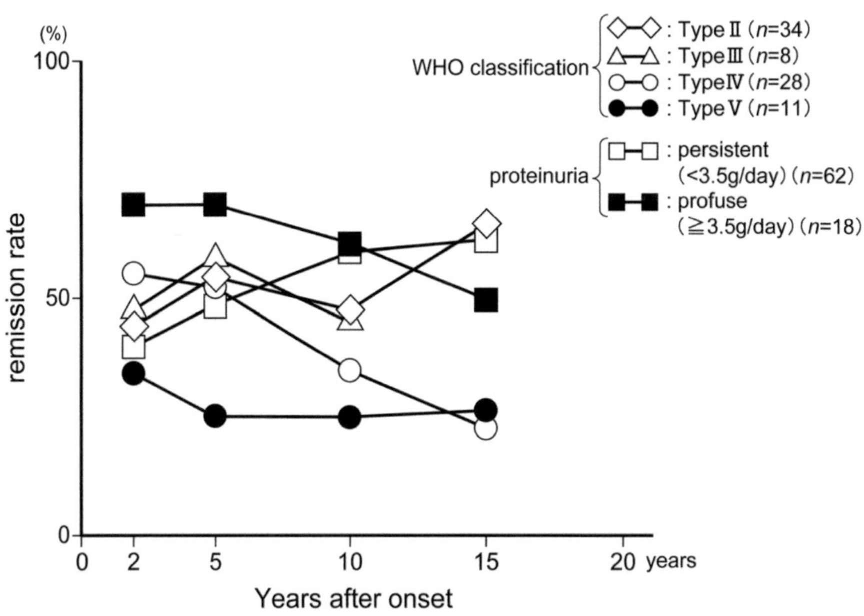

Figure 1. Remission rate of lupus nephritis according the WHO classification type and degree of proteinuria

Figure 1 shows the remission rate after onset according to the WHO classification type and degree of proteinuria. The remission rates of patients with Type IV (DPGN) and profuse peroteiniria or nephrotic syndrome tended to decrease during the course of the disease, while the remission rates of patients with Type II and persistent proteinuria tended to increase. Patients with Type V (MGN) had a low remission rate through out the course of the disease, but no decrease in the remission rate was observed until later on. Furthermore, in the outcome of 32 patients who were treated over the long-term for over 20 years, the complete remission rate was 27%, the incomplete remission rate was 37.8%, and the worsening rate was 21.6 %. As for the treatments used, those that contributed to remission could not be specified. This fact suggests that the underlying disease types had a greater influence on the remission rate than the treatment method.

3.2. Neuropsychiatric manifestations of SLE (NPLE)

3.2.1. Clinical analysis of NPLE

The frequencies of various neuropsychiatric manifestations of SLE (NPLE) have been reported to vary from 28 to 59%. In our study, NPLE could be observed in 47.6% of 1,125 cases as shown in Table 4.

Total SLE patients	1125
The number of patients with NPLE	535 (48%)
1. Neurological manifestations	
1) seizure, unconsciousness	146 (13%)
2) cerebrovascular disease	158 (14%)
3) neuropathy, cranial	45 (4%)
4) myelopathy	45 (4%)
5) aseptic meninngitis	45 (4%)
6) peripheral neuropathy	79 (7%)
7) headache	101 (9%)
2. Neuropsychological syndromes	236 (21%)

Table 4. Frequencies of neuropsychiatric manifestations (NPLE) in 1125 lupus patients

The American College of Rheumatology (ACR) proposed new criteria for the classification of neuropsychiatric syndrome of systemic lupus erythematosus (NPSLE) in 1999 [16]. NPLE is divided into psychiatric and neurological manifestations. The frequency of psychiatric manifestations was higher than that of neurological manifestations. The former included acute confusional state or organ brain syndrome, cognitive dysfunction, anxiety disorders and psychosis, etc., while the latter included seizure, cerebrovascular disease, myelopathy, aseptic meningitis, headache, and peripheral neuropathy, etc.

Although no single pathogenetic process could explain all these manifestations, it was assumed that other potential causes of these manifestations, such as side effects from treatment, complications including infections, etc., had been excluded except for causes due to lupus itself. Many NPLE cases were considered to be caused by lupus itself, excluding obvious causes such as antiphospholipid antibody syndrome (APS), necrotizing angiitis, and complications.

NPLE is one of the diseases that influence the prognosis of SLE as well as LN. Especially, patients with acute confusional state or organ brain syndrome (OBS), cognitive dysfunction, recurrent seizure, and cerebrovascular disease, etc., had poor prognosis. Acute OBS exhibits characteristic malfunctions such as consciousness disorders (i.e. delirium), disorientation, memory disorders, and cognitive dysfunction. Acute OBS showed an 85% correlation with SLE activity and exacerbation, which was greater than that of the psychiatric illness group (57%) and the psychosyndrome group (23%) [17].

Although acute OBS was correlated with active SLE lesions, correlations with high titers of anti-dsDNA antibodies and low complement levels, which were seen in active LN, were not necessarily observed. Serologically, acute OBS correlated with the serum anti-liposomal P antibody, interferon α and IL-6 in cerebrospinal fluid (CSF) [18-19].

On the other hand, acute neurologic syndrome has been reported to correlate with the anti-asialo GM1 antibody, anti-liposomal P antibody, anti-lymphocyte antibody, and anti-neurocyte antibody, as well as the anti-PCNA antibody and anti-Sm antibody [7,20].

Psychiatric symptoms often required differentiation from steroidal psychiatric symptoms. Differentiation from secondary psychiatric symptoms due to uremia and/or infection was also important. Although quite a number of cases were difficult to determine, the following information might have been helpful:

a. The actual incidence of steroid-induced psychosis is small, probably about 5%, which is less than that of lupus-induced psychosis [21].
b. The psychiatric side effects of steroids include, most commonly, mild to moderate mood changes such euphoria, sleeplessness, or depression rather than unconsciousness disorders, although there are also perceptual changes, hallucinations, anxiety, insomnia and confusion.
c. Steroid-induced psychosis appears half a month to one month after administration of steroids. It has been reported that the incidence of steroid-induced psychosis increases when over 40mg/day of PSL is administered [22].
d. Although lupus psychosis may not always be improved by increasing of the dosage of PSL, deterioration of lupus psychosis after increasing the dosage of PSL is rare.
e. High levels of IgG index and IL-6 in CSF can be seen in lupus psychosis [23].

The evaluation of NPLE should always include an assessment of whether SLE is active or not. In addition, patients with both focal and diffuse syndromes should have various examinations including CSF, electroencephalogram (EEG), and an imaging studies (such as computed tomography (CT) and magnetic resonance imaging (MRI)), cerebral blood flow by angiography or single photon emission computerized tomography (SPECT), etc. The more serious the NPLE, the more aggressive immunosuppressive therapy, including steroids, is needed.

3.2.2. Treatment of NPLE

If NPLE was active and there was severe major organ involvement, steroid therapy was indicated. In particular, patients with an acute confusional state or organic brain syndrome, and recurrent convulsive seizures were treated with high steroid doses (PSL 1–2 mg/kg/day) in conjunction with steroid pulse therapy. However, when improvement could not be seen within 48 hours after treatment, 250 to 500mg of hydrocortone was administered every 12 hours. If improvement could not be seen after treatment of steroids alone, IVCP pulse therapy or oral administration of CP in conjunction with steroids and/or plasmapheresis was given.

When signs of clinical manifestations were stable for more than 6 weeks and acute phase reactants or tests of organ function were improved or stable for 6 weeks, the dose of PSL was reduced by approximately 10 to 20% every two weeks. When the dose of PSL reached about 15mg/day, it was slowly tapered and reduced by 1mg every week.

When the patients showed panic or marked agitation and their hallucinations and delusions were threatening, several antipsychotic drugs in conjunction with steroids were also used.

3.2.3. *Outcome and prognosis of NPLE*

Almost all patients with NPLE improved after immunosuppressive therapies including steroids, immunosuppressive drugs and /or plasmapheresis.

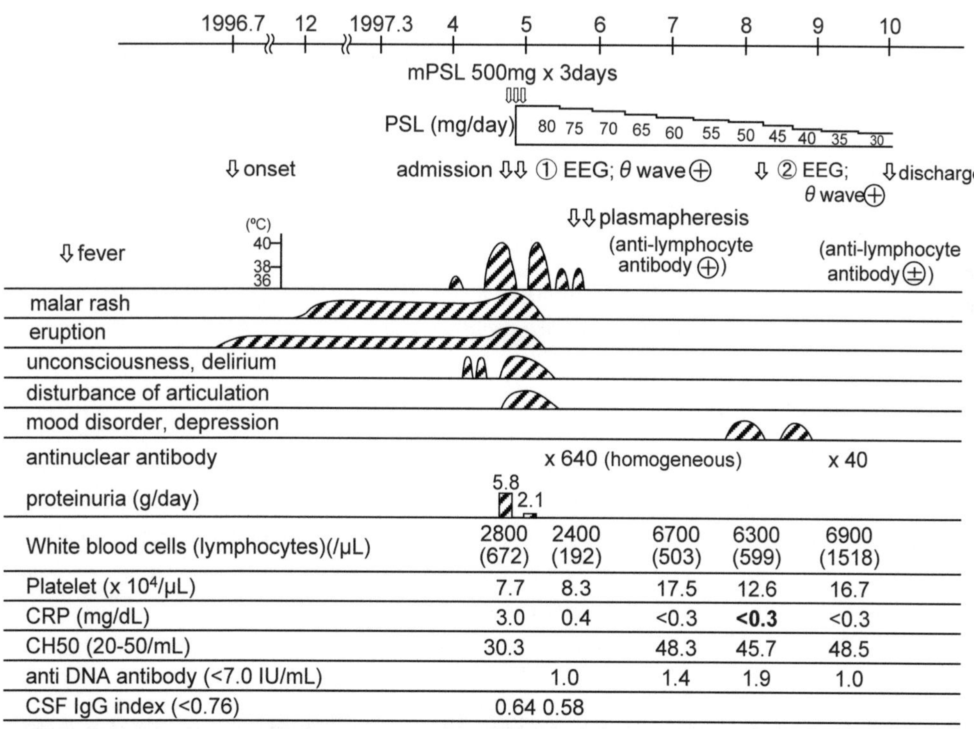

PSL: prednisolone, mPSL: methylprednisolone, EEG: electroencephalogram, CSF: cerebrospinal fluid.

Figure 2. The clinical course of SLE patient (46 years old, female) with organic brain syndrome (OBS)

Figure 2 shows the clinical course of an SLE patient with OBS who was a 46-year old female. She was diagnosed as SLE with malar rash, eruption, leucopenia, thrombocytopenia, proteinuria and positive anti-nuclear antibodies, etc. in March 1997. In April 1997, she had recurrent unconsciousness with delirium, disturbance of articulation with high fever and a worsening malar rash. Although anti-DNA antibodies and low complemetemia could not be seen, she was diagnosed as OBS or acute confusional state and treatment with steroid pulse therapy followed by a PSL dose of 80mg/day. Plasmapheresis was also conducted to remove anti-lymphocyte antibodies. Although mood disorder and depression were observed in August, 1997, her disease improved without increasing doses of steroids or additional treatment with immunosuppressive agents.

As for prognosis of lupus patients with NPLE according to the different treatment, patients treated with combined therapy of steroid pulse therapy and other therapies was significantly more favorable than those treated with steroids alone (PSL>40mg/day) and those treated with combined therapy of immunosuppressive agents and steroids.

3.3. Pulmonary manifestations

3.3.1. Pleuritis

Pleuritis is by far the most common pulmonary manifestation, occurring at some time in the course in 40 to 50% of lupus patients. However, the frequency of pleuritis in Japanese SLE patiens was lower than that in European countries and the United States. The frequency of pleuritis was 11% in this study. . Clinically, fever, chest pain, cough, dyspnea etc. could be seen in patients with pleuritis. On chest X-rays, slight to moderate pleural effusion caused by pleural inflammation could be observed bilaterally in approximately half of cases.

Pleuritis mostly improved after administration of PSL (20-40mg/day). However, in cases with a large amount of pleural effusion , thoracic drainage was needed.

3.3.2. Interstitial pneumonitis

Lupus pneumonitis is classified as acute lupus pneumonitis and chronic interstitial pneumonitis/pulmonary fibrosis. Acute lupus pneumonitis was relatively rare with an occurrence of 0.5–11.7% [24-25]. It was observed in 6 of 1,125 patients (0.5%) in this study. As clinical symptoms, fever, chest pain, dry cough, severe dyspnea, and occasional hemoptysis were noted. Bibasilar Velcro rales were noted in all instances. The majority of patients were hypoxic, requiring supplemental oxygen or intubation for assisted ventilation. Acute lupus pneumonitis was diagnosed by several examinations including X-ray, CT scan, KL-6 and/or SP-D as biomarkers, and various kinds of infectious examination to exclude infectious diseases.

All 6 patients with acute lupus pneumonitis were treated with steroid pulse therapy following 1-2mg/kg/day of PSL. Half of the patients drastically improved, but the remaining

3 patients died of pulmonary hemorrhage despite combined therapy with steroid and immunosuppressant agents and /or plasmapheresis.

Chronic interstitial pneumonitis in SLE is also rare, showing a low frequency of 3-5%. Six patients with chronic interstitial pneumonitis were observed in this study and they were treated with maintenance therapies including low doses of steroids and/or immunosuppressant agents. In one patient, chronic interstitial pneumonitis deteriorated to acute interstitial pneumonitis during the course of the disease and a large dose of steroids was needed

3.3.3. Alveolar hemorrhage

Alveolar hemorrhage in SLE is relatively rare, and it has been reported to occur in 1.4–1.7% of SLE patients in Europe and the United States [26].

It is a serious complication and results in poor prognosis. It was observed in 8 out of 1,125 patients (0.7%) in this study.

SLE patients with alveolar hemorrhage had hemoptysis and hypoxemia and rapid progression of anemia in conjunction with active LN and/or NSLE disease.

All patients with alveolar hemorrhage were treated with steroid pulse therapy following large doses of PSL, but it was also necessary to concomitantly use other immunosuppressive tharapies such as cyclophosphamide including IVCY, and plasmapheresis. Unfortunately, all of the patients with alveolar hemorrhage died, comfirming that the prognosis was very poor.

3.4. Cardiac manifestations

3.4.1. Pericarditis

The most common cardiac abnormality was pericarditis, which occured in 8-25% [27], but it was relatively rare in Japan, with a frequency of 7% (47 out of 1,125cases) in this study. Pericarditis is often one of the first manifestations. Most of the cases with pericarditis improved with administration of PSL 0.5–1 mg/day, but cases with cardiac tamponade, which was rare in this study, needed large doses of PSL over 1mg/day and/or steroid pulse therapy.

3.4.2. Myocarditis

Myocarditis was rarely observed in 2% in this study. In cases with myocarditis, positive CRP, elevated CK, IgG class anti-dsDNA antibodies, hematuria, etc., in conjunction with tachycardia, cardiac enlargement, congestive heart failure could often be observed. A myocardial biopsy was performed in order to confirm the diagnosis in one patient. The patients with myocarditis associated with congestive heart failure were treated with large-dose administration of steroids (PSL 1–1.5 mg/kg/day, divided into 3~4 dosages). All of the patients with myocarditis improved after steroid therapy.

3.4.3. Myocardial infarction and coronary artery disease

Coronary artery disease due to arteriosclerotic changes is more common in SLE patients. Death from myocardial infarction late in the course of the disease is one of the most frequent causes of death after 10 to 30 years of SLE [28]. Eleven lupus patients with myocardial infarction could be seen in this study. The average age at diagnosis of SLE was 37 years old (26–63 years old), and the average age at development of myocardial infarction was 51 years old (41–66 years old) in these patients. There were two death cases, including one case of death from cardiac rupture.

Several risk factors that cause myocardial infarction due to atherosclerosis in SLE are considered. They are renal involvement, hypertension, hyperlipidemia, long-term administration of steroids, diabetes mellitus, anti-phospholipid syndrome, smoking, etc. In this study, 4 patients had hypertension, hyperlipemia and diabetes mellitus as risk factors. Furthermore, positive antiphospholipid antibodies were observed in 5 cases. Death from myocardial infarction due to inflammation of the coronary arteries has been reported in SLE patients dying early in the course of their disease, but this is a rare event [28].

Regarding the treatment in this study, conservative medical management without large doses of steroids was used in most cases. PTCA and AC bypass procedures were also occasionally conducted.

3.5. Intestinal vasculitis

Acute abdomen caused by intestinal vasculitis is often observed. Occasionally, surgery is needed. According to a report by Zizic, et al. [29], acute abdomen was observed in 15 of 140 cases, and caused death in 53% of cases. Vasculitis was observed in 9 of 11 cases with abdominal surgery, and intestinal perforation was observed in 6 cases. In this study, 4 patients had intestinal vasculitis and 3 died of intestinal perforation. Intestinal bleeding and peritoneal bleeding due to vasculitis were often observed. In cases with mesenteric arteritis, acute abdomen with severe abdominal pain in conjunction with nausea/vomiting, diarrhea, ascites, gastrointestinal bleeding, and fever, etc., were observed. Those symptoms may be masked by steroids or immunosuppressive drugs used for treatment, thus resulting in a delayed diagnosis.

Patients with intestinal vasculitis and/or mesenteric arteritis were treated with large dose steroids including steroid pulse therapy.

When a rapid improvement was not obtained, intermittent IVCY therapy was simultaneously used. In cases associated with bowel infarction or perforation, treatment for infection was also needed.

3.6. Hematologic manifestations

Hematologic manifestations in SLE include normochromic-normocytic anemia caused by chronic inflammation, autoimmune hemolytic anemia (AIHA), iron-deficiency anemia, leukocytopenia, lymphocytopenia, thrombocytopenia, thrombocytopenic purpura (TP), thrombotic thrombocytopenic purpura (TTP), and antiphosphlipid syndrome (APS), etc. The diseases, which needed high doses of steroids were AIHA, TP, and TTP.

3.6.1. AIHA

AIHA was observed in 11% of patients in this study. AIHA is rare in Japanese SLE patients in comparison to those in Europe and the United States. Steroids were the mainstay of the treatment for AIHA and a response was achieved in about 75% of patients. PSL was given initially at a dose of 1.0 to1.5mg/kg and continued at that level for at least 4 to 6 weeks. Following a satisfactory response, the dose was reduced gradually by 10% every week. The reticlocyte count was a reliable indicator of both responsiveness to treatment and relapse. In cases of severe fulminant hemolysis, steroid pulse therapy was conducted. Patients with AIHA who failed to respond to steroids were treated with immunosuppressant agents and/or splenectomy. Plasmapheresis, high-dose intravenous gammagloburin therapy (IVIg), and danazole were also used for some refractory cases.

3.6.2. TP

Thrombocytopenia lower than 150,000 was observed in 34% of cases in this study. However, thrombocytopenia lower than 50,000 was relatively rare, and it occured in approximately 10% of cases. Thrombocytopenia in SLE is usually due to antiplatelet autoantibodies (platelet associate-IgG; PA-IgG, platelet binding-IgG; PB-IgG). In some cases, thrombocytopenia was associated with antiphospholipid antibodies. In rare case, so-called Evans syndrome, in which AIHA and TP coexist, was observed. Some cases did not tend to bleed until platelet counts were less than 20,000/ul. Patients with thrombocytopenia less than 20,000 were treated with large doses of steroids. The initial dose of PSL was usually 1-2mg /kg/day. After an increase in platelet count occurred in response to steroids, the dose was gradually reduced after 4 weeks. If thrombocytopenia did not respond to steroids with bleeding from the major organs such as gastrointestinal tract, kidney, bladder, other mucosal surface, steroid pulse therapy was used. IVIg was useful to achieve a temporary improvement in thrombocytopenia in surgical operations such as splenectomy, which was often conducted in steroid resistant cases. .In steroid resistant cases, immunosuppressive drugs such as azathioprine, cyclophosphamide, and cyclosporine, danazol, and vincristine, etc., were also used.

3.6.3. TTP

TTP usually consists of a pentad of TP, microangiopathic hemolytic anemia, fever, renal failure, and neurologic manifestations. TTP has been reported in association with various other diseases, including SLE, most of which are characterized by some degree of vasculitis of the small vessels and circulating immune complexes [30]. The main cause of acquired TTP including SLE is assumed to be an autoantibody that is an inhibitor (IgG inhibitor) of von Willebrand factor cleaving protease [31]. It has been clarified that congenital TTP is caused by a mutation in the *ADAMTS-13* gene of cleaving protease. TTP must be differentiated from DIC or catastrophic antiphospholipid syndrome, but coexistence of both are often observed.

Regarding treatment, plasmapheresis using fresh frozen plasma, and transfusion therapy of normal plasma are used. In addition, large-doses of steroids including steroid pulse therapy, immunosuppressive drugs, IVIg therapy, and anti-platelet drugs, etc. are simultaneously used.

3.7. Pregnancy and birth

When an SLE patient wished to conceive and give birth, a medical determination as to whether pregnancy would be possible was considered. Basically, there were presumed to be almost no problems in pregnancy when the patient was in remission with a maintenance dosage of steroids, and when serious organ failure was not observed. Moreover, even if the patient had active disease, pregnancy was allowed after the disease improved with treatment.

3.7.1. Treatment and management during pregnancy

It was important for the physician and the gynecologist to be in close communication for the treatment and management during pregnancy. Usually, it was unnecessary to change the maintenance dose of the steroid during pregnancy. When mild deterioration was observed in the early stage of pregnancy, an increased steroid dosage was attempted according to the clinical manifestations. If the clinical manifestations required administration of a large-dose of steroids, considering the risks to the mother and the effect of the steroids on the fetus, an artificial abortion was performed at an early stage. Although the level of serum cortisol in the fetus decreases during the steroid administration, cortisol secretion and response to ACTH are believed to remain normal [32]. If a mother is treated with prednisolone or hydrocortisone, these steroids are assumed to have a minimal effect on the fetus because they are inactivated by 11-β-dehydrogenase in the placenta. However, the use of dexamethasone and betamethasone is avoided because these steroids are difficult for the enzyme to inactivate and were assumed to have an adverse effect on the fetus.

3.7.2. Treatment and management during and after deliverly

3.7.2.1. Prevention of exacerbation

The mother was hospitalized prior to the expected delivery date for management of the mother and fetus. If pregnancy remained steady, and SLE activity was not observed, the dose of steroids was increased immediately after delivery to prevent any exacerbation of SLE. The dose of steroids was usually increased to two or three times the pre-delivery dose. The dose was reduced by 10% every 4 to 7 days while confirming no exacerbation, and continually observed until eventually reducing it to the dosage at the time of delivery. If an exacerbation of SLE such as active LN or serositis was observed in the late stage of pregnancy, the delivery of the fetus was attempted as early as possible in order to start treatment of the mother's clinical manifestations.

3.7.2.2. Breast-feeding

Because the amount of steroids was increased upon delivery, breast-feeding was prohibited until the dose was reduced to less than 20 mg of PSL, considering the rate of transfer of steroids (0.1–0.3%/day) to the mother's milk [33].

3.8. Adverse effects and complications due to steroid treatment

Side effects of prolonged treatment with oral steroids are well known. Changes in the physical appearance could usually be seen. They were acne, hirsutism, moon face, buffalo hump, obesity, and abdominal striae, etc. Although reversible with a discontinuation or reduction in dose, hypertension, peptic ulcer, diabetes mellitus, pancreatitis, osteoporosis, psychosis, etc. were also induced. Thinning of the skin, cataracts, glaucoma, osteoporosis, and osteonecrosis could be observed as irreversible side effects.

Infections were major complications in SLE and one of the major causes of death. Susceptibility to infection, particularly bacterial infection, was increased with steroid use. Staples et al. found that the infection rate in hospitalized patients increased from 0.43 to 1.63 per 100 hospital days with an increase in steroid dose from zero to more than 50mg/day [34]. Although infection rarely occurs with a small dose of PSL (2–10 mg/day), the SLE patients treated with PSL of more than 20mg/day have a higher risk of infection due to the higher dose of PSL, especially after 14 days of administration. PSL was also noted to be a major risk factor for the development of opportunistic infection, with the most common organisms including Salmonella, Candida, Strongyloides, and Aspergillus.sp according to a case controlled study of 797 SLE patients [35].

It has been noted that systemic administration of steroids could be linked to the higher occurrence of vascular diseases such as coronary artery disease, stroke, peripheral vascular disease than the expected occurrence in SLE. However, it is unclear whether this reflects pro-atherogenic effects of the underlying disease process or adverse metabolic effects associated with steroid use [36]. Recently, the number of patients with complications such as myocardial infarction/angina pectoris, cerebral infarction, diabetes mellitus, hypertension, and aseptic bone necrosis, has tended to increase over a long-term observation period due to a favorable SLE prognosis.

Table 5 shows the frequencies of these complications at the time of occurence in 97 SLE patients who had been observed for over 20 years. The number of patients with myocardial infarction/angina pectoris, diabetes, cerebral infarction increased from the ninth year of the observation period. Hypertension and aseptic osteonecrosis were seen from the onset of SLE. Most of the above complications were thought to be due to treatment including steroids, as well as aging. It was also noted that GC-associated damage accumulated over time to constitute most of the damage at 15 years, although disease –activity related damage occurred early [37].

Years after diagnosis (yrs)	1-2	3-4	5-8	9-12	13-16	17-20	>21
Myocardial infarction				1			3
Angina pectoris			1		1		2
Diabetes mellitus				3	1	3	5
Cerebral infarction				1	3	3	4
Hypertension	10	9	5	8	4	5	10
Aseptic osteonecrosis	1	3	5	1	4	3	3

yrs: years, number: cases

Table 5. Frequencies of complications related to vascular diseases according to the year (s) of the occurrence in 97 SLE patients who had been observed for over 20 years

Steroid use contributes significantly to risk of osteoporosis in women with SLE. Ramsey-Goldman et al. surveyed the frequency of fractures and associated risk factores in702 women with SLE who had been followed for 5951 person-years and found that fractures occurred in 12.3% of patients, an almost fivefold increase compared with a background population [38]. Older age at diagnosis and longer duration of steroid use were important valuables. Sinigaglia, et al. reported that osteoporosis in 22.6% of 84 premenopousal patients with SLE according to bone mineral density (BMD) was observed, and both disease duration and glucocorticoids were associated risks [39]. Steroid–induced osteoporosis leading to fracture, particularly vertebral collapse, was a major problem.

Aseptic osteonecrosis (AON) was observed in approximately 10% of SLE, with the femoral head being a common site. It also appeared in the femoral condyle, caput humeri, proximal end and distal end of the tibia, etc.. It has been suggested that increased doses of steroids (especially in the first year of treatment) and the duration of steroid therapy are correlated with a grater risk of AON in SLE patients [40]. In a prospective survey of SLE patients with administration of high-dose steroids (more than 30 mg/day of PSL for more than one month), AON occurred in 15% (9/62 patients) and the average period from the administration of a large dose of steroids to onset of AON was 640 days [41].

4. Conclusion

In this paper, steroid therapy for SLE based on the clinical analysis of 1,125 cases, especially for principal organ involvement that required large doses of steroids, was evaluated. Although there is no doubt that steroids contribute to a significant improvement in the prognosis in SLE, the effectiveness and usefulness of steroids are limited because of severe side effects, unresponsiveness and resistance to steroids.

Now, new biological agents that target B cells, T-B cell interaction, co-stimulatory pathways, intracellular molecules, etc. are being developed and are going to begin to revolutionize nonspecific therapy to a more specific pathophysiological tharapy in SLE.

Author details

Hiroshi Hashimoto
Professor Emeritus,
Aiwakai Medical Corporation, Bajikouen Clinic, Rheumatology, Tokyo, Japan

5. References

[1] Wallace DJ, Dubois EL (1987) Prognostic subsets, natural course, and causes of death in systemic lupus erythematosus, In: Wallace DJ, Dubois EL editors. Dubois' Lupus Erythematosus, 3rd ed. Lea & Febiger, Philadelphia, pp580

[2] Hochberg MC (1997) Updating the American College of Rheumatology revised criteria for the classification of systemic lupus erythematosus. Arthritis Rheum 40:1725 (letter)

[3] Wallace DJ (2007) The clinical presentation of systemic lupus erythematosus. In: Wallece DJ, Hahn BH editors. Dubois' Lupus Erythematosus. 7th ed. Lippincott Williams & Willkins, Philadelphia, pp638

[4] McGehee HA, Shulman LE, Tumulty AP, et al (1954) Systemic lupus erythematosus: review of the literature and clinical analysis of 138 cases. Medicine 33: 291-437

[5] Dubois EL, Tuffanelli DL (1964) Clinical manifestations of systemic lupus erythematosus. Computer analysis of 520 cases, JAMA 190: 104-111

[6] Pistiner M, Wallace DJ, Nessim S, et al (1991) Lupus erythematosus in the 1980s: a survey of 570 patients. Semin Arthritis Rheum 21: 55-64

[7] Hashimoto, H, Hirose S, Kano S, et al (1992) Studies on clinical subsets and severity of systemic lupus erythematosus based on a 1987 questionnaire conducted in Japan- Clinical analysis of the outcome and treatments in clinical subsets. Rhumachi 32: 27-38

[8] Wilder BL (1997) Glucocorticoids, In: Koopman WJ, editor. Arthritis and Allied Conditioins. 13th ed. Wiliams & Willkins, Baltimore, pp731

[9] Seki M, Ushiyama C, Seta N, et al (1998) Apoptosis of lymphocytes induced glucocorticoids and relationship to therapeutic efficacy in patients with systemic lupus erythematosus. Arthritis Rheum 41: 823-830

[10] Navarra SV, Guzman RM, Gallacher AE, et al (2011) Efficacy and safety of belimumab in patients with active systemic lupus eryhematosus: a randomized, placebo-controlled, phase 3 trial. Lancet 9767: 721-731

[11] Gladman DD, Urowitz MB (2007) Prognosis, mortality and morbidity in systemic lupus erythematosus. In: Wallace DJ, Hahn BH, editors. Dubois' Lupus Erythematosus, 7th ed. Lippincott Williams & Willkins, Philadelphia, pp1333

[12] Hashimoto H, Shiokawa Y (1978) Changing pattern of clinical features and prognosis in systemic lupus erythematosus. Scand J Rheumatol 7: 219-224

[13] Hashimoto H, Sugawara M, Tokano Y, et al. (1993) Follow up study on the changes in the clinical features and prognosis of Japanese patients with systemic lupus erythematosus during the past 3 to 4 decades. J Epidemiol 3:19-27

[14] D'Agati VD, Appel GB (2007) Lupus nephritis: pathology and pathogenesis. In: Wallace DJ, Hahn BH, editors, Dubois' Lupus Erythematosus, 7th ed.Lippincott Williams & Wilkins, Philadelphia, pp1094

[15] Weening JJ, D'Agati VD, Schwartz MM, et al (2004) The classification of glomerulonephritis in systemic lupus erythematosus revisited. Kidney Int 65: 521-530

[16] ACR Ad Hoc Committee on Neuropsychiatric Lupus Nomenclature (1999) The American College of Rheumatology nomenclature and case definitions for neuropsychiatric lupus syndromes. Arthritis Rheum 42: 599-608

[17] Akazawa S (1986) Psychiatric syndrome in systemic lupus erythematosus-study on 82 cases. Seishinigaku 28: 661-670(in Japanese)

[18] Schneebaum AB, Singleton JD,West SG, et al(1991)Association of psychiatric manifestations with antibodies to ribosomal-P proteins in systemic lupus erythematosus. Am J Med 90: 54-62

[19] Hirohata S, Iwamoto S, Sugiyama H, et al(1988) A patient with systemic lupus erythematosus presenting both central nervous system lupus and steroid induced psychosis. J Rheumatol 15: 706-710

[20] Bertsias G, Loannidis JPA, Bombardieri S, et al. (2008) EULAR recommendations for the management of systemic lupus erythematosus. Report of a task force of the EULAR standing committee for international clinical studies including therapeutics. Ann Rhum Dis 67:195-205

[21] Hall RCW, Popkin MK, Kirkpatrick B, et al (1978) Tricyclic exacerbation of steroid psychosis. J Nerv Ment Dis 166: 738-742

[22] Hall RCW, Popkin MK, Stickney SK, et al (1979) Presentation of steroid psychosis. J Nerv Ment Dis 167:229-236

[23] Hirohata S, Kanai Y, Mitsuo A, et al.(2009) Accuracy of cerebrospinal fluid IL-6 testing for diagnosis of lupus psychosis. A multienter retrospective study. Clin Rheumatol 28: 1319-1323

[24] D'Cruz D, Khamashta MA, Hughes G (2007) Pulmonary manifestations of systemic lupus erythematosus. In: Wallace DJ, Hahn BH, editors. Dubois' Lupus Erythematosus, 7th ed. Lippincott Williams & Wilkins, Philadelphia, pp678

[25] Matthay RA, Schwartz MI, Petty TL, et al (1975) Pulmonary manifestations of systemic lupus erythematosus: review of twelve cases of acute lupus pneumonitis. Medicine 54:397-409

[26] Baulware DW, hedgpeth MT (1989)Lupus pneumonitis and anti-SSA(Ro) antibodies . J Rheumatol 16: 479-481

[27] Bulkley BH, Roberts WC (1975) The heart in systemic lupus erythematosus and the changes induced in it by corticosteroid therapy. A study of 36 necropsy patients. Am J Med 58: 243-264

[28] Rothfield NF (1996) Cardiac aspects. In; Shur PH, ed. The Clinical Management of Systemic lupus Erythematosus, 2nd ed. Lippincott-Raven, Philadelphia, pp83

[29] Zizic TM, Classen JN, Stevens MB (1982) Acute abdominal complications of systemic lupus erythematosus and polyarteritis nodosa. Am J Med 73: 525-531

[30] Shoenfeld Y, Ehrenfelt M(1996) Hematological manifestations. In;Shur PH, ed.The Clinical Management of Systemic lupus Erythematosus, 2nd ed. Lippincott-Raven, Philadelphia, pp95

[31] Tsai HM, Lian ECY(1998) Antibodies to von Willebrand factor-cleaving protease in acute thrombotic thrombocytopenic purpura. N Eng J Med 339: 1585-1594

[32] Blanford AT, Murphy BE (1977) In vitro metabolism of prednisolone, dexamethasone, betamethasone, and cortisol by the human placenta. Am J Obstet Gynecolo 127: 264-267

[33] Katz FH, Duncan BR (1975)Letter: entry of prednisone into human milk. N Engl J Med 293:1154

[34] Staples PJ, Gerding DN, Decker JL, et al (1974) Incidence of infection in systemic lupus erythematosus. Arthritis Rheum 17: 110

[35] Ritchin C, Dobro J, Senie R, etl. (1989) Opportunistic infections in patients with systemic lupus erythematosus (abstract). Arthritis Rheum 32(Suppl):S115

[36] Wei L, MacDonald T, Walker B (2004) Taking glucocorticoids by prescription is associated with subsequent cardiovascular disease. Ann Intern Med 141:764-770,

[37] Gladman DD, Urowitz MB, Rahman P, et al. (2003) Accrual of organ damage over time in patients with systemic lupus erythematosus. J Rheumatol 30:1955-1959

[38] Ramsey-Goldman R, Dunn JE, Huang CF, et al (1999) Frequency of fractures in women with systemic lupus erythematosus: comparison with United States population data. Arthritis Rheum 42: 882-890

[39] Sinigaglia L, Varenna M, Binelli L, et al (1999) Determinations of bone mass in systemic lupus erythematosus: a cross sectional study on premenopausal women. J Rheumatol 26: 1280-1284

[40] Weiner ES, Abeles (1989) Aseptic necrosis and glucocorticosteroids in systemic lupus erythematosus: reevaluation. J Rheumatol 16: 604-608,

[41] Ono K, Tohjima T, Komazawa T(1992) Risk factors of avascular necrosis of the femoral head in patients with systemic lupus erythematosus under high-dose corticosteroid therapy. Clin Orthop 277: 89-97

Chapter 19

The Use of Glucocorticoids in the Treatment of Acute Asthma Exacerbations

Abdullah A. Alangari

Additional information is available at the end of the chapter

http://dx.doi.org/10.5772/53221

1. Introduction

1.1. Pathophysiology of asthma and acute asthma exacerbations: Brief overview

Asthma is a chronic respiratory disease that is prevalent worldwide. It is considered as a major cause of morbidity and a main contributor to the high health care expenditure especially in developed countries (Subbarao et al, 2009). There are two major pathological features in asthmatics' airways, inflammation and hyperresponsiveness. These features are interrelated but not totally dependent on each other. Airway inflammatory changes include increased airway mucus secretions, airway wall edema, inflammatory cellular infiltrates, epithelial cell damage, smooth muscle hypertrophy, and submucosal fibrosis (Bergeron et al, 2009). The cellular infiltrates are mainly composed of eosinophils, neutrophils, mast cells, lymphocytes, basophils and macrophages. The ratio of these cells may widely vary between patients pointing to asthma heterogeneity (Holgate, 2008). Overall, asthma can be divided into eosinophilic, neutrophilic, and pauci-granulocytic phenotypes. The eosinophilic phenotype is characterized by predominant eosinophilic infiltration of the airways. Patients tend to be allergic, have asthma triggered by exposure to allergens and tend to respond well to glucocorticoids. The neutrophilic phenotype is characterized by predominant neutrophil infiltration of the airways. Patients tend to have severe, more aggressive, poorly controlled asthma, or acute asthma triggered by viral infection. They usually do not respond to glucocorticoids as good as the eosinophilic type. In the pauci-granulocytic phenotype neutrophils and eosinophils are almost absent (Holgate, 2008).

Triggers of acute asthma exacerbation include allergens like pollens, animal dander, dust mites and mold; viral respiratory tract infections; irritants like smoke and dust; cold air and exercise. When pollens, for instance, are inhaled by an allergic individual, the allergenic protein is taken up by antigen presenting cells (dendritic cells) in the airway. It is then presented to naïve T-helper (Th) cells that develop into Th2 cell phenotype. These cells respond by secreting Th2 cytokines like IL-4 and IL-13 that cause allergen specific B-cells to switch from IgM producing to IgE producing cells. These cytokines could also contribute to epithelial cell damage, increased mucus secretion and airway hyperresponsiveness. Th2 cells also secrete IL-5 that stimulates eosinophil development, release from the bone marrow and their recruitment to the site of inflammation. IgE antibodies bind to their receptors on the surface of mast cells. Cross linking of adjacent IgE molecules leads to degranulation and release of mediators like histamine and tryptase that are key to features of immediate hypersensitivity reaction. Activation of mast cells and eosinophils will also stimulate the synthesis and release of lipid derived mediators like prostaglandins and cysteinyl leukotrienes that are very potent bronchoconstrictors. Moreover, activation of eosinophils leads to the release of mediators like eosinophil cataionic protein and major basic protein, which can cause airway epithelial cell damage and submucosal fibrosis. New evidence suggests that Th1 cells contribute to chronic changes in the airways including epithelial cells damage and smooth muscle cells activation. Regulatory T cells (Treg) inhibit Th2 cells by secreting IL-10 and tansforming growth factor β (TGFβ). Also, antigen specific Th17 cells were found to play an important role in neutrophilic airway inflammation and the process of airway remodeling (fixed changes to the airway) through the secretion of IL-17A and IL-17F (figure 1). This is a very quick overview, but many other changes take place during this process that are beyond the scope of this chapter.

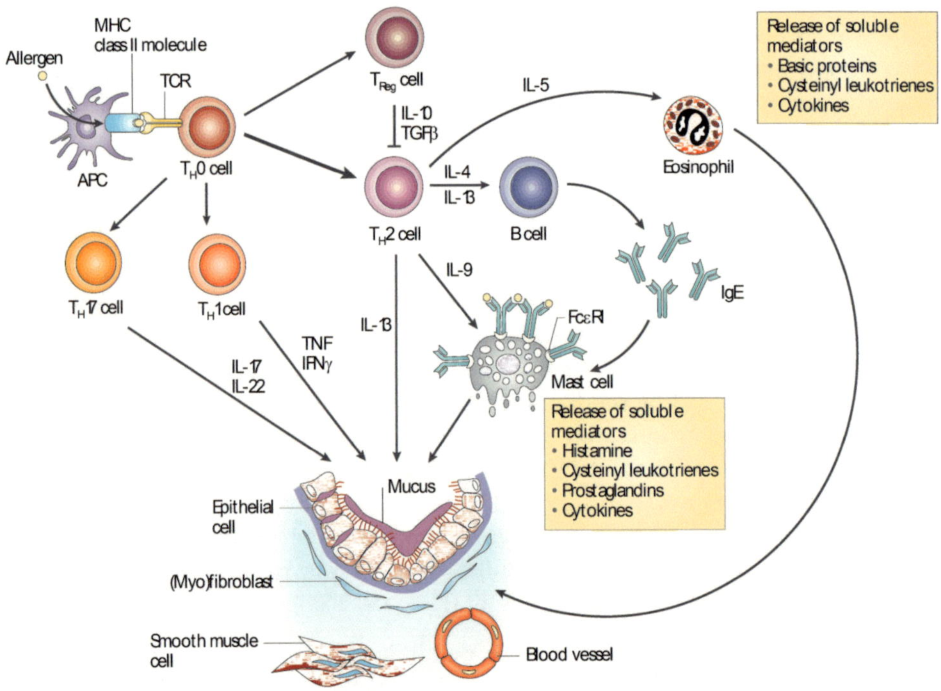

Figure 1. Major immunopahtologic processes that take place in the bronchial airways of patients with asthma. Please see the text for detailed description. FcεRI, high-affinity receptor for IgE; IFNγ, interferon-γ; TCR, T-cell receptor; TNF, tumour-necrosis factor. Reprinted by permission from Macmillan Publishers Ltd: Nature Reviews Immunology. Stephen T. Holgate and Riccardo Polosa. Treatment strategies for allergy and asthma. Vol. 8(3):Page 220, Copyright 2008.

The most common cause of acute asthma exacerbation in both adults and children, but more in children, is viral respiratory tract infections. Viruses may be responsible for up to 80% of wheezing episodes in children and 50-75% of episodes in adults (Jackson et al, 2011b). Many viruses can cause exacerbation of asthma symptoms, the most important and most common is rhinovirus (Khetsuriani et al, 2007). Respiratory syncycial virus and influenza virus also cause significant proportion of exacerbations. The pathology of virally induced asthma exacerbation is more related to the airway epithelial cells which, in response to infection secret chemokines like IL-8 and CCL-5 that can attract inflammatory cells including neutrophils and lymphocytes and augment allergic inflammation (Gern & Busse, 2002). This finding is supported by epidemiological observations that allergen sensitization and respiratory viral infections can synergize to cause asthma exacerbation (Green et al, 2002). Children who are atopic are more likely to have virally induced wheezing and respiratory distress than non-atopic children (Jackson et al, 2011a).

1.2. Treatment of acute asthma exacerbation: general overview

Acute asthma exacerbations are defined as "episodes of progressive increase in shortness of breath, cough, wheezing, or chest tightness, or some combination of these symptoms" (EPR3, 2007; GINA, 2011). Most recently an expert group formed by the NIH agreed to define acute asthma as "a worsening of asthma requiring the use of systemic corticosteroids to prevent a serious outcome" (Fuhlbrigge et al, 2012). Acute exacerbation of asthma symptoms is a common complication of the disease. The frequency in which exacerbations happen vary widely depending on the severity of disease (Moore et al, 2007), the degree of control with prophylactic medications (Peters et al, 2007), and exposure to triggers. In a multicenter study from the US (Pollack et al, 2002) the admission rate of all comers to the ER with acute asthma was 23%. On the other hand, a European study showed that only about 7% of all patients with acute asthma exacerbation required hospitalization (Rabe et al, 2000). We have a similar experience in Saudi Arabia where about 8% of all asthmatics with acute exacerbation are hospitalized, but if we look at only the severe group the rate goes up to 40% (unpublished data). These epidemiological data underscores the importance of effective treatment of asthma exacerbations and their prevention.

Patients with acute asthma exacerbation usually present with increasing cough, and dyspnea. On examination patients may have increased respiratory rate, retractions (accessory respiratory muscle use), wheezing, oxygen desaturation on pulse oxymetry and, in more severe cases, inability to speak, silent chest, with reduced respiratory lung volumes, cyanosis and change in mental status. Asthma exacerbations can be classified as mild, moderate, or severe based on the level of severity of the signs and symptoms as illustrated in Table 1. (Adams et al, 2011)

Different asthma scoring systems have been developed to assess the severity of asthma exacerbations more objectively, which is more useful for research purposes. An example is shown in table 2. (Qureshi et al, 1998). This scoring system is becoming more widely used because of its high reliability and objectivity.

Severity	Mild	Moderate	Severe
PEFR*	≥ 70%	40-69%	<40%
Speech	Sentences	Phrases	Words
Mental Status	Anxious	Agitated	Distressed
Accessory muscle use	No	Sometimes	Commonly
Oxygen saturation	≥ 95%	90-95%	<90%

Table 1. General classification of asthma severity. * PEFR: Peak Expiratory Flow Rate

Other frequently used scoring systems in the literature include; the Pulmonary Index Score (Scarfone et al, 1993) (table 3), and to a lesser degree the Preschool Respiratory Assessment Measure (PRAM) (Ducharme et al, 2008)(table 4), and the Pediatrics Asthma Severity Score (PASS) (Gorelick et al, 2004) (table 5).

Variable	Asthma score		
	1 point	2 points	3 points
Respiratory rate (breaths/min)			
2-3 years	≤ 34	35 - 39	≥ 40
4-5 years	≤ 30	31 - 35	≥ 36
6-12 years	≤ 26	27 - 30	≥ 31
>12 years	≤ 23	24 - 27	≥ 28
Oxygen saturation (%)	> 95 with room air	90 - 95 with room air	<90 with room air or supplemental oxygen
Auscultation	Normal breathing or end-expiratory wheezing	Expiratory wheezing	Inspiratory and expiratory wheezing, diminished breath sounds, or both
Retractions	None or intercostal	Intercostal and substernal	Intercostal, substernal, and supraclavicular
Dyspnea	Speaks in sentences or coos and babbles	Speaks in partial sentences or utters short cries	Speaks in single words or short phrases or grunts

Table 2. Asthma severity score (Qureshi et al). Score interpretation: Mild asthma 5-7, Moderate 8-11, Severe 12-15

In patients with mild asthma exacerbation, inhaled β2-agonists like albuterol (salbutamol) is usually sufficient to resolve symptoms. The dose can be repeated 3 times every 15-20 minutes. Levalbuterol, the (R)-enantiomer of albuterol is the effective form of the drug, but clinical trials did not show any advantage of using it over albuterol in terms of efficacy or side effects (Kelly, 2007). Most patients with mild asthma exacerbation will not require systemic glucocoricoids. However, it is recommended that patients who take them regularly or patients who fail initial treatment with albuterol should be given systemic glucocorticoids.

Score	0	1	2	3
Respiratory Rate* (breaths/min)	< 30	31-45	46-60	> 60
Wheezing	None	End expiration	Entire expiration	Inspiration and expiration without stethoscope
Inspiratory / Expiratory Ratio	5/2	5/3 - 5/4	1/1	<1/1
Accessory Muscle Use	0	+	++	+++

Table 3. Pulmonary Index Score. * For patients aged 6 years or older: <20 = 0; 21-35 = 1; 36-50 = 2; >50 = 3

Signs	0	1	2	3
Suprasternal retractions	Absent		Present	
Scalene muscle contraction	Absent		Present	
Air entry*	Normal	Decreased at bases	Widespread decrease	Absent/minimal
Wheezing*	Absent	Expiration only	Inspiratory and expiratory	Audible without stethoscope/silent chest with minimal air entry
O_2 saturation	≥95%	92%-94%	<92%	

Table 4. The Preschool Respiratory Assessment Measure (PRAM). *If asymmetric findings between right and left lungs, the most severe side is rated.

Current guidelines recommend that patients with mild-moderate or moderate exacerbation should receive 3 doses of inhaled or nebulized β2-agonist every 15-20 minutes in the first hour (Camargo et al, 2003). Additional doses may be repeated in the next 2-3 hours every 30-60 minutes. All those patients should be treated with systemic glucocorticoids at a dose of 2mg/kg or a maximum dose of 80 mg early in the course of management as it takes at least 4 hours to start working (Rowe et al, 2004). Doses more than 80 mg will not confer any additional benefit. Systemic glucocorticoids were found to speed resolution of symptoms, decrease the rate of admission and decrease the rate of relapse if administered for 3-5 days after the acute exacerbation. More detailed discussion about the use of systemic glucocoricoids in the treatment of acute asthma can be found below in section 2.1.

Clinical Finding	Definition	0	1	2
Wheezing	High-pitched expiratory sound heard by auscultation	None or mild	Moderate	Severe wheezing due to poor air exchange
Air entry	Intensity of inspiratory sounds by auscultation	Normal or mildly diminished	Moderately diminished	Severely diminished
Work of breathing	Observed use of accessory muscles, retractions, or in-breathing	None or mild	Moderate	Severe
Prolongation of expiration	Ratio of duration of expiration to inspiration	Normal or mildly prolonged	Moderately prolonged	Severely prolonged
Tachypnea	Respiratory rate above normal for age	Absent	Present	
Mental status	Observation of the child's state of alertness	Normal	Depressed	

Table 5. The Pediatrics Asthma Severity Score (PASS)

Patients with severe asthma exacerbation should obviously be treated more aggressively. High dose inhaled (8-12 puffs) or nebulized β2-agonist should be given every 15-20 minutes at least in the first hour, which could be repeated for up to 4 hours then as required. The data are conflicting whether continuous nebulization using β2-agonist is superior to intermittent nebulaization or not (Camargo et al, 2003; Rodrigo & Rodrigo, 2002). Practically, continuous high dose nebulization could be used for the first hour and then intermittent nebulization thereafter as required. Ipratropium bromide has been shown to decrease the rate of hospitalization and shorten the stay in the emergency room in patients with severe or moderate to severe asthma exacerbation in many clinical trials (Qureshi et al, 1998; Rodrigo & Castro-Rodriguez, 2005; Zorc et al, 1999). Therefore, it is recommended to add it to each treatment of β2-agonist at least in the first hour of therapy. Its use in patients after admission to the hospital was not shown to make a difference. Systemic steroids should be used as mentioned in patients with moderate exacerbation. Other treatment modalities may be considered like magnesium sulfate and helium oxygen (heliox) therapy in the more severe and non-responsive patients. Subcutaneous or intravenous β2-agonists (Travers et al, 2002), intravenous aminophylline (Parameswaran et al, 2000), intravenous montelukast (Camargo et al, 2010; Morris et al, 2010), or oral montelukast added to standard therapy in the ER (Todi et al, 2010) were not shown to be helpful in the treatment of patients with severe asthma exacerbation and therefore are not recommended. Moreover, oral montelukast given to patients post discharge for 5 days was also shown not to be helpful (Schuh et al, 2009).

β2-agonists can be delivered via a nebulizer or by metered dose inhaled (MDI) with a holding chamber. An MDI dose of 4-8 puffs depending on age is equivalent to a nebulized dose of 2.5-5 mg of albuterol (Cates et al, 2006). Nebulizer is preferable in cases of severe symptoms when patients are unable to use the MDI effectively or if other nebulized medications are needed to be mixed with albuterol at the same time or if the patient is requiring oxygen supplementation. Oxygen therapy should be given to maintain saturation ≥ 90% in adults and ≥95% in pregnant women or children.

Patients who maintain normal oxygen saturation, have no or minimal wheezing on chest auscultation, and have no or mild intercostal retractions can be discharged home after 1 hour of assessment on no additional medications in the emergency room. However, these patients should have a step up in their maintenance medications to prevent relapse. Patients who fail to achieve improvement after 4 hours of treatment should be admitted to the hospital for further aggressive therapy.

1.3. Introduction and evolution of glucocorticoids in the management of asthma: Historical background

Shortly after the discovery of the structure of adrenal steroid hormones, Hench and his colleagues examined using cortisone to treat arthritis in 1949. The effect was remarkable and that work won the Nobel Prize the next year. It also started a series of trials of corticosteroids in various inflammatory conditions. The first use of corticosteroid to treat acute asthma exacerbation occured in 1956 (Subcommittee on clinical trials in asthma, 1956). Development of corticosteroids that have less mineralocorticoid activity, like prednisone, and later those that have no mineralocorticoid activity, like dexamethasone, made glucocorticoids more attractive therapies to use in asthma. In 1972, Clerk et. al. showed for the first time that inhaled beclomethasone was effective in the management of asthma with less adverse effects than systemic steroids (Clark, 1972). Numerous reports came afterwards describing the efficacy of oral prednisone and prednisolone, intravenous methylprednisolone and inhaled glucocorticoids (IGC) like triamcinolone, budesonide, and fluticasone in the management of asthma. Table 3 shows some common systemic glucocorticoids and their relative potency.

Preparation	Potency relative to hydrocortisone	Relative sodium retention potency	Biological half life (h)
Hydrocortisone	1	1	8-12
Prednisone/Prednisolone	4	0.8	12-36
Methylprednisolone	5	0.5	12-36
Dexamethasone	25	0	36-72

Table 6. Common types of systemic glucocorticoids and their relative properties

1.4. Adverse effects of glucocorticoids

There are many adverse effects that may result from the use of oral or IGC in the treatment of asthma especially in high doses. I will summarize here the most pertinent ones.

a. Suppression of the hypothalamic-pituitary-adrenal axis. Soon after the commencement of high dose oral glucocorticoids adrenal suppression may be noticeable. It also occurs with longer use of lower doses. IGC can also be systemically absorbed in their active form through particle deposition in the orophaynx or the lungs (particles deposited in the stomach usually undergo first pass hepatic metabolism where they are deactivated). High doses of IGC, more than 400 mcg of becloemthasone and 200 mcg of fluticasone or budesonide per day, could cause systemic adverse effects especially in children (Gulliver & Eid, 2005). Patients who undergo a stressful situation like major surgery should receive systemic steroid coverage to avoid symptoms of adrenal crises. These symptoms include lethargy, vomiting, change in mental status, and electrolyte disturbances. The hypothalamic-pituitary-adrenal axis can be evaluated by measuring early morning cortisol level.
b. Osteoporosis. A common and serious complication of prolonged oral or high dose IGC therapy. Patients on such treatment, especially women and those with limited physical activity or who are taking medications that increase vitamine D metabolism in the liver, should undergo bone densitometry evaluation because this complication cannot be detected clinically. In one specialized center in the US, 40% of adolescent females admitted with severe asthma had osteopenia (Covar et al, 2000).
c. Growth suppression. Glucocorticiods have been consistently shown to suppress growth in children. This seems to be independent from the growth suppression caused by the disease itself (Covar et al, 2000). The degree of growth suppression may reach 1 cm especially in the first year after starting IGC treatment. However, children eventually reach their expected height as adults (Agertoft & Pedersen, 2000; Sharek & Bergman, 2000).
d. Ophthalmologic adverse effects. Long-term administration of oral glucocorticoids or high doses IGC can lead to the development of posterior capsular cataract (Cumming et al, 1997). Some patients may need lens replacement surgery. Another ophthalmic complication is glaucoma that also may result from prolonged therapy with high dose IGC (Garbe et al, 1997). However, short-term treatment for less than 2 years or the use of moderate doses of IGC was found to be safe (Li et al, 1999; Pelkonen et al, 2008).
e. Local adverse effects: Chronic use of IGC can be associated with the development of oral thrush (candidiasis), which could be minimized by washing the mouth with water after the inhalation. It may also be associated with hoarseness of voice and dysphonia due probably to laryngeal edema. These effects can be managed by changing the mode of inhalation (e.g: from dry powder inhaler to MDI) and the use of a holding chamber.
f. Other adverse effects: These include immune suppression, metabolic changes like hyperglycemia, acne, hirsutism, skin thinning, delayed wound healing, myopathy, psychosis or mood changes.

2. Clinical evidence of the effect of glucocorticoids in acute asthma

2.1. Systemic glucocorticoids

Systemic glucocorticoids given early in the course of treatment of acute asthma exacerbations in the emergency room were overall shown to be effective and are recommended by different asthma guidelines like GINA and EPR3. Littenberg et al. initially showed that they decrease hospital admission rate (Littenberg & Gluck, 1986). Five subsequent studies had, however, conflicting results. Rodrigo & Rodrigo reviewed all these six studies and concluded that there was no improvement in hospital admission rate or lung function (Rodrigo & Rodrigo, 1999). They, however, reported a trend of improvement in lung function only with medium or high doses systemic glucocorticoids. So data in terms of lung function are more encouraging (Fanta et al, 1983; Lin et al, 1999). In terms of effect on exacerbation relapse after discharge from the emergency room, most studies showed less relapse with systemic glucocorticoids (Schneider et al, 1988; Subcommittee on clinical trials in asthma, 1956) although others did not (Rodrigo & Rodrigo, 1994). One important issue with all these studies is the low number of patients recruited. Almost all had subject number less than 100 per study and all were performed in adults. On the other hand, Krishnan et al recently reviewed 9 published studies in the use of systemic glucocorticoids in acute asthma in adults and concluded "systemic corticosteroids provide clinically meaningful benefits in patients presenting with acute asthma" (Krishnan et al, 2009). In children, more limited data showed benefit of systemic steroids used early in the emergency room with decreased rate of admission (Scarfone et al, 1993). A Cochrane database review by Rowe et al showed decrease rate of admission in patients with acute asthma with the use of systemic glucocorticoids in adults and children especially those with severe asthma and those not currently receiving steroids (Rowe et al, 2001).

There is no significant difference in efficacy of systemic glucocorticoids at doses above 60-80 mg/d or 2 mg/kg/d in regards to pulmonary function, rate of admission, or length of stay in the hospital. For example, Marquette et al compared 1 mg/kg/d to 6 mg/kg/d methylprednisolone in 47 adults hospitalized with severe acute asthma and found no benefit of the high dose over the low dose (Marquette et al, 1995). Manser et al performed a systematic review of randomized controlled studies of patients with acute severe asthma comparing different doses of glucocorticoids with a minimum follow up of 24 hours. They divided the different doses used in the trials included into 3 groups as equivalent dose of methylprednisolone in 24 hours; low dose (≤80 mg), medium dose (>80 mg and ≤360 mg), and high dose (>360 mg). Nine trials were included with a total of 344 adults. They found no difference between the different doses (Manser et al, 2001).

Studies also showed no difference in efficacy between oral or intravenous administration or in their onset on action. Fifty-two adults with severe acute asthma were treated with either IV hydrocortisone or PO prednisolone. There was no difference in their peak flow measurements 24 hours after admission (Harrison et al, 1986). Ratto et al compared four different doses of methylprednisolone; 160 or 320 mg given orally, or 500 or 1000 mg given IV in four divided doses in adults with acute asthma and found no difference in their FEV_1, days of hospitalization (Ratto et al, 1988). In children oral prednisolone was found equivalent to IV methylprednisolone in regards to patients' length of hospital stay (Becker et al, 1999). In addition, oral treatment was cost saving. GINA and the EPR3 guidelines prefer oral administration because it is less invasive except in patients with absorption problems or those who are not able to take orally due to the severity of their respiratory distress or because they are vomiting.

Prescribing oral glucocorticoids for the treatment of acute asthma exacerbations for longer than 5 days was not found to provide any additional benefit (Hasegawa et al, 2000; Jones et al, 2002). In children, a single dose of dexamethasone 0.6 mg/kg (max. 18 mg) was found to be equivalent to prednisolone 2 mg/kg/d in two divided doses for 5 days in terms of symptoms resolution (Altamimi et al, 2006). There is also no benefit from using a dose taper over fixed-dose regimen (Krishnan et al, 2009). Because of poor compliance on oral prednisone after discharge from the emergency, intramuscular injection of methylprednisolone was studied as an alternative but was not found superior, plus there was an evidence of injection-site adverse reaction (see last reference).

2.2. Inhaled glucocorticoids

IGC were studied in the treatment of acute asthma in 4 contexts: as compared to placebo, as compared to systemic glucocorticoids, as add on therapy to systemic steroids for up to few weeks after discharge from the ER, or as add on therapy to systemic steroids in the ER only.

In the first context, a review that looked at 8 randomized and blinded studies comparing the efficacy of IGC to placebo in acute asthma exacerbation suggested that IGC are superior to placebo especially when given at high doses (> 1mg of budesonide or fluticasone) and to patients with severe exacerbations (Rodrigo, 2006). It is important to note that those studies were quite heterogeneous in terms of the severity of asthma in recruited patients, the dose and frequency of IGC administered, and in the outcome measures that included clinical symptoms, pulmonary function, oxygen saturation, admission rate, or relapse rate. A recent study found that preemptive use of high dose fluticasone (750 mcg BID) at the onset of an upper respiratory tract infection in children with recurrent virus induced wheezing and continuing it for 10 days, reduced the use of rescue oral glucocorticoids (Ducharme et al, 2009).

When IGCs were compared with systemic glucocorticoids in randomized and blinded studies the data were more controversial. Some studies reported superiority of systemic steroids in reducing admission rate (Schuh et al, 2000), some reported equal efficacy in relation to admission rate as well (Lee-Wong et al, 2002; Levy et al, 1996; Scarfone et al, 1995), and some reported clear superiority of IGC (Devidayal et al, 1999; Rodrigo, 2005). A study compared high dose fluticasone in the ER and for 5 days post discharge to systemic glucocorticoids in the same period in patients with mild to moderate asthma found that oral steroids lead to faster improvement in FEV_1 at 4 hours in the ER and less relapse rate at 48 hours post discharge (Schuh et al, 2006). One recent study showed that in patients who were given systemic glucocorticoids plus IGC post discharge from the ER, stopping the systemic glucocorticoids after 1 week resulted in rebound in the level of exhaled NO 2 weeks post discharge despite continuing IGC with no effect on the use of rescue medications or on FEV_1 (Khoo & Lim, 2009). GINA guideline state that "IGC are effective as part of therapy for asthma exacerbations….and can be as effective as oral glucocorticoids at preventing relapses"(GINA, 2011), while the EPR3 guidelines state that "high doses of IGC may be considered in the ER, although current evidence is insufficient to permit conclusions about using IGC rather than oral systemic corticosteroids in the ER"(EPR3, 2007).

When IGC were used as add on therapy to systemic glucocorticoids in the ER and continued after discharge for few weeks, Rowe et al found decrease in relapse rate when 1600 mcg/d budesonide for 21 days was added to a course of 50 mg/d prednisone for 7 days as compared to placebo (Rowe et al, 1999). On the other hand, Brenner et al found no difference in the peak expiratory flow rate between high dose flunisolide used for 24 days added to prednisone 40 mg/d for 5 days as compared to placebo (Brenner et al, 2000). A systematic review of ten trials concluded no benefit of adding inhaled to systemic glucocorticoids in reducing the relapse rate of acute asthma (Edmonds et al, 2000).

There are few randomized and blinded studies examining only the short-term effect of IGC in the ER as add on therapy to systemic glucocorticoids plus other standard acute asthma therapy. One study looked at the addition of high dose beclomethasone versus placebo to methylprednisolone in 60 adults and found no difference in FEV_1 or symptoms between the two groups (Guttman et al, 1997). One study looked at the addition of budesonide nebulizations to methylprednisolone in a population of 26 children with moderate asthma (Nuhoglu et al, 2005) and found no difference in the primary outcome of pulmonary index score but there was an improvement in the PEFR in the budesonide group compared to placebo. However, the patient number included is very small and PEFR is generally not reliable in young children. The two other randomized and blinded studies that were larger and more rigorous examined the effect of adding 2 mg of budesonide nebulization to prednisone in children with moderate to severe asthma (Sung et al, 1998; Upham et al, 2011). In the study by Sung et al, 44 children with moderate to severe asthma were included. Both groups had no difference in the pulmonary index score. In the Upham et al study, 180 children with moderate to severe asthma were included. There was no difference in the asthma score (adopted form (Qureshi et al, 1998)) at 2 hours after intervention or in the admission rate or time to discharge from the ER between the two groups. Collectively, all these studies, although small in subjects number, indicate that the addition of IGC to systemic steroid is not helpful in patients with moderate to severe acute asthma. We are conducting a larger study that will hopefully shed more light on that question, the results of which should be available quite soon.

3. A brief overview of the use of glucocorticoids in asthma prophylaxis

3.1. Inhaled glucocorticoids

IGCs are the main stay of asthma management. They were shown to very consistently change many of the pathologic inflammatory features of asthma in the lung airways. They lead to decrease cellular infiltrates including T-lymphocytes, mast cells, eosinophils, and macrophages. Also, epithelial damage, goblet cell hyperplasia, and vascular blood flow significantly decreases with IGC therapy (Fanta, 2009). Consistent with the histological changes, clinical changes are observed. Compliant use of IGC is associated with decreased airway hyperresponsiveness and improved asthma symptomatology (CAMP, 2000; Haahtela et al, 1991). Most patients will also have improved lung function demonstrated by increased FEV_1. In addition, the risk of patients' hospitalization from asthma exacerbations is decreased by up to 50% (Donahue et al, 1997). Moreover, the risk of death from asthma is decreased, an effect that is dependent on the patients' compliance on IGC and the duration of their use (Suissa et al, 2000).

It is important here to note several points. First, the local anti-inflammatory effect of IGC usually plateaus after reaching low to moderate dosages, except probably for the most severe patients. However, the other systemic effects of IGC increase steeply after exceeding the low to moderate dose (Szefler et al, 2005). Therefore, efforts should be made to maintain patients on the lowest possible dose of IGC and, in cases of inappropriate response, long acting beta-agonists (LABA) or leukotriene receptor antagonists (LTRA) or both should be added before doubling the dose of IGC (Fanta, 2009). Second, there is great heterogeneity among asthmatics in their response to IGC. This variability can be attributed to several factors, most importantly are genetic variations between individuals (Lima et al, 2009). Third, multiple studies have shown that IGC therapy over the years do not change the natural history of the disease or prevent decline in lung function. They may have little effect on some features of remodeling but not all of them. Also, IGC, even when used in high risk infants who are very likely to develop asthma, were not able to prevent its development (Murray, 2008).

3.2. Systemic glucocorticoids

Systemic glucocorticoids are only occasionally used for long-term asthma control. There use is limited to the most severe patients who are difficult to control using other common modalities (EPR3, 2007). This is due to their side effects that can be very serious as stated above. The side effects are dose and duration dependent. Prolonged low dose therapy (<7.5 mg prednisone-equivalent in adults/day) is usually associated with mild adverse effects. Moderate doses (7.5 mg – 30 mg/day) are usually associated with significant adverse effects, and high doses (30 mg – 100 mg) may be associated with serious adverse effects (Stahn & Buttgereit, 2008).

4. Mechanism of action of glucocorticoids in asthma

Discussion of the mechanism of action of glucocorticoids in asthma is beyond the scope of this chapter and was recently reviewed (Alangari, 2010). Glucocorticoids act either by altering the rate of transcription of certain genes at the DNA level or through non-genomic pathways. Some of these effects could lead to the desirable anti-inflammatory action and some may result in adverse reactions.

4.1. Genomic action

The main mechanism whereby glucocorticoids deliver their anti-inflammatory action involves genomic action. This mechanism entails binding of glucocorticoids to their cytoplasmic receptors forming complexes that then translocate to the nucleus, where they either homo-dimerize then bind to their glucocorticoid response elements (GRE) in the DNA, or bind to different transcription factors (protein-protein interaction) as monomers (Ito et al, 2006; Lowenberg et al, 2008). Because of this, the genomic action of glucocorticoids takes at least 4 hours to start showing an effect and the duration of action is also prolonged and may exceed 24 hours.

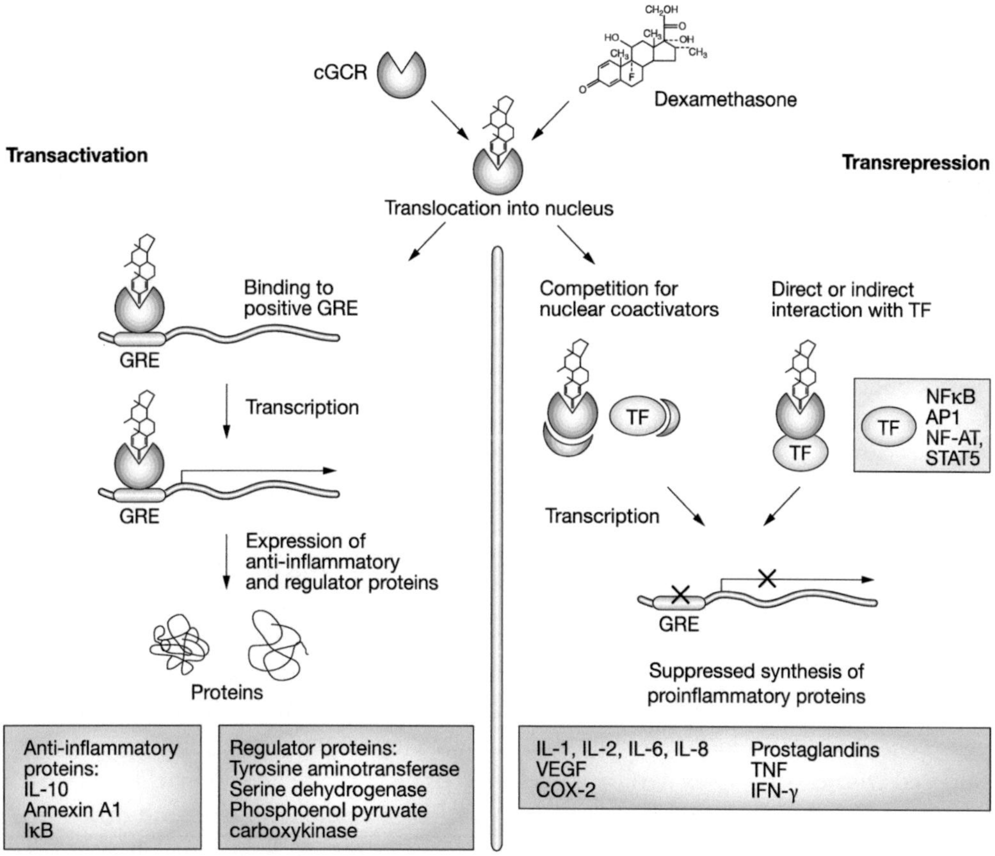

Figure 2. The genomic effect of glucocorticoids is in the form of transactivation or transrepression. In transactivation, the transcription of genes encoding certain anti-inflammatory or regulatory proteins is upregulated, while in transrepression the transcription of certain genes encoding proinflammatory proteins is up regulated. Abbreviations: AP1, activator protein 1; cGCR, cytosolic glucocorticoid receptor; COX-2, cyclooxygenase 2; GRE, glucocorticoid response element; IkB, inhibitor of NFkB; IFNγ interferon IL, interleukin; NF-AT, nuclear factor of activated T cells; NFkB, nuclear factor kB; STAT5, signal transducer and activator of transcription 5; TF, transcription factor; TNF, tumor necrosis factor; VEGF, vascular endothelial growth factor. Reprinted by permission from Macmillan Publishers Ltd: Nature Reviews Rheumatology. Cindy Stahn and Frank Buttgereit. Vol. 4(10):Page 529, copyright 2008.

Binding of glucocorticoid receptors to their GRE activates the transcription of certain genes encoding anti-inflammatory proteins, like IL-10 and IkB, and regulatory proteins. This process is called *transactivation* (figure 2). Some of the glucocorticoids adverse effects like glaucoma and hyperglycemia are mediated through this pathway (Schacke et al, 2002). On the other hand, binding of glucocorticoid receptors to pro-inflammatory transcription factors like nuclear factor kappa B (NFkB) or activator protein 1 (AP-1), or their competition for nuclear coactivators; down regulates the transcription of certain genes encoding pro-inflammatory proteins like IL-1, IL-2, IL-6, and TNF. This process is called *transrepression* (De Bosscher et al, 2003) (figure 2). Most of the desired genomic actions of glucocorticoids in asthma are mediated through this pathway.

4.2. Non-genomic action

Non-genomic action of glucocorticoids includes all actions that do not directly alter gene expression and are not blunted by inhibitors of gene transcription (Losel & Wehling, 2003). This mode of action is characterized by its rapid onset (seconds to minutes) and short duration (60-90 min). These actions are dose dependent (Wanner et al, 2004). There are four types of non-genomic action of glucocorticoids (Alangari, 2010). Firstly, acting through the inhibition of the extraneuronal monoamine transporter-mediated uptake of norepinephrine. Asthmatic patients have increased blood flow in their airways (Kumar et al, 1998). IGC were shown to decrease blood flow in the airways within few minutes. This effect will last for 90 minutes only and therefore, cannot be explained by the genomic action (Kumar et al, 2000; Mendes et al, 2003). The proposed mechanism is that IGCs by a topical effect can block the extraneuronal monoamine transporter on the membrane of vascular endothelial cells, preventing their uptake of norepinephrine and thus making it more available in the synaptic cleft (Horvath & Wanner, 2006). Secondly, in high doses, glucocorticoids can induce physiochemical changes in the cell membrane by directly incorporating into the membrane. This can result in immune cell suppression (Buttgereit & Scheffold, 2002). Thirdly, glucocorticoids may interact with membrane bound GRs on mononuclear cells. These receptors are variants of cytosolic GRs and can mediate inhibition of Lck/Fyn kinases down stream form the T-cell receptor leading to immune suppression (Lowenberg et al, 2005; Lowenberg et al, 2007). Lastly, few in vitro studies showed that some protein components associated with GRs complex, which are released upon GR ligation can inactivate cytosolic phospholipase 2 and therefore inhibit the production of arachidonic acid and downstream components like prostaglandins and leukotriens (Croxtall et al, 2000; Croxtall et al, 2002). However this action was not shown to be of clinical significance.

5. Future directions and recommendations

We have seen through this chapter that glucocorticoids play an extremely important role in the current prophylactic treatment of patients with persistent asthma, in the treatment of acute asthma exacerbations post discharge from the ER and possibly in the acute management in the ER. The introduction of IGC has revolutionized the way we manage asthma and it seems that those medications will stay with us for a long while. Further research is greatly needed to shed more light on the use of IGC in the ER in patients coming with acute asthma exacerbation and on the safety of dispensing oral glucocorticoids for home use in case of asthma exacerbation. Training physicians to follow asthma management guidelines as well as education of patients and their families cannot be over emphasized and will save a lot of money.

Our improved understanding of the tertiary structure of glucocorticoids and their receptors and their mechanisms of action has led to the discovery and development of selective glucocorticoid receptor modulators (SGRM). Those are new agents that have the transrepression but little or no transactivation properties of glucocorticoids, which means that those compounds could deliver the desired anti-inflammatory action of glucocorticoids while avoiding most of their adverse effects (De Bosscher et al, 2010). Still under investigation, those agents could hold a lot of promise in the future. Moreover, it was recently shown that simultaneous activation of GRα and peroxisome proliferator-activated receptor alpha (PPARα), which are cytosolic receptors with many immunomodulatory functions and multiple natural ligands, can block the GRE mediated transactivating effects of glucocorticoids while potentiating their anti-inflammatory effects in mice (Bougarne et al, 2009). If this holds true in humans, combination therapy of a glucocorticoid and a PPARα agonist could be very promising.

Author details

Abdullah A. Alangari
Department of Pediatrics, College of Medicine, King Saud University, Saudi Arabia

Acknowledgement

I am very grateful to Prof. Dale Umetsu for reviewing this manuscript. This work was supported by a grant form the Program of Strategic Technologies of the National Plan for Science and Technology and Innovation, Saudi Arabia. Grant number 08-MED520-02.

6. References

Adams JY, Sutter ME, Albertson TE (2011) The Patient with Asthma in the Emergency Department. *Clin Rev Allergy Immunol*

Agertoft L, Pedersen S (2000) Effect of long-term treatment with inhaled budesonide on adult height in children with asthma. *N Engl J Med* 343(15): 1064-1069

Alangari AA (2010) Genomic and non-genomic actions of glucocorticoids in asthma. *Ann Thorac Med* 5(3): 133-139

Altamimi S, Robertson G, Jastaniah W, Davey A, Dehghani N, Chen R, Leung K, Colbourne M (2006) Single-dose oral dexamethasone in the emergency management of children with exacerbations of mild to moderate asthma. *Pediatr Emerg Care* 22(12): 786-793

Becker JM, Arora A, Scarfone RJ, Spector ND, Fontana-Penn ME, Gracely E, Joffe MD, Goldsmith DP, Malatack JJ (1999) Oral versus intravenous corticosteroids in children hospitalized with asthma. *J Allergy Clin Immunol* 103(4): 586-590

Bergeron C, Al-Ramli W, Hamid Q (2009) Remodeling in asthma. *Proc Am Thorac Soc* 6(3): 301-305

Bougarne N, Paumelle R, Caron S, Hennuyer N, Mansouri R, Gervois P, Staels B, Haegeman G, De Bosscher K (2009) PPARalpha blocks glucocorticoid receptor alpha-mediated transactivation but cooperates with the activated glucocorticoid receptor alpha for transrepression on NF-kappaB. *Proc Natl Acad Sci U S A* 106(18): 7397-7402

Brenner BE, Chavda KK, Camargo CA, Jr. (2000) Randomized trial of inhaled flunisolide versus placebo among asthmatic patients discharged from the emergency department. *Ann Emerg Med* 36(5): 417-426

Buttgereit F, Scheffold A (2002) Rapid glucocorticoid effects on immune cells. *Steroids* 67(6): 529-534

Camargo CA, Jr., Gurner DM, Smithline HA, Chapela R, Fabbri LM, Green SA, Malice MP, Legrand C, Dass SB, Knorr BA, Reiss TF (2010) A randomized placebo-controlled study of intravenous montelukast for the treatment of acute asthma. *J Allergy Clin Immunol* 125(2): 374-380

Camargo CA, Jr., Spooner CH, Rowe BH (2003) Continuous versus intermittent beta-agonists in the treatment of acute asthma. *Cochrane Database Syst Rev*(4): CD001115

CAMP T (2000) Long-term effects of budesonide or nedocromil in children with asthma. The Childhood Asthma Management Program Research Group. *N Engl J Med* 343(15): 1054-1063

Cates CJ, Crilly JA, Rowe BH (2006) Holding chambers (spacers) versus nebulisers for beta-agonist treatment of acute asthma. *Cochrane Database Syst Rev*(2): CD000052

Clark TJ (1972) Effect of beclomethasone dipropionate delivered by aerosol in patients with asthma. *Lancet* 1(7765): 1361-1364

Covar RA, Leung DY, McCormick D, Steelman J, Zeitler P, Spahn JD (2000) Risk factors associated with glucocorticoid-induced adverse effects in children with severe asthma. *J Allergy Clin Immunol* 106(4): 651-659

Croxtall JD, Choudhury Q, Flower RJ (2000) Glucocorticoids act within minutes to inhibit recruitment of signalling factors to activated EGF receptors through a receptor-dependent, transcription-independent mechanism. *Br J Pharmacol* 130(2): 289-298

Croxtall JD, van Hal PT, Choudhury Q, Gilroy DW, Flower RJ (2002) Different glucocorticoids vary in their genomic and non-genomic mechanism of action in A549 cells. *Br J Pharmacol* 135(2): 511-519

Cumming RG, Mitchell P, Leeder SR (1997) Use of inhaled corticosteroids and the risk of cataracts. *N Engl J Med* 337(1): 8-14

De Bosscher K, Haegeman G, Elewaut D (2010) Targeting inflammation using selective glucocorticoid receptor modulators. *Curr Opin Pharmacol* 10(4): 497-504

De Bosscher K, Vanden Berghe W, Haegeman G (2003) The interplay between the glucocorticoid receptor and nuclear factor-kappaB or activator protein-1: molecular mechanisms for gene repression. *Endocr Rev* 24(4): 488-522

Devidayal, Singhi S, Kumar L, Jayshree M (1999) Efficacy of nebulized budesonide compared to oral prednisolone in acute bronchial asthma. *Acta Paediatr* 88(8): 835-840

Donahue JG, Weiss ST, Livingston JM, Goetsch MA, Greineder DK, Platt R (1997) Inhaled steroids and the risk of hospitalization for asthma. *JAMA* 277(11): 887-891

Ducharme FM, Chalut D, Plotnick L, Savdie C, Kudirka D, Zhang X, Meng L, McGillivray D (2008) The Pediatric Respiratory Assessment Measure: a valid clinical score for assessing acute asthma severity from toddlers to teenagers. *J Pediatr* 152(4): 476-480, 480.e471

Ducharme FM, Lemire C, Noya FJ, Davis GM, Alos N, Leblond H, Savdie C, Collet JP, Khomenko L, Rivard G, Platt RW (2009) Preemptive use of high-dose fluticasone for virus-induced wheezing in young children. *N Engl J Med* 360(4): 339-353

Edmonds ML, Camargo CA, Saunders LD, Brenner BE, Rowe BH (2000) Inhaled steroids in acute asthma following emergency department discharge. *Cochrane Database Syst Rev*(3): CD002316

EPR3 (2007) Expert Panel Report 3: Guidelines for the Diagnosis and Management of Asthma

Fanta CH (2009) Asthma. *N Engl J Med* 360(10): 1002-1014

Fanta CH, Rossing TH, McFadden ER, Jr. (1983) Glucocorticoids in acute asthma. A critical controlled trial. *Am J Med* 74(5): 845-851

Fuhlbrigge A, Peden D, Apter AJ, Boushey HA, Camargo CA, Jr., Gern J, Heymann PW, Martinez FD, Mauger D, Teague WG, Blaisdell C (2012) Asthma outcomes: exacerbations. *J Allergy Clin Immunol* 129: S34-48

Garbe E, LeLorier J, Boivin JF, Suissa S (1997) Inhaled and nasal glucocorticoids and the risks of ocular hypertension or open-angle glaucoma. *JAMA* 277(9): 722-727

Gern JE, Busse WW (2002) Relationship of viral infections to wheezing illnesses and asthma. *Nat Rev Immunol* 2(2): 132-138

GINA (2011) Global Initiative for Asthma (GINA): Global Strategy for Asthma Management and Prevention.

Gorelick MH, Stevens MW, Schultz TR, Scribano PV (2004) Performance of a novel clinical score, the Pediatric Asthma Severity Score (PASS), in the evaluation of acute asthma. *Academic emergency medicine* 11(1): 10-18

Green RM, Custovic A, Sanderson G, Hunter J, Johnston SL, Woodcock A (2002) Synergism between allergens and viruses and risk of hospital admission with asthma: case-control study. *BMJ* 324(7340): 763

Gulliver T, Eid N (2005) Effects of glucocorticoids on the hypothalamic-pituitary-adrenal axis in children and adults. *Immunol Allergy Clin North Am* 25(3): 541-555, vii

Guttman A, Afilalo M, Colacone A, Kreisman H, Dankoff J (1997) The effects of combined intravenous and inhaled steroids (beclomethasone dipropionate) for the emergency treatment of acute asthma. The Asthma ED Study Group. *Acad Emerg Med* 4(2): 100-106

Haahtela T, Jarvinen M, Kava T, Kiviranta K, Koskinen S, Lehtonen K, Nikander K, Persson T, Reinikainen K, Selroos O, et al. (1991) Comparison of a beta 2-agonist, terbutaline, with an inhaled corticosteroid, budesonide, in newly detected asthma. *N Engl J Med* 325(6): 388-392

Harrison BD, Stokes TC, Hart GJ, Vaughan DA, Ali NJ, Robinson AA (1986) Need for intravenous hydrocortisone in addition to oral prednisolone in patients admitted to hospital with severe asthma without ventilatory failure. *Lancet* 1(8474): 181-184

Hasegawa T, Ishihara K, Takakura S, Fujii H, Nishimura T, Okazaki M, Katakami N, Umeda B (2000) Duration of systemic corticosteroids in the treatment of asthma exacerbation; a randomized study. *Intern Med* 39(10): 794-797

Holgate ST (2008) Pathogenesis of asthma. *Clin Exp Allergy* 38(6): 872-897

Horvath G, Wanner A (2006) Inhaled corticosteroids: effects on the airway vasculature in bronchial asthma. *Eur Respir J* 27(1): 172-187

Ito K, Chung KF, Adcock IM (2006) Update on glucocorticoid action and resistance. *J Allergy Clin Immunol* 117(3): 522-543

Jackson DJ, Evans MD, Gangnon RE, Tisler CJ, Pappas TE, Lee WM, Gern JE, Lemanske RF, Jr. (2011a) Evidence for a Causal Relationship between Allergic Sensitization and Rhinovirus Wheezing in Early Life. *Am J Respir Crit Care Med* 185(3): 281-285

Jackson DJ, Sykes A, Mallia P, Johnston SL (2011b) Asthma exacerbations: origin, effect, and prevention. *J Allergy Clin Immunol* 128(6): 1165-1174

Jones AM, Munavvar M, Vail A, Aldridge RE, Hopkinson L, Rayner C, O'Driscoll BR (2002) Prospective, placebo-controlled trial of 5 vs 10 days of oral prednisolone in acute adult asthma. *Respir Med* 96(11): 950-954

Kelly HW (2007) Levalbuterol for asthma: a better treatment? *Curr Allergy Asthma Rep* 7(4): 310-314

Khetsuriani N, Kazerouni NN, Erdman DD, Lu X, Redd SC, Anderson LJ, Teague WG (2007) Prevalence of viral respiratory tract infections in children with asthma. *J Allergy Clin Immunol* 119(2): 314-321

Khoo SM, Lim TK (2009) Effects of inhaled versus systemic corticosteroids on exhaled nitric oxide in severe acute asthma. *Respir Med* 103(4): 614-620

Krishnan JA, Davis SQ, Naureckas ET, Gibson P, Rowe BH (2009) An umbrella review: corticosteroid therapy for adults with acute asthma. *Am J Med* 122(11): 977-991

Kumar SD, Brieva JL, Danta I, Wanner A (2000) Transient effect of inhaled fluticasone on airway mucosal blood flow in subjects with and without asthma. *Am J Respir Crit Care Med* 161(3 Pt 1): 918-921

Kumar SD, Emery MJ, Atkins ND, Danta I, Wanner A (1998) Airway mucosal blood flow in bronchial asthma. *Am J Respir Crit Care Med* 158(1): 153-156

Lee-Wong M, Dayrit FM, Kohli AR, Acquah S, Mayo PH (2002) Comparison of high-dose inhaled flunisolide to systemic corticosteroids in severe adult asthma. *Chest* 122(4): 1208-1213

Levy ML, Stevenson C, Maslen T (1996) Comparison of short courses of oral prednisolone and fluticasone propionate in the treatment of adults with acute exacerbations of asthma in primary care. *Thorax* 51(11): 1087-1092

Li JT, Ford LB, Chervinsky P, Weisberg SC, Kellerman DJ, Faulkner KG, Herje NE, Hamedani A, Harding SM, Shah T (1999) Fluticasone propionate powder and lack of clinically significant effects on hypothalamic-pituitary-adrenal axis and bone mineral density over 2 years in adults with mild asthma. *J Allergy Clin Immunol* 103(6): 1062-1068

Lima JJ, Blake KV, Tantisira KG, Weiss ST (2009) Pharmacogenetics of asthma. *Curr Opin Pulm Med* 15(1): 57-62

Lin RY, Pesola GR, Bakalchuk L, Heyl GT, Dow AM, Tenenbaum C, Curry A, Westfal RE (1999) Rapid improvement of peak flow in asthmatic patients treated with parenteral methylprednisolone in the emergency department: A randomized controlled study. *Ann Emerg Med* 33(5): 487-494

Littenberg B, Gluck EH (1986) A controlled trial of methylprednisolone in the emergency treatment of acute asthma. *N Engl J Med* 314(3): 150-152

Losel R, Wehling M (2003) Nongenomic actions of steroid hormones. *Nat Rev Mol Cell Biol* 4(1): 46-56

Lowenberg M, Stahn C, Hommes DW, Buttgereit F (2008) Novel insights into mechanisms of glucocorticoid action and the development of new glucocorticoid receptor ligands. *Steroids* 73(9-10): 1025-1029

Lowenberg M, Tuynman J, Bilderbeek J, Gaber T, Buttgereit F, van Deventer S, Peppelenbosch M, Hommes D (2005) Rapid immunosuppressive effects of glucocorticoids mediated through Lck and Fyn. *Blood* 106(5): 1703-1710

Lowenberg M, Verhaar AP, van den Brink GR, Hommes DW (2007) Glucocorticoid signaling: a nongenomic mechanism for T-cell immunosuppression. *Trends Mol Med* 13(4): 158-163

Manser R, Reid D, Abramson M (2001) Corticosteroids for acute severe asthma in hospitalised patients. *Cochrane Database Syst Rev*(1): CD001740

Marquette CH, Stach B, Cardot E, Bervar JF, Saulnier F, Lafitte JJ, Goldstein P, Wallaert B, Tonnel AB (1995) High-dose and low-dose systemic corticosteroids are equally efficient in acute severe asthma. *Eur Respir J* 8(1): 22-27

Mendes ES, Pereira A, Danta I, Duncan RC, Wanner A (2003) Comparative bronchial vasoconstrictive efficacy of inhaled glucocorticosteroids. *Eur Respir J* 21(6): 989-993

Moore WC, Bleecker ER, Curran-Everett D, Erzurum SC, Ameredes BT, Bacharier L, Calhoun WJ, Castro M, Chung KF, Clark MP, Dweik RA, Fitzpatrick AM, Gaston B, Hew M, Hussain I, Jarjour NN, Israel E, Levy BD, Murphy JR, Peters SP, Teague WG, Meyers DA, Busse WW, Wenzel SE (2007) Characterization of the severe asthma phenotype by the National Heart, Lung, and Blood Institute's Severe Asthma Research Program. *J Allergy Clin Immunol* 119(2): 405-413

Morris CR, Becker AB, Pinieiro A, Massaad R, Green SA, Smugar SS, Gurner DM (2010) A randomized, placebo-controlled study of intravenous montelukast in children with acute asthma. *Ann Allergy Asthma Immunol* 104(2): 161-171

Murray CS (2008) Can inhaled corticosteroids influence the natural history of asthma? *Curr Opin Allergy Clin Immunol* 8(1): 77-81

Nuhoglu Y, Atas E, Nuhoglu C, Iscan M, Ozcay S (2005) Acute effect of nebulized budesonide in asthmatic children. *J Investig Allergol Clin Immunol* 15(3): 197-200

Parameswaran K, Belda J, Rowe BH (2000) Addition of intravenous aminophylline to beta2-agonists in adults with acute asthma. *Cochrane Database Syst Rev*(4): CD002742

Pelkonen A, Kari O, Selroos O, Nikander K, Haahtela T, Turpeinen M (2008) Ophthalmologic findings in children with asthma receiving inhaled budesonide. *J Allergy Clin Immunol* 122(4): 832-834

Peters SP, Jones CA, Haselkorn T, Mink DR, Valacer DJ, Weiss ST (2007) Real-world Evaluation of Asthma Control and Treatment (REACT): findings from a national Web-based survey. *J Allergy Clin Immunol* 119(6): 1454-1461

Pollack CV, Jr., Pollack ES, Baren JM, Smith SR, Woodruff PG, Clark S, Camargo CA (2002) A prospective multicenter study of patient factors associated with hospital admission from the emergency department among children with acute asthma. *Archives of pediatrics & adolescent medicine* 156: 934-940

Qureshi F, Pestian J, Davis P, Zaritsky A (1998) Effect of nebulized ipratropium on the hospitalization rates of children with asthma. *N Engl J Med* 339(15): 1030-1035

Rabe KF, Vermeire PA, Soriano JB, Maier WC (2000) Clinical management of asthma in 1999: the Asthma Insights and Reality in Europe (AIRE) study. *Eur Respir J* 16(5): 802-807

Ratto D, Alfaro C, Sipsey J, Glovsky MM, Sharma OP (1988) Are intravenous corticosteroids required in status asthmaticus? *JAMA* 260(4): 527-529

Rodrigo C, Rodrigo G (1994) Early administration of hydrocortisone in the emergency room treatment of acute asthma: a controlled clinical trial. *Respir Med* 88(10): 755-761

Rodrigo G (2006) Rapid Effects of Inhaled Corticosteroids in Acute Asthma: An Evidence-Based Evaluation. *Chest* 130(5): 1301-1311

Rodrigo G, Rodrigo C (1999) Corticosteroids in the emergency department therapy of acute adult asthma: an evidence-based evaluation. *Chest* 116(2): 285-295

Rodrigo GJ (2005) Comparison of inhaled fluticasone with intravenous hydrocortisone in the treatment of adult acute asthma. *Am J Respir Crit Care Med* 171(11): 1231-1236

Rodrigo GJ, Castro-Rodriguez JA (2005) Anticholinergics in the treatment of children and adults with acute asthma: a systematic review with meta-analysis. *Thorax* 60(9): 740-746

Rodrigo GJ, Rodrigo C (2002) Continuous vs intermittent beta-agonists in the treatment of acute adult asthma: a systematic review with meta-analysis. *Chest* 122(1): 160-165

Rowe BH, Bota GW, Fabris L, Therrien SA, Milner RA, Jacono J (1999) Inhaled budesonide in addition to oral corticosteroids to prevent asthma relapse following discharge from the emergency department: a randomized controlled trial. *JAMA* 281(22): 2119-2126

Rowe BH, Edmonds ML, Spooner CH, Diner B, Camargo CA, Jr. (2004) Corticosteroid therapy for acute asthma. *Respir Med* 98(4): 275-284

Rowe BH, Spooner C, Ducharme FM, Bretzlaff JA, Bota GW (2001) Early emergency department treatment of acute asthma with systemic corticosteroids. *Cochrane Database Syst Rev*(1): CD002178

Scarfone RJ, Fuchs SM, Nager AL, Shane SA (1993) Controlled trial of oral prednisone in the emergency department treatment of children with acute asthma. *Pediatrics* 92(4): 513-518

Scarfone RJ, Loiselle JM, Wiley JF, 2nd, Decker JM, Henretig FM, Joffe MD (1995) Nebulized dexamethasone versus oral prednisone in the emergency treatment of asthmatic children. *Ann Emerg Med* 26(4): 480-486

Schacke H, Docke WD, Asadullah K (2002) Mechanisms involved in the side effects of glucocorticoids. *Pharmacol Ther* 96(1): 23-43

Schneider SM, Pipher A, Britton HL, Borok Z, Harcup CH (1988) High-dose methylprednisolone as initial therapy in patients with acute bronchospasm. *J Asthma* 25(4): 189-193

Schuh S, Dick PT, Stephens D, Hartley M, Khaikin S, Rodrigues L, Coates AL (2006) High-dose inhaled fluticasone does not replace oral prednisolone in children with mild to moderate acute asthma. *Pediatrics* 118(2): 644-650

Schuh S, Reisman J, Alshehri M, Dupuis A, Corey M, Arseneault R, Alothman G, Tennis O, Canny G (2000) A comparison of inhaled fluticasone and oral prednisone for children with severe acute asthma. *N Engl J Med* 343(10): 689-694

Schuh S, Willan AR, Stephens D, Dick PT, Coates A (2009) Can montelukast shorten prednisolone therapy in children with mild to moderate acute asthma? A randomized controlled trial. *J Pediatr* 155(6): 795-800

Sharek PJ, Bergman DA (2000) The effect of inhaled steroids on the linear growth of children with asthma: a meta-analysis. *Pediatrics* 106(1): E8

Stahn C, Buttgereit F (2008) Genomic and nongenomic effects of glucocorticoids. *Nat Clin Pract Rheumatol* 4(10): 525-533

Subbarao P, Mandhane PJ, Sears MR (2009) Asthma: epidemiology, etiology and risk factors. *CMAJ* 181(9): E181-190

Subcommittee on clinical trials in asthma MRC (1956) CONTROLLED trial of effects of cortisone acetate in status asthmaticus. *Lancet* 271(6947): 803-806

Suissa S, Ernst P, Benayoun S, Baltzan M, Cai B (2000) Low-dose inhaled corticosteroids and the prevention of death from asthma. *N Engl J Med* 343(5): 332-336

Sung L, Osmond MH, Klassen TP (1998) Randomized, controlled trial of inhaled budesonide as an adjunct to oral prednisone in acute asthma. *Acad Emerg Med* 5(3): 209-213

Szefler SJ, Phillips BR, Martinez FD, Chinchilli VM, Lemanske RF, Strunk RC, Zeiger RS, Larsen G, Spahn JD, Bacharier LB, Bloomberg GR, Guilbert TW, Heldt G, Morgan WJ, Moss MH, Sorkness CA, Taussig LM (2005) Characterization of within-subject responses to fluticasone and montelukast in childhood asthma. *J Allergy Clin Immunol* 115(2): 233-242

Todi VK, Lodha R, Kabra SK (2010) Effect of addition of single dose of oral montelukast to standard treatment in acute moderate to severe asthma in children between 5 and 15 years of age: a randomised, double-blind, placebo controlled trial. *Arch Dis Child* 95(7): 540-543

Travers AH, Rowe BH, Barker S, Jones A, Camargo CA, Jr. (2002) The effectiveness of IV beta-agonists in treating patients with acute asthma in the emergency department: a meta-analysis. *Chest* 122(4): 1200-1207

Upham BD, Mollen CJ, Scarfone RJ, Seiden J, Chew A, Zorc JJ (2011) Nebulized budesonide added to standard pediatric emergency department treatment of acute asthma: a randomized, double-blind trial. *Acad Emerg Med* 18(7): 665-673

Wanner A, Horvath G, Brieva JL, Kumar SD, Mendes ES (2004) Nongenomic actions of glucocorticosteroids on the airway vasculature in asthma. *Proceedings of the American Thoracic Society* 1(3): 235-238

Zorc JJ, Pusic MV, Ogborn CJ, Lebet R, Duggan AK (1999) Ipratropium bromide added to asthma treatment in the pediatric emergency department. *Pediatrics* 103(4 Pt 1): 748-752

Chapter 20

Glucocorticoid Resistance in the Upper Respiratory Airways

Fabiana C.P. Valera, Edwin Tamashiro and Wilma T. Anselmo-Lima

Additional information is available at the end of the chapter

http://dx.doi.org/10.5772/53105

1. Introduction

The nasal mucosa is known to be the first important barrier against inhalants of the respiratory tract. In contrast to initial opinion, this tissue actively interacts with external factors, producing a wide combination of mediators in response to aggressor agents [1]. In this respect, it is easy to understand why the nasal mucosa is predisposed to the development of several chronic inflammatory diseases, with rhinitis and rhinosinusitis being the most common disorders.

According to the ARIA guideline [2], the prevalence of allergic rhinitis has increased in the last years and has been found to be around 25% in Europe [3]. The prevalence of symptoms related to chronic rhinosinusitis is about 15% in the USA, being the second most prevalent chronic condition in the American population [4].

The most common and studied cause of chronic rhinitis is allergic rhinitis (AR) [2]. AR is a nasal inflammatory disease in which the allergen induces IgE-mediated inflammation. The mediators released by the nasal mucosa will finally lead to intense inflammatory cell recruitment (predominantly eosinophils) [5], epithelial metaplasia (more pronounced in perennial AR) [6], and noticeable stromal edema, especially due to the action of matrix metalloproteinases [7]. This response to allergens will finally induce the classical symptoms of AR, such as sneezing, itching, nasal discharge and nasal obstruction. These symptoms considerably impair the quality of life, affecting sleep quality, concentration during work/school, and other daily activities [2].

Chronic rhinosinusitis can be subdivided into two forms: chronic rhinosinusitis without nasal polyps (CRSsNP) and with nasal polyps (CRSwNP). These two entities are almost clinically identical, and it is very difficult to differentiate them based only on nasal symptoms [8]. Both forms present variable degrees of facial pain, decreased sense of smell, nasal discharge and nasal congestion. Clinically, the differentiation of these two entities is made by the detection of nasal polyps by nasal endoscopy. However, the major differences between CRSsNP and CRSwNP concern histology and molecular biomarkers [9]. CRSsNP is characterized by neutrophil recruitment, light edema, increased remodelling [9] and a Th1-subset profile. In contrast, CRSwNP is characterized by an eosinophil recruitment, intense oedema, loose connective tissue and a Th1/Th2 mixed –subset profile, but with remarkable Th2 polarization [8-10].

2. Cellular and molecular knowledge in nasal inflammatory diseases

2.1. Allergic Rhinitis

The development of signs and symptoms that characterize allergic rhinitis (AR) depends on three events: sensitization to an allergen, degranulation of inflammatory mediators after re-exposure to the allergen (early phase) and infiltration of inflammatory cells into the tissue (late phase).

The respiratory nasal mucosa is continuously exposed to several particles that are deposited on the mucous blanket that covers the respiratory epithelium. These antigens are processed by antigen-presenting cells (APCs) such as Langerhans cells, that are later presented to a naïve lymphocyte through a major histocompatibility complex (MHC) class II molecule [11]. For reasons not completely elucidated, naïve lymphocytes (Th0) differentiate into Th2 lymphocytes and produce and release a pool of cytokines characteristic of the Th2 response pattern (IL-3, IL-4, IL-5, IL-9, IL-10, IL-13, GM-CSF). Moreover, the differentiated Th2 lymphocytes stimulate the production of specific IgE by plasmocytes through IL-3 and IL-4, and inhibit the differentiation of Th0 lymphocytes into Th1, as well as its messenger molecules. This selective environment polarized to a Th2 response is typically seen in allergic mechanisms, such as AR, asthma and atopic dermatitis, and in helminthic infections. B cells that recognize the processed antigen and receive appropriate contact signals (CD40-CD40) and molecular stimuli (IL-4, IL-6, IL-10, IL-13) start to produce specific IgE. In the presence of continuous antigen stimulation, B-cells switch from the production of a low-affinity IgE molecule to the production of a high-affinity one [11].

Once high-affinity IgE circulates in the plasma and interstitial fluid, it binds to the Fc receptors. These receptors are present on the surface of mast cells and basophils, and are responsible for activating these cells when exposed to the binomial antibody-pathogen. After mast cells leave the post-capillary venules, they are able to reside in the stroma of the nasal submucosa and intraepithelially, probably by the production of several proteases. Resident mast cells are also able to produce some cytokines related to Th2 polarization (IL-4, IL-5), which in turn can cause an increased cell proliferation and survival time. In allergic mucosa, for instance, mast cells proliferate at a higher rate compared to a non-allergic environment, probably by the effect of Th2 cytokines [12, 13].

In a second phase, after sensitization and priming of resident mast cells with IgE, the respiratory mucosa becomes susceptible to a new exposure. When the specific inspired allergen binds to the complex IgE-mediator cell, massive degranulation of allergic molecules (either already existent and newly synthetized) are released in the extracellular compartment. Histamine is the main molecule released and involved in the early phase of symptoms of AR, but other mediators such as leukotriene, bradykinin, prostaglandins, platelet activating factor, and even some proteases (tryptase and chymase) and cytokines (TNF-α, IL-4, IL-5) also have a role in the development of allergic symptoms [14]. These mediators lead to the classical early symptoms of sneezing, itching, rhinorrhea, and nasal congestion that occur within a few minutes after allergen exposure (5-30 minutes). These symptoms are the consequence of direct actions of these mediators on different resident cells [15]. Glands are stimulated by leukotrienes and chymases to produce and release mucous secretions. Endothelial cells of post-capillary venules are affected by histamine, bradykinin, platelet activating factor and leukotrienes, inducing vasodilatation, increased vascular permeability and cell adhesion. Peripheral sensory endings are stimulated by histamine type 1 receptors on nociceptive type C fibers that generate an uncomfortable sensation of pain and pressure, sneezing and itching [16]. As the nasal mucosa is constantly assaulted by physical and chemical agents, the disruption of some areas facilitates the exposure of allergens to allergic mediator cells.

After the IgE-mediated inflammatory burst triggered by the allergen, some individuals present total clearance of mediators and have complete resolution of symptoms after some minutes. However, a significant percentage (60-70%) of the allergic population develops the late AR response due to the recruitment of inflammatory cells into the nasal mucosa. The increased vascular permeability added to the expression of adhesion molecules (ICAM-1) and production of chemokines, recruits a variety of inflammatory cells that include eosinophils and basophils and, to a lesser extent, neutrophils and other leukocytes.

The late phase typically occurs 4-6 hours after the allergen contact and is clinically represented by the nasal obstruction and congestion caused by mucosal edema. Toxic products of eosinophils, such as eosinophil cationic protein (ECP), major basic protein (MBP), eosinophil-derived neurotoxin and eosinophil peroxidase, are evident during the late phase and are proportional to the eosinophil recruitment. These highly charged proteins bind to proteoglycans and hyaluronic acid and cause cell damage and epithelial detachment. Other important inflammatory mediators involved in the late phase are leukotrienes, histamine, and cytokines of the Th2 response (IL-5, IL-6, GM-CSF) [17, 18]. Interestingly, the recruited eosinophils are able to promote an auto-positive feedback to prolong their survival and recruitment into the tissue, which ultimately leads to an independent eosinophilic inflammation (Figure 1). IL-3, IL-5, and GM-CSF are Th2 cytokines that reduce apoptosis and prolong eosinophil cell survival. Besides, IL-5, eotaxin and RANTES produced by eosinophils and other infiltrated cells recruit even more eosinophils to the inflammatory site, explaining the reason why a chronic allergic inflammation can be seen even when the allergen is not present [19].

Lymphocytes are another group of cells that may play an important role in the late phase of AR. Memory T cells, T-cytotoxic and B cells have been demonstrated to be increased in AR compared to other forms of non-allergic rhinitis and to controls [20].

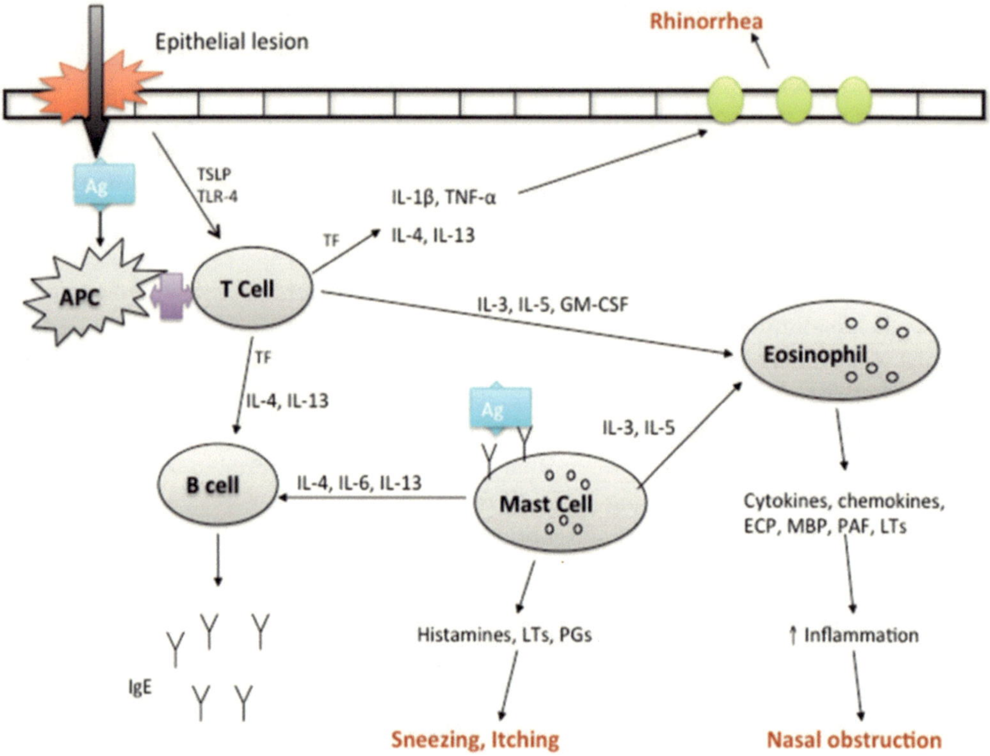

Figure legend: Ag: antigen; APC: antigen presenting cell; TSLP: thymic stromal lymphopoietin; TLR: toll-like receptor; IL: interleukin; TNF: tumor necrosis factor; TF: transcriptor factor; Ig: immunoglobulin; GM-CSF: granulocyte macrophage colony-stimulating factor; LT: leukotriene; PG: prostaglandin; ECP: eosinophil cationic protein; MBP: major basic protein; PAF: platelet activating factor

Figure 1. Cellular and molecular events involved in the early and late phase response of AR. Initially, the antigen invades the cell, and either binds to the APC (antigen presenting cell) or activates innate immune response through TSLP or TLR-4. These mechanisms together will activate adaptative immune response, and T cells are triggered to Th2 response, producing cytokines as IL-4, IL-5 and IL-13. These cytokines will induce epithelial cells to produce rhinorrhea and will recruit inflammatory cells (as eosinophils) to nasal mucosa. Eosinophils will produce several cytokines that will lead to nasal obstruction. B cells are activated and produce IgE, which, among the antigen itself, will induce the mast cell to secrete histamine, leukotrienes and prostaglandins, among others, finally leading to the symptoms of sneezing and itching.

Resident cells may also participate in the late phase and development of chronic allergic inflammation. Nasal epithelial cells express an increased number of pro-inflammatory cytokines such as IL-1α, IL-1β, IL-6, IL-8 and GM-CSF in allergic patients [21, 22]. Also, epithelial cells are the main source of thymic stromal lymphopoietin (TSLP) on the nasal mucosa, an important cytokine that drives T cells to produce Th2 cytokines [23] and is increased in AR patients compared to controls [24]. Submucosal glands located in the lamina propria are substantially increased in allergic patients (25%) compared to non-allergic individuals (15%), consistent with the chronic state of increased production of nasal secretions [25]

In summary, the cellular and molecular mechanisms of AR involve B cell production of IgE and mast cell/basophil priming, activation of resident cells, recruitment of inflammatory cells and, in some circumstances, induction of a persistent inflammatory reaction maintained by a positive feedback.

2.2. Chronic Rhinosinusitis (CRS)

Chronic Rhinosinusitis (CRS) is clinically defined as the persistence of signs and symptoms such as nasal obstruction, nasal congestion, rhinorrhea, facial pain, cough, and loss of smell for more than 12 weeks, confirmed by nasal endoscopy or computed tomography. It is related to an inflammatory process of the mucoperiosteal pavement of the sinonasal cavity, whose etiology can be clearly defined in a few subgroups of patients, involving mechanical obstruction, immunodeficiency, cystic fibrosis, and ciliary dyskinesia. However, in the majority of cases, the etiology of CRS cannot be determined. Some investigators have raised different hypotheses for the pathogenesis of CRS such as disruption of the epithelial barrier, allergy, exposure to pollutants, maintenance of mucosal inflammation due to underlying osteitis, persistence of bacterial biofilms, and overreaction to staphylococcal superantigens or fungus. It is interesting to note that individually these theories do not apply to all patients but may explain the pathogenicity in some cases. Despite the unrevealed etiopathogenesis, recent advances have been made in the elucidation of the cellular and molecular events involved in different situations of CRS. Based on molecular phenotyping studies, the classification of CRS into two different clinical subsets has been currently accepted: CRS without nasal polyps (CRS *sine* NP, CRSsNP) and CRS with nasal polyps (CRSwNP) [8, 26]. Clinically, the symptoms of both types are very similar to each other, with slight differences in the severity of nasal congestion, nasal obstruction, rhinorrhea, postnasal drip, change in the sense of smell, cough, and facial pain. In terms of physical examination, they differ by the presence or absence of nasal polyps extruding from the middle meatus of the nasal cavity. This simple difference noted by nasal endoscopy involves profound differences in cellular and molecular aspects that might be related to the prognosis and treatment of these two subsets of CRS.

Histologically, both forms of CRS are marked by niches of denuded respiratory epithelium with associated metaplasia, basal membrane thickening, and goblet cell hyperplasia. The histology of submucosal stroma demonstrates clear differences between CRSwNP and CRSsNP. In CRSwNP, the submucosal stroma usually is found with robust edema and low cellularity, in contrast to CRSsNP that characteristically involves more pronounced fibrosis and less edema [9].

In CRSwNP, eosinophilic infiltration is the hallmark of chronic inflammation. For reasons not fully elucidated, there is an increased expression of pro-inflammatory cytokines (IL-1β) mediated by transcription factors. These cytokines mediate the recruitment of inflammatory cells (eosinophils, lymphocytes, neutrophils, mast cells) through the up-regulation and expression of adhesion molecules (ICAM-1, VCAM-1) and chemokines (IL-8, eotaxin, and RANTES). In CRSwNP, the striking influx of inflammatory cells, especially eosinophils, into the stroma, leads to a positive feedback recruitment similar to allergic rhinitis [27]. In the

Caucasian CRS population, nasal polyps are remarkably characterized by a mixed expression of Th1 (INF-γ, IL-8) and Th2 cytokines, with an imbalance favoring the Th2 response. Th2 cytokines (IL-3, IL-5, GM-CSF) are produced by eosinophils and Th2 cells and increase eosinophil recruitment and survival, creating an autonomous inflammatory cycle even after the removal of the initial trigger. (Figure 2)

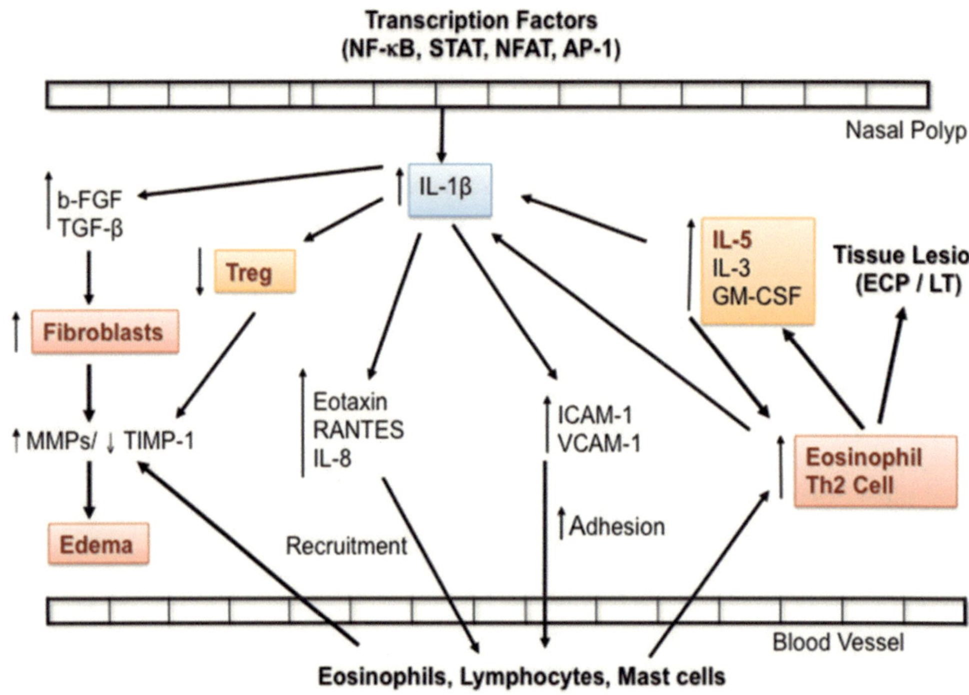

Figure legend: NF-κB: nuclear factor- κB; STAT: signal transducers and activators of tranascription; NFAT: nuclear factor of activated T-cells; AP: activator protein; IL: interleukin; FGF: fibroblast growth factor; TGF: transforming growth factor; Treg: regulatory T cell; GM-CSF: granulocyte-macrophage colony-stimulating factor; ECP: eosinophil cationic protein; LT: leukotriene; MMP: matrix metalloproteinase; TIMP: tissue inhibitor of metalloproteinase; RANTES: regulated on activation, normal T cell expressed and secreted; ICAM: intercellular adhesion molecule; VCAM: vascular cell adhesion molecule; Th: T helper cell

Figure 2. Cellular and molecular events involved in the pathogenesis of CRSwNP.

Despite the similarities to allergic rhinitis and contrary to some speculations raised in the first studies, the eosinophilic infiltration and activation found in CRSwNP is not dependent on allergic mechanisms mediated by IgE [28, 29]. In the Chinese population, however, CRSwNP has been characterized by a different Th pattern of inflammation. A mixed Th1/Th17 has been found instead of the Th1/Th2 pattern, with a significantly lower GATA-3 (Th2 specific) expression and higher IL-17 levels in the polyp tissue. The Th17 response drives a more neutrophilic infiltration rather than an eosinophilic recruitment [30].

Another important feature of CRSwNP is the impaired regulatory modulation promoted by Treg cells, which balances the T helper cell response. Low levels of Treg cell biomarkers (transforming growth factor-β1 -TGF-β1- and forkhead box protein P3 -FOXP3) together with high expression of T-bet (Th1) and GATA-3 (Th2) demonstrate the deficiency of Treg control in CRSwNP patients [31].

In terms of molecular markers, among Caucasians, IL-5 is the most important cytokine found in CRSwNP. IL-5 is related to eosinophil infiltration and activation, and is significantly related to recurrence of nasal polyps after surgical removal [32]. Activated eosinophils also release several inflammatory mediators, such as leukotrienes, and other toxic products (Eosinophil Cationic Protein – ECP, Major Basic Protein – MBP, neurotoxin eosinophil protein). Besides the damage induced by infiltrated inflammatory cells, resident fibroblasts also play a role in the structural modification of the stroma. Stimulated by fibroblast growth factor (FGF) and TGF-β, fibroblasts are recruited, proliferate, and express matrix metalloproteinases (MMP), which degrade extracellular proteins (collagen, laminin, fibronectin, elastin) and favor tissue edema and albumin deposition. Other cells such as eosinophils and neutrophils are also able to produce MMP and may play a role in tissue remodeling [33]. Furthermore, fibroblasts suppress the expression of tissue inhibitors of metalloproteinases (TIMP) which increase the activity of MMP. Taken together, these features explain the main histopathological and molecular findings in CRSwNP, i.e., eosinophilic infiltration, tissue edema, and Th2 skewing polarization.

On the other hand, CRSsNP present some different features compared to CRSwNP. Although mixed inflammatory cells are found in CRSsNP, neutrophils are the predominant cells in this subset of CRS and, together with Th1 cells. seem to play the main cellular role in the pathogenesis of the disease. Neutrophil markers of activation such as myeloperoxidase and IL-8 are found in high levels in CRSsNP compared to controls and CRSwNP. Besides, the levels of Th1 cytokines (INF-γ, IL-8) found in CRSsNP are unbalanced with Th2 cytokines, revealing Th1 polarization. In contrast to CRSwNP, FOXP3 and TGF-β are not decreased in CRSsNP, demonstrating that Treg function is not altered in CRSsNP [31]. The up-regulated TGF- β signaling pathways are believed to be an important marker that reflects the fibrosis/albumin deposition remarkably seen in CRSsNP. (Figure 3)

In conclusion, in contrast to CRSwNP, the cellular and molecular findings in CRSsNP are characterized by neutrophilic infiltration, tissue fibrosis, and Th1 skewing polarization.

3. Glucocorticoid action on nasal mucosa

Glucocorticoid (GC) has a broad anti-inflammatory effect, regulating both innate and adaptive immune responses in a wide variety of cells, such as epithelial cells, fibroblasts, eosinophils and T cells [1, 12, 34]. This is the main reason why GC is considered to be the medication of choice to treat chronic rhinitis [2] and rhinosinusitis [8].

This wide anti-inflammatory effect of GC is explained by several events induced by it, from the signaling event to post-translational mechanisms. Basically, GC is a lipophilic compound which diffuses though the membrane and binds to its cytoplasmic receptor, called glucocorticoid receptor (GR) [35].

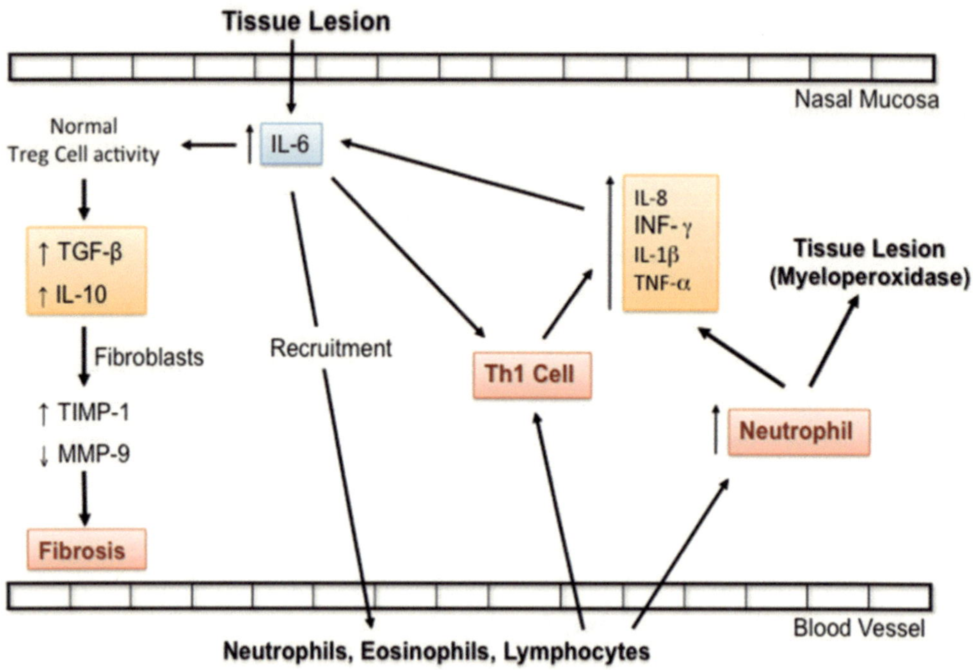

Figure legend: Treg: regulatory T cell; IL: interleukin; INF: interferon; TNF: tumor necrosis factor; Th: T helper cell; TGF: transforming growth factor; TIMP: tissue inhibitor of metalloproteinase; MMP: metalloproteinase

Figure 3. Cellular and molecular events involved in the pathogenesis of CRSsNP.

GR belongs to a large superfamily of steroid receptors. When inactivated, this receptor stays in the cytosol bound to heat shock proteins (hsp) [36]. When GC binds to GR, phosphorylation occurs to this receptor, which dissociates GR from hsp. The dimer GC-GR is able to translocate into the nucleus and then act as a transcription factor. In this respect, the GC-GR dimer can bind directly to a specific palindromic DNA consensus sequence, called glucocorticoid response elements (GREs), and consequently induces or inhibits (in case of nGREs) the transcription of several genes [35]. Nevertheless, it is recognized that the main anti-inflammatory action of GC at the transcriptional level is mediated by a direct interaction of GC-GR with other transcription factors (TF), inhibiting their action. This inhibition, called "DNA-independent transrepression" affects several pro-inflammatory TF, the most important ones being activator protein-1 (AP-1) and nuclear fator-κB (NF-κB) [1, 35-39] (Figure 4). This connection inhibits gene transcription by direct binding to DNA or by inducing histone deacetylation. Although the non-genomic effect of GC is widely known in the literature [2, 17], there is no report on its effect on chronic upper respiratory diseases, and only few studies have reported controversial results regarding asthma [40, 41].

The final effect of GC on nasal diseases is the inhibition of pro-inflammatory cytokines (IL-1β, TNF-α, GM-CSF, IL-3, IL-5, IL-6), chemokines (IL-8, RANTES, eotaxin) and adhesion molecules (VCAM-1, ICAM-1) [1, 13, 42]. Glucocorticoids also have a favorable effect on tissue remodeling (reducing MMP expression) [43, 44], reduce mucin production [45], increase cell apoptosis [46, 47], and decrease mast cell recruitment and activation [48].

Finally, glucocorticoids inhibit the expression of some cytokine receptors, among them IL-2 and IL-4 receptors.

Due to its holistic action, GC is considered to be the best medication for the treatment of chronic inflammatory diseases of the upper respiratory airways.

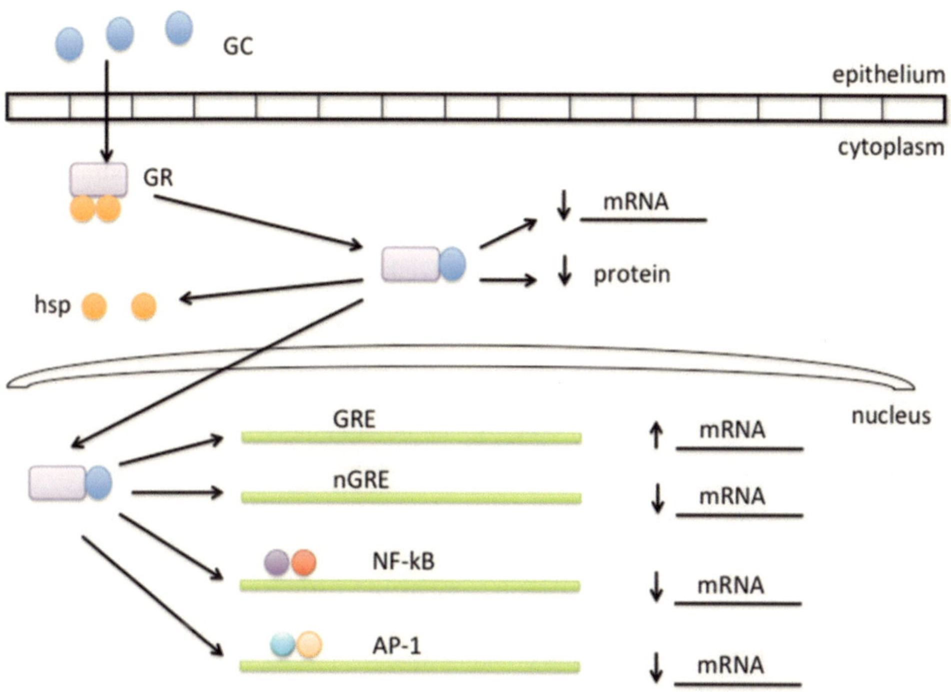

Figure 4. GC mode of action: binding to its cytoplasmic GR, and then translocating into the nucleus. GC: glucocorticoid; GR: glucocorticoid receptor; hsp: heat shock protein; GRE: glucocorticoid response element; NF-κB: nuclear factor κB; AP-1: activator protein-1

4. GR splicing

The GR gene is located in chromosome 5 and is composed of 9 exons. Alternative splicing in the ninth exon (hormone-binding domain) gives raise to several alternative GRs, GRα and GRβ being the most common [35-39].

GRα is the predominant GR isoform. It is transcriptionally active and, when ligated to GC, it can translocate into the nucleus, induce expression by binding to GRE, or repress expression by either binding to nGRE or by interacting with AP-1 and NF-κB [1, 35, 36].

For instance, GRβ is expressed at much lower rates than GRα. It cannot bind to GC, and although it can bind to GRE, nGRE, AP-1 and NF-κB, it does not activate their transcriptional action. Some authors have shown that, when overexpressed, GRβ inhibits the effect of GRα on both transactivation and on AP-1 and NF-κB repression [49-51]. GRβ is thus considered to be the dominant negative of GRα; instead, a recent study has shown that a glucocorticoid antagonist, named RU-486, has the ability to bind to GRβ, regulating gene expression even in the absence of GRα [52].

There is no previous study regarding the influence of GRγ on nasal mucosa.

5. Resistance to GC

Although GC is the medication of choice in chronic upper respiratory diseases in general, the rate of CG therapy failure in CRSwNP is reported to be between 60 and 80% [8]. Although there is no report on GC resistance in chronic rhinitis, resistance is believed to be identical to that occurring in CRSwNP. The main reasons for GC failure are: limited action of topical GC in extensive diseases [53], poor compliance with treatment [54] , and cellular/molecular resistance to GC [36, 55]. Among cellular and molecular mechanisms of GC resistance, the main lines investigated are GRα- GRβ interaction and TF influence.

One of the most studied mechanisms is the GRα-GRβ imbalance. Although GRβ is able to interact directly with GRα within the nucleus, it has a low capacity to bind to GC. This is why GRβ is considered to be an endogenous inhibitor of GRα [36, 56]. GRα-GRβ imbalance has been reported to increase cell resistance in chronic immune-mediated diseases, among those affecting the upper [37, 57] and lower airways [58, 59].

Increased expression of GRβ has been widely reported in the literature on inflammatory respiratory diseases such as CRSwNP and asthma, when compared to control mucosa [36, 55, 60, 61]. This has led to the hypothesis that increased GRβ expression could impair the action of GC. Decreased expression of GRα has also been recently reported in CRswNP with the use of a more reliable quantitative method of analysis [56, 62, 63]. More important than the expression of each individual isoform, GRα-GRβ imbalance might be the most relevant determinant of GC resistance. It is important to mention that some studies have demonstrated that CG therapy in CRSwNP does not change GR isoform expression or the GRα-GRβ relation [56, 63, 64].

Higher expression of TF could also lead to GC resistance, because TF (mainly AP-1 and NF-κB) repress the binding of the translocated GC-GR complex to GRE. This mechanism of GC resistance has been reported in several inflammatory diseases, such as inflammatory bowel diseases. Nevertheless, this mechanism has been poorly reported in respiratory diseases.

AP-1 is a dimer predominantly consisting of c-Fos/c-Jun heterodimers. As is the case for most TF, they are located in the cytoplasm and, when activated, translocate into the nucleus and induce the expression of several pro-inflammatory genes which regulate cell inflammation, proliferation, differentiation and apoptosis [65]. Conflicting results have been reported regarding the presence of AP-1 in CRSwNP. c-Fos expression has been studied in two reports because it is more important regarding the transcriptional action. One study [66] has reported an increased presence of c-Fos in patients with CRSwNP than in control mucosa using qualitative PCR, while the other [56] has observed a similar expression in the two groups using quantitative RT-PCR. The latter study also did not observe any influence of c-Fos expression on the outcome of GC treatment.

NF-κB is also a heterodimer, mainly consisting of p50 and p65 isoforms. When activated, NF-κB translocates into the nucleus, and p65 directly binds to DNA, inducing gene expression of pro-inflammatory and anti-apoptotic genes [37, 65]. NF-κB is considered pivotal to the regulation of immune and inflammatory genes, and its absence is incompatible with life. It is important to mention that the most important pro-inflammatory cytokines (IL-1β and TNF-α), whose expression is considerably influenced by NF-κB, also activate NF-κB translocation, inducing perpetuation of the inflammatory process.

Two studies have reported increased expression of both isoforms (p50 and p65) of NF-κB in patients with CRSwNP when compared to control nasal mucosa [56, 67]. Also, a high expression of p65 was related to a poor clinical outcome in response to medical treatment in CRSwNP patients [56]. This finding suggests that NF-κB may also have a pivotal effect on GC resistance.

6. Conclusions

Chronic inflammatory nasal diseases are highly prevalent in the population, and therefore nasal TGC has been widely prescribed by physicians. Considering that a high percentage of these patients only partially benefit from TGC, or do not respond to TCG treatment at all, the understanding of possible mechanisms of GC resistance is essential for future treatments.

Today, it has been accepted that cellular and molecular mechanisms of resistance do exist in nasal mucosa. Future investigations are still required to recognize affected individuals and how this would influence medical treatment. This will be essential to develop new drugs that would replace or act synergistically with CG, in order to improve the clinical outcome.

Author details

Fabiana C.P. Valera, Edwin Tamashiro and Wilma T. Anselmo-Lima
Division of Otorhinolaryngology, Departament of Ophthalmology, Otorhinolaryngology, and Head and Neck Surgery. Faculty of Medicine of Ribeirao Preto-University of São Paulo, Ribeirao Preto-SP, Brazil

7. References

[1] Stellato, C., Glucocorticoid actions on airway epithelial responses in immunity: Functional outcomes and molecular targets. J Allergy Clin Immunol 2007. 120(6): p. 1247-63.

[2] Bousquet J, K.N., Cruz AA, Denburg J, Fokkens WJ, Togias A, et al, Allergic Rhinitis and its impact on asthma (ARIA) 2008. Allergy 2008. 63: p. 8-160.

[3] Bauchau V, D.S., Prevalence and rate of diagnosis of allergic rhinitis in Europe. Eur R Espir J, 2004. 24: p. 758-764.

[4] Collins, J., Prevalence of selected chronic conditions: United States 1990-1992. Vital Health Stat, 1997. 194: p. 1-89.

[5] Bentley AM, J.M., Cumberworth V, Barkans JR, Moqbel R, Schwartz LB, et al. , Immunohistology of the nasal mucosa in seasonal allergic rhinitis: increases in activated eosinophils and epithelial mast cells. J Allergy Clin Immunol, 1992. 89: p. 877– 883.

[6] Laliberte F, L.M., Lecart S, Bousquet J, Klossec JM, Mounedji N, Clinical and pathologic methods to assess the long-term safety of nasal corticosteroids. French Triamcinolone Acetonide Study Group. . Allergy, 2000. 55(718-722).

[7] Shaida A, K.G., Devalia J, Davies RJ, MacDonald TT, Pender SL, Matrix metalloproteinases and their inhibitors in the nasal mucosa of patients with perennial allergic rhinitis. J Allergy Clin Immunol 2001. 108(5): p. 791–796.

[8] Fokkens WJ, L.V., Mullol J, Bachert C, Cohen N, Cobo R, et al. European Position Paper on Nasal Polyps 2007. Rhinology 2007, 20: 1-139., European Position Paper on Nasal Polyps 2007. Rhinology, 2007. 20: p. 1-139.

[9] Huvenne W, v.B.N., Zhang N, van Zele T, Patou J, Gevaert P, et al, Chronic Rhinosinusitis With and Without Nasal Polyps: What Is the Difference? Curr Allergy Asthma Rep, 2009. 9: p. 213–220.

[10] Jankowski R, B.F., Coffinet L, Vignaud JM, Clinical factors influencing the eosinophil infiltration of nasal polyps. Rhinology, 2002. 40: p. 173-8.

[11] Pawankar R, M.S., Ozu C, Kimura S, Overview on the pathomechanisms of allergic rhinitis. Asia Pac Allergy, 2011. 1(3): p. 157-167.

[12] Bradding P, O.Y., Howarth PH, Church MK, Holgate ST, Heterogeneity of human mast cells based on cytokines content. J Immunol, 1995. 155: p. 297-307.

[13] Kawabori Y, K.N., Tosho T, Proliferative activity of mast cells in allergic nasal mucosa. Clin Exp Allergy 1995. 25: p. 173-8.

[14] Baraniuk, J., Pathogenesis of allergic rhinitis. J Allergy Clin Immunol 1997. 99: p. S763-S772.

[15] Eccles, R., Pathophysyology of Nasal Symptoms. Am J Rhinol 2000. 14(5): p. 335-338.

[16] McDonald, D., Neurogenic inflammation in the respiratory tract: actions of sensory nerve mediators on blood vessels and epithelium of the airway mucosa. Am Rev Respir Dis, 1987. 136(6 Pt 2): p. S65-S72.

[17] Gosset P, M.F., Delnest Y, et al., Interleukin 6 and interleukin-1α production is associated with antigen induced late nasal response. J. Allergy Clin. Immunol., 1993. 94(11777-11783).

[18] Naclerio RM, B.F., Kagey-Sobotka A, Lichtenstein LM, Basophils and eosinophils in allergic rhinitis. J Allergy Clin Immunol, 1994. 94(6 Pt 2): p. 1303-1309.

[19] Moqbel R, L.-S.F., Kay AB, Cytokine generation by eosinophils. J Allergy Clin Immunol 1994. 94(6 Pt 2): p. 1183-9.

[20] Pawankar RU, O.M., Okubo K, Ra C, Lymphocyte subsets in the nasal mucosa in perennial allergic rhinitis. Am J Respir Crit Care Med, 1995. 152(6 Pt 1): p. 2049-58.

[21] Nonaka M, N.R., Jordana M, Dolovich J, GM-CSF, IL-8, IL-1R, TNF-alpha R, and HLA-DR in nasal epithelial cells in allergic rhinitis. Am J Respir Crit Care Med, 1996. 153(5): p. 1675-81.

[22] Kenney JS, B.C., Welch MR, Altman LC, Synthesis of interleukin-1 alpha, interleukin-6, and interleukin-8 by cultured human nasal epithelial cells. J Allergy Clin Immunol, 1994. 93(6): p. 1060-7.

[23] Ziegler SF, A.D., Sensing the outside world: TSLP regutates barrier immunity. Nat Immunol, 2010. 11: p. 289-293.

[24] Miyata M, N.Y., Shimokawa N, Ohnuma Y, Katoh R, Matsuoka S, Okumura K, Ogawa H, Masuyama K, Nakao A, Thymic stromal lymphopoietin is a critical mediator of IL-13-driven allergic inflammation. Eur J Immunol, 2009. 39(11): p. 3078-83.

[25] Masuda, S., Quantitative histochemistry of mucus-secreting cells in human nasal mucosa. . Pract Otol (Kyoto), 1990. 83: p. 1855-63.

[26] Van Zele T, C.S., Gevaert P, Van Maele G, Holtappels G, VanCauwenberge P, Bachert C, Differentiation of chronic sinus diseases by measurement of inflammatory mediators. Allergy 2006. 61(11): p. 1280–1289.

[27] Bachert C, G.P., Holtappels G, Cuvelier C, van Cauwenberge P, Nasal polyposis: from cytokines to growth. Am J Rhinol, 2000. 14(279–290).

[28] Min YG, L.C., Rhee CS, Kim KH, Kim CS, Koh YY, Min KU, Anderson PL, Inflammatory cytokine expression on nasal polyps developed in allergic and infectious rhinitis. Acta Otolaryngol, 1997. 117(2): p. 302-6.

[29] Lee CH, R.C., Min YG, Cytokine gene expression in nasal polyps. Ann Otol Rhinol Laryngol 1998. 107(8): p. 665-70.

[30] Zhang N, H.G., Claeys C, Huang G, van Cauwenberge P, Bachert C, Pattern of inflammation and impact of Staphylococcus aureus enterotoxins in nasal polyps from southern China. Am J Rhinol, 2006. 20(4): p. 445–450.

[31] Van Bruaene N, P.-N.C., Basinski TM, Van Zele T, Holtappels G, De Ruyck N, Schmidt-Weber C, Akdis C, Van Cauwenberge P, Bachert C, et al, T-cell regulation in chronic paranasal sinus disease. J Allergy Clin Immunol, 2008. 121(6): p. 1435–1441, 1441. 1441.e1–e3.

[32] Bachert C, W.M., Hauser U, Rudack C, IL-5 synthesis is upregulated in human nasal polyp tissue. J Allergy Clin Immunol, 1997. 99: p. 837–842.

[33] Delclaux C, D.C., D'Ortho MP, Boyer V, Lafuma C, Harf A, Role of gelatinase B and elastase in human polymorphonuclear neutrophil migration across basement membrane. Am J Respir Cell Mol Biol, 1996. 14: p. 288-295.

[34] Holm AF, F.W., Godthelp T, Mulder PG, Vroom TM, Rjintejes E, Effect of 3 month's nasal steroid therapy on nasal T cells and Langerhans cells in patients suffering from allergic rhinitis. Allergy 1995. 50: p. 204-209.

[35] Liberman AC, D.J., Perone MJ, Arzt E, Glucocorticoids in the regulation of transcription factors that control cytokine synthesis. Cytokine Growth Factor Rev, 2007. 18(1-2): p. 45-56.

[36] Pujols L, M.J., Picado C, Alpha and beta glucocorticoid receptors: relevance in airway diseases. Curr Allergy Asthma Rep, 2007. 7(2): p. 93-99.

[37] Adcock IM, C.G., Cross-talk between pro-inflammatory transcription factors and glucocorticoids. Immunol Cell Biol, 2001. 79: p. 376-384.

[38] Li Q, V.I., NF-[kappa]B regulation in the immune system. Nat Rev Immunol, 2002. 2: p. 725-734.

[39] McKay LI, C.J., Molecular control of immune/inflammatory responses: interactions between nuclear factor-kappaB and steroid receptor-signaling pathways. Endocr Rev, 1999. 20(4): p. 435-459.

[40] Stellato, C., Post-transcriptional and nongenomic effects of glucocorticoids Proc Am Thorac Soc, 2004. 1(3): p. 255-263.

[41] Urbach V, V.V., Grumbach Y, Bousquet J, Harvey BJ, Rapid anti-secretory effects of glucocorticoids in human airway epithelium. Steroids, 2006. 71(4): p. 323-328.

[42] Valera FCP, B.M., Castro-Gamero AM, Cortez MA, Rosane GP Queiroz, Luiz G Tone, Anselmo-Lima, In vitro effect of glucocorticoids on nasal polyps. Braz J Otorhinolaryngol, 2011. 77(5): p. 605-610.

[43] Kyo Y, K.K., Asano K, Hisamitsu T, Suzaki H, Supressive effect of fluticasone propionate on MMP expression in the nasal mucosa of allergic rhinitis patients in vivo. . In Vivo 2006. 20: p. 439-444.

[44] Yigit O, A.E., Gelisgen R, Server EA, Azizli E, Uzun H, The effect of corticosteroid on metalloproteinase levels of nasal polyposis. Laryngoscope 2011. 121(3): p. 667-673.

[45] Bal CH, S.S., Kim YD, Effect of glucocorticoid on the MUC4 gene in nasal polyps. Laryngoscope 2007. 117: p. 2169-2173.

[46] Bobic S, v.D.C., Callebaut I, Hox V, Jorissen M, Fokkens WJ, et al, Dexamethasone-induced apoptosis of freshly isolated human nasal epithelial cells concomitant with abrogation of IL-8 production. Rhinology 2010. 48: p. 401-407.

[47] Hirano S, A.K., Namba M, Kanai K, Hisamitsu T, Suzaki H, Induction of apoptosis in nasal polyps fibroblasts by glucocorticoids in vitro. Acta Otolaryngol, 2003. 123(1075-1079).

[48] Juluisson S, A.F.E.L.P.c.o.m.c.o.n.m.e.o.n.a.a.o.l.c.t.A., 50:15-22, Protease content of mast cells of nasal mucosa: effects of natural allergen and of local corticosteroid treatment. . Allergy 1995. 50: p. 15-22.

[49] Lu NZ, C.J., Grissom SF, Cidlowski JA, Selective regulation of bone cell apoptosis by translational isoforms of the glucocorticoid receptor. Mol Cell Biol, 2007. 27(20): p. 7143–7160.

[50] Bamberger CM, B.A., de Castro M, Chrousos GP, Glucocorticoid receptor β, a potential endogenous inhibitor of glucocorticoid action in humans. J Clin Invest, 1995. 95: p. 2435–2441.

[51] Gougat C, J.D., Gagliardo R, Henriquet C, Bousquet J, Demoly P, Mathieu M, Overexpression of the human glucocorticoid receptor α and β isoforms inhibits AP-1 and NF-κ B activities hormone independently. J Mol Med, 2002. 80: p. 309–318.

[52] Lewis-Tuffin LJ, J.C., Bienstock RJ, Collins JB, Cidlowski JA Human glucocorticoid receptor beta binds RU-486 and is transcriptionally active. Mol Cell Biol, 2007. 27(2266-2282).

[53] Valera FCP, A.-L.W., Evaluation of efficacy of topical corticosteroid for the clinical treatment of nasal polyposis: searching for clinical events that may predict response to treatment. . Rhinology 2007. 45(1): p. 59-62.

[54] Badia L, L.V., Topical corticosteroids in nasal polyposis. Drugs 2001. 61: : p. 573-578.

[55] Hamilos DL, L.D., Muro S, Kahn AM, Hamilos SS, Thawley SE, et al., GRβ expression in nasal polyp inflammatory cells and its relationship to the anti-inflammatory effects of intranasal fluticasone. J Allergy Clin Immunol, 2001. 108: : p. 59-68.

[56] Valera FCP, Q.R., Scrideli C, Tone LG, Anselmo-Lima WT, NF-κB expression predicts clinical outcome for nasal polyposis. Rhinology 2010. 48(4): p. 408-414.

[57] Valera FCP, Q.R., Scrideli C, Tone LG, Anselmo-Lima WT, Evaluating budesonide efficacy in nasal polyposis and predicting the resistance to treatment. Clin Exper Allergy, 2009. 39(1): p. 81-88.

[58] Gagliardo R, C.P., Vignola AM, Bousquet J, Vachier I, Godard P, Bonsignore G, Demoly P, Mathieu M, Glucocorticoid Receptor α and β in glucocorticoid dependent asthma. Am J Respir Crit Care Med, 2000. 162: p. 7-13.

[59] Barnes, P., Corticosteroid resistance in airway disease. Proc Am Thorac Soc 2004(1): p. 264-268.

[60] Pujolsa L, M.J., Picado C, Glucocorticoid Receptor in Human Respiratory Epithelial Cells. Neuroimmunomodul, 2009. 16(5): p. 290–299.

[61] Sousa AR, L.S., Cidlowski JA, Staynov DZ, Lee TH, Glucocorticoid resistance in asthma is associated with elevated in vivo expression of the glucocorticoid receptor β-isoform. J Allergy Clin Immunol, 2000. 105(5): p. 943-950.

[62] Li P, L.Y., Zhang X, Zhang G, Ye J, Sun Y, et al., Detection of glucocorticoid receptor-alpha mRNA expression using FQ-RT-PCR in nasal polyp. Lin Chuang Er Bi Yan Hou Ke Za Zhi, 2005. 19(769-771).

[63] Pujols L, A.I., Benítez P, Martínez-Antón A, Roca-Ferrer J, Fokkens WJ, Mullol J, Picado C, Regulation of glucocorticoid receptor in nasal polyps by systemic and intranasal glucocorticoids. Allergy 2008. 63(10): p. 1377-1386.

[64] Choi BR, K.J., Gong SJ, Kwon MS, Cho JH, Kim JH, et al, Expression of glucocorticoid receptor mRNAs in glucocorticoid-resistant nasal polyps. Exp. Mol. Med, 2006. 38: p. 466-473.

[65] Necela BM, C.J., Mechanisms of glucocorticoid receptor action in noninflammatory and inflammatory cells. Proc Am Thorac Soc, 2004. 1(3): p. 239-246.

[66] Baraniuk JN, W.G., Ali M, Sabol M, Troost T, Glucocorticoids decrease c-fos expression in human nasal polyps in vivo. Thorax 1998. 53: p. 577- 582.

[67] Takeno S, H.K., Ueda T, et al, Nuclear factor-kappa B activation in the nasal polyp epithelium: relationship to local cytokine gene expression. Laryngoscope 2002. 112(1): p. 53-58

Chapter 21

The Role of Corticosteroids in Today's Oral and Maxillofacial Surgery

Mohammad Zandi

Additional information is available at the end of the chapter

http://dx.doi.org/10.5772/48655

1. Introduction

Corticosteroids are group of hormones with similar chemical formulas which are secreted by adrenal cortex. The very slight differences in molecular structure of various corticosteroids give them very different functions. The hormonal steroids are classified according to their biologic effects as glucocorticoids, which mainly affect intermediary metabolism and the immune system, and mineralocorticoids , which have principally a salt-retaining activity. Of large number of steroids released into the circulation by adrenal cortex, two are of greater importance – aldosterone, which is a mineralocorticoid, and cortisol, which is a glucocorticoid.

Mineralocorticoids promote sodium and water retention, and potassium loss by kidney, but have no anti-inflammatory or anti-allergic effect.

Cortisol, also known as hydrocortisone, is the major glucocorticoid in humans. It is synthesized by the cells of the zona fasciculata and zona reticularis of adrenal cortex; its secretion is regulated by the adrenocorticotropic hormone (ACTH) from anterior pituitary gland. Cortisol has a wide range of physiologic actions such as influencing carbohydrate, protein, and fat metabolism; regulation of blood pressure and cardiovascular function; and affecting immune system.

Corticosteroid drugs are the synthetic analogs of cortisol hormone. They bind to specific intracellular receptors upon entering target tissues, and mimic the effects of the naturally occurring hormones; the main differences are the relative glucocorticoid versus mineralocorticoid potency and the long half-life that the synthetic analogs have. The relative potencies and duration of action of representative corticosteroids are presented in Table 1.

Compound	Glucocorticoid potency	Mineralocorticoid potency	Duration of action
Cortisol	1	1	short
Cortisone	0.8	0.8	short
Fludrocortisone	10	125	Intermediate
Prednisone	4	0.8	Intermediate
Prednisolone	4	0.8	Intermediate
Methylprednisolone	5	0.5	Intermediate
Triamcinolone	5	0	Intermediate
Betamethasone	25	0	Long
Dexamethasone	25	0	Long

Short: 8-12 hours biologic half-life; Intermediate: 12-36 hours biologic half-life; Long: 36-72 hours biologic half-life.
Adapted and modified from [1]

Table 1. Relative potencies and equivalent doses of representative corticosteroids

Glucocorticoids are used, either singly or in combination with other drugs, in the treatment of a wide variety of medical disorders. Some therapeutic indications for these drugs are as follows:

- Musculoskeletal and connective tissue diseases (rheumatoid arthritis, polymyositis, systemic lupus erythematosus, and vasculitis)
- Respiratory diseases (sarcoidosis and chronic bronchitis)
- Gastrointestinal diseases (ulcerative colitis and crohn's disease)
- Allergic disorders (asthma, hay fever, and allergic rhinitis)
- Skin conditions (pemphigus, eczema, and dermatitis)
- Eye diseases (conjunctivitis, uveitis, and optic neuritis)
- Oral and maxillofacial diseases (lichen planus, keloid formation, and Bell's palsy)

Although corticosteroids are widely used for treatment of diseases and conditions affecting oral and maxillofacial region, the scientific literature on this topic is limited and scattered throughout numerous journals and books. By gathering this scattered information, this chapter presents a concise review of various uses of corticosteroid drugs in the treatment of diseases affecting oral and maxillofacial region, and the role they have in reducing post-operative morbidities such as pain, edema and trismus after various maxillofacial surgical procedures. The relation between maternal corticosteroid use and congenital maxillofacial deformities are explained. Also discussed is the perioperative management of patients receiving long-term therapeutic doses of corticosteroids.

2. Uses of corticosteroids in the treatment of oral and maxillofacial diseases

Corticosteroids are widely used in the treatment of diseases, disorders and conditions affecting the oral and maxillofacial area and the adjacent and associated structures. The diseases of the oral and maxillofacial region may be either local or the manifestation of a systemic problem. Corticosteroids have their widest application in the management of acute and chronic conditions which have an allergic, immunologic, or inflammatory basis. Therefore, a group of corticosteroids which have predominantly a glucocorticoid activity and little or no mineralocorticoid action such as betamethasone, dexamethasone, triamcinolone, and prednisolone are used.

The following are the main therapeutic indications for glucocorticoids in oral and maxillofacial diseases.

2.1. Temporomandibular disorders (TMDs)

TMDs are clinical problems involving the temporomandibular joints (TMJs), the masticatory muscles, or both. TMDs affect a significant number of individuals, and are the most common musculoskeletal disorders that cause orofacial pain. [2] Trauma to the joint structures, especially microtrauma, accounts for the majority of patients who develop TMJ problems. However, a small number of joint diseases are caused by nontraumatic etiologic factors including benign and malignant neoplasms (osteoma, chondroma, and synovial sarcoma), congenital or developmental anomalies (condylar agenesis and heperplasia), arthritides (rheumatoid arthritis), and systemic diseases. The most common signs and symptoms of TMDs are pain, altered mandibular movements, and the elicitation of joint noise.

Treatment of TMDs varies according to their etiologic basis. Conservative managements (splint therapy, thermal application, pharmacotherapy, and physiotherapy), surgical treatments, or a combination of them may be required. A variety of medications have been used to relieve pain, inflammation, muscle spasm and other signs and symptoms associated with TMDs. They include nonsteroidal anti-inflammatory drugs (NSAIDs), corticosteroids, analgesics, and muscle relaxants.

Various glucocorticoids are used in the treatment of TMDs (Table 2). These drugs have dramatic effects on pain, hypomobility, and inflammation associated with acute TMJ problems. Oral corticosteroids are used mainly for treatment of acute TMJ discomforts or for diagnostic purposes. They should be used in a short term basis (tapering dose lasting 5 to 7 days), and repeated as infrequently as possible. Long term use of corticosteroids for the treatment of TMDs is contraindicated; it can result in a cushing's- like disease process, acute adrenal crisis, hypertension, electrolyte abnormalities, diabetes, and formation of osteoporosis including the TMJ. [2]

Drug	Alternative name	Usual dose
Hydrocortisone	Hydrocortone	20-240 mg/day
Prednisone	Deltasone, Orasone	5-60 mg/day
Prednisolone	Delta-Cortef	5-60 mg/day
Dexamethasone	Decadron	0.75-9.0 mg/day
Betamethasone	Celestone	0.6-7.2 mg/day

Adapted and modified from [2]

Table 2. Oral corticosteroids used in TMDs

Intracapsular injection of glucocortcoids has been reported to decrease pain in patients with both pain and limited mouth opening secondary to inflammatory disorders of the joint, such as arthritis and capsulitis. [3-5]

A number of mechanisms have been described for the anti-inflammatory actions of glucocorticoids. These drugs inhibit inflammatory mediator release from many cell types involved in inflammation such as macrophages, T-lymphocytes, mast cells, dendritic cells, and neutrophilic leukocytes. Glucocorticoids also reduce prostaglandin production by blocking the phospholipase A_2 enzyme.

The most striking effect of glucocorticoids is to inhibit the expression of multiple inflammatory genes encoding cytokines, chemokines, inflammatory enzymes, receptors and adhesion molecules. [6] Changes in gene transcription are regulated by proinflammatory transcription factors, such as nuclear factor-κB (NF-κB) and activator protein-1 (AP-1). These proinflammatory transcription factors switch on inflammatory genes via a process involving recruitment of transcriptional coactivator proteins and changes in chromatin modifications such as histone acetylation. Glucocorticoids exert their anti-inflammatory effect on responsive cells by binding and activating a cytoplasmic glucocorticoid receptor. The interaction between the activated glucocorticoid receptor and proinflammatory transcription factors may result in deacetylation of histones and repression of inflammatory genes. [7]

In chronic inflammatory disorders of TMJ, macrophages, T-lymphocytes, and other cell types involved in inflammation release many cytokines and chemokines which will induce expression of adhesion molecules, release of variable enzymes from fibroblasts and osteoclasts and result in bone erosion. IL-8, which is a chemokine, is known to cause the infiltration of neutrophils into synovial fluid and promote joint inflammation. It was detected in 80% of the synovial tissue specimens taken from the TMJs with internal derangement. Similarly, IL-11 has been involved in the pathogenesis of osteoarthritis and rheumatoid arthritis. It has been found in synovial fluids of diseased temporomandibular joint and other joints. [8]

Cytokines participate in various inflammatory processes and induce protease synthesis; their effects can be either synergic or inhibitory. In synovial joints, IL-1 α, IL-1 β and TNF-α induce synovitis and promote the production of proteinases resulting in degradation of cartilage, while IL-1ra works to block IL-1α and IL-1 β from binding to other cell receptors and has many beneficial effects on inflammatory diseases. [9] In a study by Nordahl et al. it was found that the local production of tumor necrosis factor-*alpha* (TNF-α) occured in the TMJ synovium of patients with chronic inflammatory connective tissue disease, and the severity of pain and tenderness of the TMJ was related to the level of TNF-α. [10] In a study by Frediksson et al., it was shown that the presence of TNF-α in the synovial fluid of TMJ predicted a positive treatment response to intra-articular glucocorticoid injection in patients with chronic TMJ inflammatory disorders. [11]

Long-term complications associated with intra-articular glucocorticoid injection cannot be determined from the limited investigations done to date and thus remained unclear. Wenneberg et al. in a study evaluating the long-term prognosis of intra-articular glucocorticoid injections for TMJ arthritis observed that this treatment modality was helpful, and there were no radiographically demonstrable side effects of the treatment. [12] In contrast, Haddad IK showed that intra-articular injections of corticosteroids (triamcinolone acetonide) cause damage to fibrous layer, cartilage, and bone of TMJ. [13]

Juvenile idiopathic arthritis (JIA) is a chronic rheumatologic disease of children which may involve TMJ region, and cause significant craniofacial growth disturbances. The treatment of TMJ arthritis is controversial. It has been shown that glucocorticoid injection of the TMJ reduces pain and inflammation, and improves the function of TMJ in children with JIA. [14] Other studies also confirmed that corticosteroid injection of the TMJ can be safely performed in children with JIA, and is effective. [15-18] Few studies have evaluated TMJ corticosteroid injection in JIA. In these studies the volume of corticosteroid injected was chosen empirically. Treatment protocols such as injection of 1 cc (40 mg) of triamcinolone acetonide, 1 cc (20 mg) of triamcinolone hexacetonidein, and 0.5 to 1 cc of the diluted (with 1% lidocaine HCL) triamcinolone hexacetonidein into each of the involved TMJs, all have been used in previous studies. [14-16] The peak effect occurs after approximately 6 weeks of treatment, and the expected duration is 6-17 months. The children may receive a second injection approximately 6 months after the first. [16]

Side effects of intra-articular steroid injection in children include immediate reactions, such as pain and headache, or delayed side effects, such as joint infection and loss of subcutaneous fat. [16] Because the mandibular endochondral growth zone is located at the head of condyle (at the site of corticosteroid injection), the concern is whether intra-articular corticosteroid injection per se may cause growth retardation. Stoustrup et al., in an animal study demonstrated that intra-articular glucocorticoid injection may result in even more pronounced mandibular growth reduction than that caused by the arthritis alone. [19] Schindler et al. reported a case of severe temporomandibular dysfunction and joint destruction after intra-articular injection of triamcinolone, and El-Hakim et al. showed TMJ resorption with active osteoclastic activity after intra-articular injection of a single dose of dexamethasone in rats. [20,21]

intra-articular corticosteroid injection has been used to improve mouth opening in patients with anterior disk displacement without reduction (ADDWOR), i.e., closed lock. [22]

2.2. Oral ulcerative and vesiculobullous lesions

Corticosteroids are successfully used for the treatment of several ulcerative and vesiculobullous lesions involving the oral cavity and perioral areas including recurrent aphthous stomatitis (RAS), Behcet's syndrome, pemphigus vulgaris, bullous pemphigoid, mucous membrane pemphigoid, erythema multiforme and Stevens-Johnson syndrome (Tables 3-5). [23]

Recurrent aphthous stomatitis: These superficial painful ulcers occur commonly in the oral cavity. Minor form of the disease has 1 to 5 ulcers at one episode. The ulcers which are under 1 cm in diameter persist 8 to 14 days, and heal spontaneously without sequelae. The major aphthous ulcers are larger than 1 cm, and persist for weeks to months. Corticosteroids either alone or in combination with other drugs have been used for treatment of these lesions. [24-28] Topical steroids, such as triamcinolone acetonide and prednisolone (2 times/day), are formulated as oral pastes. Therapeutic benefit can be derived from a mouthwash containing betamethasone. It should be noted that the long-term use of topical steroids may predispose patient to developing oral candidiasis. [28]

Topical and injectable (intralesional) corticosteroids are useful for large and painful lesions. Systemic administration of corticosteroids is reserved for severe cases to prevent lesion formation or to reduce the number of lesions. Systemic corticosteroids should be prescribed in short courses, and only for severe outbreaks or cases that don't respond to topical or injectable corticosteroids. [23]

Behcet's syndrome: The treatment of oral lesions of Behcet's syndrome is similar to the treatment of severe or major RAS. [23]

Pemphigus vulgaris: Pemphigus vulgaris is a severe, potentially life-threatening vesiculobullous disease that may affect skin and mucous membranes. Oral cavity is involved in nearly 80% of patients. In the past, corticosteroid therapy was the treatment of choice but later, combination therapy involving the use of systemic corticosteroids with immunosuppressive agents was introduced, in an attempt to achieve disease control with lower doses of steroids. [29-31]

The principal treatment of pemphigus vulgaris is systemic administration of corticosteroids at doses of 1 to 2 mg/kg/day. Maintenance of remission may be achieved with topical corticosteroids, allowing reduction of systemic drugs. Isolated lesions can be treated with injectable corticosteroids. [23]

Bullous and mucous membrane pemphigoid: The choice of drugs used for the treatment of pemphigoid is based upon the sites of involvement, clinical severity, and disease progression. For more severe disease, or with rapid progression, systemic corticosteroids are the agents of choice for initial treatment, combined with steroid-sparing agents for long-term maintenance. [32] Topical and injectable corticosteroids are useful for treatment of mild or localized oral lesions. [23]

Erythema multiforme (EM) and *Stevens-Johnson syndrome (SJS):* It has been shown that corticosteroids have a favorable influence on the outcome of EM and SJS, if administered in high doses, over a short period of time, early in the course of the disease, and with proper tapering of medication. [33-37] However, the dosing and route of administration that provides the most benefit for EMM and SJS patients is in question. Treatment protocols such as early therapy with systemic prednisone (0.5 to 1.0mg/kg/day) or pulse methylprednisolone (1mg/kg/day for 3 days), intravenous pulsed dose methylprednisolone (3 consecutive daily infusions of 20–30mg/kg to a maximum of 500mg given over 2 to 3 hours), and dexamethasone pulse therapy (1.5mg/kg IV over 30 to 60 minutes on 3 consecutive days), all have been shown to be effective. [33-35,37-39]

Drug	Triamcinolone (10 mg/ml)	Dexamethasone (4 mg/ml)
Indications	Severe recurrent aphthous stomatitis, major aphthous stomatitis, erosive lichen planus	
Usual dosage	Inject 0.1 cc/cm lesion	
Contraindications	Hypersensitivity to corticosteroids, systemic fungal infection, live vaccines, active tuberculosis	
Common side effects	Candidiasis, hyperglycemia	
Unusual side effects	Peptic ulceration with perforation, osteoporosis, impaired wound healing, mucosal atrophy	

Adapted and modified from [23].

Table 3. Injectable (intralesional) corticosteroids used for treatment of oral lesions

Drug	Beclomethasone	Betamethasone	Clobetasol	Halobetasol	Fluocinonide
Indications	Severe recurrent aphthous stomatitis, Behcet's syndrome, pemphigus vulgaris, pemphigoid				
Administration	Inhaler spray topically to mucosal lesions	Topical intraoral cream or gel, soluble tablets as mouth wash	Topical intraoral cream or gel	Topical intraoral cream or ointment	Topical intraoral cream
Usual dosage	50-100 μg sprayed onto oral lesion	0.1% cream or 0.05% gel applied thinly bid; 0.5 mg 2-4 times daily as mouth wash	0.05% cream or gel applied thinly bid	0.05% cream or ointment applied thinly bid	0.05% cream applied thinly bid
Contraindications	Untreated infections				
Common side effects	Oral candidiasis				
Unusual side effects	Adrenal suppression if doses exceeded				

Adapted and modified from [23].

Table 4. Topical corticosteroids used for treatment of oral lesions

Drug	Prednisone (tablets)
Indications	Severe recurrent aphthous stomatitis, Behcet's syndrome, pemphigus vulgaris, pemphigoid, erythema multiforme
Usual dosage	1. 30-40 mg daily after breakfast for 4-5 days 2. 1-2 mg/kg/day after breakfast until disease controlled 3. 1-2 mg/kg/day, then maintenance of 2.5-15 mg daily 4. 20-40 mg daily for 7-10 days at onset of lesions or until lesions resolve 5. 60 mg daily for 2 days, 50 mg daily for 2 days, 40 mg daily for 2 days, 30 mg daily for 2 days, 20 mg daily for 2 days, 10 mg daily for 2 days
Contraindications	Hypersensitivity to corticosteroids, systemic infection (unless specific antimicrobial therapy given), peptic disease (unless proton pump inhibitor given), live vaccines
Common side effects	Dyspepsia, candidiasis, myopathy, osteoporosis, adrenal suppression, Cushing's syndrome, euphoria, depression
Unusual side effects	Peptic ulceration with perforation, Cushingoid side effects increasingly likely with doses above 7.5 mg daily

Adapted and modified from [23].

Table 5. Systemic corticosteroids used for treatment of oral lesions

2.3. Keloid and hypertrophic scars

Keloid and hypertrophic scar (HS) represent pathologic overhealing conditions which are caused by excessive production of fibrous tissue following healing of skin injuries. Keloid produces significantly more collagen than HS. Their exact cause is unknown but inflammation, tension, and genetic background are mentioned as contributing factors. Keloid and HS have different clinical features. Keloids extend beyond the confines of the original wound, develop months after injury, and rarely regress. HS is a raised scar that remains confined to the area of the injury, usually form within weeks, and may regress without intervention.

Various treatment modalities have been used for prevention and treatment of keloid and HSs such as pressure therapy, silicone gel sheeting, topical flavonoids, corticosteroid therapy, radiotherapy, and surgery.

Topical and intralesional glucocorticoids are frequently used to treat existing keloid and HS or, prophylactically, to prevent their formation or recurrence after surgical removal. Topical administration of steroids doesn't appear to be as efficacious as intralesional injection of the drug. Intralesional steroid injection, either on its own or in combination with other treatment modalities is the most common treatment used for keloid and HSs. Glucocorticoids have a multiplicity of effects on scars including suppressive effects on the inflammatory process in the wound, diminishing collagen and glycosaminoglycan synthesis, inhibition of fibroblast growth, and enhancing collagen and fibroblast degeneration. [40,41] Triamcinolone acetonide is the most commonly used steroid for the treatment of HS and keloid. It is used in a concentration of 10-20 mg/ml, though it can be given at a dose of 40 mg/ml for a tough bulky lesion; the concentration depends upon the size and site of the lesion and age of the individual. [42] Side effects of steroid injection include hypopigmentation, dermal atrophy, telangiectasia, and cushingoid effects from systemic absorption. [41] Cushing's syndrome secondary to injection of triamcinolone acetonide for the treatment of keloids have been reported by several investigators. [43,44]

2.4. Central giant cell granuloma

Central giant cell granuloma of the jaws is a benign tumor which occurs most often in children and young adults. This tumor is made up of loose fibrous connective tissue stroma with many interspersed proliferating fibroblasts, aggregations of multinucleated giant cells, and foci of hemorrhage.

Various surgical and nonsurgical treatments have been advocated for this lesion. One of the nonsurgical treatments proposed is intralesional corticosteroid injections. Intralesional injection of triamcinolone acetonide has been shown to induce partial and in some cases complete resolution of central giant cell granuloma. However, there is no reasonably strong consensus in the literature regarding optimal dosage and duration of treatment that provides the most benefit. The mechanism of action of corticosteroids in the treatment of central giant cell granuloma is unknown. A rationale for its use has been the histologic resemblance of central giant cell granuloma to sarcoid. Because corticosteroids have been effective in the treatment of sarcoid, it was thought that they may have a similar therapeutic effect on central giant cell granuloma. In addition, corticosteroids may act by suppressing any angiogenic component of the lesion. [45]

2.5. Bell's palsy

Bell's palsy is an idiopathic inflammation of the facial nerve (the seventh of twelve paired cranial nerves) which occurs almost always on one side only. It is characterized by facial muscle weakness, hyperacusis, decreased tearing, and loss of taste on the anterior two thirds of the tongue. Because Bell's palsy results from inflammation and edema of the facial nerve, corticosteroids constitute the standard medicine in the treatment of this condition. [46-48] For adults, prednisolone at doses of 1 mg/kg/day for 7 to 10 days, taken in divided doses in the morning and evening, is suggested.

2.6. Management of post-operative morbidities associated with maxillofacial surgeries

Facial pain, edema, ecchymosis and limitation of mouth opening are the expected sequelae of oral and maxillofacial surgeries. These post-operative complications affect the ability of patient to interrelate and to return to the daily life and activities, and deteriorate the quality of life of patient. [49,50]

Many modalities are used to abate sequelae in the oral and maxillofacial surgery including use of ice pack, pressure dressing, surgical drain, and drugs.

Corticosteroids are commonly used to control post-operative morbidities and to provide comfort for patients. However, there are no definite protocols relative to molecules, doses, schedules, and routes of administration. [51] The most commonly administered types of corticosteroids are betamethasone, dexamethasone, and methylprednisolone, administered intravenously, orally or by injection into the masseter muscle. The morbidity-management protocol also varies depending upon the type of surgery being performed.

To decrease post-rhinoplasty edema, the administration of corticosteroids has been advocated for many years. In a study by Gurlek et al., it was shown that high dose methylprednisolone was effective in preventing and reducing both the periorbital ecchymosis and edema in open rhinoplasty. [52] In the same line, Kargi et al., and Kara and Gokalan showed that the perioperative use of corticosteroids reduced edema and ecchymosis associated with rhinoplasty surgery. [53,54] In contrast, Hoffmann et al. did not observe any increase either in the edema or the ecchymosis after rhinoplasty surgery. [55]

Regarding orthognathic surgery, several investigations demonstrated that perioperative corticosteroid administration significantly reduced post-operative inflammation and edema. [56-59] In contrast, Munro et al. did not observe any significant decrease in postoperative edema even with the highest doses and the longest durations of corticosteroid treatment. (56)

The effects of corticosteroids on post-operative edema after oral surgery have been widely investigated in the literature. Many prior studies demonstrated a significant decrease in post-operative edema after administration of corticosteroids. [60-63] In a study by Zandi, it was shown that steroids not only reduced the facial swelling, but also the severity of pain after surgery. [60] Similarly, several studies reported that corticosteroids significantly decreased post-operative edema and pain, indicating a strong correlation between edema and pain decreases. [62-64]

Even though the effects of corticosteroids on post-operative morbidities after various oral and maxillofacial surgeries have been widely investigated in the literature, methodological differences, variation in agents, doses, and routes of administration of the drugs have compromised the scientific conclusions.

2.7. Other uses of corticosteroids in oral and maxillofacial surgery

In addition to the aforementioned indications, corticosteroids are successfully used in the management of acute trigeminal nerve injuries, traumatic facial nerve paralysis, chronic facial pain, and allergic diseases involving maxillofacial area.

3. Corticosteroids contraindications

In prescribing corticosteroids, physicians must be aware that some patients are poor candidates for systemic, locally injected, or topical corticosteroid therapy.

Systemic corticosteroids must be used with the greatest of caution in patients with uncontrolled hypertension, diabetes, active peptic ulcer, heart diseases, infections, psychiatric disorders, osteoporosis, cataract, glaucoma, tuberculosis, mycobacterial diseases, herpes simplex infection, pregnancy, varicella zoster infection, immune deficiency, underactive thyroid, and mental disorders.

Injectable corticosteroid use is contraindicated in patients with hypersensitivity to corticosteroids, infections, and active tuberculosis.

Use of topical corticosteroids is absolutely contraindicated in the treatment of primary bacterial infections such as impetigo, furuncles, carbuncles, erysipelas, cellulitis, lymphangitis, and erythrasma. Topical corticosteroids are also contraindicated in patients with a history of hypersensitivity to any of the components of the preparation. Currently, little is known about the safety of topical corticosteroids in pregnancy. Although it has been reported that there is an association between very potent topical corticosteroids and congenital abnormalities including low birth weight and orofacial clefts, use of these drugs in pregnancy is not recommended unless the potential benefit justifies the potential risks to fetus. [65]

Ophthalmic use of topical corticosteroids is contraindicated in most viral, bacterial, and fungal diseases of ocular structures.

4. Corticosteroids side effects

Although corticosteroids have great potential in the treatment of various diseases and conditions affecting oral and maxillofacial region, they also carry the risk of many side effects. Therefore, benefits from corticosteroids should always be weighed against their potential risks. Side effects of corticosteroids vary depending on the type and dose of the medication, rout of administration, and length of treatment. Significant adverse effects are most likely to occur in patients using oral corticosteroids for a long period of time. These may include weight gain, impaired growth, adrenal insufficiency, electrolyte abnormalities, increased susceptibility to infection, myopathy, osteoporosis, osteonecrosis, cataract, glaucoma, psychological problems, fractures, hypertension, insomnia, moon face, diabetes, and peptic ulcer. [1,66]

Topical glucocorticoids may cause adverse effects such as skin atrophy, hypopigmentation, subcutaneous fat wasting, telangectasia, contact dermatitis, oral thrush, and cushingoid effects from systemic absorption. [28,41] Application of topical corticosteroids on eyelids has been reported to cause glaucoma. Adrenal suppression, growth retardation in children, and cushing's syndrome are rare adverse effects of long term topical corticosteroid use.

Intralesional glucocorticoids may cause sterile abscess, skin atrophy, hypopigmentation, panniculitis, and skin necrosis.

Although the frequency of side effects of inhaled corticosteroids is lower than systemic corticosteroids, high doses of inhaled corticosteroids have the potential to produce various local and systemic side effects. Systemic side effects associated with inhaled corticosteroids include osteoporosis, retarded growth in children, cataracts, glaucoma, and skin thinning. Inhaled corticosteroids may cause local side effects including oropharyngeal candidiasis, dysphonia, reflex cough, bronchospasm, and pharyngitis. [67]

5. Perioperative management of patients with adrenal insufficiency

Insufficient adrenocortical function is a rare disorder resulting from endogenous deficiency (primary) or from the administration of exogenous corticosteroids (secondary). Adrenal suppression should be suspected in those patients receiving the equivalent of 20 mg of prednisone daily for one week or the equivalent of 7.5 mg of prednisone daily for one month within the past year. [2] In adrenal suppression the body is not able to appropriately manage the challenge of stresses such as medical illness, surgery, and trauma. This may precipitate an adrenal crisis, signaled by the onset of fever, restlessness, flank and abdominal pain, vomiting, lethargy, hypotension, or coma.

Any patient suspected of having adrenal insufficiency should be evaluated with an ACTH (cortrosyn) stimulation test or be given supplemental corticosteroids empirically perioperatively. Cortrosyn stimulation test measures how well the adrenal glands respond to a synthetic ACTH administered to the patient.

The currently recommended corticosteroid coverage for various surgical procedures is based on the magnitude of stress and the known glucocorticoid production rate associated with it, and includes the following: [2,68]

- Minor surgical stress such as tooth extraction, biopsy, periodontal surgery, genioplasty, etc: 25 mg of hydrocortisone equivalent, the day of surgery
- Moderate surgical stress such as panfacial fractures, two jaw surgery, etc: 50-75 mg of hydrocortisone equivalent for 1 to 2 days.
- Major surgical stress such as extensive head and neck resection and reconstruction, etc: 100-150 mg of hydrocortisone equivalent for 2 to 3 days.

In the case of postoperative complications such as fever and pain, it is recommended that the corticosteroid administration be continued consistent with the post-operative stress response. [68]

6. Maternal corticosteroid use and the risk of orofacial clefts in infants

Orofacial clefts are the most common congenital deformity affecting maxillofacial area. The etiology of facial clefting is complex and has been extensively investigated. There are both major and minor genetic influences involved, with variable interactions from environmental factors. [69] Several environmental factors such as maternal drug intake, trauma, smoking, and exposure to x-rays during the pregnancy period have been suggested to increase the chance of cleft development in infants. [70]

Pregnant women often use topical, inhaled, or systemic corticosteroid drugs for a variety of inflammatory and allergic conditions. Several investigations have reported that the use of corticosteroids during early pregnancy is associated with a 3- to 6-fold increased risk of orofacial clefts. [71-75] Although systemic corticosteroids are associated with a higher risk of orofacial clefts than topical corticosteroids, the latter is not without risk. It has been shown that application of hydrocortisone cream on eczematous skin is associated with significant increase in the level of plasma cortisol. [76] In a study by Edwards et al., a significant association between topical corticosteroids and orofacial cleft was observed. [77] Epidemiologic data have shown that low-to-moderate doses of inhaled corticosteroids taken during the first trimester of pregnancy are safe but raise concerns about high doses. [78]

The mechanism of cleft palate production by corticosteroids is uncertain; it is a complicated interference in a complex developmental program involving many genetic and biochemical processes. Glucocorticoids may cause cleft palate deformity by delaying palatal shelf elevation. [79] Corticosteroids can reduce the collagen content of connective tissue by inhibiting collagen synthesis, which could disrupt cell-cell interaction and tissue-tissue interactions. [71]

7. Conclusion

Glucocorticoids are used, either singly or in combination with other drugs, for the treatment of various diseases affecting oral and maxillofacial area. They are also frequently used to minimize expected post-operative morbidities such as pain and edema after oral and maxillofacial surgeries. Because of anti-inflammatory and anti-allergic actions of glucocorticoids, they have their widest application in the management of acute and chronic conditions which have allergic, immunologic, or inflammatory basis. However, corticosteroids carry the risk of potential side effects which are sometimes severe and life threatening. Therefore, benefits from corticosteroids should always be weighed against their potential risks in each patient.

Prescribing the minimal dose and the least potent type of corticosteroids necessary to produce a given therapeutic effect, simultaneous use of non-steroidal agents to reduce the dose of corticosteroids, and prescribing corticosteroids for a short period of time or sporadically are some strategies to minimize corticosteroids adverse effects.

Author details

Mohammad Zandi
Department of Oral and Maxillofacial Surgery,
Hamedan University of Medical Sciences, Hamedan, Iran
Researcher, Dental Research Center,
Hamedan University of medical sciences, Hamedan, Iran

Acknowledgement

The author wishes to express his deep appreciation to Dr. Mojgan Ahmadian for her extensive assistance in the preparation of this chapter.

8. References

[1] Brunton LL, Lazo JS, Parker KL (2005) Goodman & Gilman's The pharmacological basis of therapeutics. Eleventh edition. New York: McGraw-Hill.

[2] Fonseca RJ, Marciani RD, Turvey TA (2009) Oral and maxillofacial surgery. Second edition. Saunders.

[3] Kopp S, Akerman S, Nilner M (1991) Short-term effects of intra-articular sodium hyaluronate, glucocorticoid, and saline injections on rheumatoid arthritis of the temporomandibular joint. J Craniomandib Disord. 5: 231-238.

[4] Alstergren P, Appelgren A, Appelgren B, Kopp S, Lundeberg T, Theodorsson E (1996) The effect on joint fluid concentration of neuropeptide Y by intra-articular injection of glucocorticoid in temporomandibular joint arthritis. Acta Odontol Scand. 54: 1-7.

[5] Fredriksson L, Alstergren P, Kopp S (2005) Serotonergic mechanisms influence the response to glucocorticoid treatment in TMJ arthritis. Mediators Inflamm. 2005:194–201.

[6] Barnes PJ (1998) Anti-inflammatory actions of glucocorticoids: molecular mechanisms. Clin Sci. 94: 557–572.

[7] Adcock IM, Ito K, Barnes PJ (2004) Glucocorticoids: effects on gene transcription. Proc Am Thorac Soc. 1: 247-254.

[8] Gulen H, Ataoglu H, Haliloglu S, Isik K (2009) Proinflammatory cytokines in temporomandibular joint synovial fluid before and after arthrocentesis. Oral Surg Oral Med Oral Pathol Oral Radiol Endod. 107: e1-4.

[9] Kardel R, Ulfgren AK, Reinhold FP, and Holmlund A (2003) Inflammatory cell and cytokine patterns in patients with painful clicking and osteoarthritis in the temporomandibular joint. Int J Oral Maxillofac Surg. 32: 390-396.

[10] Nordahl S, Alstergren P, Kopp S (2000) Tumor necrosis factor-alpha in synovial fluid and plasma from patients with chronic connective tissue disease and its relation to temporomandibular joint pain. J Oral Maxillofac Surg. 58: 525–530.

[11] Fredriksson L, Alstergren P, Kopp S (2006) Tumor necrosis factor- alpha in temporomandibular joint synovial fluid predicts treatment effects on pain by intra-articular glucocorticoid treatment. Mediators Inflamm. 2006: 59425.

[12] Wenneberg B, Kopp S, Gröndahl HG (1991) Long-term effect of intra-articular injections of a glucocorticosteroid into the TMJ: a clinical and radiographic 8-year follow-up. J Craniomandib Disord 5: 11-18.

[13] Haddad IK (2000) Temporomandibular joint osteoarthrosis. Histopathological study of the effects of intra-articular injection of triamcinolone acetonide. Saudi Med J. 21: 675-679.

[14] Arabshahi B, Dewitt EM, Cahill AM, Kaye RD, Baskin KM, Towbin RB, Cron RQ (2005) Utility of corticosteroid injection for temporomandibular arthritis in children with juvenile idiopathic arthritis. Arthritis Rheum. 52: 3563-3569.

[15] Stoll ML, Good J, Sharpe T, Beukelman T, Young D, Waite PD, Cron RQ (2012) Intra-articular corticosteroid injections to the temporomandibular joints are safe and appear to be effective therapy in children with juvenile idiopathic arthritis. J Oral Maxillofac Surg. (Article in press).

[16] Cahill AM, Baskin KM, Kaye RD, Arabshahi B, Cron RQ, Dewitt EM, Bilaniuk L, Towbin RB (2007) CT-guided percutaneous steroid injection for management of inflammatory arthropathy of the temporomandibular joint in children. AJR Am J Roentgenol. 188: 182-186.

[17] Ringold S, Torgerson TR, Egbert MA, Wallace CA (2008) Intraarticular corticosteroid injections of the temporomandibular joint in juvenile idiopathic arthritis. J Rheumatol. 35: 1157-1164.

[18] Parra DA, Chan M, Krishnamurthy G, Spiegel L, Amaral JG, Temple MJ, John PR, Connolly BL (2010) Use and accuracy of US guidance for image-guided injections of the temporomandibular joints in children with arthritis. Pediatr Radiol. 40: 1498- 1504.

[19] Stoustrup P, Kristensen KD, Küseler A, Gelineck J, Cattaneo PM, Pedersen TK, Herlin T (2008) Reduced mandibular growth in experimental arthritis in the temporomandibular joint treated with intra-articular corticosteroid. Eur J Orthod. 30: 111-119.

[20] Schindler C, Paessler L, Eckelt U, Kirch W (2005) Severe temporomandibular dysfunction and joint destruction after intra-articular injection of triamcinolone. J Oral Pathol Med. 34: 184-186.

[21] El-Hakim IE, Abdel-Hamid IS, Bader A (2005) Temporomandibular joint (TMJ) response to intra-articular dexamethasone injection following mechanical arthropathy: a histological study in rats. Int J Oral Maxillofac Surg 34: 305-310.

[22] Samiee A, Sabzerou D, Edalatpajouh F, Clark GT, Ram S (2011) Temporomandibular joint injection with corticosteroid and local anesthetic for limited mouth opening. J Oral Sci. 53: 321-325.

[23] Greenberg MS, Glick M, Ship JA (2008) Burket's oral medicine. Eleventh edition. Hamilton: BC Decker Inc.

[24] Rodriguez M, Rubio JA, Sanchez R (2007) Effectiveness of two oral pastes for treatment of recurrent aphthous stomatitis. Oral Diseases. 13: 490-494.

[25] Holbrook WP, Kristmundsdottir T, Loftsson T (1998) Aqueous hydrocortisone mouthwash solution: clinical evaluation. Acta Odontol Scand. 56: 157-160.

[26] Lo Muzio L, Della Valle A, Mignogna MD, Pannone G, Bucci P, Bucci E, Sciubba J (2001) The treatment of oral aphthous ulceration or erosive lichen planus with topical clobetasol propionate in three preparations: a clinical and pilot study on 54 patients. J Oral Pathol Med. 30: 611-617.

[27] Gonzalez-Moles MA, Morales P, Rodriguez-Archilla A, Isabel IR. Gonzalez-Moles S (2002) Treatment of severe chronic oral erosive lesions with clobetasol propionate in aqueous solution. Oral Surg Oral Med Oral Pathol Oral Radiol Endod. 93: 264-270.

[28] Altenburg A, Zouboulis CC (2008) Current concepts in the treatment of recurrent aphthous stomatitis. Skin Therapy Lett. 13: 1-4.

[29] Chams-Davatchi C, Esmaili N, Daneshpazhooh M, Valikhani M, Balighi K, Hallaji Z, Barzegari M, Akhyani M, Ghodsi SZ, Seirafi H, Nazemi MJ, Mortazavi H, Mirshams-Shahshahani M (2007) Randomized controlled open-label trial of four treatment regimens for pemphigus vulgaris. J Am Acad Dermatol. 57: 622-628.

[30] Ionnides D, Chrysomallis F, Bystryn JC (2000) Ineffectiveness of cyclosporine as an adjuvant to corticosteroids in the treatment of pemphigus. Arch Dermatol 136: 868- 872.

[31] Beissert S, Werfel T, Frieling U, Böhm M, Sticherling M, Stadler R, Zillikens D, Rzany B, Hunzelmann N, Meurer M, Gollnick H, Ruzicka T, Pillekamp H, Junghans V, Luger TA (2006) A comparison of oral methylprednisolone plus azathioprine or mycophenolate mofetil for the treatment of pemphigus. Arch Dermatol 142: 1447- 1454.

[32] Neff AG, Turner M, Mutasim DF (2008) Treatment strategies in mucous membrane pemphigoid. Ther Clin Risk Manag. 4: 617-626.

[33] Michaels B (2009) The role of systemic corticosteroid therapy in erythema multiforme major and stevens-johnson syndrome: a review of past and current opinions. J Clin Aesthet Dermatol. 2: 51-55.

[34] Kardaun SH, Jonkman MF (2007) Dexamethasone pulse therapy for Stevens-Johnson syndrome/toxic epidermal necrolysis. Acta Derm Venereol. 87: 144–148.

[35] Patterson R, Dykewicz MS, Gonzalzles A, Grammer LC, Green D, Greenberger PA, McGrath KG, Walker CL (1990) Erythema multiforme and Stevens-Johnson syndrome. Descriptive and therapeutic controversy. Chest. 98: 331–336.

[36] Kakourou T, Klontza D, Soteropoulou F, Kattamis C (1997) Corticosteroid treatment of erythema multiforme major (Stevens-Johnson syndrome) in children. Eur J Pediatr. 156: 90–93.

[37] Martinez AE, Atherton DJ (2000) High-dose systemic corticosteroids can arrest recurrences of severe mucocutaneous erythema multiforme. Pediatr Dermatol. 17: 87–90.

[38] Scully C, Bagan J (2008) Oral mucosal diseases: erythema multiforme. Br J Oral Maxillofac Surg. 46: 90–95.

[39] Schneck J, Fagot JP, Sekula P, Sassolas B, Roujeau JC, Mockenhaupt M (2008) Effects of treatments on the mortality of Stevens-Johnson syndrome and toxic epidermal necrolysis: a retrospective study on patients included in the prospective EuroSCAR Study. J Am Acad Dermatol. 58: 33–40.

[40] Gauglitz GG, Korting HC, Pavicic T, Ruzicka T, Jeschke MG (2011) Hypertrophic scarring and keloids: pathomechanisms and current and emerging treatment strategies. Mol Med. 17: 113-25.

[41] Donkor P (2007) Head and neck keloid: treatment by core excision and delayed intralesional injection of steroid. J Oral Maxillofac Surg. 65: 1292-1296.

[42] Gupta S, Sharma VK (2011) Standard guidelines of care: Keloids and hypertrophic scars. Indian J Dermatol Venereol Leprol. 77: 94-100.

[43] Langston JR, Kolodny SC (1976) Cushing's syndrome associated with the intradermal injection of triamcinolone diacetate. J Oral Surg 34: 846–9.

[44] Ritota PC, Lo AK (1996) Cushing's syndrome in postburn children following intralesional triamcinolone injection. Ann Plast Surg 36: 508–511.

[45] Ferretti C, Muthray E (2011) Management of central giant cell granuloma of mandible using intralesional corticosteroids: case report and review of literature. J Oral Maxillofac Surg. 69: 2824-2829.

[46] Sheikh SB, Jacobus C (2012) Are steroids effective for treating Bell's palsy? Ann Emerg Med. 59: 33-34.

[47] Sherbino J (2010) Evidence-based emergency medicine: clinical synopsis. Do antiviral medications improve recovery in patients with Bell's palsy? Ann Emerg Med. 55: 475-476.

[48] Gilden D (2009) Treatment of Bell's palsy--the pendulum has swung back to steroids alone. Lancet Neurol, 7: 976-977.

[49] McGrath C, Comfort MB, Lo EC, Luo Y (2003) Changes in life quality following third molar surgery--the immediate postoperative period. Br Dent J. 194: 265-8.

[50] Colorado-Bonnin M, Valmaseda-Castellón E, Berini-Aytés L, Gay-Escoda C (2006) Quality of life following lower third molar removal. Int J Oral Maxillofac Surg. 35: 343-347.

[51] Sortino F, Cicciù M (2011) Strategies used to inhibit postoperative swelling following removal of impacted lower third molar. Dent Res J (Isfahan). 8: 162-171.

[52] Gürlek A, Fariz A, Aydoğan H, Ersöz-Oztürk A, Evans GR (2009) Effects of high dose corticosteroids in open rhinoplasty. J Plast Reconstr Aesthet Surg. 62: 650-655.

[53] Kargı E, Hosnuter M, Babuccu O, Altunkaya H, Altinyazar C (2003) Effect of steroids on edema, ecchymosis, and intraoperative bleeding in rhinoplasty. Ann Plast Surg. 51: 570-574.

[54] Kara CO, Gokalan I (1999) Effects of single-dose steroid usage on edema, ecchymosis, and intraoperative bleeding in rhinoplasty. Plast Reconstr Surg 104: 2213-2218.

[55] Hoffmann DF, Cook TA, Quatela VC, Wang TD, Brownrigg PJ, Brummett RE (1991) Steroids and rhinoplasty. A double-blind study. Arch Otolaryngol Head Neck Surg. 117: 990-993.

[56] Weber CR, Griffin JM (1994) Evaluation of dexamethasone for reducing postoperative edema and inflammatory response after orthognathic surgery. J Oral Maxillofac Surg. 52: 35-9.

[57] Peillon D, Bubost J, Roche C, Bienvenu J, Breton P, Carry PY, Freidel M, Banssillon V (1996) Do corticotherapy and hemodilution decrease postoperative inflammation after maxillofacial surgery?]. Ann Fr Anesth Reanim. 15: 157-61.

[58] Schaberg SJ, Stuller CB, Edwards SM (1984) Effect of methylprednisolone on swelling after orthognathic surgery. J Oral Maxillofac Surg 42: 356-361.

[59] Munro IR, Boyd JB, Wainwright DJ (1986) Effect of steroids in maxillofacial surgery. Ann Plast Surg 17: 440-444.

[60] Zandi M (2008) Comparison of corticosteroids and rubber drain for reduction of sequelae after third molar surgery. Oral Maxillofac Surg. 12: 29-33.

[61] Buyukkurt MC, Gungormus M, Kaya O (2006) The effect of a single dose prednisolone with and without diclofenac on pain, trismus and swelling after removal of mandibular third molars. J Oral Maxillofac Surg. 64: 1761-1766.

[62] Graziani F, D'Aiuto F, Arduino PG, Tonelli M, Gabriele M (2006) Perioperative dexamethasone reduces post-surgical sequelae of wisdom tooth removal. A split-randomized double-masked clinical trial. J Oral Maxillofac Surg. 35: 241-246.

[63] Esen E, Tasar F, Akhan O (1999) Determination of the antiinflammatory effects of methylprednisolone on the sequelae of third molar surgery. J Oral Maxillofac Surg. 57: 1201–1206.

[64] Dan AE, Thygesen TH, Pinholt EM (2010) Corticosteroid administration in oral and orthognathic surgery: a systematic review of the literature and meta-analysis. J Oral Maxillofac Surg. 68: 2207-2220.

[65] Chi CC, Wang SH, Kirtschig G, Wojnarowska F (2010) Systematic review of the safety of topical corticosteroids in pregnancy. J Am Acad Dermatol. 62: 694-705.

[66] Manson SC, Brown RE, Cerulli A, Vidaurre CF (2009) The cumulative burden of oral corticosteroid side effects and the economic implications of steroid use. Respir Med. 103: 975-994.

[67] Dahl R (2006) Systemic side effects of inhaled corticosteroids in patients with asthma. Respir Med. 100: 1307-1317.

[68] Salem M, Tainsh RE Jr, Bromberg J, Loriaux DL, Chernow B (1994) Perioperative glucocorticoid coverage. A reassessment 42 years after emergence of a problem. Ann Surg. 219: 416-25.

[69] Zandi M, Miresmaeili A (2007) Study of the cephalometric features of parents of children with cleft lip and/or palate anomaly. Int J Oral Maxillofac Surg. 36: 200-206.

[70] Zandi M, Heidari A (2011) An epidemiologic study of orofacial clefts in hamedan city, iran: a 15-year study. Cleft Palate Craniofac J. 48: 483-489.

[71] Carmichael SL, Shaw GM, Ma C, Werler MM, Rasmussen SA, Lammer EJ; National Birth Defects Prevention Study (2007) Maternal corticosteroid use and orofacial clefts. Am J Obstet Gynecol. 197: 585.e1-7.

[72] Pradat P, Robert-Gnansia E, Di Tanna GL, Rosano A, Lisi A, Mastroiacovo P (2003) First trimester exposure to corticosteroids and oral clefts. Birth Defects Res Clin Mol Teratol. 67: 968-970.

[73] Kallen B (2003) Maternal drug use and infant cleft lip/palate with special reference to corticoids. Cleft Palate Craniofac J. 40: 624-628.

[74] Park-Wyllie L, Mazzotta P, Pastuszak A, Moretti ME, Beique L, Hunnisett L, Friesen MH, Jacobson S, Kasapinovic S, Chang D, Diav-Citrin O, Chitayat D, Nulman I, Einarson TR, Koren G (2000) Birth defects after maternal exposure to corticosteroids: prospective cohort study and meta-analysis of epidemiological studies. Teratology. 62: 385-392.

[75] Edwards MJ, Agho K, Attia J, Diaz P, Hayes T, Illingworth A, Roddick LG (2003) Case-control study of cleft lip or palate after maternal use of topical corticosteroids during pregnancy. Am J Med Genet. 120: 459-463.

[76] Turpeinen M (1991) Absorption of hydrocortisone from the skin reservoir in atopic dermatitis. Br J Dermatol. 124: 358-360.

[77] Edwards MJ, Agho K, Attia J, Diaz P, Hayes T, Illingworth A, Roddick LG (2003) Case-control study of cleft lip or palate after maternal use of topical corticosteroids during pregnancy. Am J Med Genet A. 120: 459-463.

[78] Blais L, Beauchesne MF, Lemière C, Elftouh N (2009) High doses of inhaled corticosteroids during the first trimester of pregnancy and congenital malformations. J Allergy Clin Immunol. 124: 1229-1234.

[79] Goldman AS (1984) Biochemical mechanism of glucocorticoid-and phenytoin-induced cleft palate. Curr Top Dev Biol. 19: 217-239.

Chapter 22

Assessment of Glucocorticoids – Induced Preclinical Atherosclerosis

Amr Amin and Zeinab Nawito

Additional information is available at the end of the chapter

http://dx.doi.org/10.5772/52889

1. Introduction

In 1948, the US rheumatologist Philip Hench and his associates at the Mayo Clinic first administered hydrocortisone to a patient with rheumatoid arthritis and discovered its clinical benefits [1]. Two years later, Hench, together with biochemists Edward Kendall and Tadeus Reichstein, shared the Nobel Prize in Medicine. Today, glucocorticoids are among the most frequently prescribed class of anti-inflammatory medications [2]. They are part of the standard treatment for a wide range of disorders which feature inflammation and/or immune activation, such as asthma, chronic obstructive pulmonary disease, hypersensitivity reactions, autoimmune diseases, and in organ transplantation. However, even early on, the euphoria generated by the discovery of corticosteroids was rapidly tempered by the realization that clinicians were, in a sense, engaging in a Faustian pact between its impressive anti-inflammatory benefits and its potentially devastating Cushingoid side effects [3, 4].

From a cardiovascular standpoint, the propensity of glucocorticoids to produce hyperglycemia, hypertension, dyslipidemia, and central obesity has long produced concern regarding possible adverse cardiovascular events [5]. Glucocorticoids administration increases blood pressure in a dose dependent fashion. The mechanisms of glucocorticoids-mediated hypertension are incompletely understood but appear to be principally related to increased peripheral vascular resistance rather than to mineralocorticoid receptor mediated effects of increased sodium retention and plasma volume expansion [6]. Dyslipidemia in the context of long term glucocorticoids use is characterized by increased total cholesterol, low density lipoprotein cholesterol, and triglycerides. Corticosteroid treatment increases the risk of glucose intolerance in patients without known diabetes and is associated with deterioration of glycaemic control in diabetic patients [7]. Glucocorticoids treatment therefore contributes to the exacerbation of a cluster of cardiovascular risk factors that are central to the metabolic syndrome. However, as inflammation plays a central role in the pathogenesis of atherosclerosis [8], it is also possible that glucocorticoids may exert some anti-atherosclerotic effects.

There was a significant association between ever use of oral glucocorticoids and any cardiovascular or cerebrovascular outcome. The association was stronger for current use of oral glucocorticoids than for recent or past use. Among current users, the highest odds ratios were observed in the group with the highest average daily dose, although the dose–response relation was not continuous. Current use was associated with an increased risk of heart failure, which was consistent between patients with rheumatoid arthritis, patients with chronic obstructive pulmonary disease, and patients without either of the two conditions. Also, current use was associated with a smaller increased risk of ischaemic heart disease [9].

RA population has an increased cardio-vascular mortality and premature death rate, but why does these patients have a higher incidence of atherosclerosis? There are several factors which are known risks in the development of atherosclerosis. Steroids may play a role in the increased mortality from vascular disease. Some reports have suggested that prolonged treatment with steroids accelerates the development of atherosclerosis. Steroids have atherogenic properties that are known to enhance the development of atherosclerosis and they induce vascular injury. In addition, they produce a state of hypercoagulability. In Moreland and O'Dell study, they found an increased atherosclerotic burden in the patients who were on long-term steroids. This suggests that steroid treatment may be a contributor to the higher rate of atherosclerosis seen in them [10]. Del Rincón et al. studied the carotid and lower-limb arteries in a sample of RA patients, and found that the extent of cumulative glucocorticoids dose was significantly associated with arterial incompressibility. This association displayed a gradient in which the proportion of incompressible arteries increased with higher glucocorticoids exposure. This pattern was independent of age at RA onset, sex, disease duration, CV risk factors, and manifestations of RA [11].

2. Historical background

Calcification of the arterial atheroma occurs in the coronary tree as it does in the remainder of the arterial tree. Such calcified coronary arteries are occasionally noted on routine chest radiographs but are difficult to distinguish from normal mediastinal structures and are confused with calcification in the chest wall, lungs, or other intracardiac structures [12]. Calcification of the coronary arteries is a common autopsy finding and is generally present in 80 to 90% of post-mortem studies. Despite this common pathologic finding, description of coronary calcification was rare until the work of Lenk [13] in 1927, who noted calcification of the left coronary artery on a posteroanterior chest radiograph in a 61-year-old male with left ventricular aneurysm. In 1964 Beadenkopf et al. [14] reported their findings in 904 consecutive autopsies; their results indicated that as the number of coronary arteries with calcification increased, coronary artery wall thickness increased. Tampas and Soule [15] in 1965 using radiographs in 1097 patients over the age of 40 found an incidence of 15% coronary calcification with a male to female ratio of 3 to 2 that was associated with increasing age. They suggested that coronary calcification might be an alarm signal of potential ischemic heart disease. Currently, it is generally recognized that the incidence of Coronary artery disease (CAD) was greater in patients with coronary calcification and atherosclerosis than in those without calcification [16].

3. Value of assessment of preclinical atherosclerosis

The presence of preclinical atherosclerosis increases global cardiovascular risk; therefore, it can be considered an emerging determinant in assessing such a risk. Single or multiple risk factors increase cardiovascular risk in an exponential manner, meanwhile the presence of one or more risk factors for atherosclerosis is associated with the development of cardiovascular disease. *A specific issue is defined as risk factor when it is possible, on the basis of a strong statistical association, to relate it to the incidence of new cases of disease and if it is clinically demonstrated that new disease cases can be reduced by correcting the same risk factor.*

Atherosclerosis is defined as a progressive structural remodeling of a vessel wall towards definitive plaque formation and possible related complications. According to new data, the disease begins as an endothelium functional disorder [dysfunction] inducing loss of vascular homeostasis and related functional reserve that initially can become clinically evident only in conditions in which there is a need to increase tissue metabolic requirements (as for instance effort Angina, transient Ischemic Attack, intermittent Claudication) while, after more time, they can become symptomatic at rest because even basal perfusion [blood flow] is impaired (acute coronary syndrome, stroke, critical leg ischemia, and even cardiovascular death) [12].

Coronary atherosclerosis is the leading cause of death in industrialized western countries. In up to 50% of its victims the first manifestation of CAD is sudden death or acute myocardial infarction. The cost of lost human value and approximate dollars spent ($90 billion annually) due to coronary artery disease in the western society is of great concern and is the reason for increased efforts for its prevention and its consequences as well. The detection of CAD in its asymptomatic stage is highly desirable because it is an increasingly treatable disease, but till now it has been hindered by the lack of sensitive and specific tests [13].

4. Methodology of assessment

4.1. Clinical background and limitations

In evaluating atherosclerosis the following demographic and clinical data are needed; sex, age, cigarette smoking, alcohol consumption, physical activity and life style, socioeconomic status, previous diseases, family history, BMI, WHR [waist to hip ratio] and blood pressure assessments in the standard way.

Chronic subclinical inflammation is thought to be part of the metabolic syndrome [MetSyn]. The latter is characterized by a clustering of atherosclerotic CVD risk factors. The WHO definition of MetSyn [14] requires the presence of insulin resistance plus 2 other of central obesity, hypertension, or dyslipidemia. Insulin resistance is thought to be the most prominent pathophysiological process underlying MetSyn. Recent studies of coronary artery calcification (CAC) in asymptomatic samples have shown an association of MetSyn and insulin resistance with the burden of coronary atherosclerosis [13]. Lakka et al. [15] found a 2- to 4-fold increased risk of cardiovascular death with MetSyn in a sample of 1209 Finnish men free from diabetes and CVD at baseline. MetSyn predicted atherosclerosis progression and CVD events in 888 subjects in the Bruneck study, whereas most individual components of the syndrome were not significantly associated with CVD out-comes [16] supporting the concept that MetSyn provides information that is "more than the sum of its parts."[17].

4.2. Laboratory methods

In more than 15 large prospective studies, C-reactive protein (CRP) has emerged as an independent predictor of an incident cardiovascular event in initially healthy subjects and outcome after acute coronary syndrome [18]. More importantly, its high levels have been demonstrated to be an even stronger predictor of cardiovascular events than LDL cholesterol levels. CRP represents only one of several new inflammatory biomarkers to be associated, independent of lipid profile, with future cardiovascular events. Among these, serum amyloid A (SAA), soluble vascular cell adhesion molecule-1 (VCAM-1), soluble intercellular adhesion molecule 1 (ICAM-1), lipoprotein associated phospholipase A2 (Lp-PLA2), homocysteine and monocyte chemoattractant protein-1 (MCP-1) are the best characterized. Interestingly, from the most recent epidemiological trials, evidence has consistently emerged that these biomarkers are independent from cholesterol levels, but also unrelated to each other. For instance, in healthy middle-aged men, CRP levels were found to correlate only marginally to Lp-PLA2 and MCP-1. The direct evidence that inflammatory biomarkers contribute to atherogenesis would be validated from the utilization of novel specific inhibitors for each of the soluble molecules which should prevent atherogenesis and coronary artery disease [18].

4.3. Sonographic modalities

Atherosclerosis is a chronic inflammatory disorder that often progresses silently for decades before becoming clinically evident. In this section we will preview sonographic noninvasive imaging of the vascular changes that occur in the atherosclerosis disease process including assessment of its inflammatory component. Because inflammation participates in plaque initiation and progression, a method capable of imaging the extent of vascular inflammation could potentially provide powerful predictive information on both early disease presence and future risk for disease progression.

4.3.1. Intima-Media Thickness (IMT) or Asymptomatic Carotid Plaque (ACP)

Echocolordoppler scanning evaluation of the carotid wall is a non invasive, low cost, and highly reproducible procedure even if, like most parts of the echographic analysis, it is strongly operator dependent. The Doppler mode permits the visualization of vessels and an evaluation of flow disturbance that helps to quantify stenosis severity. It measures the IMT and size and number of atheromatous plaques. According to the European Society of Cardiology; 2007-Guidelines on the Management of arterial Hypertension, normal IMT is the distance between the media-adventitia and the intima-media interfaces and is interpreted as follows:

- under 0,9 mm of the entire vascular wall; normal
- between 0.9 and 1.5 mm is an increased IMT,
- While all conditions in which it is greater than 1.5 mm can be considered an ACP.

Increased IMT (or ACP) is related to the presence, number, intensity and duration of atherosclerosis risk factors as well as endothelial dysfunction [24, 25]. Also, IMT is a potent and independent predictor of future cerebro- and cardiovascular events, as proven by several studies (Finnish, American Rotterdam groups) [17].

4.3.2. Ankle Brachial Pressure Index (ABI)

Normally, ankle systolic arterial pressure (posterior or anterior tibial artery) is just a little higher than brachial pressure measurements so that their ratio always is always > 1.0. This parameter is called the Ankle-Brachial pressure Index (ABI) and can reflect altered pressure values. It is reduced < 0.90 if atherosclerosis induced arterial system impairment is present; hence the patient is considered to have an asymptomatic peripheral artery disease. It is a simple, non-expensive procedure and can also be practiced by general practitioners [17]. Several population trials evidenced an important correlation between decreased ABI, carotid or coronary atherosclerosis and future cardiac or cerebrovascular events (27).

4.3.3. Endothelial function evaluation

A new, non-invasive technique was introduced to evaluate brachial artery flow-mediated dilatation (FMD). The evaluation through a sonographic assessment of brachial artery in basal condition and after 5 minutes of occlusion using pneumonic cuff (250 mm Hg) determined a reactive hyperemia and therefore, FMD. A low FMD is a marker of multifocal atherosclerosis and severity of the disease where the progressive reduction of FMD is associated with more extensive coronary tree involvement and future cardiovascular events [28, 29].

4.3.4. Targeted Ultrasound Detection of Vascular Cell Adhesion Molecule-1 (VCAM-1)

VCAM-1 is expressed by activated endothelial cells and participates in leukocyte rolling and adhesion primarily by interacting with its counterligand VLA-4 ($\alpha 4\ \beta 1$) on monocytes and lymphocytes. VCAM-1 expression on the vessel endothelial surface or the underlying vasa vasorum plays an important role in atherosclerotic plaque development by monocyte and T-lymphocyte recruitment. It is an ideal target for molecular imaging because there is little constitutive expression and its upregulation occurs at the earliest stages of atherogenesis. It was hypothesized that molecular imaging with *targeted contrast enhanced ultrasound* **[CEU]** could be used to evaluate the degree of vascular inflammation in atherosclerosis. CEU have multiple practical considerations; low cost, short duration [10 Minutes], good sensitivity and balance between spatial resolution and sensitivity for targeted contrast agent detection. It can potentially be useful in the early diagnosis of atherosclerosis and in monitoring the efficacy of therapeutic interventions.

4.4. Radiological modalities

4.4.1. Fluoroscopy

The detection of coronary calcification on chest films is not easy and the accuracy is only 42% compared with fluoroscopy, which itself is not sensitive. Fluoroscopy has frequently been used to detect calcification in the coronary arteries [31]. Data from the Duke registry of 800 patients by Margolis et al. [32] showed that patients with fluoroscopic evidence of calcium in the coronary arterial tree had a remarkably high prevalence of significant disease (94%). Only 6% of patients with coronary calcification had normal coronary angiograms. Among those without demonstrable calcification, 87% survived for more than 5 years compared to 58% with coronary calcification. Hence the latter implies a greater risk of future cardiac events. Fluoroscopy is widely available but it has several disadvantages [18]:

1. Although it can detect moderate to large calcifications; its ability to identify small calcifications is low.
2. Fluoroscopic detection of calcification is dependent on the skill and experience of the operator as well as the number of views studied.
3. Other important factors include variability of the equipment, patient's body habitus, and calcifications in other structures such as valves and vertebrae and overlying anatomic structures.
4. Finally with fluoroscopy, quantification of calcium is not possible and film documentation is not commonly obtained.

4.4.2. Computed tomography (CT)

Conventional CT is extremely sensitive in detecting vascular calcification. CT showed 50% more calcified vessels than did fluoroscopy. Its limitations are slow scan times resulting in motion artifacts, breathing misregistration, and inability to quantify amount of plaque. *Helical CT* has considerably faster scan times than conventional CT and overlapping sections improves calcium detection. *Double-helix CT scanners* appear to be more sensitive and now termed *electron beam (EBCT)* to distinguish them from conventional CT scanners.

Only *EBCT* can quantitate the amount or volume of calcium. The absence of calcific deposits on an EBCT scan implies the absence of significant angiographic coronary narrowing; however, it does not imply the absence of atherosclerosis, including unstable plaque. One of the most appealing features of EBCT is the potential to detect progression or regression of coronary atherosclerotic disease non-invasively and quantification with the use of calcium-volume score. Although the ACC/AHA [American College of Cardiology (ACC) and the American Heart Association (AHA)] guidelines affirm the strong negative predictive value of a normal EBCT they are not supportive for its widespread use in asymptomatic patients [18].

4.4.3. Magnetic Resonance Imaging [MRI]

Imaging techniques are needed that allow earlier and more refined diagnosis, guide targeted treatment in individual patients and monitor response to that treatment. MRI is well-suited to these tasks as it can provide anatomical, structural, and functional data of the arterial wall. Its capabilities are further enhanced by the use of a range of increasingly sophisticated contrast agents that target specific molecules, cells, and biological processes. Currently, it is considered to identify biologically relevant targets involved in the pathogenesis of atherosclerosis along its different stages [33].

For assessment of lesions that encroach on the vessel lumen inducing ischemia as in angina; angiography provides excellent resolution for the affected vascular territory with possible therapeutic intervention. However, atherosclerosis commonly develops within the walls of arteries without impinging on the vessel lumen; even established disease can be concealed from lumenographic methods. Unfortunately, even these non-stenotic lesions can rupture or erode precipitating intra-arterial thrombosis and acute ischemic events.

Distinct from alternative imaging modalities, MRI can provide data on a large range of vascular parameters that includes measures of vascular physiology (compliance, pulse wave velocity, and flow-mediated vasodilatation), cellular imaging, molecular imaging [adhesion molecule expression (VCAM-1), fibrin and platelets targeting] and functional anatomical data such as wall sheer stresses and density of neovascularization [33].

4.5. Radionuclide evaluation

4.5.1. Tc-99m sestamibi lower extremity muscle scan

Amin et al. [34] stated that Tc-99m sestamibi lower extremity muscle scan is a technique that can be effectively used to diagnose preclinical atherosclerosis in rheumatoid arthritis disease by measuring the so called perfusion reserve [PR]. They reported that it has a place as a screening tool considering the fact; whenever the diagnosis, the better it is the result, however, it could be used for detecting preclinical atherosclerosis even in apparently healthy subjects.

4.5.2. Technique

Prior to the administration of Tc-99m sestamibi for measurement of PR in lower limbs, each subject moved her right foot to produce maximal dorsal and plantar flexion 30–40 times in the sitting position (exercising side). 185 mBq of Tc-99m sestamibi was injected through intravenous line at least 10 sec before exercise termination. Posterior images of each calf were obtained 10 min post-injection. The processing phase was carried out by drawing symmetrical and equal regions of interest (ROI) over both exercising and resting calves. The total counts (Cts) in each (ROI) were obtained through a closed program inherent to the computer system [figure 1]. The percentage of increase of Cts in the exercising right calf was calculated, and the percentile increase obtained was considered as the perfusion reserve using the following formula [normal PR is approx. 50%]:

Perfusion reserve (%) =

[Cts in the exercising calf - Cts in the resting calf/ Cts in resting calf] x 100

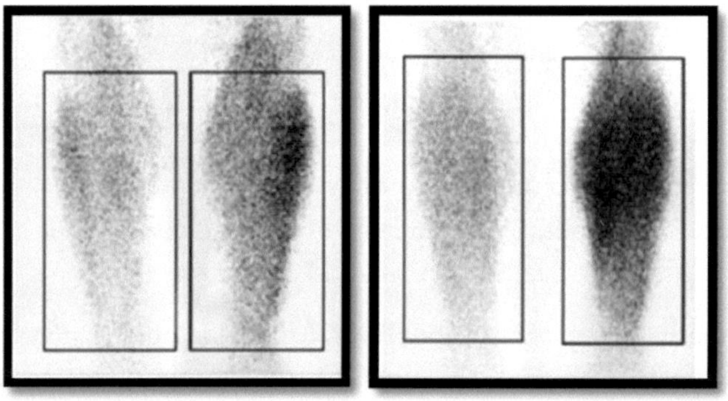

Figure 1. Tc-99m sestamibi muscle scans of an RA patient (PR 29.4%) [Left panel] and a control subject (PR 85%) [Right panel]

4.5.3. Myocardial sestaMIBI Gated-SPECT

Also, in our center a study was designed to evaluate usefulness of Dipyridamole pharmacological stress test in conjunction with Tc-99m sestamibi Gated-SPECT to screen the prevalence of subclinical coronary vascular dysfunction [SCED] in asymptomatic Egyptian Behçet's disease patients and to identify those at higher risk for the presence of such abnormalities as a predictor for preclinical atherosclerosis [*data are not published yet*]. Dipyridamole is an indirect coronary vasodilator that works by increasing intravascular adenosine through inhibition of phosphodiesterase that prohibits reuptake of endogenously produced adenosine into endothelial and red blood cells leading to arteriolar vasodilatation. This increases coronary arterial flow to approximately three times resting values in healthy endothelial state, however it is attenuated in diseased coronary arteries that cannot further dilate in response to adenosine. So, Dipyridamole infusion produces relative flow heterogeneity throughout coronary arteries, resulting in relatively more coronary blood flow in healthy arteries compared with the diseased-arteries inducing ischemia via a "*coronary steal phenomenon*" with subsequent perfusion defects ± abnormal left ventricular wall motion during radionuclide imaging. Hence, we used Dipyridamole stress in conjunction with Tc-99m sestamibi Gated-SPECT as a screening tool for SCED [Figure 2 and 3].

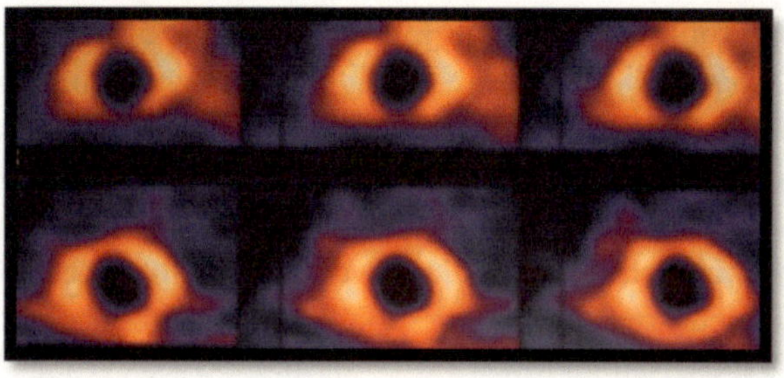

Figure 2. A 35-year-old male with stress induced reduced flow in LAD [anterior wall] and RCA vascular territories [inferior wall] with Complete recovery in the rest phase Coronary angiography was normal; [Stress; Upper row and Rest; Lower row- Short axis slices]

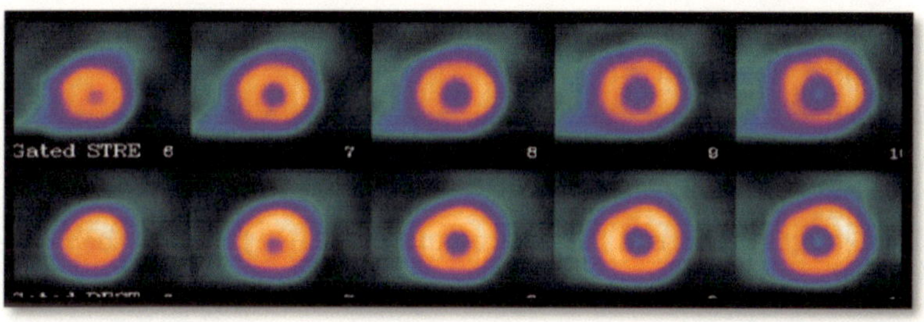

Figure 3. A 33-year-old negative Case for SCED [Stress; Upper row and Rest; Lower row-Short axis slices]

5. Special consideration

5.1. Premature lower limb atherosclerosis

Symptomatic lower extremity arterial occlusive disease in young adults is presumably rare provided that atherosclerosis is a natural consequence of ageing process. Several factors contribute to the "neglect" of premature lower extremity atherosclerosis (*PLEA*) among young population in clinical practice; including low public health awareness of this pathology, absence of large-scale epidemiologic studies, and overall low index of suspicion for vascular etiology of effort-induced lower extremity symptoms. A number of small clinical studies published in the last decade have strongly suggested that PLEA is the major cause for peripheral arterial disease (PAD) in young patients [35].

Levy report in 2002 identified 3 major clinical presentations of PLEA; the majority of patients had typical symptoms of effort-induced claudication, frequently misdiagnosed and attributed to arthritides, muscle spasms, and trauma. Approximately 20-25% present with "blue toe syndrome" caused by atheromatous embolization, most frequently originating from a segmental aortoiliac atherosclerotic lesion. The rest of patients presents with rapidly progressive symptoms of limb-threatening ischemia secondary to atherothrombosis. Also, they observed that many younger patients with isolated aortoiliac atherosclerotic disease had prolonged lower back pain on ambulation involving the spinal muscles who have been treated for several years for chronic low back pain by orthopedic surgeons, or neurosurgeons and some of them even had "unsuccessful" laminectomies before the diagnosis of PAD. In PLEA patients, clinical atherosclerotic disease was present in more than one anatomic location in approximately 60% including the coronary tree. Noninvasive studies are a mainstay of the PLEA diagnosis including ABI measurement and standardized lower extremity treadmill testing that has been developed to assess hyperemic blood flow response to exercise with repeat ABIs compared to the resting ABI with pulse-wave recordings. Also, Tc-99m sestamibi lower extremity muscle scan is suggested as a diagnostic test in PLEA patients [35].

6. Summary and conclusions

In summary, improved understanding of atherogenesis allowed the identification of a large number of molecules and processes. This will provide functional insights to aid diagnosis and to guide treatment with the introduction of new molecular imaging approaches that hold much promise for translation to the clinical practice. In fact, inflammatory biomarkers and imaging will combine structural and functional information to provide a comprehensive evaluation of vascular status at an early stage; hoping to be reversible.

Author details

Amr Amin
Nuclear Medicine, Cairo University, Egypt

Zeinab Nawito
Rheumatology & Rehabilitation, Cairo University, Egypt

Acknowledgement

To our parents and families for their patience, time and support they give all through our life time.

7. References

[1] Hench PS, Kendall EC, Slocumb CH, et al. The effect of a hormone of the adrenal cortex (17-hydroxy-11-dehydrocorticosterone, compound 8E) and of pituitary adrenocorticotrophic hormone on rheumatoid arthritis. Proc Staff Meet Mayo Clin 1949;24:181–97.

[2] Schacke H, Docke WD, Asadullah K. Mechanisms involved in the side effects of glucocorticoids. Pharmacol Ther 2002;96:23–43.

[3] Plotz CM, Knowlton AI, Ragan C. The natural history of Cushing's syndrome. Am J Med 1952;13:597–614.
[4] Plotz CM, Knowlton AI, Ragan C. Natural course of Cushing's syndrome as compared with the course of rheumatoid arthritis treated by hormones. Ann Rheum Dis 1952;11:308–9.
[5] Sholter DE, Armstrong PW. Adverse effects of corticosteroids on the cardiovascular system. Can J Cardiol 2000; 16:505–11.
[6] Kelly JJ, Mangos G,Williamson PM, et al. Cortisol and hypertension. Clin Exp Pharmacol Physiol Suppl 1998; 25:S51–6.
[7] Andrews RC, Walker BR. Glucocorticoids and insulin resistance: old hormones, new targets. Clin Sci (Lond) 1999;96:513–23.
[8] Libby P. Inflammation in atherosclerosis. Nature 2002; 420:868–74.
[9] Rheumatoid arthritis and macrovascular diseasJ. K. Alkaabi, M. Ho1 ,R.Levison,T.Pullar andJ.J.F.Belch Rheumatology 2003;42:292–297.
[10] Moreland LW, O'Dell JR. Glucocorticoids and Rheumatoid Arthritis Back to the Future? Arthritis Rheum. 2002; 46: 2553–63
[11] Del Rincón I, O'Leary DH, Haas RW, Escalante A. Effect of glucocorticoids on the arteries in rheumatoid arthritis. Arthritis Rheum. 2004; 50:3813-22.
[12] McCarthy JH, Palmer FJ: Incidence and significance of coronary artery calcification. Br Heart J 1974, 36:499–506.
[13] Lenk R: Rontgendiagnose der Koronarsklerose in vivo. Fortschr ad Geb D Rontgenstrahlen 1927, 35:1265–1268.
[14] Beadenkopf WG, Daoud AS, Love BM: Calcification in coronary arteries and its relationship to arteriosclerosis and myocardial infraction. Am J Roentgenol 1964, 92:865–871.
[15] Tampas JP, Soule AB: Coronary arterial calcification: its incidence and significance in patients over forty years of age. Am J Roentgenol 1966, 97:369–376.
[16] Fuseini M, Goodwin WJ, Ferris EJ, Mehta JL. Does electron beam computer tomography provide added value in the diagnosis of coronary artery disease? Curr Opin Cardiol. 2003; 18:385-93.
[17] Novo S, Amoroso G, Novo G. Cardiovascular Disease Prevention - Risk Assessment and Management. European society of cardiology 2007: Vol 6, No 10.
[18] Fuseini M, Goodwin WJ, Ferris EJ, Mehta JL. Does electron beam computer tomography provide added value in the diagnosis of coronary artery disease? Curr Opin Cardiol. 2003; 18:385-93.
[19] Alberti KG, Zimmet PZ. Definition, diagnosis and classification of diabetes mellitus and its complications, II: diagnosis and classification of diabetes mellitus provisional report of a WHO consultation. Diabet Med.1998;15:539–553.
[20] Lakka HM, Laaksonen DE, Lakka TA, Niskanen LK, Kumpusalo E, Tuomilehto J, et al. The metabolic syndrome and total and cardiovascular disease mortality in middle-aged men. JAMA. 2002;288:2709–2716.

[21] Bonora E, Kiechl S, Willeit J, Oberhollenzer F, Egger G, Bonadonna RC, et al. Carotid atherosclerosis and coronary heart disease in the metabolic syndrome: prospective data from the Bruneck study. Diabetes Care. 2003;26:1251–1257.

[22] Reilly MP, Rader DJ. The metabolic syndrome: more than the sum of its parts? Circulation. 2003; 108:1546–1551.

[23] Ferri N, Paoletti R, Corsini A. Biomarkers for atherosclerosis: pathophysiological role and pharmacological modulation. Curr Opin Lipidol. 2006; 17:495-501.

[24] Novo S, Pernice C, Barbagallo C M, Tantillo R, Caruso R, Longo B. Influence of risk factors and aging on asymptomatic carotid lesions. In: Advances in Vascular Pathology 1997, A. N. Nicolaides and S. Novo (Eds.), Elsevier Science, Excerpta Medica, Amsterdam, 1997, pp. 33-44.

[25] Corrado E, Bonura F., Tantillo R, Muratori I, Rizzo M, Vitale G, Mansueto S, Novo S. Markers of infection and inflammation influence the outcome of patients with baseline asymptomatic carotid lesions in a 5 years follow-up. Stroke 2006; 37: 482-6.

[26] Corrado E, Muratori I, Tantillo R, Contorno F, Coppola G, Strano A, Novo S. Relationship between endothelial dysfunction, intima media thickness and cardiovascular risk factors in asymptomatic subjects. Int Angiol. 2005; 24:52-8.

[27] Diehm C, Lange S, Darius H, Pittrow D, von Stritzky B, Tepohl G, Haberl RL, Allenberg JR, Dasch B, Trampisch HJ. Association of low ankle brachial index with high mortality in primary care. Eur Heart J. 2006; 27: 1743-9.

[28] Corrado E, Rizzo M, Coppola G, Muratori I, Carella M, Novo S. Endothelial dysfunction and carotid lesions are strong predictors of clinical events in patients with early stages of atherosclerosis: a 24-month follow-up study. Coron Artery Dis. 2008; 19(3):139-44.

[29] Landmesser U, Hornig B, Drexler H Endothelium Function: A Critical Determinant in Atherosclerosis. Circulation. 2004; 109 (suppl. II): II-27-II-33.

[30] Kaufmann BA, Sanders JM, Davis C, Xie A, Aldred P, Sarembock IJ, Lindner JR. Molecular imaging of inflammation in atherosclerosis with targeted ultrasound detection of vascular cell adhesion molecule-1. Circulation. 2007; 116:276-84.

[31] Souza AS, Bream PR, Elliot LP: Chest film detection of coronary artery calcification: the value of the CAC triangle. Radiology 1978, 129:7–10.

[32] Margolis JR, Chen JTT, Kong Y, et al.: The diagnostic and prognostic significance of coronary artery calcification. Radiology 137:609–616.

[33] Choudhury RP. Atherosclerosis and thrombosis: identification of targets for magnetic resonance imaging. Top Magn Reson Imaging. 2007 Oct;18(5):319-27.

[34] Amin AM, Nawito ZO, Atfy RA, El-Hadidi KT. Tc-99m sestamibi lower extremity muscle scan, is it a useful screening tool for assessment of preclinical atherosclerosis in rheumatoid arthritis patients? Rheumatol Int. 2012 Jul;32(7):2075-81.

[35] Levy PJ. . Premature lower extremity atherosclerosis: clinical aspects. Am J Med Sci. 2002; 323:11-6.

Chapter 23

Steroids in Asthma: Friend or Foe

Mahboub Bassam and Vats Mayank

Additional information is available at the end of the chapter

http://dx.doi.org/10.5772/50536

1. Introduction

Asthma is a common chronic inflammatory disease of the respiratory tract characterized by episodic exacerbations with a heterogeneous population distribution. The prevalence of asthma has increased substantially over the past 5 decades throughout the globe, yet the reasons for this increase remain unknown. The disease represents a substantial burden, not only in terms of morbidity, mortality and reduced quality of life of patients, but also imposing a huge cost on the healthcare facilities in all countries.

2. Burden of asthma

Approximately 300 million people worldwide currently have asthma, and its prevalence increases by 50% every decade, seeing a rise to 400 million by year 2025 (Braman, 2006; Masoli et al., 2004) The increasing number of hospital admissions for asthma, which are most pronounced in young children, reflect an increase in severe asthma, poor disease management, and poverty. Worldwide, approximately 180,000 deaths annually are attributable to asthma. Most asthma deaths occur in those >45 years old and are largely preventable, frequently being related to inadequate long-term medical care or delays in obtaining medical help during the attack.

The financial burden on patients with asthma in different western countries ranges from $300 to $1,300 per patient per year, disproportionately affecting those with the most severe disease. It is the most common chronic disorder in children and adolescents, with more than 3 million asthma attacks occurring in more than 5% of all children each year.

Asthma is a cause of concern due to under diagnosis, under investigated, under control and non-adherence to treatment (Barreto, 2006, National Institutes of Health, Bethesda, 2006, Woolcock, 1989, Bassam, 2012). A recent report from WHO suggests that 50% of patients from developed world with chronic diseases do not take their medications as recommended. In developing countries, the situation may be even worse when considering together all the issues related with poor access to health care, lack of appropriate diagnosis, and limited access to medicines. Poor adherence seriously threatens any effort to tackle such chronic illness (WHO, 2003, Horne, 2003).

Steroids V/S No Steroids in asthma: If ever there was a magic potion that should resolve the symptoms of an affliction, it is the use of glucocorticoids in asthma. Since their first clinical application, there has been uniform agreement that the anti-inflammatory activities of the corticosteroids make them ideal agents to stabilize asthma during all stages of asthma symptomatology ranging from chronic persistent phase to acute severe life threatening exacerbations.

Pathophysiology of asthma: Asthmatic inflammatory process results from inappropriate immune responses to common environmental antigens in a genetically susceptible individual (Wills-Karp 1999). These inappropriate immune responses are orchestrated by a subset of CD4+ T helper cells termed T helper 2 (Th2) cells.

Cytokines play a pivotal role in the development of asthma by regulating the expansion of Th2 cells and by mediating many of the Th2 effector functions that underlie the pathogenic events of an asthmatic response. Much effort has recently been placed in elucidating the pathways used by cytokines to mediate their actions. These studies have revealed that cytokine-mediated signals are primarily transduced by the Janus Kinase- Signal Transducer and Activator of Transcription (JAK-STAT) signaling cascade (Darnell, 1997). Recent advances have shown the important roles of JAK-STAT signaling pathway in the pathogenesis of asthma.

3. JAK-STAT signaling in Th1 and Th2 differentiation:

The two major subsets of CD4+ T helper cells, Th1 and Th2, secrete mutually distinct profiles of cytokines and thereby coordinate different classes of immune response. The cytokines IL-12 and IL-4 direct the differentiation of Th1 and Th2 cells, respectively, from naive T helper cells. Th1 cells secrete IL-2, IFN-γ, and TNF-β, whereas Th2 cells produce IL-4, IL-5, IL-6, IL-10, and IL-13.

Th1 cells are critically involved in the generation of delayed-type hypersensitivity responses, whereas Th2 cells can direct B cells to mount strong humoral responses. Polarization of immune response toward a Th2 phenotype and when directed against an otherwise innocuous environmental antigen result in the pathogenesis of allergic diseases like asthma.

The Th2 cytokines (IL-4, IL-5, and IL-13) control all the major components that characterize an inflammatory asthmatic response, including IgE isotype switching, mucus production, and the recruitment and activation of eosinophils and have been corroborated by studies in humans. The population of Th2 cells is notably expanded in the airways of asthmatic subjects, and presence of these cells correlates with airway hyper responsiveness (AHR) and airway eosinophilia (Rengarajan et al., 2000, Murphy et al., 2000).

IL-4 and IL-12 activate the Jak-Stat signaling cascade discussed elsewhere in this Perspective series. In this signaling pathway, binding of a cytokine to its receptor leads to the activation of members of the JAK family of receptor associated kinases. These kinases subsequently activate, via tyrosine phosphorylation, preexistent cytoplasmic factors termed Stats (signal transducer and activator of transcription). Tyrosine phosphorylation allows the Stat proteins to dimerize and translocate to the nucleus, where they mediate changes in gene expression by binding specific DNA elements. Although both IL-4 and IL-12 follow this basic signaling framework, the two cytokines differ in the specific Jak and Stat components that they activate (Wurster, A.L. et al 2000). IL-4 stimulates Jak1 and Jak3 to activate Stat6. In contrast, interaction of IL-12 with its receptor leads to the activation of Jak2 and Tyk2 and the subsequent phosphorylation of Stat4. Activation of Stat6 and Stat4 are thus critical events in the signaling cascades of IL-4 and IL-12, respectively.

Mechanism of Action of steroids: Glucocorticoids (GC's) are potent anti-inflammatory agents and are useful in the treatment of both allergic and idiosyncratic asthma. Although the mechanisms of corticosteroid action in asthma are poorly understood, several possible sites of action have been proposed which help reverse the pathologic process of bronchial asthma.

Glucocorticoid receptors (GRs) are specific cytoplasmic transcription factors that mediate the biological actions of corticosteroids (Beato M et al *1995*). On ligand binding, GR translocates into the nucleus and binds to DNA at glucocorticoid response elements (GREs) in the promoter region of corticosteroid-responsive genes that induce transcription (Barnes PJ & Adcock IM 1998). GR activation may also influence antiinflammatory events by nongenomic pathways, forming inhibitory interactions within the nucleus with proinflammatory DNA-binding transcription factors, such as activator protein (AP)-1 or nuclear factor (NF)–_B, or by recruitment of co-repressors, and thereby repressing the actions of these important inflammatory proteins (Karin M. 1998, Ito K et al. 2000). GR nuclear translocation is, therefore, essential and necessary for corticosteroid action.

It has been well investigated that the novel mechanism of GC action is by blocking cytokine signaling via the JAK-STAT signaling pathway. Dexamethasone inhibited IL-2-induced DNA binding, tyrosine phosphorylation, and nuclear translocation of Stat5 in primary T cells. Inhibition of Stat5 correlated with inhibition of expression of IL-2-inducible genes and T cell proliferation. The mechanism of inhibition involved suppression of IL-2 receptor and Jak3 expression. Signaling by IL-4, IL-7, and IL-15, which use IL-2 receptor components, also was inhibited, indicating a block in T cell responses similar to that seen in immunodeficient patients lacking the IL-2 receptor gamma chain or Jak3.

IL-2 signaling also was blocked in patients after treatment with GC's, suggesting that inhibition of cytokine signaling contributes to the clinical efficacy of GC's. Hence inhibition of both cytokine production and Jak- stat signaling contribute to their therapeutic potency (Bianchi, 2000).

Corticosteroids enhance the beta-adrenergic response to relieve the muscle spasm. They also act by reversing the mucosal edema, decreasing vascular permeability by vasoconstriction, and inhibiting the release of Leukotrienes (LT) LT-C4 and LT-D4. Corticosteroids reduce the mucus secretion by inhibiting the release of secretagogue from macrophages. Corticosteroids inhibit the late phase reaction by inhibiting the inflammatory response and interfering with chemotaxis due to the inhibition of LT-B4 release. The eosinopenic effect of corticosteroids may help to prevent the cytotoxic effect of the major basic protein and other inflammatory mediators released from eosinophils. Corticosteroids have no effect on the immediate hypersensitivity reaction and have no direct role in bronchial reactivity. By blocking the late reaction, they prevent the increased airway reactivity observed with late bronchial reactions, all of which aid in the resolution of bronchospasm in asthmatic patients **(Figure 1)**

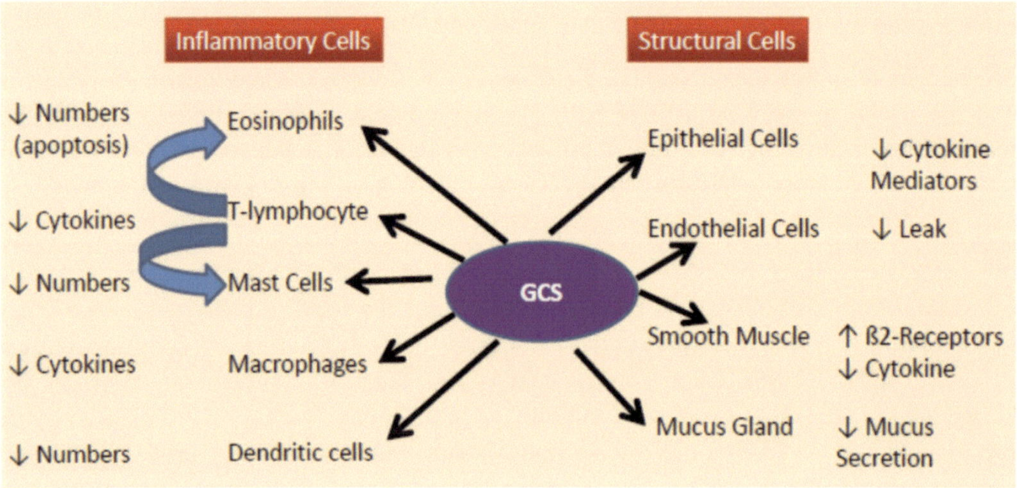

Figure 1. Mechanism of Action of Corticosteroids in asthma

Mode of Delivery: All levels of persistent asthma require daily anti-inflammatory treatment (with additional doses of oral or intravenous steroid based on the severity of symptoms). Inhaled corticosteroids (ICS's) are the safest and most effective anti-inflammatory treatment for patients with persistent asthma of all severity having a significant positive impact on outcomes. Although steroids may be given orally or systemically, and numerous non-steroidal medications are available for treating persistent asthma, ICS's are the treatment of choice considering their risk-benefit and cost-effectiveness ratio. Even when ICS's are given daily over prolong period of time, they have less toxicity than oral or systemic steroids administered only occasionally. A wide range of ICS's are available & the choice depends upon the availability, cost, physician and patient's preference, however it is important to use the equipotent doses of various ICS's while switching over the ICS's for control of asthma **(Table-1)**

In cases of acute severe asthma or patients requiring maintenance therapy with steroids for chronic persistent asthma intravenous or oral routes are to be preferred, it's important to know the equipotent doses of various type of steroid while starting or switching from one form to another or from one steroids to another in order to get the equivalent response and to avoid worsening of symptoms (if underdosing done) or side effects (if overdosing done). **Table 2** summarizes the equivalent doses of various types of intravenous or oral steroids. (http://www.globalrph.com/corticocalc.htm)

Drug	Low Daily dose (µgm)	Medicum Daily dose (µgm)	High Daily dose (µgm)
Beclomethasone Dipropionate	200-500	500-1000	1000-2000
Budesonide	200-400	400-800	800-1600
Ciclesonide	80-160	10-320	320-1280
Flunisolide	500-1000	1000-2000	>2000
Fluticasone Propionate	100-250	250-500	500-1000
Mometasone Furoate	200	400	800
Triamcinolone acetonide	400-1000	1000-2000	>2000

Table 1. Estimated Equipotent daily doses of all formulations of ICS in adults

Glucocorticoid	Approximate Equivalent dose (mg)	Half-life(Biologic) hours
	Short-Acting	
Cortisone	25	8-12
Hydrocortisone	20	8-12
	Intermediate-Acting	
Methylprednisolone	4	18-36
Prednisolone/ Prednisone	5	18-36
Triamcinolone	4	18-36
	Long-Acting	
Betamethasone	0.6 - 0.75	36-54
Dexamethasone	0.75	36-54

Table 2. Estimated Equipotent daily doses of all formulations of glucocorticoids in adults

Steroids in Children: ICS are the first-line therapy for persistent asthma in children. Major safety concerns of long-term ICS therapy in children include suppression of adrenal function and impaired growth and bone development. Dosage, type of inhaler device used, patient technique, and characteristics of the individual drug influence systemic effects of ICS's. Systemic side effects can occur when continuous high-dose treatment is required for severe asthma or when prescribed dosage is excessive and compliance is unusually good.

It is very important to know that uncontrolled or severe asthma adversely affects growth and final adult height in children & no long-term controlled studies have reported any statistically or clinically significant adverse effects on growth of 100-200 µg/ day of ICS's however it may be seen with all ICS's when a high dose is administered for prolonged periods (dose dependent effect). Different age groups seem to differ in their susceptibility to the growth-retarding effects of ICS's, children aged 4 to 10 are more susceptible than adolescents, however Children with asthma treated with ICS's attain normal adult height (predicted from family members) but at a later age(Pedersen, 2001, Agertoft & Pedersen, 2000,. Sharek, & Bergman 2000). No studies have reported any statistically significant increase in risk of fracture in children taking ICS's.

Oral or systemic steroids increases the risk of fracture in children with a 32 % increase in 4 courses ever, however ICS's are safe in this regard. Controlled longitudinal studies of 2-5 yrs duration and several cross sectional studies found no adverse effect of ICS on bone mineral density (Agertoft & Pedersen , 1998, Hopp et al., 1995).

Suppression of Hypothalamic-pituitary-adrenal (HPA) axis: Though differences exist between the various ICS's and inhaler devices, treatment with ICS's doses of less than 200 μg budesonide or equivalent daily is normally not associated with any significant suppression of the HPA axis in children. At higher doses, small changes in HPA axis function can be detected with sensitive methods. The clinical relevance of these findings is not known, since there have not been reports of adrenal crisis in clinical trials of ICS's in children. However, adrenal crisis has been reported in children treated with excessively high doses of ICS's (Roux et al., 2003).

Recent studies confirm that benefits of ICS, properly prescribed and used, clearly outweigh not only their potential adverse effects but also the risks associated with poorly controlled asthma.

Benefits of oral corticosteroids for asthma include reduction in mucus production, chest tightness, coughing, and wheezing. Other non-asthma related conditions, such as sinus conditions and psoriasis, may also improve due to the anti-inflammatory properties of oral steroids.

Side effects of steroids: Side effects of short-term oral steroids include fluid retention, stomach upset, excessive hunger, and blurred vision. Difficulty concentrating, insomnia, and mood changes can also occur as a result of taking oral corticosteroids. The systemic side-effects of long-term treatment with high doses of ICS's may include cataracts, osteoporosis, easy bruising, and hair loss, Weight gain, an increase in facial hair in women, and muscle weakness. Long term use of oral corticosteroids may also increase the risk of diabetes, high blood pressure, and certain infections. Systemic effects of inhaled glucocorticosteroids are not a problem in adults at doses of ≤ 400 mg budesonide or equivalent daily.

Factors affecting response of ICS's: Three most important factors that appear to have significant impact on the effectiveness of inhaled corticosteroid (ICS) treatment are:

1.) **Patient compliance with inhaled anti-asthma therapy:** The term "Compliance" is defined as the extent to which a patient's behavior matches the prescriber's advice but recently it has mostly been superseded by the term adherence, a similar concept but having fewer negative connotations from physician/patient relationship point of view (Haynes, 1979). Adherence is defined as the extent to which the patient's behavior matches agreed recommendations from the prescriber.

The issue of noncompliance is complicated by different patterns of noncompliance and a variety of measurements of noncompliance. Cochrane GM 1996 identified several patterns of noncompliance, including taking only half of the medications at the prescribed times, taking the medication regularly for a period and stopping, and skipping prescribed doses. Compliance with preventive therapy such as ICSs whose effect is seen over a period of weeks may be less than compliance with drugs that relieve asthma symptoms more rapidly. Patient adherence to medication is influenced by a number of factors relating to how the individual judges the necessity of their treatment relative to their concerns. These factors can be categorized as follows:

1. Treatment factors:
   - Dosing schedule too frequent
   - cost / non-availability of medicine
   - Complexity or inconvenience of treatment regimen
   - Need to use proper inhaler technique
   - Discomfort of drug administration (eg, bad taste, dry throat, hoarseness, fungal infections)
   - Physician's Inertia / Attitude/ lack of communication
   - Proper education about the disease not given by physician
2. Behavioral factors
   - Belief that medication is not really needed (esp. Controller medicine (ICS)
   - Belief that medication would not work
   - Poor perception of the impact of the disease (symptoms, experience, expectations & interpretation of illness)
   - Fear of adverse effects or dependence/ negative orientation to medicines
   - Steroid phobia
   - Forgetting to take medication
   - Volitional non-adherence: voluntarily not taking medication
   - Non-volitional non-adherence: from failure to take medication properly (e.g. ICS± LABA)
3. Contextual issues: Past experiences, Cultural issues/ Social beliefs/ Poor pt /View of others/ Practical difficulties

It is important to keep the medication regimen as simple as possible, prioritize recommendations, educate the patient regarding disease management, and individualized the dosing and schedule of ICS as per patient's requirment.

2.) **Inhalation technique.** The effectiveness of inhaler therapy depends not only on compliance, but also on the inhaler technique. Various types of inhaler devices are available including trubohaler, discus etc however they can be broadly categorized based on the form of drugs used as dry powder inhalers (DPI) and Metered Dose inhalers (MDI). Although both types of inhalers are equally effective but While prescribing ICS to patient due consideration should be given to the age of the patient, comorbid conditions, coordination between the hands & mouth & the educational level of patient, otherwise the inhaled ICS will get deposited in the oropharynx & produce local side effects(such as change in voice, Oropharyngeal candidiasis). Use of Spacer with MDI can largely reduce the deposition of the ICS in throat & hence avoid local side effects of the steroids.

3.) **Impact of inhalation technique and device on drug deposition in the lungs:** For ICSs, the efficacy depends on the topical activity of the drug that reaches the target area, whereas the adverse events depend both on oral deposition and systemic activity. Systemic activity of the drug depends on the amount of the drug absorbed either through the GI tract or through the lungs, as well as on the first-pass metabolism for drug absorbed through the GI tract.

The amount of drug delivered to the lungs depends on the inhalation technique,(Dolovich, 1981, Jackson & Lipworth , 1995) as well as on the type of inhaler used and the fine particle size (respirable particle diameter between 1- 4 μm) of the drug. **Table -3** shows the Estimates of the Lung to Systemic Bioavailability Ratios for different types of ICS's.

Product	% Dose Deposited in the Lungs	% Dose Reaching the Systemic Circulation after Absorption from the Gastrointestinal Tract	Lung/Systemic Bioavailability Ratio
BDP via CFC propellant	5.5	14.7	0.27
BDP (non-CFC propellant)	56.1	5.5	0.92
Budesonide via MDI	15	7.7	0.66
Budesonide via DPI	30	5.3	0.85

BDP-beclomethasone dipropionate. CFC-chlorofluorocarbon. MDI-metered-dose inhaler, DPI- dry powder inhaler.

Table 3. Estimates of the Lung to Systemic Bioavailability Ratios for Inhaled Corticosteroids

Recent Recommendations about the delivery device for ICS from American College of Chest Physicians/American College of Asthma, Allergy, and Immunology states that:

1. For the treatment of asthma in the outpatient setting, both the MDI with a spacer/holding chamber and the DPI are appropriate devices for the delivery of ICS's.
2. For outpatient asthma therapy, the selection of an appropriate aerosol delivery device for ICS's includes the patient's ability to use the device correctly, the preferences of the patient for the device, the availability of the drug/device combination, the compatibility between the drug and delivery device, the lack of time or skills to properly instruct the patient in the use of the device or monitor the appropriate use, the cost of therapy, and the potential for reimbursement(Dolovich, 2005). **Table -4** summarizes the advantages & disadvantages of all the devices available for the delivery of ICS's

Type	Advantages	Disadvantages
Small-volume jet nebulizer (Respiratory solution, Respules, nebules)	Patient coordination not required Effective with tidal breathing High dose possible Dose modification possible Can be used with supplemental oxygen Can deliver combination therapies if compatible	Lack of portability Pressurized gas source required Lengthy treatment time Device cleaning required Contamination possible Not all medication available in solution form Does not aerosolize suspensions well Device preparation required Performance variability Expensive when compressor added
Ultrasonic nebulizer	Patient coordination not required High dose possible Dose modification possible Small dead volume small and portable Faster delivery than jet nebulizer No drug loss during exhalation (breath actuated devices)	Expensive Need for electric power source Contamination possible Not all medication available Device preparation required before treatment Does not nebulize suspensions well Possible drug degradation airway irritation with some drugs
Pressurized MDI (CFC/ HFA as propellant) accuhaler, Evohalers	Portable and compact Treatment time is short No drug preparation required No contamination of contents Dose-dose reproducibility high Some can be used with breath actuated mouthpiece	Coordination of breathing and device actuation needed High pharyngeal deposition Upper limit to unit dose content Remaining doses difficult to determine Potential for abuse Not all medications available
Holding chamber, reverse flow spacer, or spacer (Zerostat, Zerostat-v **spacer**)	Reduces need for coordination Reduces pharyngeal deposition	Inhalation can be more complex for some patients Can reduce dose available if not used properly More expensive/Less portable Integral actuator devices may alter aerosol properties compared to native actuator
DPI (Turbohaler, Diskus, Rotahaler, Handihaler, aerolizer)	Breath-actuated Less coordination required No Propellant required Small and portable Short treatment time Dose counters	Requires moderate to high inspiratory flow Can result in high pharyngeal deposition Not all medications available

CFC-Cloro-fluor-Carbon, HFA- hydro-fluoro-alkane, MDI- Metered dose inhaler, DPI- Dry Powder inhaler

Table 4. Advantages and Disadvantages of Aerosol-Generating Device or System

In short, effective asthma treatment requires a combination of pharmacology and psychology. Effective prescribing needs to take account of patients' beliefs, expectations, and adherence behavior.

Goal of Asthma Management: According to Global Initiative for Asthma (**GINA 2010**) Guidelines issued by the National Heart Lung & Blood institute, the goals for successful management of asthma are to:

- Achieve and maintain control of symptoms
- Maintain normal activity level including exercise
- Maintain pulmonary functions as close to normal as possible
- Prevent asthma exacerbations
- Avoid side effects from asthma medications
- Avoid asthma mortality

Therefore, for successful management of asthma and optimum control of asthma , patients should always be assessed to know their status of asthma control , Following classification of asthma by level of control is more relevant and **useful** (Figure 2).

Characteristic	Controlled (All of the following)	Partly Controlled (Any measure present in any week)	Uncontrolled
Daytime symptoms	None (twice or less/week)	More than twice/week	Three or more features of partly controlled asthma present in any week
Limitations of activities	None	Any	
Nocturnal symptoms/ awakening	None	Any	
Need for reliever/ rescue treatment	None (twice or less/week)	More than twice/week	
Lung function (PEF or FEV_1)‡	Normal	< 80% predicted or personal best (if known)	
Exacerbations	None	One or more/year*	One in any week†

Adopted from Global Initiative for Asthma (GINA 2010) Guidelines
* Any exacerbation should prompt review of maintenance treatment to ensure that it is adequate.
† By definition, an exacerbation in any week makes that an uncontrolled asthma week.
‡ Lung function testing is not reliable for children 5 years and younger.

Figure 2. Classification of asthma by level of control

To reach this goal, four interrelated components of therapy are required:

Component 1: Develop patient/doctor partnership: In order to help in the effective management of asthma so that the asthmatic patient can learn how to: avoid risk factors, take medications correctly, understand the difference between "controller" and "reliever" medications, monitor their status using symptoms and, if relevant Peak expiratory Flow (PEF) recognize signs that asthma is worsening and take action, seek medical help as appropriate.

Component 2: Identify and Reduce Exposure to Risk Factors: To improve control of asthma and reduce medication needs, despite physical activity is a common cause of asthma symptoms however patients should not avoid exercise. Common strategies for avoiding allergens and pollutants include the followings; Stay away from tobacco smoke, patients and parents should not smoke, avoid drugs, foods, and additives if they are known to cause symptoms, reduce or, preferably, avoid exposure to occupational sensitizers.

Component 3: Assess, Treat, and Monitor Asthma: Each patient is assigned to one of five treatment "steps" based on the frequency and severity of symptoms, PFT values and the exacerbations. At each treatment step, asthma education, environmental control & vaccination are important component of asthma control. Rescue medication should be provided for quick relief of symptoms as needed. As the severity of disease increases, from Steps 2- 5, patients should be given one or more regular controller medications (*ICS*) in order to keep asthma under control & to avoid the morbidity & mortality related with asthma and to prevent the long term consequences of the disease. Regular use of ICS has *demonstrated* high efficiency in reducing asthma symptoms, reducing frequency & severity of exacerbations, reducing mortality, improving quality of life, improving lung function, decreasing airway hyper-responsiveness & controlling airway inflammation.

Component 4: Managing asthma exacerbations: Exacerbations of asthma are characterized by episodes of progressive increase in shortness of breath, cough, wheezing or chest tightness, or some combination of these symptoms. Mamgement of asthma exacerbation requires close objective monitoring (both clinical and using PEF), repetitive administration of rapid-acting inhaled bronchodilators, early introduction of systemic glucocorticosteroids and oxygen supplementation. It is very important to use systemic steroids early in case of exacerbation in order to control the underlying inflammation earliest possible. GINA guidelines have simplified the recognition of severity of acute exacerbation of asthma and management in acute care setting base on the severity of symptoms & response to treatment (For details: www.ginasthma.org)

Stepwise approach for asthma Management: GINA guidelines have simplified the management of asthma at all stages in stepwise manner starting from rescue medicines to regular controller medicine. (**Figure 3**)

4. Glucocorticoid resistance

Although glucocorticoids are highly effective in the control of chronic inflammation or immune dysregulation occurring in asthma pts however a small proportion of patients displays persistent immune activation and airway inflammation and fail to respond despite high doses of oral corticosteroids imposing a big challenge for the physicians. (Barnes, 1995, 1995, Sze¯er, 1997). This group of patients has been classified as "steroid-resistant"

Step 1	Step 2	Step 3	Step 4	Step 5
Asthma education Environmental control				
As needed rapid-acting β_2-agonist	As needed rapid-acting β_2-agonist			
Controller options	Select one	Select one	Add one or more	Add one or both
	Low-dose inhaled ICS*	Low-dose ICS plus long-acting β_2-agonist	Medium-or high-dose ICS plus long-acting β_2-agonist	Oral glucocorticosteroid (lowest dose)
	Leukotriene modifier**	Medium-or high-dose ICS	Leukotriene modifier	Anti-IgE treatment
		Low-dose ICS plus leukotriene modifier	Sustained release theophylline	
		Low-dose ICS plus sustained release theophylline		

* ICS=inhaled glucocorticosteroids
** =Receptor antagonist or synthesis inhibitors

Adopted from Global Initiative for Asthma (GINA 2010) Guidelines

Figure 3. Stepwise approach for asthma Management

Steroid resistant asthma: American Thoracic Society (ATS) defined Steroid resistant patients as characterized by a pre-bronchodilator Force expiratory volume in 1 sec (FEV1) of less than 70% predicted with a maintained bronchodilator response. Steroid resistance is defined by administering a course of oral prednisone e.g. 40 mg/d (divided doses) for 7 days or preferably 2 wk, and observing the effect on morning pre-bronchodilator FEV1 (Lee, 1996). If the FEV1 fails to increase by 15% (and 200 ml), the patient is considered steroid resistant (Sally et al., 2000). These patients show the typical diurnal variability in peak expiratory flow and bronchodilatation with inhaled B-2 agonists. This type of trial can also assess the possibility of poor adherence to the maintenance regimen.

Patients with steroid resistance can be grouped into two broad categories,

Type 1 steroid resistance: is either immune-mediated or acquired as the result of environmental triggers or lifestyle. Clinically, such patients will develop steroid side effects, including adrenal gland suppression, osteoporosis, and cushingoid features from pharmacologic doses of systemic steroids. This is because there is only one (glucocorticoid resistant) GR gene and these patients have steroid resistance only at the level of their immune/inflammatory cells (i.e., T cells). The rest of the tissues in their body remain sensitive to the deleterious effects of systemic steroids.

Type 2 steroid resistances: is rare but involves a generalized primary cortisol resistance that affects all tissues and is likely associated with a mutation in the GR gene or genes that modulate GR function. This form is not associated with the development of steroid's side effects or suppression of morning cortisol levels (**Table 5**). It is analogous to genetically inherited familial cortisol resistance. When patients present with a history of no side effects after high doses of prednisone, it is critical to confirm that they are taking the oral prednisone by checking their morning serum cortisol after a course of therapy under strict supervision. Such individuals need alternative approaches to control their pulmonary inflammation.

Features	Type 1 steroid resistances	Type 2 steroid resistances
AM cortisol levels	Suppressed	No
Cushingoid side effects	Yes	No
Cause	Cytokine induced(May be genetic), Allergy, Microbes	Genetic
GCR ligand and DNA binding affinity	Reduced	Normal
GCR numbers	Normal or High	Low
Reversibility of GCR defect	Yes	No

Table 5. Summarizes difference in both Types of steroid resistance

It is imperative to exclude confounding factors when trying to make the diagnosis of steroid-resistant asthma in a patient. These factors include non-adherence with asthma medication, inadequate inhalation technique, incorrect diagnosis, unrecognized concomitant diagnoses, and ongoing exposure to environmental allergens, abnormal corticosteroid pharmacokinetics, and psychosocial disturbances. Low dose methotrexate, cyclosporine, Intravenous immunoglobulin, leukotriene antagonists, such as zafirlukast and montelukast and Nedocromil sodium has been used in steroid resistant patients with varying success rates and with associated side effects.

5. Clinical features of glucocorticoid-resistant asthma

Glucocorticoid resistance in asthma was first described in six patients with asthma who did not respond clinically to high doses of systemic glucocorticoids and in whom there was also a reduced eosinopenic response (Schwartz et al .,1968). Larger groups of patients with chronic asthma who were glucocorticoid resistant were subsequently identified (Carmichael et al ., 1981). These patients were not Addisonian and did not suffer from the abnormalities in sex hormones described in familial glucocorticoid resistance (see below). Plasma cortisol and adrenal suppression in response to exogenous cortisol is normal (Lane et al., 1996). Complete glucocorticoid resistance in asthma is very rare, but reduced responsiveness is more common, so that oral glucocorticoids are needed to control asthma adequately (steroid-dependent asthma).

Mechanisms of glucocorticoid resistance: There may be several mechanisms for resistance to the effects of glucocorticoids. Although a family history of asthma is more common in patients with GCR than GCS asthma, little is known about its inheritance. It is possible that a certain proportion of the population has glucocorticoid resistance which only becomes manifest when they develop a severe immunological or immune disease that requires glucocorticoid therapy. Resistance to the inflammatory and immune effects of glucocorticoids should be distinguished from the rare familial glucocorticoid resistance, where there is an abnormality of glucocorticoid binding to GR.

Glucocorticoid resistance may be *primary* (inherited or acquired of unknown cause) or *secondary due to* reduced glucocorticoid responsiveness (glucocorticoids themselves, cytokines, b-adrenergic agonists).

Primary glucocorticoid resistance: There are several possible mechanisms for a reduced anti-inflammatory response to glucocorticoids.

a. Pharmacokinetic abnormalities.
b. Antibodies to lipocortin-1.
c. Cellular abnormalities.
d. Abnormality in GR function.
e. Interaction between GR and transcription factors.

Secondary glucocorticoid resistance: various probable mechanisms include:

a. Down-regulation of GR.
b. Effects of cytokines.
c. Effect of B2 agonists.

6. Factors contributing to corticosteroid resistance

A variety of factors known to contribute to immune activation and pulmonary disease have been found to alter corticosteroid responsiveness (**Table 6**).

Clinical allergy and allergen exposure
Infection
Smoking
Obesity
Stress
Ethnicity
Low vitamin D level

Table 6. Factors Contributing to Corticosteroid Insensitivity

6.1. Allergen exposure

Allergen exposure in vivo reduces GR binding affinity in PBMCs from atopic asthmatics. In vitro treatment with cat allergen of peripheral blood mononuclear cell (PBMC) from cat-allergic asthmatics was also observed to reduce GR binding affinity and T-cell proliferation induced by allergens compared with control antigens. The induction of these GR binding abnormalities was found to be IL-2 and IL-4 dependent.

6.2. Infection

Infection is a common trigger for pulmonary disease. An analysis of the T-cell repertoire in patients whose asthma was poorly controlled (FEV_1 <75% predicted despite use of high-dose corticosteroids) revealed that their T cells were activated by a microbial superantigen. To determine whether microbial super antigens could alter corticosteroid sensitivity, the capacity of corticosteroids to inhibit the activation of T cells from normal subjects with super antigens as compared with the mitogen, phytohemagglutinin, was studied. While corticosteroids caused a 99% inhibition of phytohemagglutinin-induced PBMC proliferation, there was only 19% inhibition of super antigen-induced T-cell proliferation. The mechanism by which super antigens induce corticosteroid resistance of human T cells is via activation of the Mitogen-Activated protein Kinase Kinase/Extracellular signal-Regulated Kinase (MEKK-ERK) pathway (Li et al., 2004, Goleva et al., 2004). Viruses can also alter response in corticosteroids. In particular, rhinovirus has been reported to reduce GR nuclear translocation and thereby reduce corticosteroid response.

6.3. Neutrophilia

The nature of the inflammatory infiltrate will also determine whether the particular pulmonary disease being treated is likely to resolve with corticosteroid therapy. Pulmonary diseases associated with infiltration of neutrophils are likely to be Steroid resistant. To determine the potential mechanism of corticosteroid resistance in neutrophils, Strickland et al.,2001 examined relative amounts of GRα and GRβ in freshly isolated neutrophils and observed increased GRβ, but not GRα, protein and mRNA expression in neutrophils at baseline and after IL-8 exposure (Strickland et al. 2001). High constitutive expression of GR-β by neutrophils may provide a mechanism by which these cells escape corticosteroid-induced cell death.

6.4. Other factors contributing to steroid resistance

Other factors contributing to steroid resistance include smoking, stress, obesity, ethnicity, and vitamin D deficiency. In smokers, oxidative stress results in reduced levels of histone deacetylase-2 (Barnes, Adcock, 2009). Stress may induce steroid resistance via multiple mechanisms, including the chronic elevation of the stress hormone, cortisol, which downregulates expression of the GR (Haczku , Panettieri, 2010). The association of steroid resistance with obesity may be related to the systemic inflammation found in this condition, leading to chronic elevation of TNF and mitogen-activated protein kinase (MAPK) activation that causes GR dysfunction (Sutherland et al., 2008) Black patients with asthma have also been found to have reduced steroid responsiveness compared with white asthmatics (Federico, 2005), although the reason for this is not known, but it could be due to a combination of genetic and environmental factors.

Several recent studies on asthmatics have now shown that low vitamin D levels are associated with increased corticosteroid requirements, and there is a potential role for vitamin D in the enhancement of corticosteroid response (Sutherland et al., 2010)

7. Management of corticosteroid resistance

The management of steroid resistant (SR) asthma poses a significant challenge to the clinician. Identification of the SR patient early in the course of illness is important to prevent tissue remodeling and irreversible changes in lung pathology. Definitions of clinical response to steroid therapy will be dictated by the pulmonary disease being treated and time frame for improvement of clinical disease before unacceptable steroid side effects occur. In the case of asthma, clinical studies have suggested that favorable response to inhaled steroids is associated with high levels of exhaled nitric oxide, high bronchodilator response, and a low FEV_1/FVC ratio prior to treatment (Barnes,2008)

A systematic, stepwise approach is important for a successful outcome (Leung and Bloom, 2003). **Table 7** lists factors to be considered in the evaluation of patients with a history of steroid resistance.

Correct diagnosis
Comorbid conditions- rhinosinusitis, congestive heart failure, COPD, Gastro Esophageal reflex
Drug adherence
Drug delivery
Drug interactions causing enhanced metabolism of steroids
Alternative anti-inflammatory therapies

Table 7. Considerations in Treating Steroid Resistance

Step 1. Complete Evaluation including history, physical examination, pulmonary function testing, and appropriate laboratory tests to confirm the diagnosis and rule out concomitant medical disorders such as vocal cord dysfunction, Gastroesophageal reflux/aspiration, chronic rhinosinusitis, allergic bronchopulmonary aspergillosis, heart failure, COPD & broncholitis etc.(**Figure 4**)

Step 2. Try to find out psychological & social factors including adherence to therapy and take corrective measures for them.

Step 3. Observe the inhalational technique of patient, reeducate, reinforce about the proper technique especially in patients requiring high doses of ICS for severe persistent asthma. Spacer devices should be used to maximize ICS dose delivery and reduce adverse effects.

Step 4. Strict environmental control at home, in school, and at work including finding the source of allergens & eliminating the same because persistent allergen exposure will increase the symptoms of asthma & reduces steroid responsiveness.

Step 5. Search for concomitant bacterial/ mycobacterial/ fungal infection of the tracheobronchial tree especially in patients taking high doses of ICS or chronic oral steroids. Chronic colonization with *Mycoplasma pneumoniae* or *Chlamydia pneumoniae,* can trigger airway inflammation in chronic asthmatics and thus poor responsiveness to steroids.

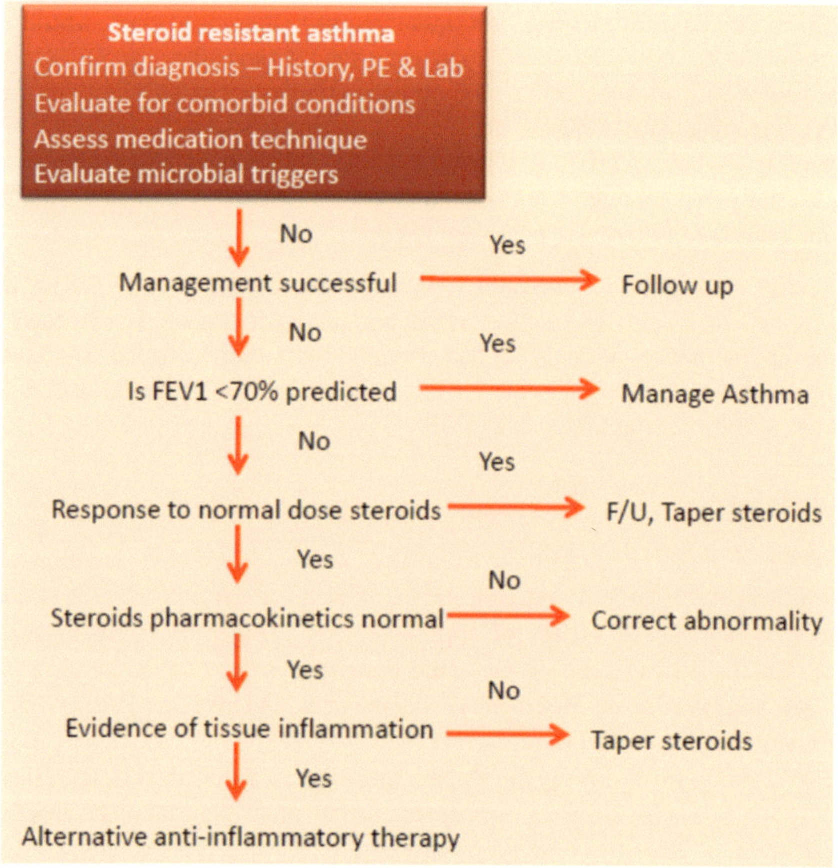

Figure 4. Flow diagram to manage steroid resistant asthma

Step 6. Search for factors affecting lifestyle and steroid responsiveness. Patients with Vitamin D deficiency have increased steroid requirements. Other cofactors, including obesity, smoking, no or little exposure to sunlight and pigmented skin are well known to lower vitamin D levels.

Step 7. Combination therapy can be used to maximize clinical response. Inhaled long-acting β_2-agonists (LABA) have been found to enhance Glucocorticoid receptor (GR) nuclear translocation and reduced corticosteroid requirements. Consider addition of other steroid-sparing drugs such as leukotriene modifiers, anticholinergic drugs, nidocromil sodium(Marin, 1996) and theophylline.

Step 8. In very difficult case, studies to identify systemic steroid pharmacokinetics and receptors to assess the basis for corticosteroid resistance to determine whether there is incomplete corticosteroid absorption, failure to convert corticosteroids to an active form, or rapid elimination of steroids (frequently as a result of interactions with other medications). Patients with poor absorption of prednisone usually respond well to oral liquid steroid preparations. In patients with rapid corticosteroid elimination, a split dosing regimen (morning & afternoon) is suggested.

Step 9. Consider Steroid sparing anti-inflammatory therapies that would enhance corticosteroid action including cyclosporine (Alexander et al., 1992), IV Immunoglobulin (Mazer , 1991), methotrexate (Mullarkey et al. 1998, Erzurum et al., 1991), mycophenolate mofetil, azathioprine, Macrolides, trolendamycin and gold, depending on the severity of asthma and the potential of significant side effects. Omalizumab (recombinant anti IgE antibody) is useful in patients with primarily allergic asthma & with severe persistent allergic rhinitis.

Further Studies are needed to determine whether cytokine antagonism—TNF-α, IL-2, IL-4, or IL-13—could restore steroid responsiveness because such cytokines have been found to induce steroid resistance. Vitamin D has recently been demonstrated to induce IL-10-producing regulatory T cells (Xystrakis et al., 2006) and enhance steroid action, and may therefore be steroid sparing(Zhang et al., 2010)

8. Novel steroids

Steroids, either systemic or inhaled, are exquisitely active and effective in asthma, but their mechanism of action is broad, and concern for toxicity—even with topical steroids—has limited their wider use. A variety of approaches are being pursued to maximize local activity within the airways and at the same time to minimize systemic absorption and toxicity. One approach is development of on-site-activated steroids such as ciclesonide, which is a nonhalogenated ICS prodrug that requires endogenous cleavage by esterases for activity. Soft steroids are also being developed; these have improved local, topical selectivity and have much less steroid effect outside the target area. They may be inactivated by esterases or other enzymes (for example a lactone–glucocorticosteroid conjugate).

Dissociated glucocorticoids: The recognition that most of the anti-inflammatory effects of glucocorticoids are mediated by repression of transcription factors (transrepression), whereas the endocrine and metabolic effects of steroids are likely to be mediated via glucocorticoid response element binding (transactivation) has led to a search for novel corticosteroids that selectively transrepress, thus reducing the potential risk of systemic side effects. These dissociated steroids which favor monomeric glucocorticoid receptor complexes (i.e., they produce transrepression) and avoid dimerization or transactivation, which is undesirable in asthma would make the treatment of asthma more effective without the current fear of steroid's side effects. Agents from each of these categories are undergoing clinical trials.

Steroid sparing : The combination of long acting beta agonist (LABA) with inhaled corticosteroid (ICS) is used frequently in asthma and a benefit from adding LABA to ICS has been described. One review compared reduced dose (mean 60% reduction in inhaled steroid) ICS/LABA combination to either a fixed moderate/high dose ICS or a reduced/tapering ICS dose. In adults with asthma, who use moderate to high maintenance doses of ICS, the addition of LABA has an ICS-sparing effect. LABA permit a reduction of 37% (253 mcg BDP) in subjects on minimum maintenance ICS and up to 60% (300 mcg FP) in subjects on maintenance ICS without deterioration in asthma control. They are most effective when combined with ICS, and this combination therapy is the preferred treatment when a medium dose of ICS alone fails to achieve control of asthma (Gibson, 2005). The addition of a LABA to a daily regimen of ICS improves symptom scores, decreases nocturnal symptoms, improves lung function, decreases the use of relief medication, reduces the number of exacerbations and achieves clinical control of asthma in more patients, more rapidly, and at a lower dose of ICS, than ICS given alone(Greening,1994, Pauwel, 1997).

Certain case reports have documented tiotropium as a useful steroid sparing agent however future clinical trials are warranted that explore the use of tiotropium as a potential 'steroid-sparing agent' in severe refractory asthma (Kapoor, 2009).

9. Immunomodulator therapy as steroid sparing

Methotrexate: Methotrexate may have a small steroid sparing effect in adults with asthma who are dependent on oral corticosteroids. However, the overall reduction in daily steroid use is probably not large enough to reduce steroid-induced adverse effects. This small potential to reduce the impact of steroid side-effects is probably insufficient to offset the adverse effects of methotrexate (Davies, 1998)

Azathioprine : Currently there is a clear lack of evidence to support the use of azathioprine in the treatment of chronic asthma as a steroid sparing-agent. Large, long-term studies with pre-defined steroid reducing protocols are required before recommendations for clinical practice can be made (Dean, 2004)

Cyclosporine: The improvement in asthma with cyclosporin are small and of questionable clinical significance. Given the side effects of cyclosporin, the evidence available does not recommend routine use of this drug in the treatment of oral corticosteroid dependent asthma (Evans, 2001)

Chloroquine : There is insufficient evidence to support the use of chloroquine as an oral steroid-sparing agent in chronic asthma. Further trials should optimise oral steroid dosage before addition of the steroid-sparing agent (Dewey, 2003)

Troleandomycin : There is insufficient evidence to support the use of troleandomycin in the treatment of steroid dependent asthma.(Evans ,2001)

Gold: Gold has limited clinically significanct benefits as steroid sparing agent & given the side effects of gold and necessity for monitoring the use of gold as a steroid sparing agent in asthma cannot be recommended.(Evans , 2001)

10. Conclusion

Inhaled Corticosteroids are the most effective first line of therapeutic intervention to control the primary immunologic mechanism of the disease and to avoid the devastating consequences of this disease with resultant cost- effectiveness and risk benefits analysis leading to best control of asthma. As far as steroids are concerned, there is over fear of its side effects in the patients as well as physicians which has to be removed. It should be make clear that steroids are friends of asthma pts if optimally used but if overused it may turned out to be foe, hence emphasis should be given on the optimized and appropriate use of steroids based on the asthma severity, Hence physicians should try to use the both edges of this **"double edged sword"** for the benefit of patients.

In addition to pharmacological intervention, emphasis should always be given on the patient's education about asthma including its pathogenesis, medications, inhalation technique and strict environmental control on every visit of the patient. Definitively the safety issues of the use of

Steroids in asthma has to be taken in to consideration in order to address the instructions of Hippocrates, **"first do no harm"** in relation to the steroids, however steroids continue to be the most potent and the most effective controller medication for asthma, and their use in the appropriate clinical setting remains invaluable for the control & management of asthma in clinical practice.

Author details

Mahboub Bassam and Vats Mayank
Department of Pulmonology and Allergy & Sleep Medicine , Rashid Hospital, Dubai

11. References

Agertoft L, Pedersen S. (1998). Bone mineral density in children with asthma receiving long-term treatment with inhaled budesonide. *Am J Respir Crit Care Med*; 157(1):178-83.

Agertoft L, Pedersen S. (2000).Effect of long-term treatment with inhaled budesonide on adult height in children with asthma. *N Engl J Med*;343(15):1064-9.

Alexander AG, Barnes NC, Kay AB.(1992). Trial of cyclosporin in corticosteroid dependent chronic severe asthma. *Lancet*,339:324–328.

Barnes PJ, Adcock IM. (1995). Steroid-resistant asthma. Q J Med, 88: 455-468.

Barnes PJ, Greening AP, Crompton GK. (1995). Glucocorticoid resistance in asthma. *Am J Respir Crit Care Med*, 152: 125-140.

Barnes PJ, Adcock IM.(1998) Transcription factors and asthma. *Eur Respir J*;12:221–234.

Barnes PJ. (2008). Emerging pharmacotherapies for COPD. *Chest*, 134(6):1278-1286.

Barnes PJ, Adcock IM. (2009). Glucocorticoid resistance in inflammatory diseases. *Lancet*, 373(9678):1905-1917.

Barreto M. L., Cunha S. S., Alcˆantara-Neves N et al., (2006). Risk factors and immunological pathways for asthma and other allergic diseases in children: background and methodology of a longitudinal study in a large urban center in Northeastern Brazil (Salvador-SCAALA study). *BMC Pulmonary Medicine*, vol. 6, article 15.

Bassam M, Vats M, Afzal S, Sharif W, Iqbal MN. (2012). Environmental Exposure and nonadherence with Medicines directly correlate with Exacerbations and Hospitalization for

Asthma: A Population-Based Survey from UAE. ISRN Pulmonology, Volume 2012.

Beato M, Herrlich P, Schutz G. Steroid hormone receptors: many actors in search of a plot. *Cell* 1995;83:851–857.

Bianchi M, Meng C, Ivashkiv BL (2000). Inhibition of IL-2-induced Jak-STAT signaling by glucocorticoids. PNAS, vol. 97, no. 17, pg 9573–9578. www.pnas.orgycgiydoiy10.1073ypnas.160099797

Braman SS.(2006). The global burden of asthma. *Chest,*130(suppl 1):4S-12S

Carmichael J, Paterson IC, Diaz P, Crompton GK, Kay AB, Grant IWB. (1981) Corticosteroid resistance in chronic asthma. *Br Med J,* 282: 1419-1422.

Cochrane GM. (1996) Compliance and outcomes in patients with asthma. *Drugs,* 52:12–19

Darnell, J.E. (1997). STATs and gene regulation. *Science.* 277:1630–1635.

Davies HRH R, Olson LLG, Gibson PG. (1998). Methotrexate as a steroid sparing agent for asthma in adults. *Cochrane Database of Systematic Reviews*, Issue 3. Art. No.: CD000391

Dean TP, Dewey A, Bara A, Lasserson TJ, Walters EH. (2004)Azathioprine as an oral corticosteroid sparing agent for asthma. *Cochrane Database of Systematic Reviews*, Issue 1. Art. No.: CD003270

Dewey A, Bara A, Lasserson TJ, Walters EH.(2003) Chloroquine as a steroid sparing agent for asthma. *Cochrane Database of Systematic Reviews*, Issue 4. Art. No.: CD003275.

Dolovich M, Ruffin RE, Roberts R, et al. (1981)Optimal delivery of aerosols from metered dose inhalers. *Chest;* 80(suppl): 911–915,

Dolovich MB, Ahrens CR, Hess DR et al . (2005)Device Selection and Outcomes of Aerosol Therapy: Evidence-Based Guidelines : American College of Chest Physicians/American College of Asthma, Allergy, and Immunology *Chest,*127;335-371

Erzurum Sc, Leff JA, et al. (1991). Lack of benefit of methotrexate in severe, steroid dependent

asthma. *Ann Intern Med.,*114:353–360.

Evans DJ, Cullinan P, Geddes DM, Walters EH, Milan SJ, Jones P. (2001)Gold as an oral corticosteroid sparing agent in stable asthma. *Cochrane Database of Systematic Reviews,* Issue 2. Art. No.: CD002985

Evans DJ, Cullinan P, Geddes DM, Walters EH, Milan SJ, Jones P. (2001)Troleandomycin as an oral corticosteroid sparing agent in stable asthma. *Cochrane Database of Systematic Reviews,* Issue 2. Art. No.: CD002987

Evans DJ, Cullinan P, Geddes DM, Walters EH, Milan SJ, Jones P. (2001)Cyclosporin as an oral corticosteroid sparing agent in stable asthma. *Cochrane Database of Systematic Reviews,* Issue 2. Art. No.: CD002993

Federico MJ, Covar RA, Brown EE, Leung DY, Spahn JD. (2005). Racial differences in T-lymphocyte response to glucocorticoids. *Chest,*127(2):571-578.

Gibson P.G. Powell H, Ducharme FM.(2005) Long-acting beta2-agonists as an inhaled corticosteroid-sparing agent for chronic asthma in adults and children. *Cochrane Database of Systematic Reviews,* Issue 4. Art. No.: CD005076

Global Strategy for Asthma Management and Prevention. Global INitiative for Asthma (GINA), 2010. Available from www.ginasthma.org Date last updated, 2010.www.ginasthma.org

Greening AP, Ind PW, Northfield M, Shaw G. (1994)Added salmeterol versus higher-dose corticosteroid in asthma patients with symptoms on existing inhaled corticosteroid. Allen & Hanburys Limited UK Study Group. *Lancet*; 344: 219-224.

Goleva E, Hall CF, Ou LS, Leung DY. (2004)Superantigen-induced corticosteroid resistance of human T cells occurs through activation of the mitogen-activated protein kinase kinase/extracellular signal-regulated kinase (MEK-ERK) pathway. *J Allergy Clin Immunol.*,114(5):1059-1069

Haczku A, Panettieri RA Jr. (2010). Social stress and asthma: the role of corticosteroid insensitivity. *J Allergy Clin Immunol*,125(3):550-558.

Haynes RB, Taylor DW, Sackett DL, eds. (1979) Compliance in health care. Baltimore, MD: Johns Hopkins University Press.

Hopp RJ, Degan JA, Biven RE, Kinberg K, Gallagher GC.(1995) Longitudinal assessment of bone mineral density in children with chronic asthma. *Ann Allergy Asthma Immunol*;75(2):143-8.

Horne R, (2003). *Concordance and Medicines Management in the Respiratory Arena*, Hayward Medical Publications, London, UK.

Ito K, Barnes PJ, Adcock IM.(2000) Glucocorticoid receptor recruitment of histone deacetylase 2 inhibits interleukin-1beta-induced histone H4 acetylation on lysines 8 and 12. *Mol Cell Biol* 20:6891–6903.

Jackson C, Lipworth B. (1995)Optimizing inhaled drug delivery in patients with asthma. *Br J Gen Pract*; 45:683–687)

Kapoor AS, Olsen SR , CO'Hara C , et al. (2009). The efficacy of tiotropium as a steroid-sparing agent in severe asthma. *Can Respir J* Vol 16; No 3.

Karin M. (1998). New twists in gene regulation by glucocorticoid receptor: is DNA binding dispensable? *Cell*;93:487–490.

Kirkham B, Corkill MM, Davison SC, Panayi GS. (1991) Response to glucocorticoid treatment in rheumatoid arthritis: *in vitro* cell mediated immune assays predicts *in vivo* response. *J Rheumatol* 18: 1130-1133.

Lane SJ, Atkinson BA, Swimanathan R, Lee TH. (1996) Hypothalamic pituitary axis in corticosteroid-resistant asthma. *Am J Respir Crit Care Med*, 153: 1510 -14.

Lee TH, Brattsand R, Leung DYM, editors (1996). Corticosteroid action and resistance in asthma. *Am J Respir Cell Mol Biol*; 154(Suppl): S1–S79.

Leung DYM, Martin RJ, Sze¯er SJ, et al. (1995) Dysregulation of interleukin 4, interleukin 5, and interferon c gene expression in steroid-resistant asthma. *J Exp Med*, 181: 33±40.

Leung DY, Bloom JW.(2003). Update on glucocorticoid action and resistance. *J Allergy Clin Immunol.* 111(1):3-22.

Li LB, Goleva E, Hall CF, Ou LS, Leung DY. (2004).Super antigen-induced corticosteroid resistance of human T cells occurs through activation of the mitogen-activated protein kinase kinase/extracellular signal-regulated kinase (MEK-ERK) pathway. *J Allergy Clin Immunol.*;114(5):1059-1069.

Marin JM, Carrizo SJ, Garcia R, Ejea MV.(1996). Effects of nedocromil sodium in steroid-resistant asthma: a randomized controlled trial. *J Allergy Clin Immunol.*; 97:602–610.

Masoli M, Fabian D, Holt S, Beasley R.(2004). Global Initiative for Asthma (GINA) program: the global burden of asthma: executive summary of the GINA Dissemination Committee report. *Allergy,* 59:469-478.

Mazer BD, Gelfand EW. (1991). An open-label study of high-dose intravenous immunoglobulin in severe childhood asthma. *J Allergy Clin Immunol,* 87:976–983.

Mullarkey MF, Blumenstein BA, et al. (1988). Methotrexate in the treatment of corticosteroid-dependent asthma. *N Engl J Med.,*318:603–607.

Murphy, K.M., et al. (2000). Signaling and transcription in T helper development. *Annu. Rev. Immunol.* 18:451–494.

National Institutes of Health, Bethesda: (2006) National Institutes of Health/US Department of Health and Human Services; Inc., c1998. National Heart Lung and Blood Institute. Practical Guide for the Diagnosis and Management of Asthma, April, http://www.nhlbi.nih.gov/health/prof/lung/asthma/ practgde.htm.

Pauwels RA, Lofdahl CG, Postma DS, et al. (1997) Effect of inhaled formoterol and budesonide on exacerbations of asthma. Formoterol and Corticosteroids Establishing Therapy (FACET) International Study Group. N Engl J Med; 337: 1405- 1411.

Pedersen S. (2001)Do inhaled corticosteroids inhibit growth in children? *Am J Respir Crit Care Med*;164(4):521-35.

Rengarajan, J., Szabo, S.J., and Glimcher, L.H. (2000). Transcriptional regulation of Th1/Th2 polarization. *Immunol. Today.* 21:479–483.

Roux C, Kolta S, Desfougeres JL, Minini P, Bidat E. (2003)Long-term safety of fluticasone propionate and nedocromil sodium on bone in children with asthma. *Pediatrics*;111(6 Pt 1): e706-13.

Sally E. W., Fahy JV, Irvin C et al. (2000)Proceedings of the ATS Workshop on Refractory Asthma Current Understanding, Recommendations, and Unanswered Questions. *Am J Respir Crit Care Med* Vol 162. pp 2341–2351,

Schwartz, Lowell FC, Melby JC. (1968) Steroid resistance in bronchial asthma. *Am J Int Med,* 69: 493-499.

Sharek PJ, Bergman DA.(2000) Beclomethasone for asthma in children: effects on linear growth. *Cochrane Database Syst Rev*;2.

Strickland I, Kisich K, Hauk PJ, et al. (2001). High constitutive glucocorticoid receptor beta in human neutrophils enables them to reduce their spontaneous rate of cell death in response to corticosteroids. *J Exp Med.*;193(5):585-593.

Sutherland ER, Goleva E, Strand M, Beuther DA, Leung DY. (2008).Body mass and glucocorticoid response in asthma. *Am J Respir Crit Care Med.*;178(7):682-687.

Sutherland ER, Goleva E, Jackson LP, Stevens AD, Leung DY. (2010)Vitamin D levels, lung function, and steroid response in adult asthma. *Am J Respir Crit Care Med.*;181(7):699-704.

Szefler SJ, Leung DY. (1997) Glucocorticoid-resistant asthma: pathogenesis and clinical implications for management. *Eur Respir J,* 10(7): 1640-47.

Wills-Karp, M. (1999). Immunologic basis of antigen-induced airway hyperresponsiveness. *Annu. Rev. Immunol.* 17:255–281.

Woolcock A , Rubinfeld AR, Seale JP et al. (1989) Thoracic society of Australia and New Zealand. Asthma management plan, 1989. *The Medical Journal of Australia*, vol. 151, no. 11- 12, pp. 650–653,

World Health Organization.(2003). *Adherence to Long-Term Therapies: Evidence for Action*, World Health Organization, Geneva, Switzerland.

Wurster, A.L., Tanaka, T., and Grusby, M.J. 2000. The biology of Stat4 and Stat6. *Oncogene.* 19:2577–2584.

Xystrakis E, Kusumakar S, Boswell S, et al. (2006) Reversing the defective induction of IL-10-secreting regulatory T cells in glucocorticoid-resistant asthma patients. *J Clin Invest.* 116(1):146-155

Zhang Y, Goleva E, Leung DYM. (2010).Vitamin D has corticosteroid sparing effects by enhancing glucocorticoid induced mitogen-activated protein kinase phosphatase-1 [abstract]. *J Allergy Clin Immunol.*;125(2):216

Section 6

New Formula of Glucocorticoids in Clinical Treatment

Chapter 24

Corticosteroids for Skin Delivery: Challenges and New Formulation Opportunities

Taner Senyigit and Ozgen Ozer

Additional information is available at the end of the chapter

http://dx.doi.org/10.5772/53909

1. Introduction

Currently, corticosteroids are the most widely used class of anti-inflammatory drugs. The introduction of topical hydrocortisone in the early 1950s provided great advantages over previously available therapies and initiated a new era for dermatological therapy. Their clinical effectiveness in the treatment of dermatological disorders is related to their vasoconstrictive, anti-inflammatory, immunosuppressive and anti-proliferative effects. Despite their benefit in the therapy of inflammatory diseases, topical corticosteroids (TC) are associated number of side effects that limit their use. Most TC are absorbed in quantities that can produce both systemic and topical side effects [1-2]. Table 1 shows the currently used TC in various dermatological disorders according to the British classification system [3]. In general, mild and moderate TC are used for long-term treatments while the potent and very potent products especially preferred for shorter regimes.

Over the years, research has focused on strategies to optimize the potency of steroids while minimizing adverse effects due to drug absorption across the skin. In other words, research focus no longer been on the synthesis of more potent derivatives but on safer one. Several attempts have been made to increase the safety of TC treatment, including new application schedules, special vehicles and new synthesized agents [4]. However, "ideal" TC have not yet been synthesized. They should be able to permeate the stratum corneum (SC) and reach adequate concentrations in the epidermis without reaching high systemic concentrations.

One of the approaches to reduce the adverse effects of TC is to enhance their permeability so as to reduce the topically applied dose [5]. Several approaches have been attempted, such as iontophoresis, electroporation or the application of eutectic mixtures [6,7]. However, the use of chemical penetration enhancers is the most widely used approach to increase skin delivery [8].

POTENCY	DOSE % (w/w)	TC
Mild		Hydrocortisone
	1	Hydrocortisone acetate
	0.25	Methylprednisolone
	0.05	Alclometasone dipropionate
	0.01-0.1	Dexamethasone
	0.0025	Fluocinolone acetonide
	0.75	Fluocortyn butyl ester
	0.5	Prednisolone
Moderate	0.05	Clobetasone butyrate
	0.02	Triamcinolone acetonide
	0.005	Fluocinolone acetonide
Potent	0.05	Betamethasone dipropionate
	0.1	Betamethasone valerate
	0.025	Fluocinolone acetonide
	0.1	Hydrocortisone butyrate
	0.05	Halometasone monohydrate
	0.1	Diflucortolone valerate
Very potent	0.1	Halcinonide
	0.05	Clobetasol propionate

Table 1. The currently used TC in various dermatological disorders [3]

TC are formulated in a variety of conventional vehicles, including ointments, creams, lotions and gels. In addition to conventional formulations several innovative systems such as nanoparticles, liposomes, microemulsions, foams and patches have been evaluated for different dermatological conditions. Colloidal drug carrier systems, such as liposomes and nanoparticles, could target TC to the viable epidermis, where the inflammatory reactions take place. In particular, liposomal preparations showed a strong affinity for the SC. Patents filed on topical nanoparticulate formulations also claimed the importance of colloidal drug carrier systems for this type of applications [9-12].

This chapter will review major innovations and advances in TC formulations based on the published articles and patent applications. The main factors influencing the effectiveness and bioavailability of TC will be also briefly discussed before emphasizing formulation alternatives.

2. Skin structure

The skin, in Latin called cutis, is considered the largest organ of the body, accounting more than 10% of the body mass and having an average surface of approximately 2 m^2. The thickness of the skin is highly variable (average thickness of 1.5 mm), depending of several factors as the anatomic location, age and sex. The functions of the skin have been classified as protective, homeostatic, or sensorial. To maintain its characteristics, this organ is in a continual renewing process [13].

Anatomically, the skin consists on 3 basic layers: epidermis, dermis and subcutaneous tissues. Depending on the region considered, the epidermis is made of 4-5 sublayers that, from bottom to top, are: stratum basale, stratum spinosum, stratum granulosum, stratum lucidum (present only in palm and soles) and SC or horny layer. In addition to these structures, there are also several associated appendages: hair follicles, sweat glands, apocrine glands, and nails [14].

The most important skin function is permeability barrier function. The outermost layer of the epidermis, the SC, with its peculiar structure, plays an important role in permeability barrier function [15]. Due to its barrier properties, the skin membrane is equally capable at limiting the molecular transport from and into the body. Overcoming this barrier function will be the purpose of skin drug delivery.

3. Clinical limitations and side effects of TC

TC are successfully used in the treatment of several common cutaneous diseases but their major limitation is still their side effect potential. The most common side-effects occur locally in the areas of skin treated with the steroid. Probably the most well known is thinning of the skin (atrophy), which sometimes results in permanent stretch marks (striae). Fine blood vessels may swell and become prominent under the skin surface (telangiectasia), again a permanent change. In addition, there may be a temporary loss of pigment in the areas of skin treated; this may be more noticeable in dark-skinned people. Sometimes the skin may become allergic to the steroid, making the eczema appear to get worse. The skin may also bruise more easily and become more susceptible to infection.

The occurrence and severity of the side effects are depend on the duration of use, dosage, dosing regime and spesific drug used, along with individual patient variability. However, the highest risk factor seems to be prolonged use [16-18]. The concentration of corticosteroid in systemic circulation and risk of sytemic side effects are increased by prolonged therapy with TC. Systemic side-effects of TC, such as pituitary–adrenal axis suppression, should be taken into account when treating children. Children have a higher ratio of total body surface area to body weight (about 2.5- to 3-fold that of adults) and adrenal suppression may cause growth retardation.

The principle systemic side effects associated with TC are bodyweight gain, Cushing's syndrome, electrolyte imbalance, hypertension, diabetes mellitus, pseudoprimary aldosteronisim, growth retardation, osteoporosis peptic ulser and gastritis. In addition, TC are mostly capable of causing local side effects. One particularly important local side effect is epidermal thinning or atrophy [19]. This effect is characterized with the reduction in cell size and number of cell layers in epidermis. Other local side effects related to TC treatment are steroid acne, rosacea, perioral dermatitis, corticoid acne, allergic contact dermatitis, hypopigmentation, glaucoma, cataracts, worsening of cutaneous infections and hypertrichosis [2]. Table 2 represents the possible local and systemic side effects of TC which are organized in subsections for tissue-organ level.

TISSUE - ORGAN	SIDE EFFECTS
Cardiovascular system	Hypertension
Endocrin system	Adrenal insufficiency, Cushing's syndrome, diabetes mellitus, bodyweight gain, pseudoprimary aldosteronism
Eye	Glaucoma, cataract
Immune system	Increased risk of infection, re-activation of latent viruses
Gastrointestinal	Peptic ulser, gastritis
Central nervous system	Behavioural changes, loss of memory/cognition
Skeleton and muscle	Growth retardation, osteoporosis
Skin	Atrophy, striae, allergic contact dermatitis, delayed wound healing, steroid acne, perioral dermatitis, rosacea, erythema, teleangiectasia, hypertrichosis, hypopigmentation

Table 2. The possible local and systemic side effects of TC

4. Classification of TC

TC are classified in two different ways by American and British National Formulary classification systems [20-21]. The American classification system includes seven potency groups while the British National Formulary contains four groups. In the former system, the potency of a product is defined by the corticosteroid, its concentration and the nature of the vehicle. On the other hand, The British classification system is irrespective of the topical vehicle used. According to the American classification sytem, it is important to note that the greater in potency for TC result in the greater therapeutic efficacy and side effects. Therefore, low-potency formulations should be used for long term treatments by physicians while the more potent products should be chosen for short periods and sites such as palms and soles, where low potency TC are ineffective [1,2].

5. Formulations of TC

It is well known that, besides the active molecule, the potency of each topical formulation can be influenced by vehicle characteristics. Vehicles should allow adequate release of the active compound, spread easily and be aesthetically pleasant [21]. Some important rules should be considered when choosing a vehicle; the solubility, release rate and stability of the therapeutic agent in the vehicle, the ability of the vehicle to hydrate the SC, the physical and chemical interactions of the vehicle with the skin and active molecule and also the phase, localization and extent of disease [22].

TC are formulated in a variety of conventional vehicles, including ointments, creams, lotions and gels. As mentioned previously, the character of the vehicle system defines the potency of topical preparations and its selection is crucial for product performance.

Ointments are semi-solid preparations intended for application to skin or mucous membranes. There are four types of ointment bases; hydrocarbon bases, absorption bases, emulsion bases and water-soluble bases. The potential of the absorption is affected by choice of the bases. Hence, appropriate selection of the base is important for the efficacy of the dermal therapy [23].

Ointment formulations are generally more effective than creams containing the same drug and they are especially preferred for infiltrated, lichenified lesions. In a comparative study, the absorption of clobetasol propionate from ointment and cream formulations was evaluated and it was reported that a greater amount of clobetasol propionate was absorbed from the ointment [24]. Ointments including well-known and new synthesized TC were formulated and they were still first-option for treatment of dermatological diseases. However, the greasy nature and hardness of the removal from the skin due to their lack of water-washability is their disadvantages.

Mobile dispersions intended for topical application are generally described as lotions and semi-solid systems as creams. Although, creams are usually emulsions of the oil-in-water type (aqueous creams) or water-in-oil type (oily creams), lotions are mostly oil-in-water emulsions [25]. Regarding to the phase of disease, lotions and creams are generally recommended in acute and subacute dermatoses. Good compliance is obtained by prescribing creams and lotions which are easily applied by patients rather than ointments in case of large extensional dermatoses. Sequeira et al. [26] filed a patent application which provided a corticosteroid lotion formulation exhibiting high vasoconstrictor and excellent anti-inflammatory activities in steroid responsive dermatoses. The addition of propylene glycol to a hydro-alcoholic lotion base exhibited and significantly higher vasoconstrictor activity than the corresponding lotion without propylene glycol.

Gels are semi-solid systems with dispersions of small or large molecules in an aqueose vehicle with a gelling agent. The gel formulations are suitable for topical delivery of drugs for treatment of diseases due to lack of irritating components. Pharmaceutical gel formulations for topical drug delivery include drug and gelling agent [27]. Gels based on carbopol, cellulose derivatives and chitosan are commonly used in the pharmaceutical and cosmetic industries [28, 29].

Recently, new hydrogel formulation intended for cosmetic use was introduced as a novel formulation of steroids for the treatment of atopic dermatitis. The formulation was prepared with carbopol-based polymer that contained 0.05% (w/w) of micronized desonide which is a well-known synthetic corticosteroid. This formulation was easily applied for atopic dermatitis patients aged 3 months. A wide variety of studies have been performed to validate the safety and efficacy of this product and these studies supported very favourable safety, tolerability and efficacy profile [30, 31].

Senyigit et al. [32] investigated the effect of vehicles (chitosan and sodium-deoxycholate gel) on the skin accumulation and permeation of two topical corticosteroids: clobetasol propionate and mometasone furoate. Commercial cream formulations containing the same amount of drug were also used for comparison. It was reported that sodium-deoxycholate gel formulation dramatically improved the amount of drug in the skin although chitosan gel produced the same skin accumulation as commercial creams for both active agents. In addition, all of these gel formulations did not induce the permeation.

For conventional formulations it can be stated that the effectiveness of the active agent is directly related to the composition of the formulation. In general, the potency of the corticosteroids in the formulations could be listed in order such as; ointments> gels> creams> lotions. This generalization was supported with a patent filed by McCadden [33]. The brief summary about conventional TC formulations including pharmaceutical characteristics, clinical usage, benefits and disadvantages were given in Table 3.

Formulation type	Pharmaceutical characteristics	Clinical usage	Benefits	Disadvantages
Ointment	Semi-solid preparations containing different types of ointment bases	Infiltrated, lichenified lesions	Occlusive property on the skin for inducing skin hydration at the skin-ointment interface	Greasy nature and hardness of the removal from the skin due to their lack of water-washability
Cream	Oil-in-water (aqueous creams) or water-in-oil (oily creams) type of emulsion	Acute and subacute dermatoses	Easy application and good patient compliance	Difficulty of spreadability and soiling linen and clothing during treatment for oily creams
Lotion	Generally oil-in-water emulsions	Acute and subacute dermatoses	Easy application and good patient compliance	Not suitable for use on dry skin
Gel	Dispersions formulated with a gelling agent	Suitable for all types of skin diseases	Easy application, easy to attach to the skin, good patient compliance and lack of irritating components	-

Table 3. The summary about conventional TC formulations

The activity of a TC formulation can be enhanced by adding a chemical penetration enhancer which may result in an increase of drug delivery into skin. Chemical penetration enhancers have been reviewed by several researchers and the authors underline the difficulty to select rationally a penetration enhancer for a specific permeant [34-36]. Recent studies showed that terpenes appear to be promising penetration enhancers for pharmaceutical formulations with favourable properties such as low cutaneous irritancy and possess good toxicological profile [32, 37].

Recently, it has been a great interest in developing new drug carriers for TC that may contribute to reduction of side effects. Therefore, in addition to previously mentioned conventional formulations several innovative systems such as nanoparticles, liposomes, microemulsions, foams and patches have been developed for TC.

Liposomes, microemulsions, solid lipid and polymeric nanoparticles have been proposed to increase percutaneous absorption of therapeutic agents while mitigating the damage to the skin barrier function [38,39]. Besides, the drug targeting to the skin or even to its substructures could be realized by micro- and nanoparticulate systems [40,41]. These drug carrier systems could target glucocorticoids to the viable epidermis, where the inflammatory reactions take place [9]. In particular, liposomal preparations showed strong affinity for the SC [42].

The loading of therapeutic agents into nanoparticles and administration to the skin using a simple vehicle offer many advantages over other traditional topical formulations, including enhanced formulation aesthetics, protection of unstable active agents against degredation, targeting of active agents to the skin layers and prolonged active agent release [43]. As a consequence of their proposed advantages in dermal/transdermal formulations two most common types of particles have been produced: Lipid nanoparticles and polymeric nanoparticles. The uses of lipid and polymeric nanoparticles for pharmaceutical formulations applied to skin have been reviewed by several authors [40, 44-46]. Most of the data reported on TC was obtained using lipid nanoparticles of differing lipid compositions.

The inclusion of prednicarbate into solid lipid nanoparticles (SLN) of various composition appeared to increase the penetration of the drug into human skin by 30% as compared to cream, permeation of reconstructed epidermis increased even 3-fold [47]. In a subsequent report SLN were shown to induce prednicarbate targeting in the epidermal layer in excised human skin and reconstructed epidermis [9]. Epidermal targeting was evidenced also for prednisolone, the diester prednicarbate and the monoester betamethasone 17-valerate included in solid lipid nanoparticles [48]. The authors hypothesized specific interactions of the drug-carrier complex and the skin surface, possible by the lipid nature and nanosize of the carrier. On the other hand, using the appropriate lipid combination, the skin retention of betamethasone 17 valerate was increased when SLN was used as a vehicle compared to a conventional formulations [49], both using intact skin as well as barrier impaired [50].

Clobetasol propionate was included in SLN as well [51]. SLN containing cream registered significant improvement in therapeutic response (1.9 fold inflammation, 1.2 fold itching) in terms of percent reduction in degree of inflammation and itching against marketed cream.

de Vringer disclosed a stable aqueous suspension of SLNs, comprising at least one lipid and preferably also at least one emulsifier for topical application to the body. According to this invention steroidal anti-inflammatory compound such as hydrocortisone, hydrocortisone-17α-butyrate, budesonide or TA, anti-proliferatives, anti-psoriatics, anti-eczema agents and dithranol could be succesfully incorporated into the suspension of SLNs. It was stated that a combination of two or more topically effective medicaments could also be used [52]. Senyigit et al. [53] prepared lecithin/chitosan nanoparticles containing clobetasol propionate and found a preferential retention in the epidermis while no permeation across the skin was observed. In vivo studies including transepidermal water loss measurements, anti-inflammatory effect and histological evaluation of the formulations on wistar albino rats were also performed and the results were promising (Data not published).

Liposomes are lipid vesicles prepared with phospholipids which have been shown to facilitate transport of drugs into and across skin [54]. Recently, many reports have been published on percutaneous enhancing property of liposomes for both hydrophilic and lipophilic compounds [55]. Liposomes do not only enhance the drug penetration into the skin by showing slow release, but also decrease the clearence of drug by minimizing its absorption into the systemic circulation [56]. Hence, the liposomes can improve the therapeutic effectiveness of TC while reducing systemic side effects. However, many stability problems are reported for liposomes.

Mezei et al. [57, 58] applied triamcinolone acetonide (TA) in liposomes and compared it with TA in Dermabase®. In this study, four- to five fold higher TA concentrations in the epidermis and dermis, with lower systemic drug levels were observed when the drug was delivered from liposomal lotion in comparison with conventional formulations of the same drug concentration.

Lasch and Wohlrab [59, 60] studied the skin distribution of cortisol and hydrocortison after application in a cream and liposomes. As a result, improved concentration-time profile was observed in skin layers by liposomes for both drugs.

Korting et al. [61] compared the efficacy of betamethasone dipropionate encapsulated in liposomes and cream. The liposomes were prepared with egg lecithine and incorporated in a polyacrylate gel. The in vivo studies were carried out in patients with atopic eczema and psoriasis vulgaris. It was concluded that, betamethasone encapsulated in liposomes improved the antiinflammatory action, but not the antiproliferative effect.

Fresta et al. [62] prepared skin-lipid liposome formulations of different corticosteroids (hydrocortisone, betamethasone valerate and TA). They indicated that skin lipid liposomes showed a 6 and 1.3 fold higher blanching effect than control formulations of ointment and the phospholipid-based liposomes, respectively. Skin-lipid liposomes also produced a reduction in drug levels in the blood and urine. Consequently, this liposome formulation was proposed for improving the pharmacological effectiveness and reducing the systemic absorption of TC.

In order to overcome the stability problem of liposomes, new attempts have been maden and new drug carrier systems have been developed by adding some functional chemicals into the liposome structure. These systems are niosomes, transfersomes and ethosomes.

Niosomes, non-ionic surfactant vesicules, are widely studied as an alternative to liposomes for topical and transdermal drug delivery. Niosomes alleviate the disadvantages associated with liposomes, such as chemical instability, variable purity of phospholipids and high cost. In addition, they have the potential for controlled and targeted drug delivery to the skin [63-65]. Deformable liposomes (Transfersomes®) are the first generation of elastic vesicles introduced by Cevc [66]. They consist of phospholipids and an edge activator. An edge activator is often a single chain surfactant that destabilizes lipid bilayers of the vesicles and increases deformability of the bilayers [67-68].

Cevc et al. [69] investigated the regio-specificity potential of transfersomes which included different corticosteroids (hydrocortisone, dexamethasone and TA). They demonstrated that transfersomes ameliorate the targetability of all tested corticosteroids into the viable skin. They also suggested that the introduction of transfersomal corticosteroids creates new opportunities for the well controlled topical medication.

In another study performed by Fesq et al. [70], the efficacy of transfersomes was compared with commercially available cream and ointment formulations of TA in humans. According to the results of this study, 10-fold lower dose of TA in transfersome was found bioequivalent to conventional formulations as measured by erythema suppression. Ultrasonic measurements also revealed significantly reduced atrophogenic potential of transfersomes in comparison to commercial formulations.

Ethosome is another novel lipid carrier showing enhanced skin delivery and recently developed by Touitou. The ethosomal system is composed of phospholipid, ethanol and water. The use of high ethanol content was decribed for ethosomes although liposomal formulations containing up to 10% ethanol [71, 72].

Microemulsions are thermodynamically stable, transparent, isotropic, low-viscosity colloidal dispersions consisting of microdomains of oil and/or water stabilized by an interfacial film of alternating surfactant and cosurfactant molecules [73]. Microemulsions are effective formulations for the dermal and transdermal delivery of particularly lipophilic compounds like TC because of their solubilizing properties and also their components may act as penetration enhancers [74, 75].

Wiedersberg et al. [76] studied the dermato-pharmacokinetic properties of betamethasone valerate from two different formulations either in the reference vehicle consisting of medium chain triglycerides or in the microemulsion. The results showed that microemulsion significantly increased the extent of drug delivery into the SC.

In another study, the penetration behaviour of hydrocortisone from the microemulsion system and a commercialy available cream formulation containing the same amount of hydrocortisone (0.5%) was investigated. *Ex vivo* penetration studies on human breast skin were carried out and the drug contents in the different skin layers were measured. With regard to the cream, the results showed that, a higher percentage of hydrocortisone was found in the epidermis and dermis. This result pointed out the skin targeting effect achieved by microemulsion formulation [77, 78].

Formulation type	Pharmaceutical characteristics	Benefits	Disadvantages
Nanoparticles	Solid lipid nanoparticles include solid or the mixture of solid and fluid lipids Polymeric nanoparticles contain non-biodegradable and biodegradable polymers	Enhanced formulation aesthetics, protection of unstable active agents against degredation, targeting of active agents to the skin layers and prolonged active agent release	Mechanism of interaction between nanoparticles - skin structures and in vivo toxicity issues are need to be clarified
Liposomes	Lipid vesicles prepared with phospholipids	Percutaneous absorption enhancing property, slow release and decrease the clearence of drug by minimizing its absorption into the systemic circulation	Stability problems
Niosomes	Non-ionic surfactant vesicules	Alleviate the disadvantages associated with liposomes, such as chemical instability, variable purity of phospholipids and high cost. Controlled and targeted drug delivery to the skin.	Less effective drug delivery in comparison to liposomes
Transfersomes	Consist of phospholipids and an edge activator	Improved therapeutic risk-benefit ratio,due to better targeting and longer drug presence in the skin	-
Ethosomes	Composed of phospholipid, ethanol and water.	Improved dermal/transdermal delivery of lipophilic or hydrophilic molecules	The mechanism of action is not clear

Formulation type	Pharmaceutical characteristics	Benefits	Disadvantages
Microemulsions	Thermodynamically stable, transparent, isotropic, low-viscosity colloidal dispersions consisting of microdomains of oil and/or water stabilized by an interfacial film of alternating surfactant and cosurfactant molecules	Ease of manufacturing and high loading capacity. Effective formulations for the dermal and transdermal delivery of particularly lipophilic compounds.	-
Patches	Drug delivery systems intended for skin application	Provides the administration of effective and known drug amount to the skin and the occlusive effect	Skin irritation
Foams	Incorporate active agents, solvents, co-solvents, surfactants and propellants in a sealed canister under pressure	More convenient topical drug delivery with easy application and spreadability characteristics in comparision to other topical dosage forms	-

Table 4. The summary about innovative TC formulations

Patches are other innovative drug delivery systems intended for skin application in view of achieving local or systemic effect. The patch provides the administration of effective and known drug amount to the skin [79].

The occlusive effect of Actiderm® (hydrocolloid dermatological patch) has been studied on the percutaneous penetration of several drugs including corticosteroids. It was found to be effective in controlling and sustaining the localized delivery of the steroid into the skin and enhancing the healing of dermatological disorders [80, 81].

Ladenheim et al. [82] investigated the effect of occlusion on *in vitro* TA penetration using hydrocolloid containing patches by measuring transepidermal water loss. They found that the diffusion rate of TA was increased 3-4 fold when applied occluded patch in comparison with unoccluded. Same research group was also evaluated the occlusive properties of a range of hydrocolloid patches containing TA on the drug penetration *in vivo* using visual assessment and the graded multiple-measuremet procedure. They concluded that these patch formulations showed great potential for localized prolonged delivery of drugs to the skin, which would be desirable for the topical use of other corticosteroids [83].

More recently, novel foam formulations of TC have been developed and proposed as alternative therapy to conventional formulations. They offer more convenient topical drug delivery with easy application and spreadability characteristics in comparision to other topical dosage forms [84, 85].

A novel foam formulation with enhanced BMV bioavailability has been shown to be superior in efficacy when compared with a lotion in the treatment of disease, without an concomitant increase in toxicity [86]. Another study has been performed comparing the ability of a foam formulation to release the active ingredient (betamethasone benzoate) with ointment, gel, and cream formulations. It was found that the release of betamethasone benzoate from the foam formulation better than the release from the cream [87].

The thermolabile and low-residue foam formulations of corticosteroids (betamethasone valerate and clobetasol propionate) are available in USA market. These foam formulations are associated with better patient compliance and improvements in quality of life [88, 89]. Table 4 summarizes the new drug carrier formulations of TC.

6. Conclusion

Current therapy of dermatological disorders with conventional dosage forms including TC is insufficient due to the low absorption rate and the risk of side effects. Therefore, it is necessary to synthesize the new topical corticosteroid molecules with adequate anti-inflammatory activity and minimal side effects. Fluticasone propionate, mometasone furoate and prednicarbate are very promising molecules showed lower side effects and better tolerability as a member of new generation TC. Also, improved dermal absorption of established TC may be obtained by new designed vehicle system as an alternative to conventional formulation. Recently, lipid and polymeric based carriers such as liposomes, niosomes, transfersomes, ethosomes, microemulsions and nanoparticles have been studied intensively and the potential of these carrier systems have also been described. Another alternative approach for TC treatment is a combined therapy which is more effective than in case of drug alone. The combined use of TC and synthetic vitamin D analogues such as calcipotriol would be promising for the treatment of inflammatory skin diseases. I

In conclusion, due to the difficulty of synthesizing new steroid molecules, developing the novel alternative drug carrier systems which improve the risk-benefit ratio of TC would be more beneficial in topical corticosteroid treatment. Besides, more in vivo study is required to validate the ability of new formulations in enhancing topical delivery of corticosteroids.

Author details

Taner Senyigit and Ozgen Ozer
Ege University, Faculty of Pharmacy, Department of Pharmaceutical Technology, Bornova, Izmir, Turkey

7. References

[1] Wiedersberg S, Leopold CS, Guy RH (2008) Bioavailability and Bioequivalence of Topical Glucocorticoids. Eur. j. pharm. biopharm. 68:453–466.

[2] Brazzini B, Pimpinelli N. (2002) New and Established Topical Corticosteroids in Dermatology. Am. j. clin. dermatol. 3:47-58.

[3] British National Formulary (2004) London: British Medical Association and the Royal Pharmaceutical Society of Great Britain.

[4] Schackert C, Korting HC, Schafer-Korting M (2000) Qualitative and Quantitative Assessment of the Benefit-Risk Ratio of Medium Potency Topical Corticosteroids In Vitro and In Vivo Characterisation of Drugs with an Increased Benefit-Risk Ratio. BioDrugs. 13:267-277.

[5] Fang JY, Fang CL, Sung KC, Chen HY. (1999) Effect of Low Frequency Ultrasound on the In Vitro Percutaneous Absorption of Clobetasol 17-Propionate. Int. j. pharm. 191:33-42.

[6] Banga AK, Bose S, Ghosh TK (1999) Iontophoresis and Electroporation: Comparisons and Contrasts. Int. j. pharm. 179:1-19.

[7] Kaplun-Frischoff Y, Touitou E (1997) Testesterone Skin Permeation Enhancement by Menthol Through Formation of Eutectic with Drug and Interaction with Skin Lipids. J. pharm. sci. 86:1394-1399.

[8] Moster K, Kriwet K, Naik A, Kalia YN, Guy RH (2001) Passive Skin Penetration Enhancement and Its Quantification In Vitro. Eur. j. pharm. biopharm. 52:103-112.

[9] Santos-Maia C, Mehnert W, Schaller M, Korting HC, Gysler A, Haberland A, Schafer-Korting M (2002) Drug Targeting by Solid Lipid Nanoparticles for Dermal Use. J. drug target. 10:489-495.

[10] Schaller M, Preidel H, Januschke E, Korting HC (1999) Light and Electron Microscopic Findings in a Model of Human Cutaneous Candidosis Cased on Reconstructed Human Epidermis Following the Topical Application of Different Econazole Formulations. J. drug target. 6:361-372.

[11] Beumer R, Chen C, Gutzwiller H, Maillan PE, Nowotny M, Schlegel B, Vollhardt J (2008) Topical compositions comprising nanoparticles of an isoflavone. US Patent Application 20080311209.

[12] Dmowski P, Dipiano GT (2008) Topical Administration of Danazol, US Patent Application, 20080153789, (2008).

[13] Walters KA, Roberts MS (2002) The Structure and Function of Skin. In: Walters KA, editor Dermatological and Transdermal Formulations: Drugs and the Pharmaceutical Sciences New York: Marcel Dekker Inc., pp. 1-39.

[14] Menon GK (2002) New Insight into Skin Structure: Stratching the Surface. Adv. drug del. rev. 54:S3-S17.

[15] Elias P (1983) Epidermal Lipids, Barrier Function and Desquamation. J. invest. Dermatol. 80:44-49.

[16] Schoepe S, Schacke H, May E, Asadullah K (2006) Glucocorticoid Therapy-Induced Skin Atrophy. Exp. dermatol. 15:406-420.

[17] Schacke H (2002) Mechanisms Involved in the Side Effects of Glucocorticoids. Pharmacol. ther. 96:23–43.
[18] Adcock IM (2004) Corticosteroids: Limitations and Future Prospects for Treatment of Severe Inflammatory Disease. Drug dev. tech. 1:321-328.
[19] Korting HC, Kerscher MJ, Schafer-Korting M (1992) Topical Glucocorticoids with Improved Benefit/Risk Ratio: Do They Exist? J. am. acad. dermatol. 27:87–92.
[20] P.O. National Psoriasis Foundation, Steroids (1998) www.psoriasis.org.
[21] Buhse L, Kolinski R, Westenberger B (2005) Topical Drug Classification. Int. j. pharm. 295:101-112.
[22] Fang JY, Leu YL, Wang YY, Tsai YH (2002) In Vitro Topical Application and In Vivo Pharmacodynamic Evaluation of Nonivamide Hydrogels Using Wistar Rat as an Animal Model. Eur. j. pharm. sci. 15:417-423.
[23] Singh SK, Naini V. (2007) Dosage Forms: Non-parenterals. In: Swarbrick J. editor. Encyclopedia of Pharmaceutical Technology. New York: Informa Healthcare, pp. 988-1000.
[24] Harding SM, Sohail S, Busse MJ (1985) Percutaneous Absorption of Clobetasol Propionate from Novel Ointment and Cream Formulations. Clin. exp. dermatol. 10:13-21.
[25] Eccleston GM (1997) Functions of Mixed Emulsifiers and Emulsifying Waxes in Dermatological Lotions and Creams. Colloid surface physicochem. eng. aspect. 123-124:169-182.
[26] Sequeira JA, Munayyer FJ, Galeos R (1988) US4775529.
[27] Beaurline JM, Roddy PJ, Tomai MA (1998) WO1998024436.
[28] Patel NA, Patel NJ, Patel RP (2009) Formulation and Evaluation of Curcumin Gel for Topical Application. Pharm. dev. tech. 14:80-89.
[29] Ozer O, Ozcan I, Cetin EO (2006) Evaluation of In Vitro Release and Skin Irritation of Benzoyl Peroxide-Containing Products. J. drug del. sci. tech. 16:449-454.
[30] Hebert A, Cook-Bolden F, Ford R, Gotz V (2008) Early Relief of Atopic Dermatitis Symptoms with a Novel Hydrogel Formulation of Desonide 0.05% in Pediatric Subjects. J. am. acad. dermatol. AB51:614.
[31] Kerney DL, Ford R, Gotz V. (2009) Patient Assessment of Desonide Hydrogel for the Treatment of Mild to Moderate Atopic Dermatitis. J. am. acad. derm. 60:AB69.
[32] Senyigit T, Padula C, Ozer O, Santi P (2009) Different Approaches for Improving Skin Accumulation of Topical Corticosteroids. Int. j. pharm. 380:155-160.
[33] McCadden, ME (2005) US6890544.
[34] Williams AC, Barry BW (2004) Penetration Enhancers. Adv. drug. deliv. rev. 56:603-618.
[35] Thong HY, Zhai H, Maibach HI (2007) Percutaneous Penetration Enhancers: An Overview. Skin pharmacol. physiol. 20:272-282.
[36] Asbill CS, Michniak BB (2000) Percutaneous Penetration Enhancers: Local Versus Transdermal Activity. PSTT 3:36-41.
[37] El-Kattan AF, Asbill CS, Michniak BB (2000) The Effects of Terpene Enhancer Lipophilicity on the Percutaneous Permeation of Hydrocortisone Formulated in HPMC Gel Systems. Int. j. pharm. 198:179-189.

[38] Shim J, Kang HS, Park W, Han S, Kim J, Chang I (2004) Transdermal Delivery of Minoxidil with Block Copolymer Nanoparticles. J. Control. release 97:477–484.

[39] Alvarez-Roman R, Naik A, Kalia YN, Guy RH, Fessi H (2004) Skin Penetration and Distribution of Polymeric Nanoparticles. J. control. release 99:53–62.

[40] Schafer-Korting M, Mehnert W, Korting HC (2007) Lipid Nanoparticles for Improved Topical Application of Drugs for Skin Diseases. Adv. drug deliv. rev. 59:427–443.

[41] Alvarez-Roman R, Naik A, Kalia YN, Guy RH, Fessi H (2004) Enhancement of Topical Delivery from Biodegradable Nanoparticles. Pharm. Res. 21:1818–1825.

[42] Schaller M, Preidel H, Januschke E, Korting HC (1999) Light and Electron Microscopic Findings in a Model of Human Cutaneous Candidosis Based on Reconstructed Human Epidermis Following the Topical Application of Different Econazole Formulations. J. drug target. 6:361–372.

[43] Zhao Y, Brown MB, Jones SA (2010) Pharmaceutical Foams: Are They Answer to the Dilemma of Topical Nanoparticles? Nanomedicine 6:227-236.

[44] Prow TW, Grice JE, Lin LL, Faye R, Butler M, Becker W, Wurm EMT, Yoong C, Robertson TA, Soyer HP, Roberts MS (2011) Nanoparticles and Microparticles for Skin Drug Delivery. Adv. drug deliv. rev. 63:470-491.

[45] Muller RH, Radtke M, Wissing SA (2002) Solid Lipid Nanoparticles (SLN) and Nanostructured Lipid Carriers (NLC) in Cosmetic and Dermatological Preparations. Adv. drug deliv. rev. 54:131-155.

[46] Muller RH, Petersen RD, Hommoss A, Pardeike J (2007) Nanostructured Lipid Carriers in Cosmetic Dermal Products. Adv. drug deliv. rev. 59:522-530.

[47] Maia CS, Mehnert W, Schafer-Korting M (2000) Solid Lipid Nanoparticles as Drug Carriers for Topical Glucocorticoids. Int. j. pharm. 196:165-167.

[48] Schlupp P (2011) Drug Release and Skin Penetration from Solid Lipid Nanoparticles and a Base Cream: a Systematic Approach from a Comparison of Three Glucocorticoids. Skin pharmacol. physiol. 24:199-209.

[49] Zhang J, Smith E (2011) Percutaneous Permeation of Betamethasone 17-Valerate Incorporated in Lipid Nanoparticles. J. pharm. sci. 100:896-903.

[50] Jensen LB, Petersson K, Nielsen HM (2011) In Vitro Penetration Properties of Solid Lipid Nanoparticles in Intact and Barrier-Impaired Skin. Eur. j. pharm. biopharm. :79(1):68-75.

[51] Kalariya M (2005) Clobetasol Propionate Solid Lipid Nanoparticles Cream for Effective Treatment of Eczema: Formulation and Clinical Implications. Indian j. exp. biol. 43:233-240.

[52] de Vringer T (1997) US5667800.

[53] Senyigit T, Sonvico F, Barbieri S, Ozer O, Santi P, Colombo P (2010) Lecithin/Chitosan Nanoparticles of Clobetasol-17-Propionate Capable of Accumulation in Pig Skin. J. control. release 142:368-373.

[54] Schreier H, Bouwstra J (1994) Liposomes and Niosomes as Topical Drug Carriers: Dermal and Transdermal Drug Delivery. J. control. release 30:1-15.

[55] Lopez-Pinto JM, Gonzalez-Rodriguez ML, Rabasco AM (2005) Effect of Cholesterol and Ethanol on Dermal Delivery from DPPC Liposomes. Int. j. pharm. 298:1-12.

[56] Manosroi A, Kongkaneramit L, Manosroi J (2004) Stability and Transdermal Absorption of Topical Amphotericin B Liposome Formulations. Int. j. Pharm. 270:279-286.
[57] Mezei M, Gulasekharam V (1980) Liposomes: A Selective Drug Delivery System for the Topical Route of Administration. Life sci. 26:1473-1477.
[58] Mezei M, Gulasekharam V (1982) Liposomes: A Selective Drug Delivery System for the Topical Route for Administration: Gel Dosage Form. J. pharm. Pharmacol. 34: 473-474.
[59] Lasch J, Wohlrab W (1986) Liposome-Bound Cortisol: A New Approach to Cutaneous Therapy. Biomed. biochim. acta 45:1295-1299.
[60] Wohlrab W, Lasch J (1987) Penetration Kinetics of Liposomal Hydrocortisone in Human Skin. Dermatologica 174: 18-22.
[61] Korting HC, Zienicki H, Schafer-Korting M, Braun-Falco O (1990) Liposome Encapsulation Improves Efficacy of Betamethasone Dipropionate in Atopic Eczema but not in Psoriasis Vulgaris. Eur. j. clin. pharmacol. 39:349-351.
[62] Fresta M, Puglisi G (1997) Corticosteroid Dermal Delivery with Skin-Lipid Liposomes. J. control. release 44:141-151.
[63] Williams AC (2003) Physical and Technological Modulation of Topical and Transdermal Drug Delivery. In: Transdermal and Topical Drug Delivery London: Pharmaceutical Press, pp. 123-167.
[64] Uchegbu IF, Vyas SP (1998) Non-Ionic Surfactant Based Vesicles (Niosomes) in Drug Delivery. Int. j. pharm. 172: 33-70.
[65] Sinico C, Fadda AM (2009) Vesicular Carriers for Dermal Drug Delivery. Expert opin. drug deliv. 6:813-825.
[66] Cevc G, Blume G (1992) Lipid Vesicles Penetrate into Intact Skin Owing to the Transdermal Osmotic Gradients and hydration force. Biochim. biophys. acta 1104:226–232.
[67] Cevc G (1996) Transfersomes, Liposomes and Other Lipid Suspensions on the Skin: Permeation Enhancement, Vesicle Penetration, and Transdermal Drug Delivery. Crit. rev. ther. drug carrier syst. 13(3/4): 257–388.
[68] Cevc G, Blume G, Schatzlein A, Gebauer D, Paul A. (1996) The Skin: A Pathway for Systemic Treatment with Patches and Lipid-based Agent Carriers. Adv. drug deliv. rev. 18(3):349–378.
[69] Cevc G, Blume G, Schatzlein A. (1997) Transfersomes-mediated Transepidermal Delivery Improves the Regio-Specifity and Biological Activity of Corticosteroids In Vivo. J. Control. release 45(3):211-226.
[70] Fesq H, Lehmann J, Kontny A, Erdmann I, Theiling K, Rother M, Ring J, Cevc G, Abeck D. (2003) Improved Risk-benefit Ratio for Topical Triamcinolone Acetonide in Transfersome® in Comparison with Equipotent Cream and Ointment: a Randomized Controlled Trial. British j. dermatol. 149(3):611-619.
[71] Touitou E, Alkabes M, Dayan N. (1997) Ethosomes: Novel Lipid Vesicular System for Enhanced Delivery. Pharm res. S14:305–306.

[72] Touitou E, Dayan N, Bergelson L, Godin B, Eliaz M. (2000) Ethosomes—Novel Vesicular Carriers for Enhanced Delivery: Characterization and Skin Penetration Properties. J. control. release 65(3):403–418.

[73] Date AA, Naik B, Nagarsenker MS. (2006) Novel Drug Delivery Systems: Potential in Improving Topical Delivery of Antiacne Agents. Skin pharmacol. physiol. 19(1):2–16.

[74] Kreilgaard M. (2002) Influence of Microemulsions on Cutaneous Drug Delivery. Adv. drug deliv. rev. 54(S1):77–98.

[75] Santos P, Watkinson AC, Hadgraft J, Lane ME. (2008) Application of Microemulsions in Dermal and Transdermal Drug Delivery. Skin pharmacol. physiol. 21(5):246–259.

[76] Wiedersberg S, Leopold CS, Guy RH. Dermatopharmacokinetics of betamethasone 17-valerate: Influence of formulation viscosity and skin surface cleaning procedure. Eur J Pharm Biopharm 2009; 71(2): 362–366.

[77] Krause SA, Wohlrab WA, Neubert RHH. (1998) Release of Hydrocortisone from a Microemulsion and Penetration into Human Skin. The First european graduate student meeting, Frankfurt, Germany.

[78] Jahn K, Krause A, Martin J, Neubert RHH. (2002) Colloidal Drug Carrier Systems. In: Bronaugh RL, Maibach HI. editors. Topical Absorption of Dermatological Products. New York: Marcel Dekker pp. 483-493.

[79] Padula C, Nicoli S, Santi P. (2009) Innovative formulations for the delivery of levothyroxine to the skin. Int. j. pharm. 372(1/2):12-16.

[80] Queen D, Martin GP, Marriott C, Fairbrother JE. (1988) Assessment of the Potential of a New Hydrocolloid Dermatological Patch (Actiderm) in the Treatment of Steroid Responsive Dermatoses. Int. j. pharm. 44:25-30.

[81] Juhlin L. (1989) Treatment of Psoriasis and Other Dermatoses with a Single Application of a Corticosteroid Left Under a Hydrocolloid Occlusive Dressing for One Week. Acta dermatol. venereol. 69(4):355-357.

[82] Ladenheim D, Martin GP, Marriott C, Holligsbee DA, Brown MB. (1996) An In-vitro Study of the Effect of Hydrocolloid Patch Occlusion on the Penetration of Triamcinolone Acetonide Through Skin In Man. J. pharm. pharmacol. 48(8):806-811.

[83] Martin GP, Ladenheim D, Marriott C, Hollingsbee DA, Brown MB. (2000) The Influence of Hydrocolloid Patch Composition on the Bioavailability of Triamcinolone Acetonide In Humans. Drug dev. ind. pharm. 26(1):35-43.

[84] Purdon CH, Haigh JM, Surber C, Smith EW. (2003) Foam Drug Delivery In Dermatology: Beyond the Scalp. Am. j. drug deliv. 1(1):71-75.

[85] Tamarkin D, Friedman D, Shemer A. (2006) Emollient Foam In Topical Drug Delivery. Expert opin. drug deliv. 3(6):799-807.

[86] Feldman SR, Sangha N, Setaluri V. (2000) Topical Corticosteroids In Foam Vehicle Offers Comparable Coverage Compared with Traditional Vehicles. J. am. acad. dermatol. 42(6):1017-1020.

[87] Woodford R, Barry BW. (1977) Bioavailability and Activity of Topical Corticosteroids from a Novel Drug Delivery System: the Aerosol Quick Break Foam. J. pharm. sci. 66(1):99-103.

[88] Stein L. (2005) Clinical Studies of a New Vehicle Formulation for Topical Corticosteroids in the Treatment of Psoriasis. J. am. acad. dermatol. 53(S1):39-49.

[89] Franz TJ, Parsell DA, Halualani RM, Hannigan JF, Kalbach JP, Harkonen WS. (1999) Betamethasone Valerate Foam 0.12%: A Novel Vehicle with Enhanced Delivery and Efficacy. Int. j. dermatol. 38(8):628–632.

Chapter 25

Soft Glucocorticoids: Eye-Targeted Chemical Delivery Systems (CDSs) and Retrometabolic Drug Design: A Review

Pritish Chowdhury and Juri Moni Borah

Additional information is available at the end of the chapter

http://dx.doi.org/10.5772/48380

1. Introduction

Steroids play a vital role in human physiology and medicine. Glucocorticoids have dominated the class of anti-inflammatory agents quite successfully over other drugs since their introduction to dermatology more than fifty years ago. Later they have been developed both as topical and systemic anti-inflammatory agents. From studies it has been found that glucocorticoids normally release their anti-inflammatory effects mainly through the modulation of the cytosolic glucocorticoid receptor (GR) at the genomic level [1, 2]. The activated glucocorticoid-GR complex formed *via* binding of glucocorticoid with the GR in the cytoplasm, migrates to the nucleus, where it upregulates the expression of anti-inflammatory proteins and repress the expression of pro-inflammatory proteins. In some recent work, it has been reported that the activated glucocorticoid-GR complex has also been found to initiate nongenomic effects like inhibition of vasodilation, vascular permeability and migration of leukocytes [1, 3]. Glucocorticoids also mediate anti-inflammatory activity through membrane-bound GR-mediated nongenomic effects and also through direct non specific interaction with cellular membranes [3, 4]. Since GR is involved in a plethora of signalling pathways, more than 5000 genes are expressed or suppressed following glucocorticoid exposure [4, 5]. Therefore long term use or high dosages of glucocorticoids could result in adverse drug reactions (ADRs) like increased Intraocular Pressure (IOP) [6, 7] in ocular therapeutics. Glucocorticoids- induced ocular hypertension is of great concern in ophthalmic therapeutics as it can lead to secondary iatrogenic open-angle glaucoma. Glaucoma is a group of eye diseases characterized by progressive optic nerve cupping with visual field loss leading to bilateral blindness. It has been reported that glaucoma is estimated to affect more than 50 million people worldwide as defined by the World Health Organization (WHO) [8].

However, the use of corticosteroids has become more and more restricted and unacceptable because most of these agents are found to be associated with severe side effects, including percutaneous absorption and cutaneous atrophy [9]. Also allergic contact dermatitis is an unexpected adverse effect in most of these corticosteroids. On the other hand because of their high efficacy, their use is inevitable to give them the status of life saving drugs. The severe side effects associated with these glucocorticoids, has led to the pharmaceutical industry to make a productive effort towards the introduction of new generation of topical corticosteroids with specific substituents in their parent molecules to make them safer in comparison to the old generation glucocorticoids [10].

The effectiveness of hydrocortisone was first demonstrated by Sulzberger and Witten during 1950 [11] and soon after the new and more effective fluorinated hydrocortisones were introduced in the market during 1960 [12]. Further R&D works on these glucocorticoids led to introduction of super potent corticosteroids in the 1970s and 1980s. Cornell and Stoughton [13] had proposed a potency rating of these topically applied glucocorticoids in 1984, based primarily on the vasoconstrictor assay or skin-blanching of corticosteroid preparations. Again based upon the consensus of the United States Pharmacopoeia (USP) Dermatology Advisory Panel, a classification of the potency ranking for these glucocorticoids had been done as low, medium, high and very high [14]. New generation of glucocorticoids do not cause much cutaneous atrophy or systemic absorption in human body. Molecular configuration of these new corticosteroids tends to display a rapidly declining concentration gradient in the skin. Many of these new generation glucocorticoids are developed through the concept of prodrugs – a tool for improving physiochemical, biopharmaceutical or pharmacokinetic properties of pharmacologically active agents. Thus prodrugs are bioreversible derivatives of drug molecules that undergo an enzymatic or chemical transformation *in vivo* to release the active parent drug, which could then exert the desired pharmacological effect. These new generation glucocorticoids primarily act in the top layers of the skin where the most important mediators of the inflammatory reactions are [10, 14] found.

As for these new generation glucocorticoids, the action in the deeper layer is considerably diminished making them having less systemic side effects [14]. European and North American based clinical studies have shown that the new generation corticosteroids with their improved risk- benefit ratio are as effective as products currently available in the market [15]. These new generation glucocorticoids are highly effective in treating plethora of disease including psoriasis, allergies, asthma, rheumatoid arthritis and lupus [2-8, 14,15].

Again the application of anti-inflammatory agents in ophthalmic therapeutic is a challenging task because of severe complications arising out of the currently used anti-inflammatory agents. The eye is vulnerable to damage from low level of intraocular inflammation. The blood-aqueous and blood-retinal barriers generally limit penetration of protein and cells from peripheral circulation, while regulatory molecules and cells in the eye actively suppress immunological responses [16]. The fact that ocular inflammatory conditions and surgical trauma induce changes in the blood- aqueous and blood-retinal barriers [16-18], due to which immune cells and mediators of inflammation could enter the eye, resulting in the development of symptoms of ocular inflammation such as redness, pain, swelling and itching [19]. Ocular inflammation is a serious problem, negligence of which may lead to temporary or permanent blindness [20].

Clinical studies suggest that topical glucocorticoids are effective in the management of anterior segment inflammation. They impart a number of potent anti-inflammatory effects [21]. They are found to suppress cellular infiltration, capillary dilution, proliferation of fibroblasts, collagen deposition leading to scar formation; they also stabilize intracellular and extracellular membranes. Glucocorticoids increase the synthesis of lipocortins which block *phospholipase A2* and also inhibit Histamine (**A**) synthesis in mast cells. A critical step in the inflammatory cascade is the inhibition of *phospholipase A2* that inhibits the transformation of Phospholipids (**B**) to Arachidonic acid (**C**). Glucocorticoids are also found to increase the enzyme histaminase and modulate transcription factors present in mast cell nuclei [21, 22]. The formation of cataract is also one of the severe adverse drug reactions (ADRs) associated with glucocorticoids when used for ocular problems.

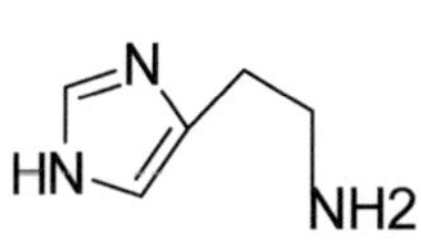

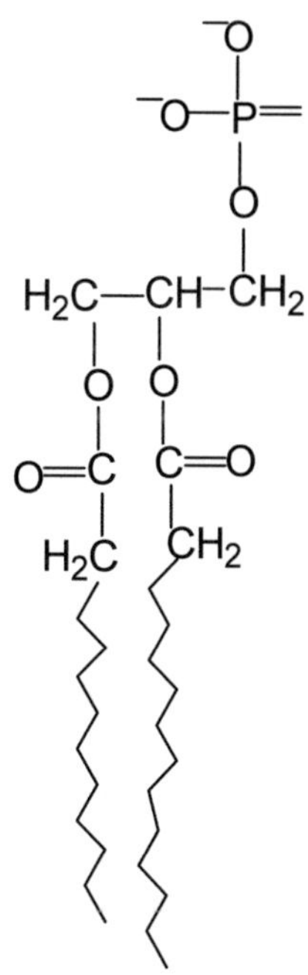

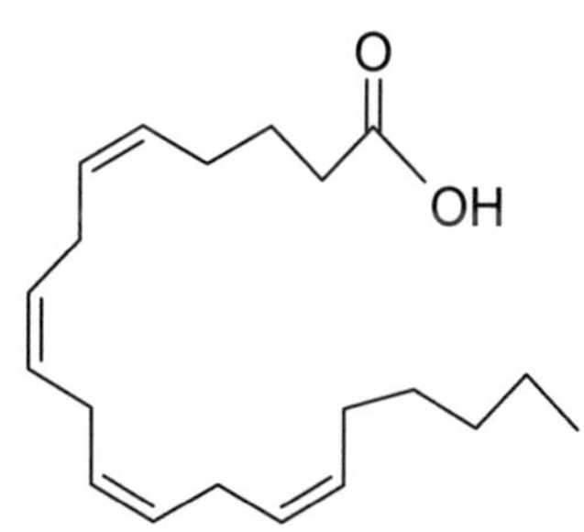

Arachidonic Acid (**C**)

Histamine (**A**) Phospholipids (**B**)

It has been reported by Manabe *et al* [23] that the mechanism of steroid-induced cataract formation is chemically based and possibly not related to the downstream effects of glucocorticoid receptor (GR) activation. At present the most accepted hypothesis of this mechanism is likely to involve non-enzymatic formation of Schiff base intermediates between the steroid C-20 ketone group and nucleophilic groups such as β -amino groups of lysine residues of proteins (**Figure 1**). Schiff base formation is followed by a Heyns rearrangement [23] involving the nearby C-21 hydroxyl group of the glucocorticoid molecule furnishing stable amine-linked adducts. This covalent binding results in the destabilization of the protein structure allowing further oxidation leading to steroid-induced cataract formation [23].

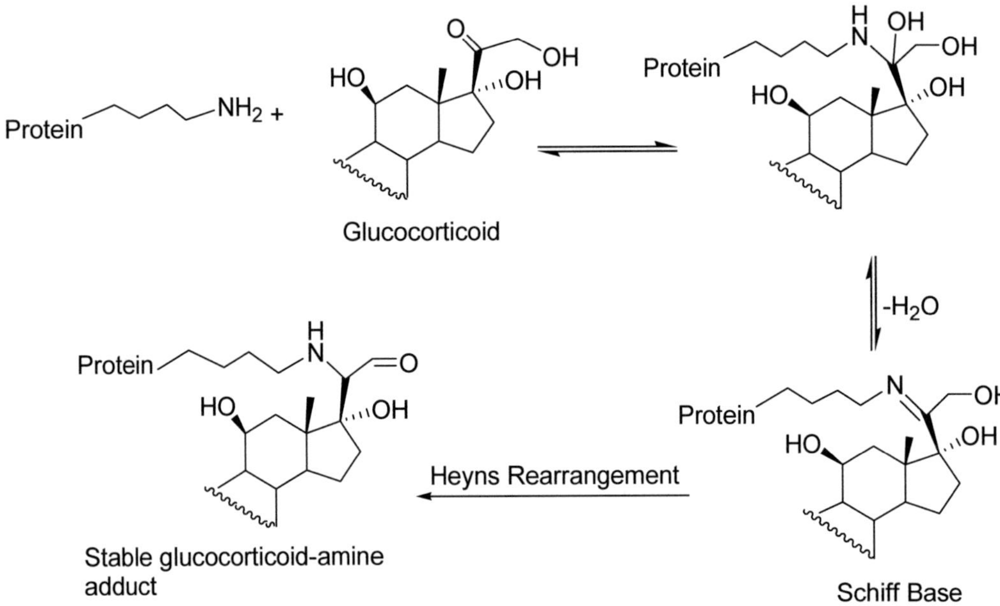

Figure 1. Mechanism of steroid-induced cataract formation due to the synthesis of the stable steroid-amine adduct between the C-20 carbonyl group of glucocorticoids and nucleophilic group such as β-amino groups of lysine residues of proteins via formation Schiff Base

R&D work in understanding the mechanism of action of steroids, both for their anti-inflammatory effects and adverse drug reactions (ADRs) has lead to the development new generation glucocorticoids mainly through prodrug design approach to find use in treating plethora of diseases as mentioned earlier. All these new generation glucocorticoids are not designed for ophthalmic therapeutics. Hence a real breakthrough in the field of ophthalmic therapeutic could be achieved only by specifically designing new drug entities to incorporate the eye targeting possibility into their chemical structure [24,25]. Chemical Delivery Systems (CDSs) and Retrometabolic drug design principles have led to development of a new but unique class of glucocorticoids which are safe and effective in treating a wide variety of ocular inflammatory conditions including giant papillary conjunctivitis, seasonal allergic conjunctivitis, and uveities as well as in the treatment of ocular inflammation and pain following cataract surgery. This new and unique class of glucocorticoids are now known as soft glucocorticoids which are associated with highly minimized ADRs to justify terming them as `soft drugs' [24, 26].

It is pertinent to note that, this important drug design based on Chemical Delivery Systems (CDSs) and Soft drug (SD) approaches integrate the specific pharmacological, metabolic, and targeting requirements for ophthalmic therapeutics. .A number of glucocorticoid soft drugs and soft β -blockers have been developed this way for clinical trials. Their potential is already documented by the results obtained with several soft drugs designed within this framework. Glucocorticoid soft drugs such as Loteprednol Etabonate, and Etiprednol Dicloacetate and β -blockers such as Betaxoxime, and Adaprolol are some of the new chemical entities developed as soft drugs for ocular applications. Besides, many of these soft drugs have already reached the clinical development phase in various ophthalmic areas and one of them Loteprednol Etabonate has already been marketed [24]. Herein we review the important aspects of the development of new generation glucocorticoids through prodrug approach with special reference to the development of the first and second generation glucocorticoid soft drugs by the application chemical delivery systems (CDSs) and retrometabolic drug design approaches towards ophthalmic therapeutics. A few examples of soft ocular β –blockers have also been cited to know more about the retrometabolic drug design approach in depth as have been put forwarded by Bodor and his co-workers (24).

2. New generation glucocorticoids: Prodrugs

As discussed earlier several numbers of new entities of glucocorticoids have been developed during the last two decades. Many of them are already in market for their high efficacy and less systemic side effects. These new generation corticosteroids were developed with modifications made in the basic glucocorticoid molecules, *viz.*, Betamethasone **1** or Dexamethasone **2** extensively used during early stage of glucocorticoids therapy. The main object of synthesizing these modified glucocorticoids was to get better skin penetration, slower enzyme degradation, and greater affinity for cytosol receptors [5].

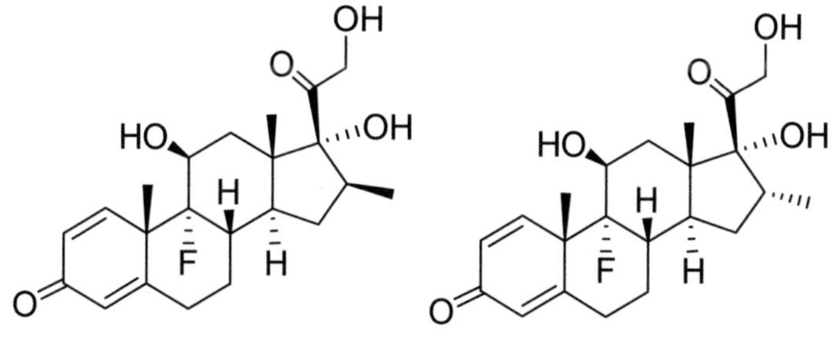

Betamethasone (**1**) Dexamethasone (**2**)

Even then in some cases it was observed that the changes that increased potency, also led sometimes to more systemic side effects. As per clinical investigations by various workers, these new generation glucocorticoids have been found to act *via* hepatic or extra hepatic biotransformation. These results in lesser systemic side effects and hence are much safer drugs to be used specially by adults and non- erythrodermic patients. However, while systemic side effects are of concern, cutaneous side effects are generally common involving problems such as striae formation, atrophy, purpura, peri-oral dermatitis, steroid rosacea, hypertrichosis and steroid acne [2,6]. Most of the side effects associated even with these new generation glucocorticoids are basically related to the duration and potency of the application, the manner of application, the presence of penetration-enhancing substances and the state of skin barrier. Besides these, the anatomic site and the age of the patient could also adversely influence the side effect profile [2, 6]. In both drug discovery and development, prodrug design approach helped to maximize the amount of an active drug to reach its target through changing the physicochemical, pharmacokinetics or biopharmaceutical properties of the drug. Therefore the term prodrug refers to a pharmacologically inactive compound which is converted to an active drug by metabolic biotransformation which may occur prior, during or after absorption or at specific target sites within the body because of their specific molecular configurations [28-30]. The labile `prodrug' corticosteroids such as 17-Prednicarbate, Alclometasone, Methylprednisolone aceponate, Fluticasone Propionate and Fluocortin butylester are some of these new generation glucocorticoids which are developed through prodrug approach [2,6]. Based on the molecular configuration of these new generation glucocorticoids, they are classified into several categories [**Table1**] [2, 6].

Molecular Configurations	**Structures**	**Names**
Asymmetric acetonides	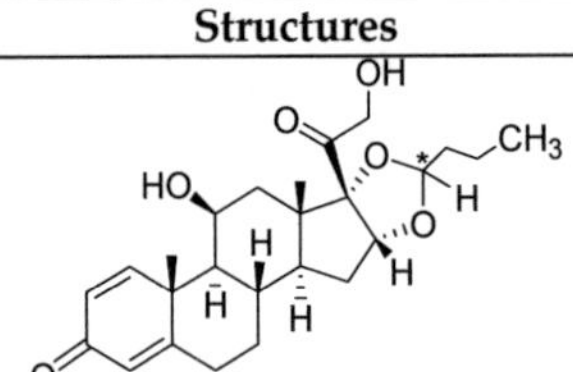 3	Budesonide (**3**)
C-21-Carboxylesters	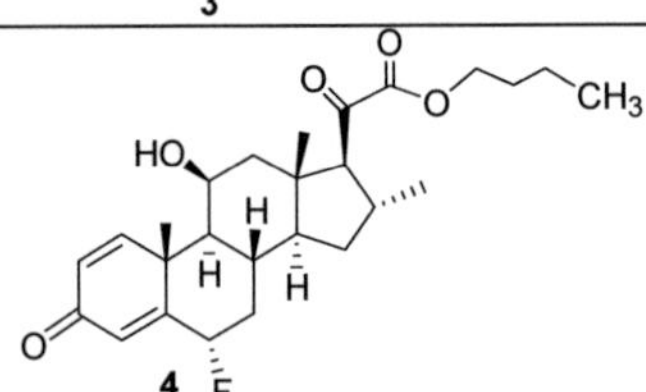 4	Fluocortin butylester (**4**)
	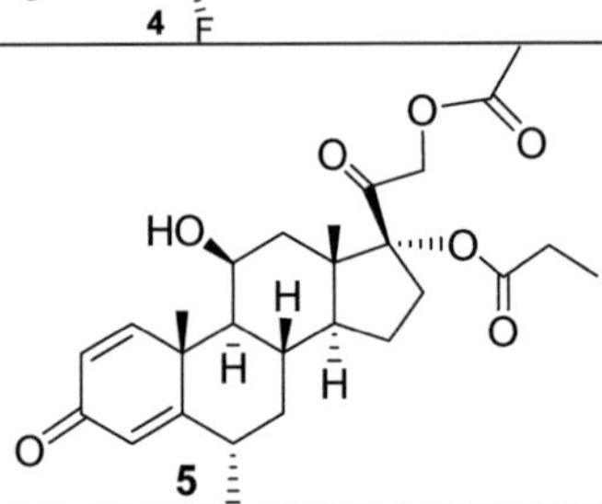 5	Methylprednisolone aceponate (**5**)
	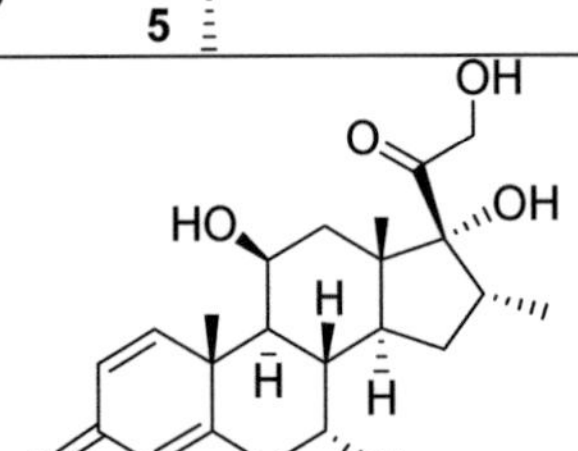 6	Alclometasone dipropionate(**6**)
	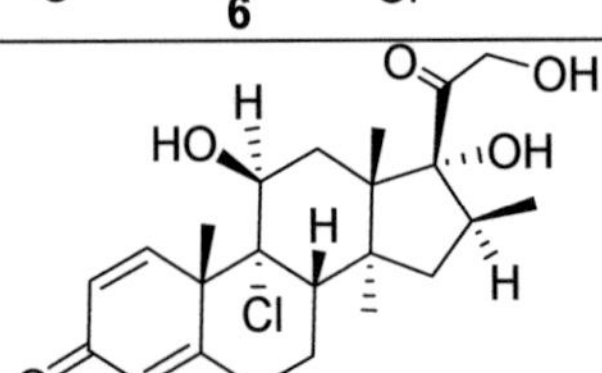 7	Beclomethasone (**7**)

	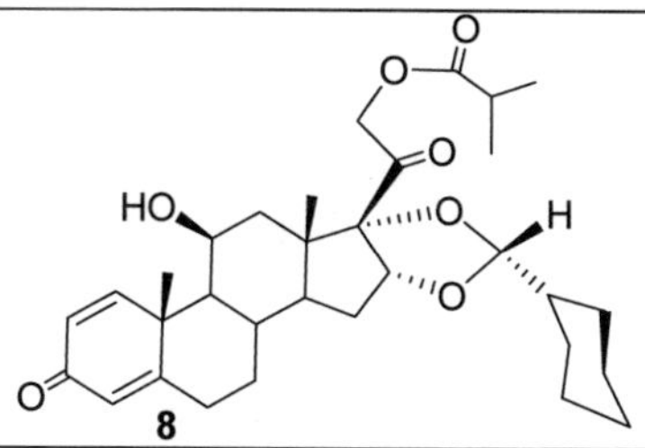 8	Ciclesonide (**8**)
C-17 –Prednicarbonates	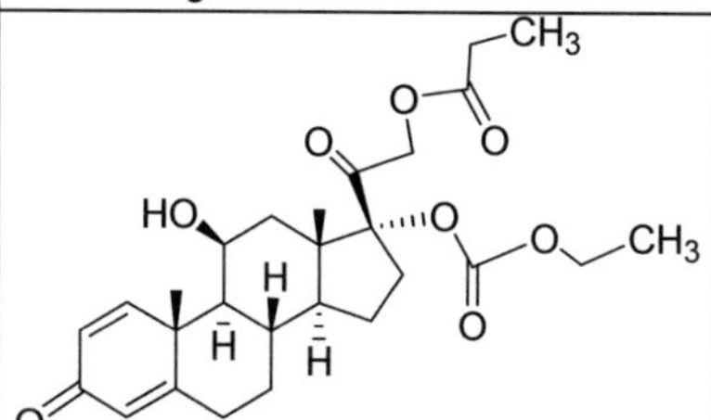 9	17-Prednicarbate (**9**)
Carbothiates	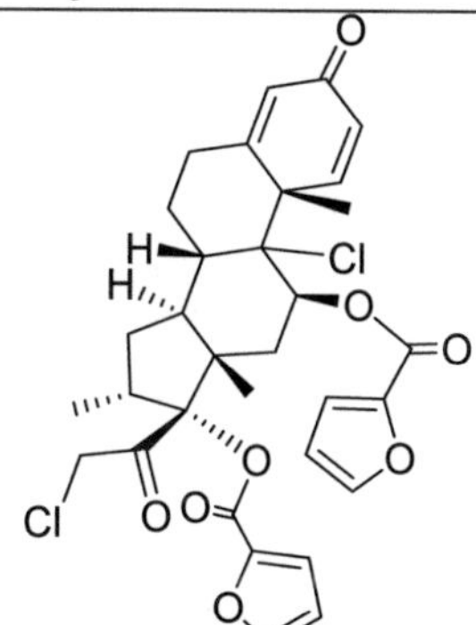 10	Mometasone furoate (**10**)
	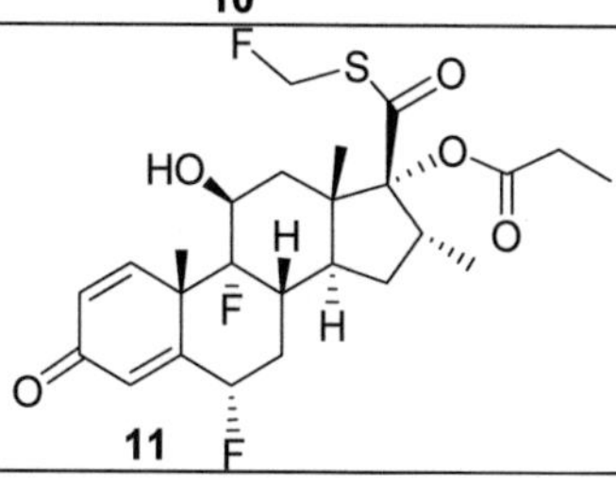 11	Fluticasone propionate (**11**)

Table 1. Classification of new generation glucocorticoids on the basis of their molecular configurations

Chemical stability is another criteria for classification of these new generation corticosteroids. Based on this, most of these newer drugs can be regarded as prodrugs because immediately after application to the system, they undergo metabolization and acyl-exchanges to form the active molecule to fight the ailment in the system. As mentioned earlier, all these glucocorticoids have been developed through prodrugs design approach in order to maximize the amount of an active drug reaching its target through changing the physicochemical, biopharmaceutical or pharmacokinetic properties of drugs. Prodrugs are bioreversible derivatives of drug molecules that undergo an enzymatic or chemical transformation *in vivo* to release the active parent drug, which can then exert the desired pharmacological effect [28-30]. Most of the new generation corticosteroids have been found belonging to the class of molecules having high potency. By introducing various substituents at different positions, changes or modifications were made on the parent hydrocortisone molecules, such as Betamethasone (**1**) and Dexamethasone (**2**) in order to get better skin penetration, slower enzymatic degradation and greater affinity for the cytosol receptor for these molecules to reduce or eliminate their systemic side effects [6]. The systemic side effects of these new corticosteroids are reduced due to rapid biotransformation while applying them for treatment of atopic dermatitis. However it is pertinent to note that there are still risks of having potential hypothalamus and pituitary axis (HPA) suppression with some of these new generation glucocorticoids while treating young children and erythrodermic patients. Clinical safety has been demonstrated in most of these newer corticosteroids with restricted duration of treatment up to six weeks [2, 6]. Even then skin atropy and some telangiectasia have been observed in some patients. A large number of reports of contact allergic reactions associated with these new generation glucocorticoids were still of great concern. To explain the increased allergenicity, data from clinical studies and literature were reviewed to define precisely some of the more important groups of cross-reacting molecules [31]. **Table2** represents the various allergy groups of these newer glucocorticoids based on their molecular structures and configurations. Clinical studies have revealed that Tixocortol pivalate (**19**) has been identified as a good screening agent for the Group A [32]. Budesonide (**3**) is infact a 1:1 mixture of two diasteriomers (R- and S- isomer). The R-isomer has been found to be a marker for the Group B while the S-isomer for the Group D. Glucocorticoid members of Group C cause minimized contact sensitivity and do not cross react with other groups. As shown in **Table2**, Group D has been divided in two sub-groups D_1 and D_2 based on recent studies [2, 33] with respect to their mode of substitutions.

Group	Molecular configuration	Characteristics of substituent
A	Hydrocortisone (12) type	No substitution in D ring, except a short chain ester on C-17 or C-21 or a thioester on C-21
B	Triamcinolone (13) type	C-16,C-17-*cis*-ketal or –diol structure
C	Betamethasone (1) type	C-16 methyl substitution, no side chain on C-17; possible side chain at C-21.
	Fluocortin Butylester (4)	
D	Hydrocortisone-17α-butyrate(14) type	Long chain ester at C-17 and/or C-21 with or without C-16 methyl substitution.
D_1	Betamethasone Dipropionate(15)	Long chain ester at C-17 and/or C-21 with C-16 methyl substitution; halogen substituent in ring B
	Betamethasone17α-Valerate (16)	
	Clobetasol 17α -Propionate (17)	
	Mometasone Furoate (10)	
	Fluticasone Propionate (11)	
D_2	Hydrocortisone-17α-butyrate(14)	Long chain ester at C-17; possibly a side chain at C-21; no methyl substitution at C-16 and no halogen substituent in ring B.
	Hydrocortisone 17α-Valerate (18)	
	17-Prednicarbate (9)	
	Methylprednisolone Aceponate (5)	

Table 2. Allergy Groups of new generation corticosteroids based on their molecular structures and configurations

To the Group D_1, belong not only the old generation glucocorticoid molecules like Betamethasone dipropionate (**15**), Betamethasone-17α-valerate (**16**) and Clobetasol 17α propionate (**17**) but also new generation corticosteroids such as Mometasone furoate (**10**) and Fluticasone propionate (**11**). These glucocorticoids are found to possess very less systemic side effects and so can be used safely even in case of patients who are allergic to other corticosteroids. To the Group D_2 belong Hydrocortisone-17α- valerate (**18**) and Hydrocortisone -17α-butyrate (**14**) as well as the labile new generation glucocorticoids like 17-Prednicarbate (**9**) and Methylprednisolone Aceponate (**5**). They are sometimes found to cause allergic reactions.

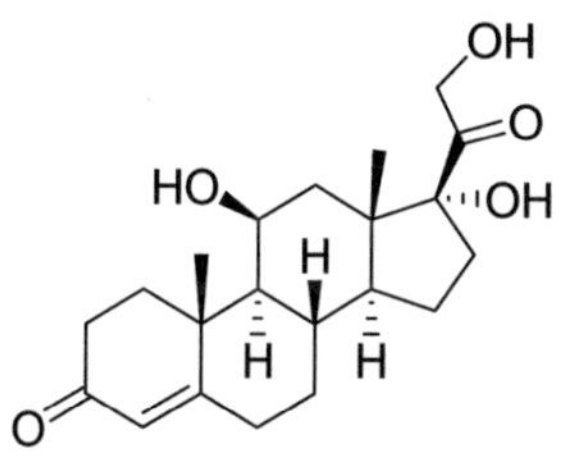

Hydrocortisone (**12**)

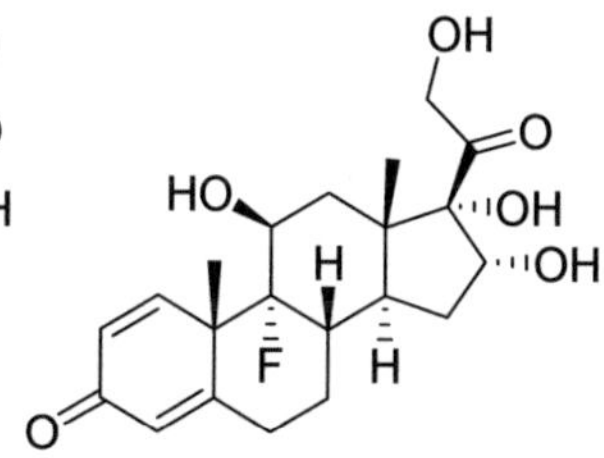

Triamcinolone (**13**)

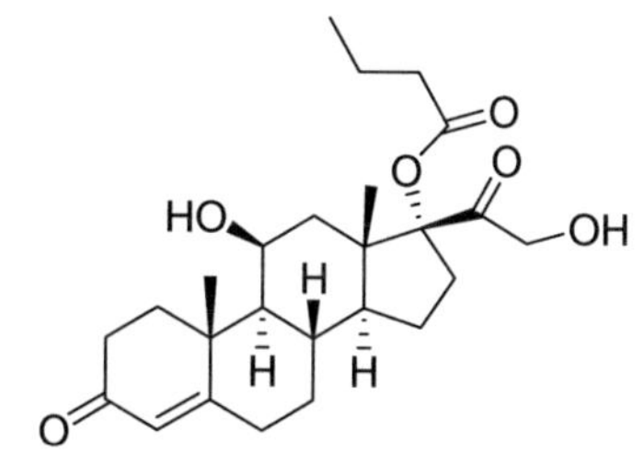

Hydrocortisone-17α-butyrate (**14**)

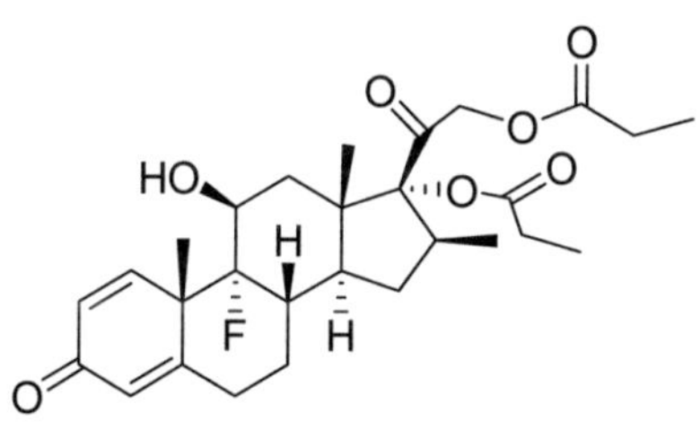

Betamethasone Dipropionate (**15**)

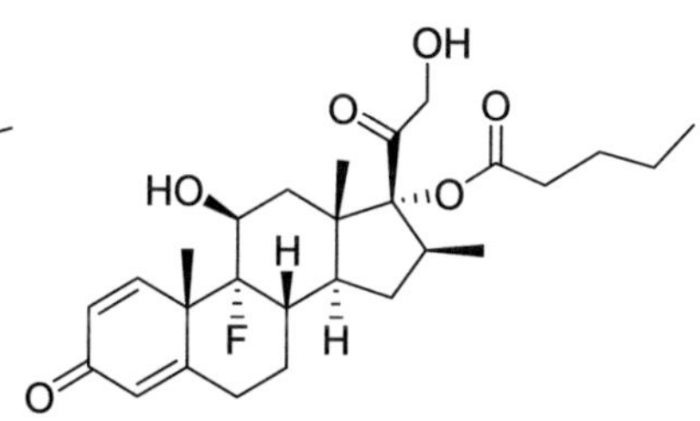

Betamethasone-17α-Valerate (**16**)

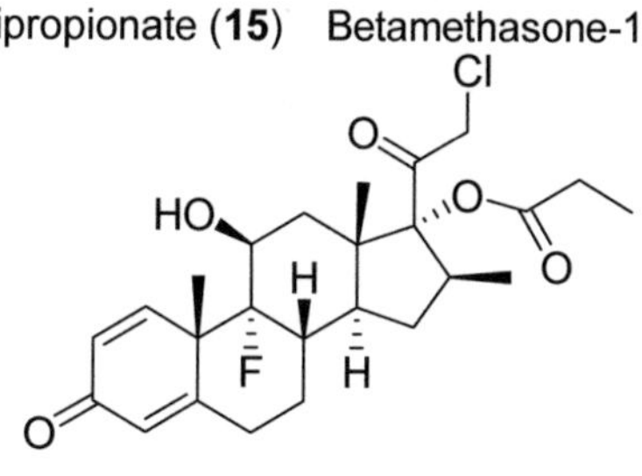

Clobetasol-17α-Propionate (**17**)

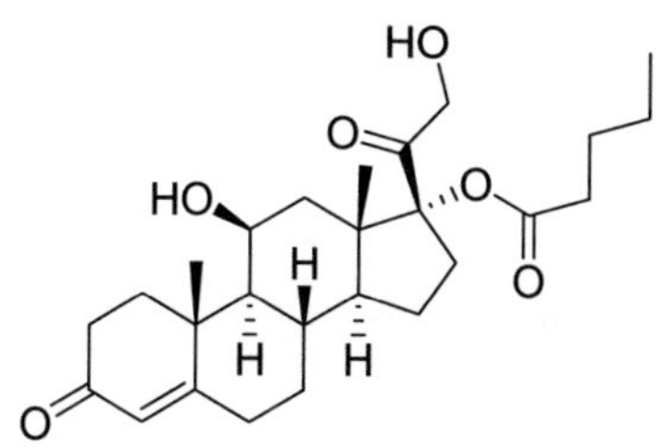

Hydrocortisone-17α-Valerate (**18**)

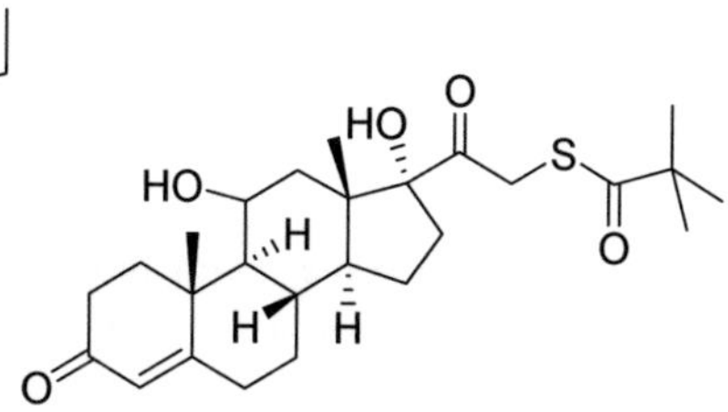

Tixocortol pivalate (**19**)

S-isomer of Budesonide (**3**) is the marker for this Group D_2, but they can cross react with the Group A. **Table 3** illustrates the safety profile, potency , side effects and allergy groups of some of the new generation glucocorticoids along with their manufactures.

Product	Manufacturer	Safety profile	Potency	Side effect	Allergygroup
Budesonide(3)	Astra, Entcort	A Stable asymmetric acetonide undergoing rapid biotransformation in liver with less systemic side effects	High potency	May be problem with contact sensitivity	B
Mometasone Furoate (10)	Schering-Plough, Elocom	A stable chlorinated topical glucocorticoid with low penetration with high biliary excretion, and also low resorption in the circulation with fast biotransformation in the liver resulting in rare local systemic side effect.	High potency	Very rare contact hypersensitivity	D_1
Fluocortin butylester(4)	Schering Corp.-Essex, Varlane	Biotransformation into the non- active fluocortolone-21-acid in skin.	Medium potency	Rare contact hyper-sensitivity	C
Alclometasone dipropionate(6)	Schering-Plough, Aclovate, Glaxo- -welcome	A labile prodrug metabolizing to inactive compound	High potency	Occasional Contact hyper-sensitivity	D_2
17-Prednicarbate(9)	Hoechst-Roussel,Dermatop Emollient	A labile prodrug glucocorticoid, converting to prednisolone in the skin	High potency	Contact hyper-sensitivity is observed. Also can cross-react with the Group A	D_2
Methylprednisolone aceponate(5)	Schering Corp. Essex, Advantan	A labile prodrug. Get transformed into methyl prednisolone in the skin and into nonactive derivatives in the liver	High potency	Contact hyper-sensitivity is not rare	D_2

Fluticasone propionate (11)	Cutivate, Glaxo Wellcome	A fluorinated topical glucocorticoid. Readily metabolized in the liver resulting in a locally potent sterid drug with a low HPA inhibitory potency	High potency	Contact hyper-sensitivity is very rare	D_1
Beclomethasone(7)	Schwitz Biotech, Havione Farmaciencies, Portugal	A chlorinated topical corticosteroid. Readily metabolized in the liver resulting in a locally potent steroid with a low HPA inhibitory potency	High potency	Contact hyper-sensitivity is very rare	D_1
Cyclesonide (8)	Brand Name: Alvesco, Taj Pharmaceuticals Ltd. India	A triamcinolone type Gluco-corticoid with low HPA inhibitory potency	High Potency	Contact hyper-sensitivity is rare	D_1

Table 3. Some of the marketed new generation glucocorticoids and their allergy groups:

Continuous efforts are still being still sought after by pharmaceutical companies worldwide to develop and market more and more safer glucocorticoids as anti-inflammatory agents, because clinical investigations on some already marketed newer glucocorticoids have revealed that many of them are still prone to cause allergic reactions and other systemic side effects specially on prolonged use. However, glucocorticoids are still regarded as life saving drugs dominating over the other anti-inflammatory agents for the treatment of a number of diseases including psoriasis, allergies, acute asthma, rheumatoid arthritis and lupus.

Eye–targeted Chemical Delivery Systems (CDSs) and retrometabolic drug design: Soft β-Blockers and Soft Glucocorticoids

Soft corticosteroids or Soft glucocorticoids can be termed as a unique class of new generation glucocorticoids that are designed specifically for ophthalmic therapeutics [24-27]. The new generation glucocorticoids developed by prodrug approach as described earlier have brought revolution in treating a plethora of disease including psoriasis, allergies, asthma, rheumatoid arthritis and lupus because of their minimized systemic side effects. However, these new generation glucocorticoids are still not useful for ophthalmic applications due to their association with adverse drug reactions (ADRs) including elevation of intraocular pressure (IOP) and steroid-induced cataract formation [23] in ophthalmic applications. For the therapeutic treatment of most of ocular problems, topical administration undoubtedly seems preferred mode, because for systemically administered drugs, only a very small fraction of the total dose will reach the eye from the general circulatory system. Even distribution for this fraction to the inside of the eye is further hindered by the blood-retinal barrier (BRB), which is almost as effective as blood-brain barrier (BBB) in restricting the passage of xenobiotics from the blood stream [34]. Therefore despite its apparent accessibility, the eye, in fact, is well protected against the absorption of foreign materials, including drug molecules, by the eyelids, by flow of tears, and also by the permeability barriers imposed by the cornea on one side and the blood-retinal barrier on the other side as mentioned above [24]. Because of this a significant portion of the applied drug is absorbed through nasolacrimal duct and the mucosal membranes of the nasal, oropharyngeal, and gastrointestinal tract to pass to the system. It has been found that no more than 2% of medication introduced topically to the eye is adsorbed [35-37]. Again clinical studies by various workers reveal that the main biological barrier for penetration to the eye is represented by the cornea. The relatively lipophilic corneal epithelium tissue having low porosity and high tortuosity due to tight annular junctions, is the primary barrier for hydrophilic drugs, where as the middle stromal layer consisting mainly of water interspersed with collagen fibrils(major thickness of cornea), is the main barrier for the lipophilic drugs [38-41]. All these facts result not only in a low net eye drug delivery, but also in substantial systemic availability of ophthalmic drugs after

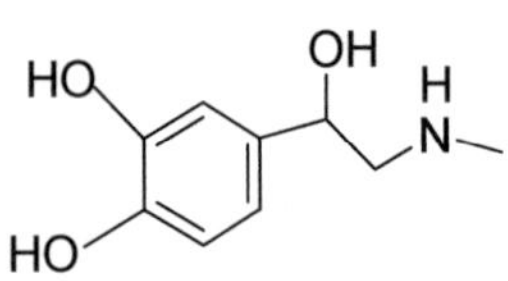

Epinephrine (**20**)

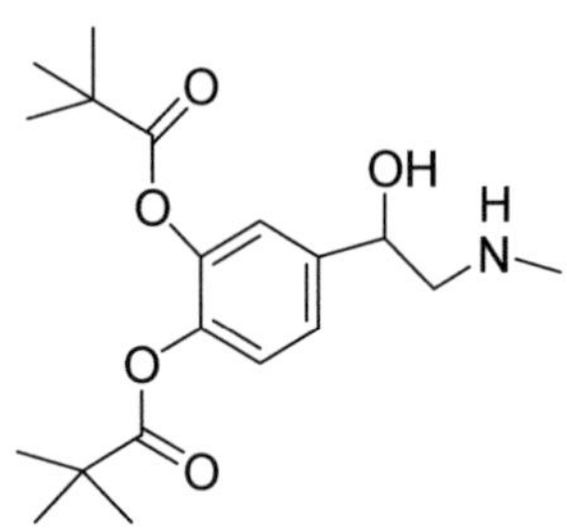

Dipivefrine (**21**)

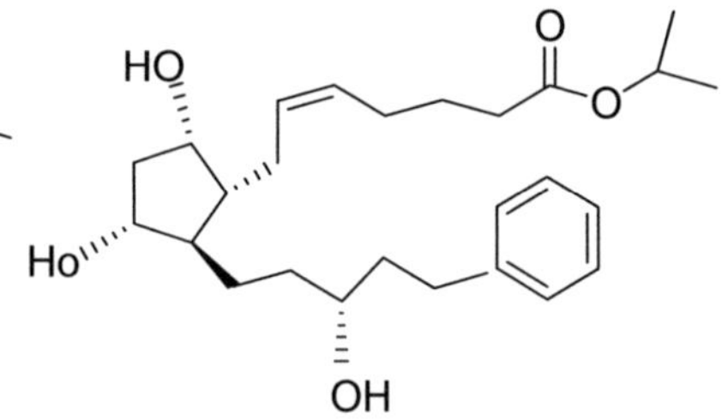

Latanoprost (**22**)

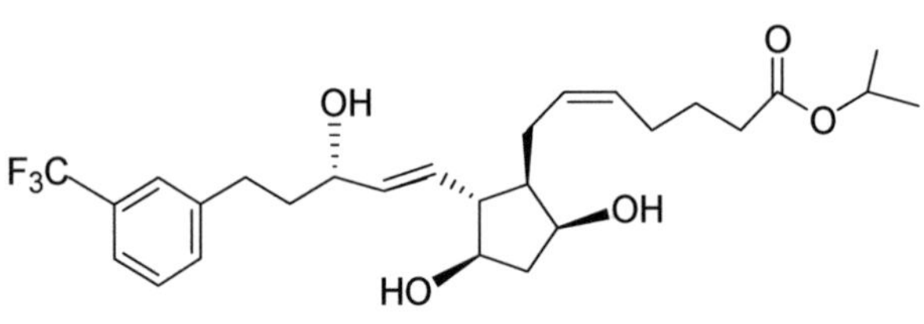

Travoprost (**23**)

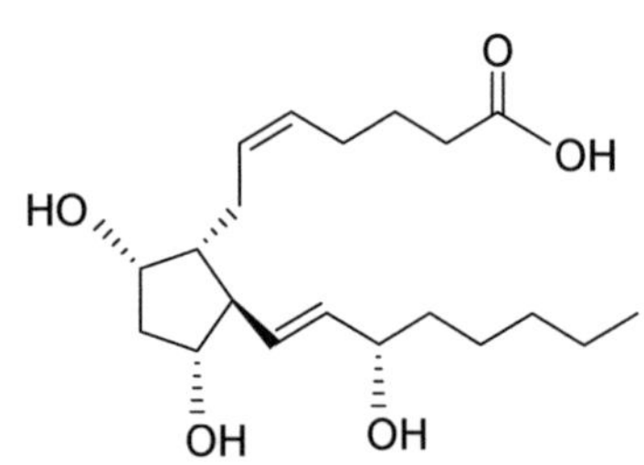

Prostaglandin $F_{2\alpha}$ (**24**)

topical administration giving systemic side effects [42]. Moreover as mentioned earlier, existing ophthalmic drugs are actually not developed for ocular applications, they were intended for other therapeutic areas which were later converted to ocular applications following their high efficacy. This further has decreased the likelihood of achieving eye-specific delivery along with reduced systemic side effects. In view of this, various drug design approaches have been tried to eliminate the problems of low ocular delivery and potential for substantial systemic side effects [6, 43]. It has been found that prodrug approach here had some limitations. Prodrugs are pharmacologically not active (or may be weakly active) compounds that results from transient chemical modifications of biologically active species, so that they are metabolically transformed into effective drugs following administration [28-30, 44-47]. Compared with the original structures, prodrug structures incorporate chemical modifications to get improvement in some deficient physiological properties, such as membrane permeability or water solubility or to overcome some other problems like rapid elimination, bad taste, a formulation difficulty etc. After administration, the prodrug because of its improved characteristics, is more systemically or locally available than the parent drug. However the prodrug must undergo chemical or biochemical conversion to the active form before exerting its biological effect. Some of the marketed ophthalmic prodrugs include Dipivefrine (**21**)-the dipivalate ester prodrug of epinephrine (**20**), latanoprost (**22**) and travoprost (**23**) -isopropyl ester prodrugs that are prostaglandin $F_{2\alpha}$ (**24**) analogs [24].

Retrometabolic Drug Design:

Because of the adverse drug reactions (ADRs) associated even with the new generation glucocorticoids in ocular treatment, the real breakthrough in the area of ophthalmic therapeutics could be achieved only by specifically designing new drugs with their ophthalmic applications in mind, so that the possibility of eye targeting with reduced systemic side effects is already incorporated in their chemical structures. In an effort to minimize ADRs and other complicacies associated with glucocorticoids, Bodor and his colleagues for the first time have developed the concept of retrometabolic drug design for ophthalmic therapeutics to introduce a new and unique class of glucocorticoids now known as soft corticosteroids or soft glucocorticoids that helped in developing glucocorticoid soft drugs for ophthalmic use [24, 48-50]. Soft β-blockers are also falling in this soft drug category. The concept of soft drugs has been originated from the pioneer work of Prof. N Bodor and his co-workers at the Center for Drug Discovery, University of Florida, Health Science Center, Gainesville, FL 32610-0497, USA [24, 48-50]. The possibility of developing these soft drugs has been extensively studied along the lines of retro- metabolic drug design for two important classes of ophthalmic drugs, β- blockers and glucocorticoids [24]. The underlying principle of retrometabolic drug design involves synthesizing analogs of lead molecules or reference molecules, starting from one of the known inactive metabolites of that lead compound. The inactive metabolite is then converted to an isosteric or isoelectronic analog with structural modifications designed for a rapid and predictable metabolism back to the original inactive metabolite after exerting the desired therapeutic effect at the site (**Figure 2**) [24, 26]. These analogs or soft drugs were predicted to have therapeutic potential similar to that of the lead compound, but because of the structural modifications provided by the design, any active drug remaining after attainment of the therapeutic effect would be metabolically deactivated, thus reducing adverse drug reactions (ADRs) [24, 26, 48-51]. According to Prof Bodor, in developing soft drugs the goal is not to avoid metabolism but rather to control and direct it. Inclusion of a metabolically sensitive moiety into the parent drug molecule can make possible the design and prediction of the major metabolic pathway preventing the formation of undesired toxic, active, or high-energy intermediates. It is desired that, If possible, inactivation should take place as the result of a single, low- energy and high- capacity step that gives the inactive species subject to rapid elimination. Most critical metabolic pathways in a biological system are mediated by *oxygenases*, a consequence of the fact that the normal reaction of an organism to a foreign material is to burn it up as food [52]. However *oxygenases* exhibit not only interspecies, but also inter individual and are subject to inhibition and induction (24) and because the rates of hepatic *mono-oxygenases* reactions are at least two orders of magnitude lower than the slowest of the other enzymatic reactions [53,54], it is usually desirable to avoid oxidative pathways as well as these slow, easily saturable *oxidase*s. In view of this, the design of soft drugs must be based on moieties activated by hydrolytic enzymes. Rapid metabolism could be more reliably performed by these ubiquitously distributed *esterases*. Bodor et al (26) suggested that it is desirable not to rely exclusively on metabolism by organs such as kidney or liver to have an additional advantage because blood flow and enzyme activities in these organs can be fatally damaged in critically ill patients. However, the increase in the therapeutic index can only be achieved if the drug is stable enough to reach its receptor site to deliver the desired effect, and any free drug remaining thereafter should be metabolized to minimize ADRs [24].

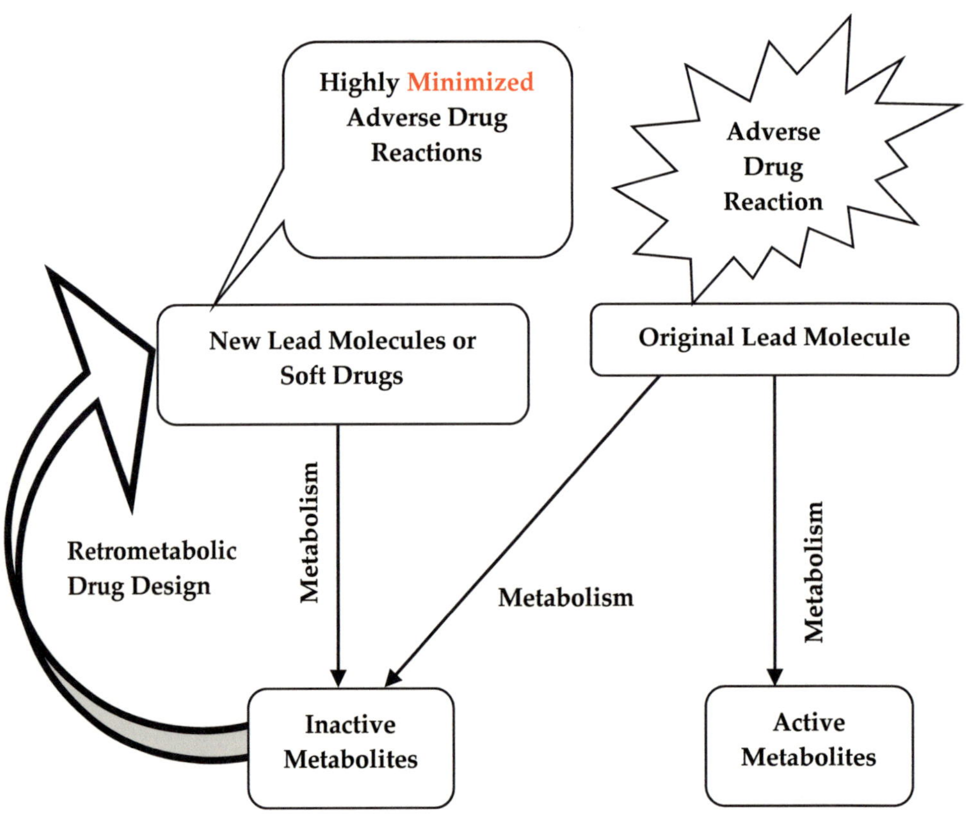

Figure 2. Retrometabolic drug design approach: Synthesis of new lead molecules (Soft drugs) based on an inactive metabolite of an original lead molecule

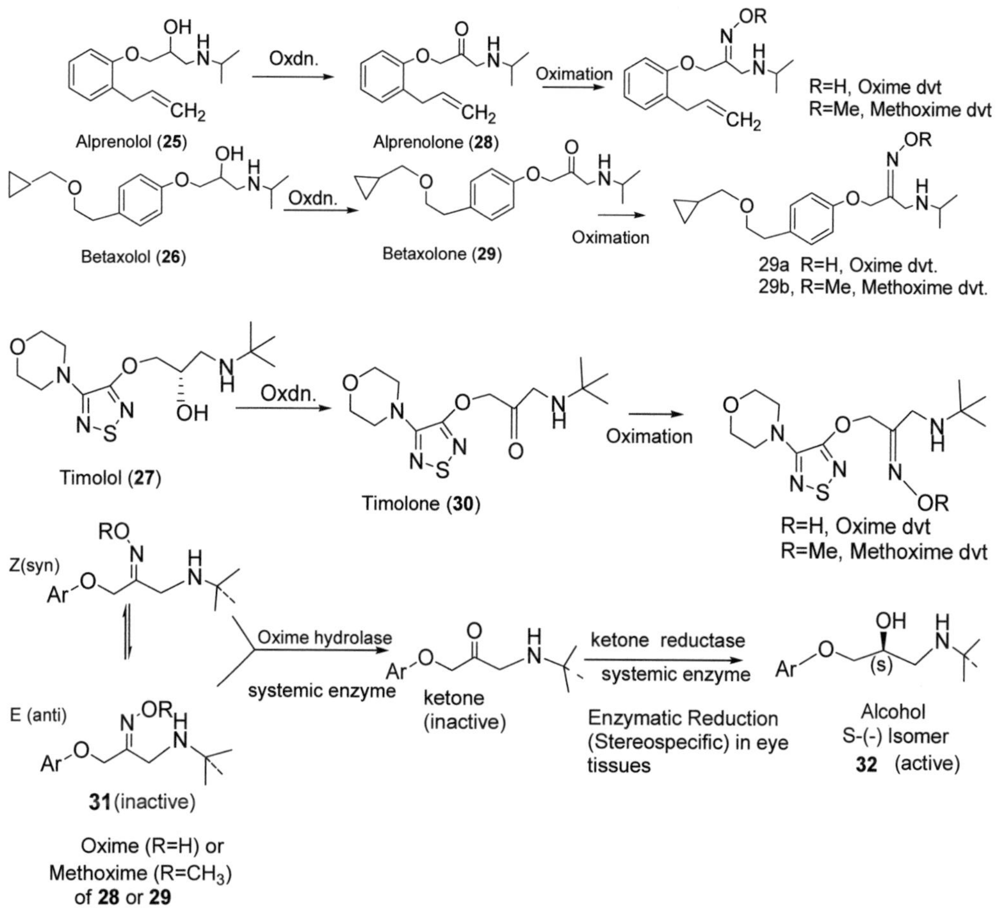

Figure 3. Site- and Stereospecific delivery of β-adrenergic antagonists to the eye through sequential activation of their oximes and alkyl oximes.

Soft- β-Blockers:

As because soft drug design is a general concept, topically applied soft drugs that show local activity with reduced systemic side effects could become potential therapeutics for any ocular diseases [24]. During the last three decades, Bodor and his colleagues have applied retrometabolic drug design to a variety of therapeutic agents such as β- blockers, antimicrobials, analgesics, and acetyl *cholinesterase* (ACE) inhibitors and were successful in developing retrometabolically designed compounds with market potential. As for example, in addition to the oxime or methoxime β -blocker analogs, the development of soft β -blockers could represent another possible route toward improved and safer antiglaucoma agents [54-62]. Several oxime and methoxime analogs of known β -Adrenergic blockers such as Alprenolol **(25)**, Betaxolol **(26)**l, Timolol **(27)** etc. were synthesized from their respective ketone derivatives, *viz.*, Alprenolone **(28)**, Betaxolone **(29)**, Timolone **(30)** and studied clinically [54-62]. They are potential drugs which have been developed applying general retrometabolic drug design principle and can be recognized as site-specific enzymatic chemical delivery systems (CDSs) [54-62]. In these compounds, a β -amino oxime or alkyloxime function replaces the corresponding β -amino alcohol pharmacore part of the original molecules (**Figure 3**). These oxime or alkyloxime derivatives (**31**) are found to exist in Z (syn) or E (anti) configuration. They are hydrolyzed within the eye by enzymes located in the iris-cillary body and subsequently again by reductive enzymes present there producing only the active S- (-) stereoisomeric alcohol (**32**) of the corresponding β-blockers [54]. For aryl β -amino alcohol-type β -adrenergic agonists and antagonists, most of the activity has been known to be

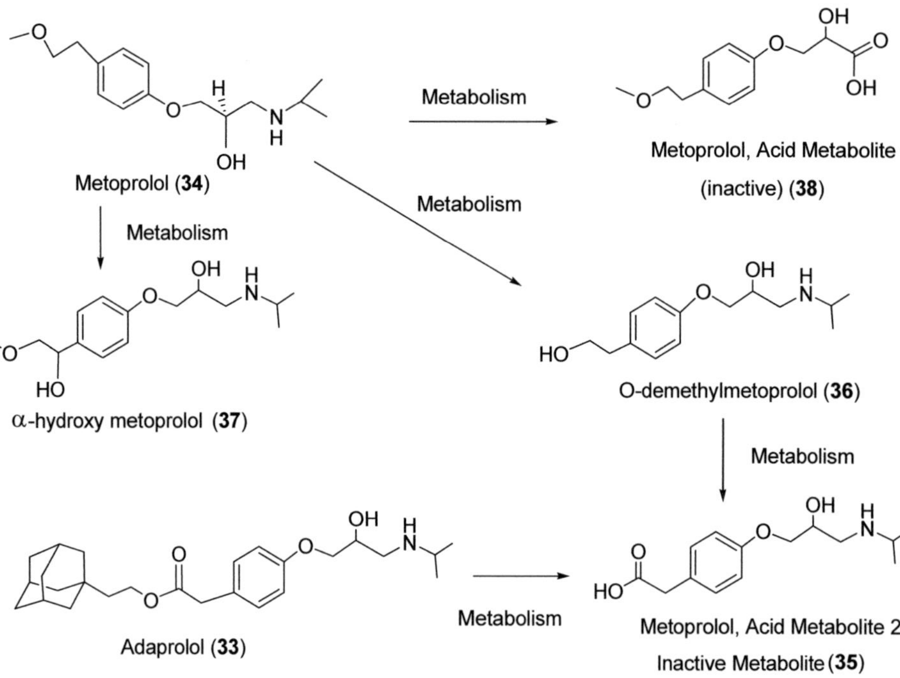

Figure 4. Inactive Metabolite-based Soft Drug Design: Comparison of the structure and metabolism of the soft β -blocker Adaprolol (23) with that of the traditional β -blocker Metoprolol(24).

present with the S- (-) stereoisomer [63-65], possibly because this isomer allows better interaction of all three important functionalities (aromatic, amino and β -hydroxyl moieties) with the β -adrenoceptor. In fact these oxime and alkyloxime derivatives have been found to exhibit significant intraocular pressure (IOP) lowering activity, but even their intravenous administration did not produce the active β -blocker metabolically; as a result they are void of any cardiovascular activity, which has been found to be a major drawback of classical antiglaucoma agents [26].

According to Bodor and his team [24], the oxime-type CDS approach clearly demonstrates the site- specific or site-enhanced drug delivery through sequential, multi-step enzymatic and/or chemical transformations through a targetor moiety that is converted into a biologically active function by enzymatic reactions which take place primarily at the site of action as a result of differential distribution of some enzymes found in the eye [24].

Again as Prof. Bodor and his team suggest [24,26], soft drugs (SDs) represent a different, conceptually opposite targeting concept; whereas eye-targeting CDSs, represented here by the above discussed oxime analogs, are inactive compounds designed to achieve the targeted effects *via* a multi-step activation process by enzymes found at their intended site of action. However soft drugs represented by β-blockers or glucocorticoids are active compounds designed to achieve the targeted effects *via* a single-step inactivation process involving enzymes found ubiquitously in the systemic circulation. Because in this class, inactive metabolite based soft drugs can be achieved introducing the hydrolytically sensitive functionality at a flexible pharmacophore region, there is considerable freedom for structural modifications. As a result, transport and metabolism properties are easier to control. From the various soft β-blockers developed along these lines by Bodor and Buchwald [24], Adaprolol (**33**), an adamantane ethyl ester was selected as a potential candidate for a new topical antiglaucoma agent [24]. The metabolism of the well-known β -blocker Metoprolol (**34**) has been compared with that of the soft β -blocker Adaprolol which has been designed starting from one of Metoprolol`s inactive acid metabolite (**35**), *viz.*, phenyl acetic acid (**Figure 4**). Its other metabolites include α-hydroxymetoprolol (**36**) and O-Dimethylmetoprolol (**37**) both of which are active. Another inactive metabolite includes the acid derivative **38.** Adaprolol was chosen because of the fact that if membrane transport (lipophilicity) and relative stability are important for pharmacological activity as they are needed to achieve right corneal permeability, then the ester goup should be relatively lipophilic and should provide ester stability [66-70]. In clinical trials Adaprolol (**33**) indeed produced prolonged and significant IOP-reduction while hydrolyzed relatively fast [67, 68]. Therefore, it was possible to separate local activity from undesired systemic cardiovascular or pulmonary activity, a characteristic highly desirable in development of antiglaucoma therapy [24]. Adaprolol (**33**) could be now a potent antiglaucoma soft β -blocker to replace the traditional β -blocker Metoprolol (**34**). Further clinical studies confirmed that Adaprolol is not only effective in reducing intraocular pressure (IOP) but also has a safer cardiovascular profile than Timolol (**27**) because unlike Timolol, Adaprolol did not reduce the systolic blood pressure [24].

Glucocorticoid Soft Drugs: Ophthalmic Therapeutics

Along the line of soft β-blockers, development of soft anti-inflammatory glucocorticoids represents a promising and successful ophthalmic drug design area initiated by Bodor and his colleagues [24,26]. Inflammation in the eye could result from surgery, injury, infection, conjunctivitis, or uvitis-conditions that can cause severe discomfort even leading to loss of vision. As mentioned earlier, topical glucocorticoids represent an important class of molecules to treat ocular inflammations and allergies as they are the most effective anti-inflammatory compounds offering the broadest range of treatment. However a number of contradictions limit their usefulness severely [12]. In addition to the general systemic side effects or adverse drug reactions (ADRs) associated with these glucocorticoids, they also cause several ocular complications such as IOP-elevation resulting steroid- induced glaucoma, induction of cataract formation and other secondary complications [12, 71]. In this context design of soft anti-inflammatory glucocorticoids has been one of the most active and productive fields of soft drug design. Ophthalmic use of glucocorticoids usually causes increased intraocular pressure (IOP) as a result of increased resistance to aqueous humour outflow. The design of soft anti-inflammatory glucocorticoids has been one of the most important and most successful areas of Soft Drug design. Although the soft nature of such drugs are mainly associated with fast hydrolytic degradation, in fact it is not necessarily be so as Bodor and his co-workers suggested [24].Too much rapid hydrolysis may in fact result in weak activity. The desired increase of therapeutic index can be obtained only if the drug is sufficiently stable to reach the receptor sites at the target organ to produce the desired effect, but the free, non-protein-bound drug undergoes facile hydrolysis to avoid undesired systemic side effects. Therefore to develop a soft drug and hence separating successfully the desired local activity from systemic toxicity, an adequate balance between intrinsic activity, solubility/lipophilicity, tissue distribution, protein binding and rate of metabolic deactivation have to be achieved. In the case of slow, sustained release to the general circulatory system from delivery site, even a relatively slow hydrolysis could result in a very low, almost steady-state systemic concentration [24]. Based on these concepts of eye-targeting chemical delivery systems (CDSs) and retrometabolic drug design approaches, Bodor and his group was successful in developing glucocorticoid soft drugs for ophthalmic therapeutics having potential market value.

First Generation Cortienic Acid (39)-based Glucocorticoid Soft Drugs: Loteprednol Etabonate (41) and its Analogs (42):

Synthesis of Dug molecules and Structure-Activity Studies:

As already mentioned, Bodor and his colleagues [24, 26] have applied retrometabolic drug design approach to a variety of therapeutic agents such as β- blockers, antimicrobials, analgesics, and acetyl cholinesterase (ACE) inhibitors and were successful in developing retrometabolically designed molecules reaching towards market application. They had designed a number of analogs starting with Δ^1-cortienic acid (**40**), the primary metabolite of prednisolone that lacks corticosteroid activity [25]. Hydrocortisone can undergo a variety of oxidative and reductive metabolic conversions [72] by local *esterases* within the system. Thus oxidation of its dihydroxyacetone side chain leads to the formation of cortienic acid *via* 21-dehydrocortisol (21-aldehyde) and cortisolic acid (21-acid) [**Figure 5**]. Cortienic acid (**39**) is an ideal lead molecule for the inactive metabolite soft drug (SD) approaches because it is lack of corticosteroid activity and therefore is major metabolite excreted in human urine. To get the new lead compounds, the pharmacophore moieties of the 17α-hydroxyl and 17β-carboxy substituents of the lead compound had to be restored by suitable isosteric/isoelectronic substitution containing esters or other types of functions that could restore the anti-inflammatory potency of the original corticosteroid while at the same time incorporating hydrolytic features to ensure metabolism. Other structural considerations included the presence or absence of double bond at C-1 position, presence of 6 α or 9 α fluorine, and 16 α & 16 β –methyl group (**Figure 6**). More than hundred possible drug molecules were synthesized and tested in pre-clinical anti-inflammatory models [5]. Structure-activity studies by Bodor and his group [24] of these molecules have confirmed that the best substituent for maximal therapeutic activity included a haloester at 17β–position and a carbonate or ether moiety at 17α– position. Incorporation of 17 α carbonates or ether was preferred over 17α– esters to increase stability and to prevent potential formation of mixed anhydrides by reaction of a 17α ester with a 17β acid functionality and subsequent potential for lens protein binding leading to steroid- induced cataract formation.

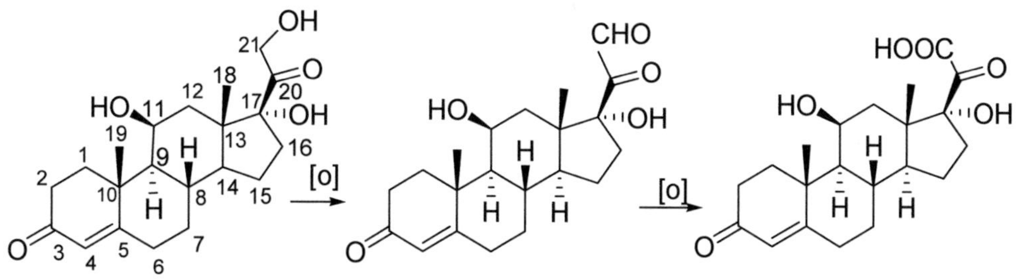

Hydrocortisone(**12**) C-21 Aldehyde C-21 Acid (Cortisolic Acid)

Figure 5. Oxidative metabolism of hydrocortisone by local esterases into C-21 Aldehyde and C-21 Acid (Cortisolic Acid)

Therefore in addition to the C-20 ketone functionality of prednisolone being replaced to eliminate the possibility of Schiff base intermediates, other chemical features associated with cataracterogenesis were also eliminated by the proposed design. The carbonates were expected to be less reactive than the corresponding esters due to the lower electrophilicity of the carbonyl carbon [24].

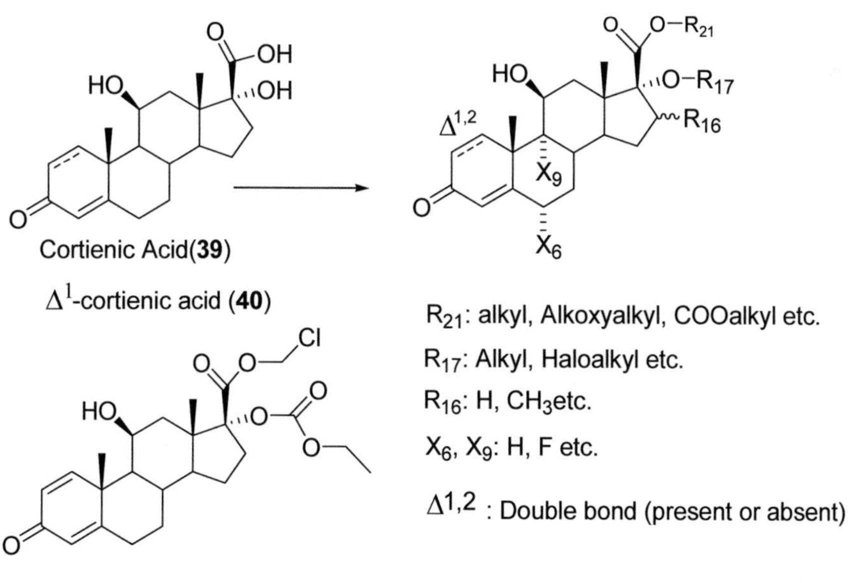

Loteprednol Etabonate(41) **1st Generation Soft Glucocorticoid Analogs (42)**

Figure 6. Design of 1st Generation Cortienic acid-based Glucocorticoid Soft Drugs (**42**) with their Glucocorticoid Soft Drug representative Loteprednol Etabonate (LE)(**41**)

Loteprednol Etabonate (LE) namely chloromethyl- 17α-[(ethoxycarbonyl) oxy]-11β-hydroxy-3-oxoandrosta-1, 4-diene-17 β -carboxylate (**41**), was the most promising drug candidate among the various cortienic acid-based derivatives synthesized by Bodor and his group (**Figure 6**)]. In Loteprednol Elaborate (**41**), a metabolically labile ester function occupies 17 β - position, while a stable carbonate group occupies 17α-position. The ester is hydrolyzed to an inactive carboxylic acid, Δ^1-cortienic acid etabonate (**43**), and then into Δ^1-cortienic acid (**40**) in biological systems after exerting the desired therapeutic effect, thereby minimizing the likelihood of toxicity [**Figure 7**]. As a result of the predictable conversion of Loteprednol Etabonate into an inactive metabolite in the eye following topical administration, this glucocorticoid has a low propensity for undesirable toxicity while possessing increased anti-inflammatory activity. In fact Loteprednol Etabonate (**41**) has been found to be 1.5 times more potent than the parent anti-inflammatory agent dexamethasone [24].

Loteprednol Etabonate (41) and its Clinical Investigations in Ophthalmic Therapeutics:

Clinical study confirmed that Loteprednol Etabonate and some of the other soft glucocorticoids synthesized, provided a significant improvement of the therapeutic index, determined as the ratio between the anti-inflammatory activity and the thymus evolution activity [24]. In addition, binding studies using rat lung cytosolic corticosteroid receptors exhibited that the receptor binding affinity of LE and some of its analogs even exceeded that of the most potent glucocorticoids known[24]. Loteprednol Etabonate (**41**) is the one of the first-generation cortienic acid-based glucocorticoid soft drugs to get approved by Food and Drug Administration (FDA), USA for use in all inflammatory and allergy-related ophthalmic disorders, including inflammation after cataract surgery, uveitis, allergic conjunctivitis, and giant papillary conjunctivitis (GPC) [73-76]. Clinical tests on LE (**41**) by various groups of workers suggest it to be a potent glucocorticoid soft drug for ocular therapeutics. LE has also been selected for development as a potent glucocorticoid soft drug based on various considerations including the therapeutic index, availability, synthesis, and `softness' (the rate and easiness of metabolic deactivation). LE is now the active ingredient of a number of ophthalmic preparations available in the market (*Lotemax, Alrex, Zylet etc.*) [73, 74, 76].

Loteprednol Etabonate (**41**) has been found to be highly lipophilic which is 10 times greater than that of Dexamethasone (**2**), a characteristic that could increase its efficacy by enhancing penetration through biological membranes [24,26]. Competitive binding studies with rat lung type II GRs confirmed that binding affinity of LE was more than 4 times that of Dexamerhasone [77]. A vasoconstriction test in humans used to assess the bioavailability exhibited that LE could produce a blanching response similar to that of Betamethasone 17α-valerate (**16**) to confirm its good penetration properties and strong potency [11]. Bodor and his group, have reported the therapeutic index of LE having more than 20-fold better than that of other glucocorticoids including Hydrocortisone 17α-butyrate (**14**), Betamethasone 17α-valerate (**16**) and Clobetasol 17α-propionate (**17**) based on their cotton pellet glaucoma test and thymolysis potency [9]. LE (**41**) has been rightly selected on the basis of considerations including Therapeutic Index (TI) which is the ratio between the median toxic dose (TD_{50}) and the median effective dose (ED_{50}), availability, synthesis and the rate and easiness of metabolic deactivation (Softness)[24]. In traditional glucocorticoids such as Hydrocortisone 17α-butyrate (**14**), Betamethasone 17α-valerate (**16**) and Clobetasol 17α-propionate (**17**), efficacy and toxicity are closely correlated (r^2 =0.996) applying the relationship between the anti- inflammatory and thymus involution activities [24] determined in the cotton pellet granuloma test (**Figure 8**). In these glucocorticoids, the reported results [24] have shown that TI have been found to be almost similar regardless of their intrinsic activities; however glucocorticoid soft drug Loteprednol Etabonate (41) owing to its softness and improved toxicity profile, provides a significant improvement(24) (**Table 4**).

Loteprednol Etabonate (LE) (**41**) →

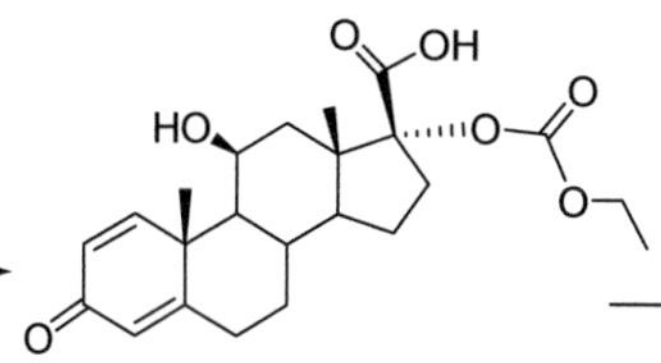

→ Δ^1-cortienic acid (**40**)
(inactive)

Δ^1-cortienic Acid Etabonate (**43**)
(inactive)

Figure 7. Metabolism of Loteprednol Etabonate (41) to Δ^1-Cortienic acid etabonate (43) and then to Δ^1-Cortienic acid(**40**).

Loteprednol Etabonate (LE) is predictably metabolized by local *esterases* into its inactive metabolite Δ^1-cortienic acid (**40**) which has been confirmed through animal studies [20]. Clinical studies by Druzgala *et al* [78] have confirmed that the highest concentration of LE was found in cornea, followed by the iris/ciliary body and aqueous humour. The cornea also showed the highest ratio of metabolite to Loteprednol Etabonate (**41**), indicating that the cornea was the prime site of metabolism, while aqueous humour concentrations of LE were nearly 100-fold lower. This finding suggested that Loteprednol Etabonate may exert a decreased IOP effect as compared to other glucocorticoids [78]. Further a comparison of the IOP-elevating activity of Loteprednol Etabonate with that of Dexamethasone (**2**) in rabbits confirmed a lack of IOP effect with LE [79, 80]. LE was found to have a terminal half- life (t1/2) of 2.8 hrs in dogs following intravenous administration [81]. Further when absorbed systemically, LE was found to be metabolized to Δ^1-cortienic acid etabonate (**43**) and then to Δ^1-cortienic acid (**40**) (**Figure 7**) and have been found to be eliminated rapidly through the bile and urine [26, 81, 82]. So far numerous preclinical tests were carried out on Loteprednol Etabonate (**41**) including more recent ones by Comstock and DeCory [20, 83]. Most of these clinical studies have confirmed that Loteprednol Etabonate achieves the required balance between the solubility/lipophilicity, ocular tissue distribution, receptor binding, and subsequent rate of metabolic deactivation as have been outlined by Bodor when he conceptualized for the first time the retrometabolic drug design.

Since the design of this glucocorticoid soft drug LE by Bodor and his group, various ophthalmic suspension formulation of LE *viz.*, a 0.2% suspension, a 0.5% suspension and a combination suspension of LE 0.5% plus tobramycin 0.3%, have been developed and clinically tested in various ocular inflammatory conditions and postoperative ocular inflammation.

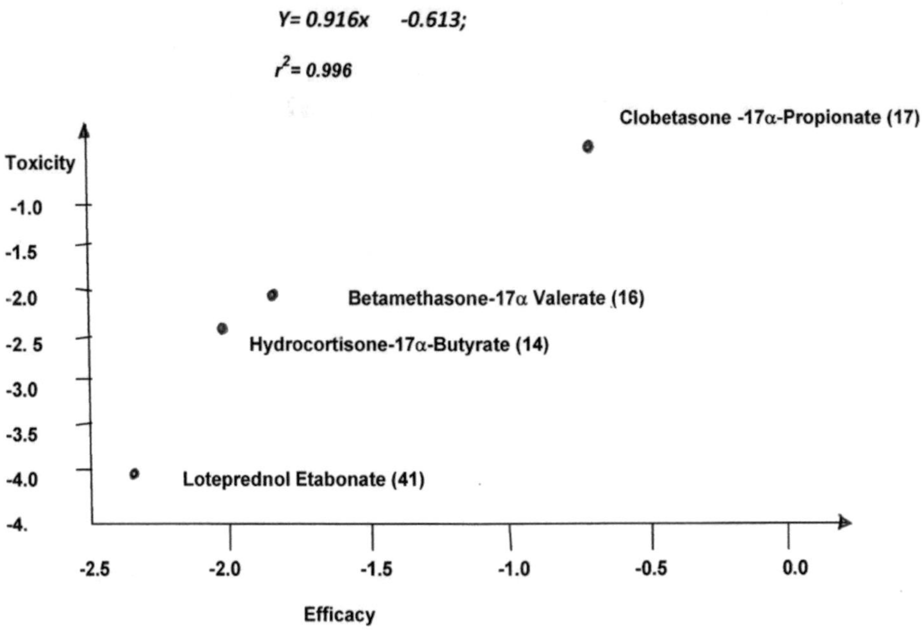

Figure 8. Literature reported [24] graph showing the relationship between the Efficacy [log 1/ED_{50} (μg/pellet)] and Toxicity [log 1/TD_{50} (μg/pellet) of Hydrocortisone-17 α-Butyrate (14: 0.1%), Betamethasone-17 α-Valerate (16: 0.12%), Clobetasone-17 α-Propionate (17: 0.1%) and Loteprednol Etabonate (41: 0.1%). Relative TI being computed with Betamethasone-17 α-Valerate (16) as reference.

Glucocorticoids	Therapeutic Index (TI) TD_{50}/ED_{50}	Relative Therapeutic Index (Rel TI) TI/TI_{BMV}
Loteprednol Etabonate (41)	56.2	22.5
Clobetasone-17α-Propionate (17)	3.8	1.5
Hydrocortisone-17 α -Butyrate (14)	3.1	1.3
Betamethasone-17 α -Valerate (BMV: 16)	2.5	1.0

Table 4. Literature reported Therapeutic Index (TI) and Relative Therapeutic Index (Rel. TI) of some glucocorticoids and Loteprednol Etabonate (**41**). Relative Therapeutic Index was computed with Betamethasone-17α -Valerate (BMV)(**16**) as the reference.

Ocular diseases against which LE formulations were clinically tested included Giant Papillary Conjunctivitis, Prophylaxis of Seasonal Allergic Conjunctivitis, Seasonal Allergic Conjunctivitis, Anterior Uveitis, Blepharokerato Conjunctivitis, and Keratoconjunctivitis sicca etc. All these studies confirmed the clinical anti-inflammatory potency of LE and lack of significant IOP after its use [20]. Again two identical placebo-controlled trials examined the safety and efficacy of LE in treating post operative inflammation following cataract surgery with intraocular lens implantation [92]. Ilyas *et al* [93] have studied the long term safety of LE 0.2% by conducting a retrospective review of more than 350 seasonal and perennial conjunctivitis patients who used LE 0.2% on a daily basis for extended periods of time. The results showed the absence of significant ADRs as there were no reports of posterior subcapsular opacification with quite insignificant IOP in most of the patients. In fact there was no observation of IOP elevation greater than 4mm Hg over base line at any period of time.

Besides, safety and efficacy of LE ophthalmic ointment 0.5% in the treatment of inflammation and pain following cataract surgery was studied in two randomized, multicentre, double-masked, parallel group, vehicle-controlled studies [20]. A very fewer LE ointment-treated patients needed rescue medication and most of them did not showed any ocular adverse event. Clinical trials on gel formulation of LE in treatment of ocular inflammation and pain after cataract surgery have been taken up more recently [20]. It is because of the high lipophilic nature of LE, gel formulation could provide improved product homogeneity over a suspension formulation to enhance its more consistent clinical response.

LE has been designed by Bodor and his group with a C-20 ester rather than a C-20 ketone and so LE is unable to form covalent adduct with lens protein, the main reason behind steroid-induced cataract formation as discussed earlier. Global market research indicates that an estimated more than 20 million LE units have been distributed globally. Clinical studies suggest the rapid metabolism of LE into inactive metabolites in conjunction with the lack of C-20 carbonyl functionality have resulted in LE – to become a unique glucocorticoid soft drug with significantly less, if any, potential for promoting steroid-induced cataract formation.[20]. LE has now been proved as a safe and effective treatment for contact lens-associated GPC, seasonal allergic conjunctivitis, postoperative inflammation or uveitis. Retrospective study established that even long time (>1 year) use of LE caused no reported adverse effects. .

Synthesis of the Side Chain of Loteprednol Etabonate (41) directly from 20-Oxopregnane (44) to furnish an Analog (45) of LE:

Based on promising results from animal studies, further clinical trials on Loteprednol Etabonate (**41**) are also going on for a safer treatment of gastrointestinal inflammation and other diseases such as asthma, rhinitis, and dermatological problems [76,82,84-86]. Success story of this retrometabolically designed glucocorticoid soft drug Loteprednol Etabonate has drawn attention to pharmaceutical industries as well as people working in steroid field worldwide. The authors of this chapter [87], recently, have reported a facile synthesis of the side chain of this potent ocular glucocorticoid soft drug, starting directly from 20-oxopregnanes, *viz.*, 3β-acetoxy-pregn-5(6),16(17)-diene-20-one (16- dehydropregnenolone acetate i.e. 16-DPA) (**44**)- a potent steroid drug intermediate, utilizing their recently developed metal mediated halogenation technique as a key reaction [88,89] to furnish the final product –an analog (**45**) of Loteprednol Etabonate (**41**) with the requisite side chain [**Scheme 1**].

The present methodology paves a useful and productive way to construct the side chain of this important glucocorticoid soft drug directly from 20-oxopregnanes *via* its C-21 functionalization in much simpler and easier way with their newly developed metal mediated halogenation technique, which avoids application of harsh and tedious reaction conditions associated with this conversion [90, 91].

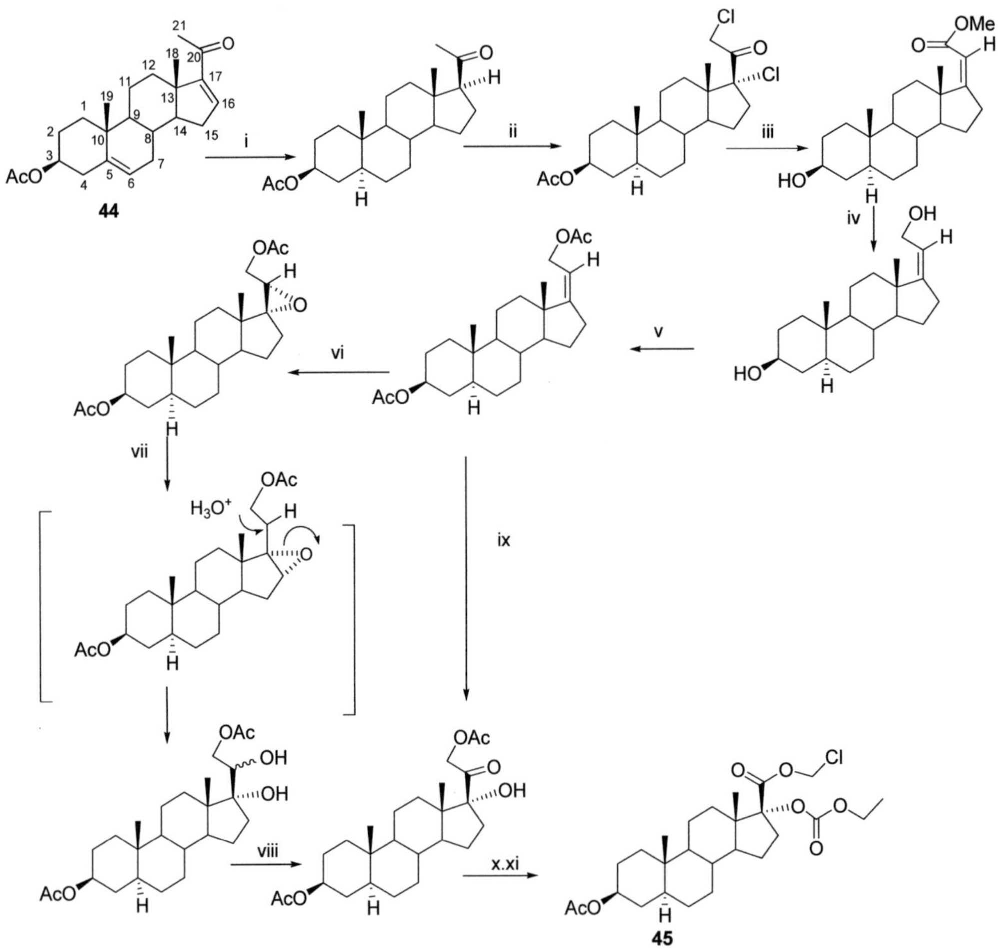

Scheme 1. Reagents and conditions: (i) H_2,Pd-C, 95% (ii) MnO_2-TMSCl/AcCl-AcOH, 81% (iii) 3% KOH, MeOH-H_2O, 75% (iv) $LiAlH_4$,THF, 88% (v) CAN, AcOH, 75% (vi) *m*-CPBA, $CHCl_3$, 62% (vii) H_2SO_4,acetone-H_2O, 48% (viii) Jones reagent, 57% (ix) OsO_4 – H_2O_2, rt., 50% (x) $NaIO_4$, Ethyl chloroformate, 70% xi) Chloromethyl iodide, 75% .

Second –generation Cortienic Acid (39)-based Glucocorticoid soft drugs: Etiprednol dicloacetate (46) and its Analogs (47):

Synthesis of Drug molecules and Structure-Activity Studies:

Based on their retrometabolic drug design approach, Nicholas Bodor [94] have more recently introduced another new class of soft glucocorticoids with 17α-dicloroester substituent. These are now known as the second generation soft glucocorticoids (**Figure 9**). This is said to be a unique design as no known glucocorticoid has been found to contain a halogen substituent at the 17α position. Nevertheless, the pharmacophore portions of these second- generation cortienic acid-based soft glucocorticoids, having the halogen atoms at 17α position, can be positioned so as to provide excellent overlap with those of the traditional glucocorticoids [24, 95]. It has been conceived the idea that dichlorinated substituents seem required for activity and sufficiently soft nature. Molecular configuration suggests that with dicholrinated substituents, one of the chlorine atom would necessarily point in the direction needed for pharmacophore overlap, whereas with monochlorinated substituents, steric hindrance might force the lone chlorine atom to point away from this desired direction. Secondly experimentally it has been found that as compared with the unsubstituted ester, dichloro substituents could cause ~20 fold increase in the second-order rate constant k_{cat}/K_M of enzymatic hydrolysis in acetate esters, on the other hand monochloro

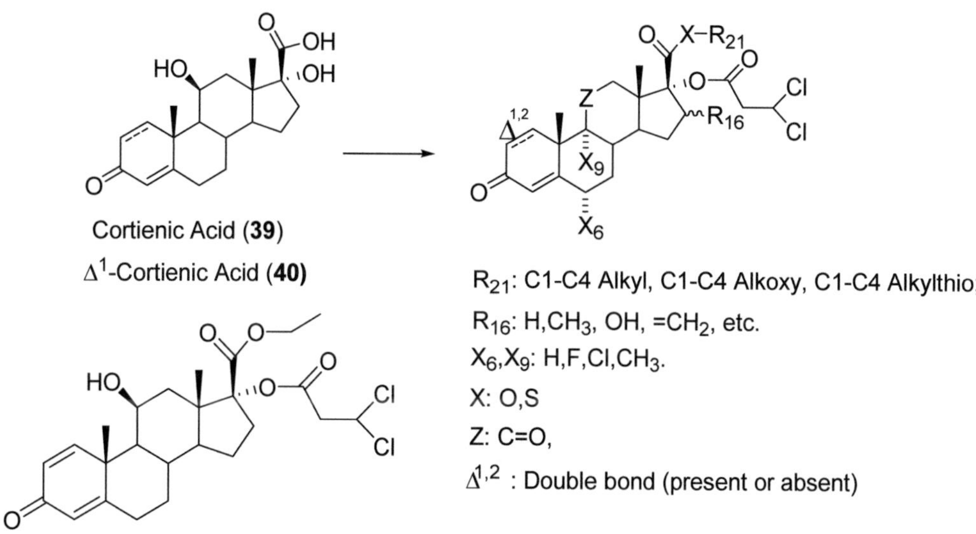

Etiprednol Dicloacetate(46) **2nd Generation Soft Glucorticoid Analogs (47)**

Figure 9. Design of 2nd Generation Cortienic Acid-based Soft Glucocorticoids Soft Drugs (**47**) and their Glucocorticoid Soft Drug representative Etiprednol Dicloacetate (ED)(**46**)

substituent did not cause any change [96]. Unlike first generation soft glucocorticoids, in the second generation of this soft steroid series, hydrolysis primarily cleaves the 17α- ester group and not the 17β-ester group. The corresponding metabolites are also not active. From large no of compounds synthesized in this series, Etiprednol Dicloacetate (ED) (**46**) had been selected for development as a potent ocular glucocorticoid soft drug [24].

Etiprednol Dicloacetate (46) and its Clinical Investigations in Ophthalmic Therapeutics:

In animal and in human clinical trials, in accordance with its soft nature, Etiprednol Dicloacetate (**46**) was found to have low systemic toxicity [94, 97-99]. Etiprednol Dicloacetate had also shown better receptor binding capacity than Loteprednol Etabonate and was found to be more effective than Budesonide (**3**) in various asthma models [24]. Further No Observable Adverse Effect Level (NOAEL) of ED after oral administration for 28 days was found to be 2mg/kg in rats and dogs, and about 40 times higher than that of Budesonide [97].

The comparison of the transrepressing and transactivating activity of Etiprednol Dicolacetate (**46**) and Budesonide(**3**) were done by measuring their inhibition in interleukin(IL)-1β production of a simulated human monocyte cell line and by evaluating glucocorticoid-induced increase in the activity of tyrosine-amino-transferase (TAT) of a rat hepatoma cell line respectively [99] and the measured activities were expressed relative to Dexamethasone (**2**) From the results it was found that ED (**46**) possesses less transactivating activity with a preserved transrepressing acivity, and hence ED is to be called as a dissociated glucocorticoid. Dissociation of transactivating (carbohydrate metabolism altering) and transrepressing (anti-inflammatory) activity found in Etiprednol Dicloacetate(ED) is a fruitful advantage in subsequent help in separating the most beneficial anti-inflammatory activity from the undesired side effects or adverse drug reactions (ADRs).A comparison of transrepression (anti-inflammatory effect) and transactivation (carbohydrate metabolism altering) effects of dexamethasone (**2**), used as 100% reference, Budesonide (**3**) and Etiprenol Dicloacette (**46**) determined on an average of two experiments for concentrations of 10 $^{-7}$ (98) is depicted in **Figure 10** [24]. Hence this productive effort in developing dissociated glucocorticoids can be termed as one of the novel and sought after mechanistic approaches towards the development of newer glucocorticoid soft drugs [24, 100,101].

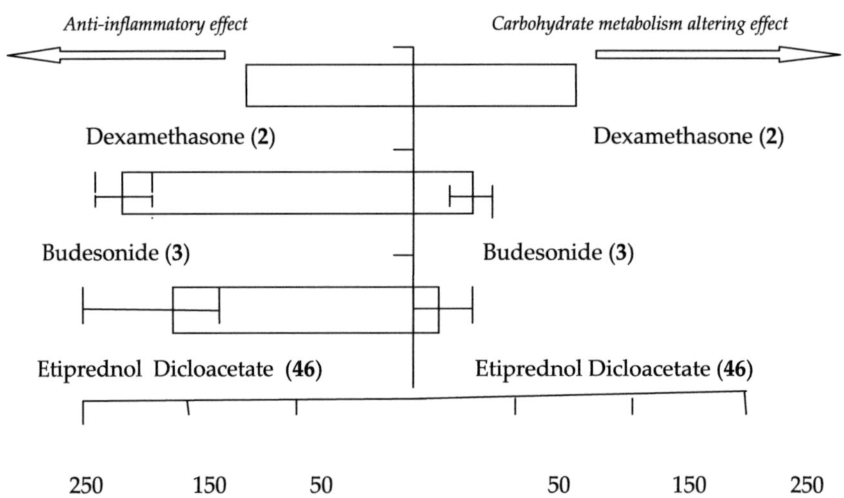

Figure 10. Literature reported [24] tentative comparison of transrepression (anti-inflammatory effect) and transactivation (carbohydrate metabolism altering) effects of dexamethasone (**2**)(used as 100% reference), Budesonide (3) and Etiprednol Dicloacetate (**46**)

3. Conclusion

Since the introduction of glucocorticoids in drug industry more than a half century ago, new series of glucocorticoids have been introduced for site specificity as well as for minimizing systemic side effects. At the initial stage, several new generation glucocorticoids were developed using prodrug design approach involving changes or modifications made in glucocorticoid molecules introducing specific substituents at various specific positions of the basic glucocorticoid skeletons to obtain better skin penetration, slower enzyme degradation and greater affinity for the cytosol receptor. The term prodrug refers to a pharmacologically inactive molecule that is converted to an active drug by metabolic biotransformations that may occur prior, during or after adsorption or at specific target sites within the body. This approach has given several potent new generation glucocorticoids such as Budesonide (**3**), 17-Prednicarbate (**9**), Fluticasone propionate (**11**), Methyl prednisolone aceponate (**5**), Beclomethasone (**7**) etc towards successful treatment of plethora of diseases including psoriasis, allergies, asthma, rheumatoid arthritis and lupus, with significantly minimized systemic side effects. However, all these old and new generation glucocorticoids are effective in reducing anterior segment inflammation only and not suitable for ophthalmic therapeutics as they are found to be associated with Adverse Drug Reactions (ADRs) including elevation of Intraocular Pressure (IOP) and steroid-induced cataract formation in case of ophthalmic therapeutics as they were not designed for ocular treatment. Successful eye-specific therapeutic agents can only be achieved by suitable drug-design approaches which thoroughly can integrate the specific pharmacological, metabolic, and targeting requirements of ophthalmic drugs. Chemical Delivery Systems (CDSs) and Retrometabolic Soft Drug Design approaches initiated by Prof.Nicholas Bodor and his group at the Center for Drug Discovery, University of Florida, Health Science Center, USA, are found to be quite successful with a major break through for this purpose providing flexible and generally applicable solutions. Their potential is indeed well illustrated by the results obtained with a number of soft β-blockers and glucocorticoid soft drugs designed within this framework towards ophthalmic therapeutics. Soft β-blockers, *viz.*, Betaxoxime (**29a**), Adaprolol (**33**) and Glucocorticoid Soft drugs *viz.,*, Loteprednol Etabonate (**41**) and Etiprednol Dicloacetate (**46**) are some of the soft drugs developed by this retrometabolic drug design approach which have already reached the clinical development phase in various ophthalmic areas and one of them Loteprednol Etabonate (LE) is already being in the market as a promising glucocorticoid soft drug in ophthalmic therapeutics. Not only that, based on clinical results from animal studies, LE now also finds place in safer treatment of gastrointestinal inflammations and other diseases such as asthma, rhinitis and dermatological problems. Moreover dissociation of transactivating and transrepressing activity found in the second generation glucocorticoid soft drug, viz., Etiprednol Dicloacetate (ED) could open up a novel and promising mechanistic pathways towards the development of more and more potent glucocorticoid soft drugs in future.

Author details

Pritish Chowdhury and Juri Moni Borah
Natural Products Chemistry Division CSIR- North East Institute of Science & Technology, Jorhat, India

Acknowledgement

We sincerely thank Prof Nicholas Bodor, Executive Director, Center for Drug Discovery, University of Florida, USA for his helpful suggestions. Department of Biotechnology (DBT), New Delhi, India is thankfully acknowledged for financial support. Thanks are also due to Ms Ashma Begum, PhD scholar, for her help in preparing the manuscript.

4. References

[1] Rhen T, Cidlowski JA (2005) Antiinflammatory Action of Glucocorticoids – New Mechanisms for Old Drugs. n..engl j. Med. 353: 1711-23.

[2] Newton R (2000) Molecular Mechanisms of Glucocorticoid Action: What is Important? thorax. 55: 603-613.

[3] Stahn C, Buttgereit F (2008) Genomic and Nongenomic Effects of Glucocorticoids. nat.clin.pract.rheumatol. 4: 525-533.

[4] Stahn C, Lowenberg M, Hommes DW, Buttgereit F (2007) Molecular Mechanisms of Glucocorticoid Action and Selective Glucocorticoid Receptor Agonists. mol.cell.endocrinol. 275: 71-78.

[5] Cidlowski JA, (2009) Glucocorticoids and their Action in Cells. retina.29: S21-23.

[6] Schake H, Docke WD, Asadullah K (2002) Mechanisms involved in the Side Effects of Glucocorticoids. pharmacol.ther. 96: 23-43.

[7] McGhee CN, Dean S, Danesh-Meyer H (2002) Locally Administered Ocular Corticosteroids: Benefits and Risks. drug safety 25: 33-55.

[8] Quigley H (2002) How Common is Glaucoma World-wide? int.glaucoma rev.[serial online]; Available at: http://www.glaucoma.com/Meetings/3-3/worldwide.php.Accessed August 16,2005.

[9] Fisher DA (1995) Adverse Effects of Topical Corticosteroid Use. west j med. 162:123-126.

[10] Degreef H (1999) New Corticosteroids. In: Maddin S editor. skin therapy letter vol.4 No.6.

[11] a) Sulzberger M B, Witten V H (1952) The effect of topically applied compound F in selected dermatoses *j. invest. dermatol.* 19: 101-102. b) Sulzberger M B, Witten V H, Smith C C (1953) Hydrocortisone (Compound F) acetate ointment in dermatological therapy. *j.a.m.a.*, 151: 468- c) Sulzberger M B, Witten V H (1954) Hydrocortisone ointment in dermatological therapy. *m. clin. north America*, 38: 321-

[12] Diassi PA, Fried J, Palmere RM, Sabo EF (1961) Fluorinated Steroids I Synthesis of 2◉-Fluorohydrocortisone j.Am.chem.soc. 83: 4249-4256.

[13] a) Cornell RC, Stoughton RB (1985) Correlation of the vasoconstrictive assay and clinical activity in psoriasis (sôrī`əsĭs), occasionally acute but usually chronic and recurrent inflammation of the skin. The exact cause is unknown, but the disease appears to be an inherited, possibly autoimmune disorder that causes the arch dermatol. 121: 63-67.

b) Stoughton RB (1992) Vasoconstrictor *n.* Assay--Specific Applications. In: Maibach HI, Surber C,editors. Topical Corticosteroids. New York: Karger. Pp.42-53. 1. causing constriction of blood vessels. 2. a nerve or agent that does th[14] Degreef H, Dooms-Goossens, A (1993) The New Corticosteroids: are they Effective and Safe? dermatol.clin.11: 155-160.

[15] Hadzija BW, Ambrose WW (1996) Comparison of Cosmetic and Physicochemical Properties of Six Topical Corticosteroid Creams. cutis. 57: S13-18.

[16] Stein-Streilein J, Streilein JW (2002) Anterior Chamber Associated Immune Deviation (ACAID): Regulation, Biological Relevance and Implications for Therapy. int. rev. immunol. 21: 123-152.

[17] Lapalus P, Moulin G, Bayer V, Fredj-Reygrobellet D, Elena PP (1986) Effects of a New Anti-allergic Agent : Magnesium Salt of N-Acetyl-Aspartyl-Glutamic Acid on Experimental Allergic Inflammation of the Rabbit Eye. curr. eye res. 5: 517-522.

[18] Ferguson VM, Spalton DJ (1991) Recovery of the Blood-Aqueous Barrier after Cataract Surgery. br. j. ophthalmol. 75: 106-110.

[19] Abelson MB, Schaefer K (1993) Conjunctivitis of Allergic Origin: Immunologic Mechanisms and Current Approaches to Therapy. surv. ophthalmol. 38: S115-132.

[20] Chambless SL, Trocme S (2004) Development in Ocular Surgery. curr. opin.allergy clin. 4: 431-434.

[21] Comstock TL, Paterno MR, Singh A, Erb T, Davis E (2011) Safety and Efficacy of Loteprednol etabonate Ophthalmic Ointment 0.5% for theTreatment of Inflammation and Pain following Cataract Surgery. clin ophthalmol. 5: 177–186.

[22] Pavesio CE, DeCory HH (2008) Treatment of Ocular Inflammatory Conditions with Loteprednol etabonate. br. j. .ophthalmol. 92 :455–459.

[23] Manabe S, Bucala R, Cerami A (1984) Nonenzymatic Addition of Glucocorticoids to Lens Proteins in Steroid-Induced Cataracts. j. clin. invest. 74: 1803-1810.

[24] Bodor N, Buchwald P (2005) Ophthalmic Drug Design Based on the Metabolic Activity of The Eye: Soft Drugs and Chemical Delivery Systems. The AAPS Journal 7: Article 79.

[25] Bodor N, Shek E, Higuchi T (1976) Improved Delivery Through Biological Membranes.1. Synthesis and Properties of 1-Methyl-1,6-Dihydropyridine-2-Carbaldoxime, A Prodrug of N-Methylpyridium-2-Carbalddoxime Chloride. j. med. chem. 19: 102-107..

[26] Bodor N, Buchwald P (2000) Soft Drug Design: General Principle and Recent Applications. med. res. rev. 20: 58-101.

[27] Bodor N, Loftsson T, Wu WM (1992) Metabolism, Distribution and Transdermal Permeation of a Soft Corticosteroid, Loteprednol etabonate pharm.res. 9: 1275-1278.

[28] Hu L (August, 2004) The Prodrug Approach to better Targeting. www.currentdrugdiscovery.com.

[29] Mueller CE (2009) Prodrug Approaches for Enhancing the Bioavailability of Drugs with Low Solubility. 6: 2071-2075.

[30] Verma A, Verma B, Prajapati SK, Tripathy K (2009) Prodrug as a Chemical Delivery System: A Review. 2: 100-102.

[31] Coopman S, Degreef H, Dooms-Goossens A (1989) Identifications of Cross Reaction Patterns in Allergic Contact Dermatitis from Topical Corticosteroids. br. j. dermatol.121: 27-34.

[32] Larochelle P, Du Souich P, Bolte E, Lelorier J, Goyer R (1983). Tixocortol pivalate, a corticosteroid with no systemic glucocorticoid effect after oral, intrarectal, and intranasal application. *clin. pharmaco. therap.* 33: 343–350

[33] Goossens A, Matura M (1999) Corticosteroids in Occupational Skin Diseases, 3rd Edition by Adams R. WB Saunders Co. Philadelphia, USA.

[34] Stewart PA, Tuor UI (1994) Blood-Eye Barriers in the Rat: Correlation of Ultrastructure with Function. j. comp. neurol. 340: 566-576.

[35] Schoenwald RD (1990) Ocular Drug Delivery: Pharmacokinetic Considerations. clin pharmacokinet . 18 : 255 - 269.

[36]. Mitra AK, Mikkelson TJ (1988) Mechanism of Transcorneal Permeation of Pilocarpine. j. pharm sci . 7: 771 - 775.

[37] Davies NM (2000) Biopharmaceutical Considerations in Topical Ocular Drug Delivery. clin exp pharmacol physiol . 27 : 558 - 562 .

[38] Schoenwald RD (1990) Ocular Drug Delivery: Pharmacokinetic Considerations. clin pharmacokinet . 18: 255 - 269.

[39] Grass GM, Robinson JR (1988) Mechanism of Corneal Penetration. *In vivo* and *in vitro* kinetics. j. pharm sci . 7: 3 - 14.

[40] Prausnitz MR, Noonan JS (1998) Permeability of Cornea, Sclera, and Conjunctiva: A Literature Analysis for Drug delivery to the eye. j pharm sci . 87: 1479 - 1488.

[41] Edwards A, Prausnitz MR (2001) Predicted Permeability of the Cornea to Topical Drugs. pharm res . 18: 1497 - 1508 .

[42] Lee VH, Robinson JR (1986) Topical Ocular Drug Delivery: Recent Developments and Future Challenges. j ocul pharmacol . 2 : 67 - 108 .

[43] Sasaki H, Yamamura K, Mukai T (1999) Enhancement of Ocular Drug Penetration. crit rev ther drug carrier syst 16 : 85 -- 146 .

[44] Bundgaard H (1985) ed. Design of Prodrugs . Amsterdam,The Netherlands : Elsevier Science .

[45] Bodor N, Kaminski JJ (1987) Prodrugs and Site-Specifi c Chemical Delivery Systems. *annu rep med chem* . 22 : 303 - 313 .

[46] Wermuth CG, Gaignault J-C, Marchandeau C (1996) Designing Prodrugs and Bioprecursors I: Carrier Prodrugs. In: Wermuth CG, ed. The Practice of Medicinal Chemistry. London, UK: Academic Press. pp 671- 696.

[47] Ettmayer P, Amidon GL , Clement B Testa B (2004) Lessons learned from Marketed and Investigational Prodrugs. j med chem . 47: 2393 – 2404.

[48] Bodor N (1994) Drug Targeting and Retrometabolic Drug Design Approaches. *adv drug deliv rev* 14 : 157 - 166 .

[49] Bodor N, Buchwald P (1997) Drug targeting *via* Retrometabolic Approaches. Pharmacol ther . 76 : 1 - 27 .

[50] Bodor N, Buchwald P (2003) Retrometabolism-Based Drug Design and Targeting. In: Abraham DJ, ed. Drug Discovery and Drug Development. Burger's Medicinal Chemistry and Drug Discovery. Vol 2. 6th ed.New York, John Wiley and Sons. pp 533-608.

[51] Bodor N (1996) Designing Safer Ophthalmic Drugs: In: Trends in Medicinal Chemistry: Proceedings of the Xth International Symposium on Medicinal Chemistry. Amsterdam, The Netherlands. Elsevier : pp 145- 164.

[52] Albert A (1985) Selective Toxicity: The Physico-Chemical Basis of Therapy. London, UK, Chapman and Hall.

[53] El-Koussi A, Bodor N (1989) Formation of Propanolol in the Iris-Ciliary Body from its Propranolol Ketoxime Precursor - A Potential Antiglaucoma Drug. *int j pharm* . 53 : 189 - 194 .

[54] Bodor N, Prokai L (1990) Site- and Stereospecific Ocular Drug Delivery by Sequential Enzymatic Bioactivation p*harm res* . 7 : 723 - 725 .

[55] Bodor N, El-Koussi A Improved Delivery through Biological Membranes. LVI. Pharmacological Evaluation of Alprenoxime - A New Potential Antiglaucoma Agent. *pharm res* . 8 : 1389 - 1395 .

[56] Simay A, Prokai L, Bodor N (1989) Oxidation of Aryloxy-β-Amino Alcohols with Activated Dimethylsulfoxide: A Novel C-N Oxidation facilitated by Neighboring Group Effect. Tetrahedron 45 : 4091 - 4102 .

[57] Simay A, Bodor N (1992) Site- and Stereospecific Drug Delivery to the Eye. In: Sarel S, Mechoulam R, Agranat I, eds. Trends in Medicinal Chemistry '90 .Oxford, UK : Blackwell Scientific Publications. pp 361- 368 .

[58] Bodor N (1995) Retrometabolic Drug Design Concepts in Ophthalmic Targetspecific Dug Delivery. adv drug deliv rev 16 : 21 - 38 .

[59] Polgar P, Bodor N (1995) Minimal Cardiac Electrophysiological Activity of Alprenoxime, A Site-Activated Ocular β -Blocker, in Dogs. life sci .56 : 1207 - 1213 .

[60] Prokai L, Wu W-M, Somogyi G, Bodor N (19950 Ocular Delivery of the β -Adrenergic Antagonist Aprenolol by Sequential Bioactivation of its Methoxime Analog. j. med. chem . 38: 2018 - 2020 .

[61] Bodor N, Farag HH, Somogyi G, Wu W-M, Barros MDC, Prokai L (1997) Ocular-Specific Delivery of Timolol by Sequential Bioactivation of its Oxime and Methoxime Analogs. *J ocul pharmacol* . 13: 389 - 403.

[62] Farag HH, Wu W-M, Barros MDC, Somogyi G, Prokai L, Bodor N (1997) Ocular-Specific Chemical Delivery System of Betaxolol for Safe Local Treatment of Glaucoma. *drug des discov* .15: 117 – 130.

[63] Nathanson JA (1988) Stereospecificity of Beta Adrenergic Antagonists: R-Enantiomers show Increased Selectivity for beta-2 receptors in ciliary process. *j pharmacol exp ther* .245 : 94 - 101 .

[64] Mehvar R, Brocks DR (2001) Stereospecifi c Pharmacokinetics and Pharmacodynamics of β-Adrenergic Blockers in Humans. *j pharm pharm sci* . 4: 185 - 200.

[65] Sharif NA, Xu SX, Crider JY, McLaughlin M, Davis TL (2001) Levobetaxolol (Betaxon) and Other β -adrenergic Antagonists: Preclinical Pharmacology, IOP-Lowering Activity and Sites of Action in Human Eyes. *j ocul pharmacol ther* .17: 305 – 317.

[66] Bodor N, Oshiro Y, Loftsson T, Katovich M, Caldwell W (1984) Soft Drugs. 6. The Application of the Inactive Metabolite Approach for Design of Soft β -Blockers. *pharm res.* 1 : 120 - 125 .

[67] Bodor N, El-Koussi A, Kano M, Khalifa MM (1988) Soft Drugs. 7. β -Blockers for Systemic and Ophthalmic Use. *j med chem* . 31 : 1651 - 1656 .

[68] Bodor N, El-Koussi A (1988) Novel 'Soft' β -Blockers as Potential Safe Antiglaucoma Agents. *curr eye res* . 7 : 369 - 374 .

[69] Polgar P, Bodor N (1991) Cardiac Electrophysiologic Effects of Adaprolol maleate, A New β -Blocker, in Closed Chest Dogs. *life sci* . 48: 1519 - 1528.

[70] Bodor N, El-Koussi A, Zuobi K , Kovacs P (1996) Synthesis and Pharmacological Activity of Adaprolol Enantiomers: A New Soft Drug for Treating Glaucoma. *j ocul pharmacol ther* . 12 : 115 - 122 .

[71] Buchman AL (2001) Side Effects of Corticosteroid Therapy. j clin gastroenterol 33: 289-294.

[72] Monder C, Bradlow HL (1980) Cortoic Acids: Explorations at the Frontier of Corticosteroid Metabolism. *Recent Prog Horm Res* . 36: 345 - 400.

[73] Noble S, Goa KL (1998) Loteprednol etabonate: Clinical Potential in the Management of Ocular Infl ammation. *bio drugs* .10 : 329 - 339 .

[74] Howes JF (2000) Loteprednol Etabonate: A Review of Ophthalmic Clinical Studies. *pharmazie* . 55: 178 - 183.

[75] Bartlett JD, Howes JR, Ghormley NR, Amos JF, Laibovitz, R, Horwitz B (1993) Safety and Efficacy of of Loteprednol Etabonate for Treatment of Papillae in Contact Lens Associated Giantpapillary Conjunctivitis. curr. eye. res. 12: 313-321.

[76] Bodor N, Buchwald P (2002) Design and Development of a Soft Corticosteroid, Loteprednol Etabonate. In: Schleimer RP, O'Byrne PM, Szefl er SJ, Brattsand R, eds. Inhaled Steroids in Asthma. Optimizing Effects in the Airways. New York, NY: Marcel Dekker. pp 541- 564.

[77] Druzgala P, Hochhaus G, Bodor N (1991) Soft Drugs – 10. Blanching Activity and Receptor Binding Affinity of aNew Type of Glucocorticoid: Loteprednol etabonate. j steroid biochem mol biol 2: 115-125.

[78] Druzgala P, Wu WM, Bodor N (1991) Ocular Absorption and Distribution of Loteprednol Etabonate, A Soft Steroid in Rabbit Eyes. curr. eye. res. 10: 933-937.

[79] Bodor N, Wu W-M (1992) A Comparison of Intraocular Pressure Elevating Activity of Loteprednol Etabonate and Dexamethasone in Rabbits. *curr eye res* .11 : 525 - 530 .

[80] Novack GD, Howes J, Crockett RS (1998) Sherwood MB . Change in Intraocular Pressure During Long-Term Use of Loteprednol Etabonate. *j glaucoma* . 7: 266 – 269.

[81] Hochhaus G, Chen LS, Ratka A, Druzgala P, Howes J, Bodor N, Derendorf H (1992) Pharmacokinetic Characterization and Tissue Distribution of the New Glucocorticoid Soft Drug Loteprednol Etabonate in Rats and Dogs. j pharm sci. 81: 1210-1215.

[82] Bodor N, Wu W-M, Murakami T , Engel S (1995) Soft drugs. 19. Pharmacokinetics, Metabolism and Excretion of a Novel Soft Corticosteroid, Loteprednol Etabonate, in Rats. pharm res 12 : 875 - 879 .

[83] Comstock TL, Usner DW (2010) Effect of Loteprednol Etabonate Ophthalmic Suspension 0.5% on Postoperative Pain and Discomfort : Presented at the American Society of Cataract and Surgery Meeting.

[84] Bodor N, Murakami T, Wu W-M(1995) Soft Drugs. 18. Oral and Rectal Delivery of Loteprednol Etabonate, A Novel Soft Corticosteroid, in Rats -for Safer Treatment of Gastrointestinal Infl ammation. pharm res 12 : 869 - 874 .

[85] Szelenyi I, Hermann R, Petzold U, Pahl A, Hochhaus G (2004) Possibilities in Improvement of Glucocorticoid Treatments in Asthma with Special Reference to Loteprednol Etabonate. pharmazie . 59: 409 - 411 .

[86] Szelenyi I, Hochhaus G, Heer S (2000) Loteprednol Etabonate: A Soft Steroid for the Treatment of Allergic Diseases of the Airways. drugs today (Barc) . 36 : 313 - 320 .

[87] Chowdhury P, Borah J.M, Goswami P, Das A.M (2011) steroids, 76: 497–501.

[88] Borah P, Ahmed M, Chowdhury P (1 998) j chem res (M) 1173–1180.

[89] Borah P, Ahmed M, Chowdhury P (1998) j chem res (S) 236–237.

[90] Djerassi C (1963) In: Steroid Reactions (An outline for Organic Chemistry). San Francisco: Holden-Day, USA.

[91] Wuts PGM, Cabaj JE, Meisto KD (1993) synth commun 23: 2199–2211.

[92]Stewart R, Horwitz B, Howes J, Novack GD, Hart K (1998) Double-Masked, Placebo-controlled Evaluation of Loteprednol Etabonate 0.5% for postoperative Inflammation. Loteprednol Etabonate Post-Operative Inflammation Study Group 1. j. cataract. refract. surg. 24: 1480—1489.

[93] Ilyas H, Slonim CB, Braswell GR, Favetta JR, Schulman M (2004) Long-term Safety of Loteprednol Etabonate 0.2% in the treatment of Seasonal and Perennial Allergic Conjunctivitis. eye contact lens 30: 10-13.

[94] Bodor N (1999) Inventor. Androstene Derivatives. US patent 5 981 517.

[95] Buchwald P, Bodor N (2004) Soft Glucocorticoid Design: Structural Elements and Physicochemical Parameters Determining Receptor-Binding Affi nity. *p harmazie* . 59: 396 - 404.

[96] Barton P, Laws AP, Page MI (1994) Structure-Activity Relationships in the *esterase*-Catalysed Hydrolysis and Transesterifi cation of esters and lactones. *j chem. soc, perkin trans 2* . pp 2021 - 2029.

[97] Miklós A , Magyar Z, Kiss É (2002) 28-Day Oral Toxicity Study with Soft Corticosteroid BNP- 166 in Rats and Dogs, followed by a 14-Day Recovery Period. *pharmazie* 57 : 142 - 146 .

[98] Kurucz I, Tóth S, Németh K (2003) Potency and Specificity of the Pharmacological Action of a New, Antiasthmatic, Topically Administered Soft steroid, Etiprednol Dicloacetate (BNP-166). *j pharmacol exp ther* .307 : 83 – 92.

[99] Kurucz I, Németh K , Mészáros S *et al* (2004) Anti-infl ammatory Effect and Soft Properties of Etiprednol Dicloacetate (BNP-166) A New, Antiasthmatic Steroid. *pharmazie* . 59 : 412 – 416.

[100] Jaffuel D, Demoly P, Gougat C (2000) Transcriptional Potencies of Inhaled Glucocorticoids. *am j respir crit care med* . 162: 57 – 63.

[101] Bhalay G, Sandham DA (2002) Recent Advances in Corticosteroids for the Treatment of Asthma. *curr opin investig drugs* . 3: 1149 - 1156.